Advanced Praise for *Convergence Mental Health*

"Mental health conditions are a key contributor to the global burden of disease and disability. The devastating impact of these conditions is even more apparent as the world faces global challenges such as the COVID-19 pandemic, climate change, societal inequity, and more. At the same time, the human brain, thought, and behavior are the most complex objects of human science. To make progress, we need a fundamental shift in our approach. Convergence science, which integrates expertise from diverse fields to form comprehensive frameworks to address specific challenges, holds promise for tackling the global mental health crisis. *Convergence Mental Health* deftly makes the case that a convergence approach is urgently needed to tackle the global mental health crisis and provides a roadmap for change."

Victor Dzau, MD
President, National Academy of Medicine

"Considering concurrent trends related to persistent and emerging mental health needs, fractured and dysfunctional systems of care, and global population aging, the sheer magnitude of the challenges before us can be daunting. *Convergence Mental Health* calls for the very type of new thinking and innovative frameworks that will enable us to deliver desperately needed technologies, services, and approaches that will improve lives, now, and well into the future. For those bold enough to think big while wise enough to appreciate the value of starting where we are, this book will serve as a welcome resource, guide, and companion."

Scott A. Kaiser, MD
Aging Services Innovation Executive and Geriatrician
Chief Innovation Officer, Motion Picture Television Fund
Director, Geriatric Cognitive Health, Pacific Neuroscience Institute
Adjunct Faculty, USC Leonard Davis School of Gerontology

"Mental health and substance-related issues affect the lives of more than a billion people worldwide. *Convergence Mental Health* explores novel financing mechanisms like social impact bonds and other blended finance vehicles to address the global shortage of providers and the lack of effective treatments. By realigning risk across the public, non-profit, and private sectors, innovative finance can help advance mental health technology to improve outcomes and the health of our society."

Tracy Palandjian
Co-founder and CEO, Social Finance
Vice Chair, U.S. Impact Investing Alliance

"*Convergence Mental Health* is a paradigm shifting book that breaks us out of the reductionistic approach to mental illness. The authors collectively show us the way forward with tools from technology integrated as an innovative bridge to a new approach to improving mental health that respects the complexity of brain function yet tackles the vexing problems that occur when illness interferes with that brain function."

Stephen M. Stahl, MD, PhD, DSc (Hon)
Professor of Psychiatry, University of California San Diego
and University of California Riverside
Honorary Fellow, University of Cambridge
Director of Psychopharmacology, California Department
of State Hospitals Editor-in-Chief, CNS Spectrums

"Fifty years since we developed the modern classification of psychiatric disorders and billions of dollars of research which followed, we still have no definitive causal mechanism, effective prevention, or curative intervention for any disorder. Business as usual, or even an incremental change, is a wholly unsatisfactory and inadequate response to this challenge. This book demonstrates, with compelling examples, that a convergence of disciplines and perspectives are needed to transform our understanding of mental health across the life course and to realize our shared goals of reducing the suffering due to mental health problems globally."

Vikram Patel, MD, FMedSci
Pershing Square Professor of Global Health and Wellcome
Trust Principal Research Fellow, Department of Global Health
and Social Medicine, Harvard Medical School
Professor, Department of Global Health and Population,
Harvard TH Chan School of Public Health
Co-Founder and Member of Managing Committee, Sangath

"As we enter an era where we are learning enough about the brain to alter its function by design, rather than by serendipity, we urgently require bold, transdisciplinary strategies that seek to bridge the chasms that currently separate understanding of the mind from understanding of its physiological substrates. *Convergence Mental Health* offers a bold step in that direction and provides an example of transdisciplinary synthesis that is sorely needed right now. From bioinformatics, through applications of artificial intelligence and advanced technology to improve efficacy and access, to establishing the social and political frameworks that will enable our society to promote the greater good, this work is audacious in its coverage—and that is exactly what we require."

Robert M Bilder PhD ABPP-CN
Michael E. Tennenbaum Distinguished Professor of Creativity Research
Semel Institute for Neuroscience & Human Behavior at UCLA
Chair, Disruptive Technology Initiative of the American
Academy of Clinical Neuropsychology

"The world is amid the Fourth Industrial Revolution that has improved quality of life in so many ways. However, we have seen limited benefits of this innovation applied to mental health, which happens to be one of the greatest sources of human suffering today. We are still today reliant on subjective diagnostics, psychotherapy, and pharmaceuticals invented decades ago. Eyre and colleagues provide a unique road map for creating a new pathway for innovation in mental health by harnessing a cross-disciplinary approach—which has already proven to work in so many other industries. *Convergence Mental Health* inspires us to see the untapped potential of innovation to transform people's lives through a unique formula of collaboration, and makes the case that we already have many of the ingredients we need to pursue major advancements."

Jeremy Kranz
Technology Investor and Mental Health Advocate
SVP & Head, Global Technology Investment Group at GIC
Co-Head, The Bridge Forum
Board Member, Treatment Advocacy Center

"The world needs evidence-based solutions that can help maximize opportunity and minimize injustice. This is particularly true for the field of mental health. The brain is the most complex object in human science and a better understanding of how it works remains key to critical improvements in fields ranging from criminal justice to education and public health. It will take cutting across silos, integrating knowledge from different fields, and implementing radical transparency to make the breakthroughs the world needs. *Convergence Mental Health* provides a roadmap for this new way of thinking, linking fresh ideas about research and funding with the potential for revolutionary outcomes."

John Arnold
Philanthropist
Co-Founder and Co-Chair, Arnold Ventures

"Equitable access to mental health care is a critical human rights priority. This is particularly true for rural, remote, Indigenous, and Tropical communities. I applaud the editors of *Convergence Mental Health* for emphasizing these issues and the impressive and diverse expertise they have brought together to explore novel solutions and inform policy for future decades."

Ian Wronski AO
Professor and Deputy Vice Chancellor of the
Division of Tropical Health and Medicine,
James Cook University Member, Asia Pacific Economic
Cooperation (APEC) Life Sciences Innovation Forum Board
Immediate Past Chair, Australian Council of Pro-Vice
Chancellors and Deans of Health Science
Past President, Australian College of Rural and Remote Medicine

"Far beyond the naïve promises of the 90s, global mental health disciplines face a dire crisis driven by fragmentation. *Convergence Mental Health* provides a conceptual turn for the field, ambitiously pursuing the integration of emergent approaches within an innovative framework. This book delves deeply into convergence mental health and its relation with translational, personalized, transdisciplinary, precision-based, implementation-based, and entrepreneurship breakthroughs applied to diverse areas of neuroscience, psychiatry, psychology, artificial intelligence, bioinformatics, innovation, multiomics, and organizational structures. The authors flesh out a bold clinical, theoretical, and research program in mental health, ranging from basic definitions to organizational considerations. The result is an ultimate vantage point to both anticipate and create the future of mental health."

Agustín Ibáñez, PhD
Director, Cognitive Neuroscience Center,
UdeSA, Argentina

"Mental disorders are among mankind's most devastating conditions and exact a tremendous personal, familial, and societal toll. Rapid advances in science and technology over the past decades have provided us with an unprecedented opportunity and the tools needed to unlock the secrets of the brain. However, these advances in knowledge have so far not been reflected in truly transformational improvements in outcomes. Part of the reason for this lack of progress is likely to have been too great a focus on developing single 'magic bullet' drugs for these very complex diseases. It is clear that—while targeting the underlying biology is indeed critical—we need a more holistic approach toward a true understanding of these disorders and the societal ecosystem that markedly impacts them. *Convergence Mental Health* provides a very thoughtful approach toward developing a strong, united, cross-disciplinary approach toward a key common goal: to improve the lives of patients. The authors also admirably highlight the key role that digital technologies may have to help address some of these deep challenges; and put forth a framework for this work to be done rigorously, collaboratively, in an ethically driven and culturally sound manner."

Husseini K Manji, MD, FRCPC
Global Head, Neuroscience, Janssen, Johnson & Johnson
Former Director of NIMH Laboratory of Molecular Pathophysiology
and Director of NIMH Mood and Anxiety Disorders Program

"This is a very exciting book of the rising utilization of mental health technology as a newly developing discipline. The authors propose a working model with insights being gained from other disciplines such as innovation diplomacy."

Professor Ian Paul Everall
Executive Dean, Institute of Psychiatry,
Psychology, & Neuroscience, King's College London

"This is a timely, highly innovative volume that discusses in great depth the new opportunities and exciting new avenues for research that arise from the convergence of various related, synergistic disciplines to bear onto brain sciences with a focus on the mechanisms of vulnerability, resilience, disease, and recovery related to mental illnesses. The editors have done a superb job to assign a great cast to tackle this ambitious task. They have succeeded in a major way. This will be a very interesting read to all in the mental health field who are curious about new possibilities and the potential revolutionary role of convergence sciences onto our field."

Jair C. Soares, MD, PhD
Professor and Chairman, Pat R. Rutherford Chair in Psychiatry
Executive Director, UT Harris County Psychiatric Center
Director, Center of Excellence on Mood Disorders
UTHealth School of Medicine

"The complexity of mental disorders deserves a strategy that goes beyond simple explanations and magic bullet solutions. *Convergence Mental Health* provides a roadmap for what a complex, transdisciplinary, transformative approach might be. An approach that includes the innovations from the technology revolution along with new insights from neuroscience and cognitive science offers unprecedented promise for people struggling with complex brain disorders. But crossing the bridge from technology and science to healthcare and health outcomes will require a new roadmap. This volume maps out that road, inviting a new generation of innovators to help a population in profound and urgent need."

Thomas R. Insel, MD
Co-Founder and Chair, NEST Health
Former Director of the National Institute of Mental Health
Former Head of Mental Health at Verily (formerly Google Life Sciences)

"Mental health issues are common and increasing in prevalence. The current standard of care is not sufficient. We must urgently innovate to empower billions of minds—to enable better mental health. The rapid spread of new technology tools offers new opportunities for scaling access to mental healthcare. The greater use of technologies in this space raises a complex web of ethical dilemmas, particularly in the areas of data privacy and individuals' rights. I commend *Convergence Mental Health* for considering the ethical adoption of technologies via robust consumer participation and innovation diplomacy."

P. Murali Doraiswamy, MBBS, FRCP
Professor of Psychiatry and Medicine, Duke University
School of Medicine Co-chair of the World Economic
Forum Global Future Council on Technology for Mental Health

"Mental health is becoming a more and more pressing issue in our time. *Convergence Mental Health* is the first to give an astute, translational overview of the progress of artificial intelligence and biobehavioral sensing technologies. I highly recommend this book for readers wanting to develop, deploy, and scale technology in an integrated approach to help millions of people with mental health issues."

Richard Socher, PhD
Artificial Intelligence Executive
Chief Scientist, SalesforceFormer Adjunct Professor,
Department of Computer Science, Stanford University

"Eyre and his colleagues have attacked a very important topic in this book. We have made immense progress in recognizing the prevalence of, and societal impact from, mental health over the last twenty years. Governments, employers, and other public figures have made mental health an important part of their agendas for human flourishing. Societies are increasingly less willing to view mental health as a stigma. However, providing appropriate mental health diagnoses and treatment programs now lag the willingness of society to engage in mental health solutions. And these solutions must be modernized. The integration of neuroscience, technological innovation, and human psychology is now joined as a priority with the need to provide greater numbers of psychiatrists, therapists, clinical doctors trained in recognizing (and making referrals related to) mental health needs and facilities. This book is an invitation for all of us to see mental health improvements as a shared duty for many disciplines. Funders, practitioners, and patients will all see something to like and to learn from in this book."

Maureen and Jim Hackett
Mental health advocates and philanthropists
Founders of the Hackett Mental Health Policy Center

"*Convergence Mental Health* is a timely and welcome idea, rich in potential to rid the world of the distressing, disabling, deadly, economically burdensome, and preventable effects of mental disorders. For this, *Convergence Mental Health* can usefully focus on specific problem-solving objectives. Prevention is one. That is, prevention of the onset of mental distress and disorder early in life and chronicity later in life and prevention of premature death triggered by suicide and hastened by depression among cardiovascular and cancer patients."

Bill Wilkerson, LLD (Hon)
Executive Chairman, Mental Health International
Industry Professor, International Mental Health, McMaster University

"We live in an era of discovery that includes the continuous presence of humans in space. The physical and psychological challenges facing astronauts on exploration-class missions to the moon and Mars requires innovative strategies to mitigate risks, including those affecting mental health. Convergence science is inherently interdisciplinary, integrated, and well-suited for tackling critical problems at the interface of space, medicine, science, and engineering. This book by Eyre and colleagues provides a nuanced and sophisticated template for addressing innovation and entrepreneurship relevant to psychiatry, space health, and other fields."

Jeffrey Sutton, MD, PhD
Founding Director and Professor, Center for Space
Medicine, Baylor College of Medicine
Former CEO, National Space Biomedical Research Institute

"Separation and isolation are features of many mental health problems. Why are they also features of our health systems' attempts to fix them? This book is a bold and informed attempt to show a new way."

Harold Mitchell, AC
Philanthropist
Founder, Harold Mitchell Foundation

"The core of *Convergence Mental Health* is "science that matters." Tremendous progress has been made in understanding brain function and the biological basis of neurologic and psychiatric illness. Advances have been made—albeit with a long way to go yet—in identifying new pharmacologic and nonpharmacologic means of assisting those with mental illness and brain disorders. The message of *Convergence Mental Health* is that we can do much more to reach those afflicted—through technology, entrepreneurship, public policy, and transdisciplinary collaboration we can reach millions of individuals whose lives can be improved if only they had access to the advances that have been achieved. *Convergence Mental Health* provides a roadmap to this goal."

Jeffrey Cummings, MD, ScD
Joy Chambers-Grundy Professor of Brain Sciences
Department of Brain Health, University of Nevada Las Vegas
Director, Center for Neurodegeneration and Translational Neuroscience
Founding Director, Cleveland Clinic Lou Ruvo Center for Brain Health

"*Convergence Mental Health* is a crucial approach to ensuring the universal coverage of mental health services. In Rwanda, a country healing from deep emotional wounds left by the 1994 Genocide against the Tutsi, mental health is included in the top health priorities of the country. One of the mechanisms used is a homegrown solution: an army of Community Health Workers (CHWs) trained to provide a comprehensive package of community health services, including sensitizing the community in the fight against stigma related to mental disorders and supporting families to detect and orient patients to the healthcare system for seeking mental healthcare. We have seen that a multidisciplinary approach to mental health involving important unconventional actors such as CHWs often yields greater results. For example, CHWs already have a rapport with community members which makes these ones more prone to following CHWs' guidance."

Yvonne Kayiteshonga, PhD
National Director of Mental Health
at Rwanda Biomedical Center Ministry of Health,
Government of Rwanda

"This important book addresses the very real need for cross-disciplinary approaches to reducing the societal and personal impact of mental health disorders, being amplified by global climate change and pandemics. Machine learning, data science, systems identification, CRISPR gene editing, and designer molecules, among others, are key technologies that can bring rapid diagnosis and solutions in cost-effective ways to patients and care givers. Bringing researchers and engineers together across seemingly unrelated fields is frequently the way to create meaningful breakthroughs and disrupt conventional thinking. *Convergence Mental Health* does an outstanding job of bringing this approach into perspective and promotes a much-needed point of view."

Mike Lyons
Managing Director, Force12 Ventures
Adjunct Professor, Stanford School of Engineering
Serial Entrepreneur

"Psychiatry is better placed than any other branch of medicine to embrace the complexity of the human condition in health and disease, including of course that which underpins the spectrum of mental illness. However, it has failed to truly face this challenge through a series of retreats into reductionism. Over the past 150 years psychiatry has flipped back and forth between biological and psychological reductionism, or suffered destructive culture wars between these two paradigms, both of which have failed people with mental illness. Psychiatry as a discipline has been handicapped by stigma, discriminated against within medicine, denied funding anywhere near proportional to the need that exists for care, and assailed by harsh and partly justified populist critique. Consequently, it has proven impossible so far to create an intellectual space and modus operandi that inspires public trust, and demands investment from governments in what is clearly a massive public health challenge facing the world: the care of the mentally ill. *Convergence Mental Health* is a potential antidote to this stasis and represents a new mindset that holds out new hope for the future of our field. Its challenge will be to translate ideas into action."

Pat McGorry, MD, PhD, AO
Executive Director, ORYGEN,
Professor of Youth Center, Centre for Youth Mental
Health, University of Melbourne

"As the next technological revolution is transforming humanity, we will see the disintegration of boundaries among the physical, digital, and biological worlds. Safeguards that ensure responsible limits on technology must be undertaken; particularly as global mental health is impacted by these changes. *Convergence Mental Health* provides a 'must-read' overview of the promises and perils of frontier technologies in mental health."

Ernestine Fu, PhD
Partner at Alsop Louie Partners Lecturer,
Stanford University
Author of *Civic Work Civic Lessons*
and *Renewed Energy*

"Sleep and mental health are closely connected. Sleep deprivation affects your psychological state and mental health. And those with mental health problems are more likely to have insomnia or other sleep disorders. The brain basis of a mutual relationship between sleep and mental health is not yet completely understood. Convergent neuroscience studies suggest that a good night's sleep helps foster both mental and emotional resilience, while chronic sleep deprivation sets the stage for negative thinking and emotional vulnerability. Biomedical engineering can help address sleep deprivation-driven mental health issues. Novel engineering solutions can develop innovation screening tools, biomarkers, therapeutics, and devices. These approaches are very much in line with *Convergence Mental Health*. Further, *Convergence Mental Health* provides a roadmap for accelerating the development, deployment, and scaling of these types of solutions."

Peter C. Farrell,
Biomedical Engineer, Entrepreneur, Executive, and Philanthropist
Founder and Chairman, ResMed Member, MIT Dean of Engineering's Advisory
Council Member, Advisory Board, Rady Business School and Jacobs Engineering
School, UCSD Member, National Academy of Engineering

Convergence Mental Health

A Transdisciplinary Approach to Innovation

Edited by

HARRIS A. EYRE, MBBS (HONS.), PHD
Co-Founder
The PRODEO Institute
San Francisco, CA, USA

MICHAEL BERK, MBBCH, MMED(PSYCH),
FF(PSYCH)SA, FRANZCP, PHD, FAAHMS
Alfred Deakin Professor
School of Medicine
Deakin University
Geelong, VIC, Australia

HELEN LAVRETSKY, MD, MS
Professor
Department of Psychiatry and Biobehavioral Sciences
University of California
Los Angeles, CA, USA

and

CHARLES F. REYNOLDS III, MD
Emeritus and Distinguished Professor of Psychiatry
University of Pittsburgh
Pittsburgh, PA, USA

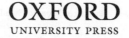

OXFORD
UNIVERSITY PRESS

OXFORD
UNIVERSITY PRESS

Oxford University Press is a department of the University of Oxford. It furthers
the University's objective of excellence in research, scholarship, and education
by publishing worldwide. Oxford is a registered trade mark of Oxford University
Press in the UK and certain other countries.

Published in the United States of America by Oxford University Press
198 Madison Avenue, New York, NY 10016, United States of America.

Library of Congress Cataloging-in-Publication Data
Names: Eyre, Harris A., editor. | Berk, Michael, editor. |
Lavretsky, Helen, editor. | Reynolds, Charles F., III, 1947– editor.
Title: Convergence psychiatry : a transdisciplinary approach to innovation/
Harris A. Eyre, Michael Berk, Helen Lavretsky, and
Charles F. Reynolds III.
Description: New York : Oxford University Press, 2021. |
Includes bibliographical references and index.
Identifiers: LCCN 2020033781 (print) | LCCN 2020033782 (ebook) |
ISBN 9780197506271 (paperback) | ISBN 9780197506295 (epub) |
ISBN 9780197506301
Subjects: LCSH: Psychiatry.
Classification: LCC RC435 .C66 2021 (print) | LCC RC435 (ebook) |
DDC 616.89—dc23
LC record available at https://lccn.loc.gov/2020033781
LC ebook record available at https://lccn.loc.gov/2020033782

DOI: 10.1093/med/9780197506271.001.0001

1 3 5 7 9 8 6 4 2
Printed by Marquis, Canada

Contents

IV CONVERGENT MENTAL HEALTH TECHNOLOGIES

V OPERATIONAL ORGANIZATIONS CULTIVATING CONVERGENCE MENTAL HEALTH

VI SPECIAL CONSIDERATIONS FOR OPERATIONALIZING CONVERGENCE MENTAL HEALTH

VII NOVEL FUNDING MODELS FOR CONVERGENCE MENTAL HEALTH

VIII CONCLUSION

Contributors

Ryan Abbott, MD, JD, MTOM, PhD
Professor
Department of Law
University of Surrey
Guildford, UK

Abdullah Al Maruf, PhD, MPharm
Research Scientist
The Mathison Centre for Mental Health
Research & Education, Hotchkiss Brain
Institute; Departments of Psychiatry and
Physiology & Pharmacology
University of Calgary
Calgary, AB, Canada

Steven M. Albert, PhD, MS
Professor
Department of Behavioral and
Community Health Sciences
University of Pittsburgh
Pittsburgh, PA, USA

Anjali Albuquerque, MSc, BA
Organizational Consultant and Behavioral
Health Writer
Global Health UCSF; Political Science
Stanford University
Stanford Brainstorm Lab
Palo Alto, CA, USA

Cara M. Altimus, PhD
Director
Center for Strategic Philanthropy
Milken Institute
Chevy Chase, MD, USA

Gowri G. Aragam, MD
Psychiatrist
Department of Psychiatry
Massachusetts General Hospital
San Francisco, CA, USA

Amanda Arnold, MSc
Executive Director
Federal Research Relations
Knowledge Enterprise
Arizona State University
Tempe, AZ, USA

Michael Berk, MBBCh,
MMed(Psych), FF(Psych)SA,
FRANZCP, PhD, FAAHMS
Alfred Deakin Professor
School of Medicine
Deakin University
Geelong, VIC, Australia

Supriya Bhavnani, PhD
Co-Principal Investigator
Child Development Group
University of Sangath
Ahmedabad, GJ, India

Chad Bousman, MPH, PhD
Associate Professor
Medical Genetics
University of Calgary
Calgary, AB, Canada

Katherine Bowman, PhD
Senior Program Officer
Board on Life Sciences
National Academies of Sciences,
Engineering, and Medicine
Washington, DC, USA

Lisa C. Brown, PhD
Medical Science Liaison
Medical Affairs
Myriad Genetics
Brooklyn, NY, USA

Jessica Carson
Director of Innovation
Strategy Office
Major Mental Health Organization
Lancaster, PA, USA

Steven Chan, MD, MBA
Clinical Assistant Professor (Affiliated)
Department of Psychiatry
Stanford University School
of Medicine
Stanford, CA, USA

Donald D. Chang, PhD
Medical Student
School of Medicine
Ochsner Medical Center
Jefferson, LA, USA

Wendy Charles, PhD
Chief Scientific Officer
Life Sciences Division
BurstIQ
Centennial, CO, USA

Neha P. Chaudhary, MD
Child & Adolescent Psychiatrist and
Clinical Faculty
Department of Psychiatry
Massachusetts General Hospital and
Harvard Medical School
San Francisco, CA, USA

Chelsea L. Cockburn, BS, MD, PhD
Candidate
School of Medicine
Virginia Commonwealth University
Richmond, VA, USA

Walter Dawson, DPhil
Professor
Department of Neurology
Oregon Health & Science University
Portland, OR, USA

Maira Okada de Oliveira, MSc
Neuropsychologist
Department of Neurology
University of Sao Paulo
Sao Paulo, SP, Brazil

Joao L. de Quevedo, MD, PhD
Professor
Faillace Department of Psychiatry and
Behavioral Sciences
The University of Texas Health
Science Center
Houston, TX, USA

Juliet B. Edgcomb, MD, PhD
Child and Adolescent Psychiatry Fellow
Department of Psychiatry
University of California
Los Angeles, CA, USA

Juan Enriquez, MBA
Managing Director
Excel Venture Management
Newton, MA, USA

Harris A. Eyre, MBBS (Hons.), PhD
Co-Founder
The PRODEO Institute
San Francisco, CA, USA

Laís Fajersztajn, PhD
Research Associated
Department of Pathology
University of Sao Paulo School of Medicine
Sao Paulo, SP, Brazil

Malcolm Forbes, MBBS, MPM, GCEpi
Clinical Senior Fellow
Department of Psychiatry
University of Melbourne
Parkville, VIC, Australia

William D. Freeman, MD, FNCS, FAAN
Professor of Neurology and Neurosurgery
Departments of Neurologic Surgery,
Neurology, and Critical care
Mayo Clinic
Jacksonville, FL, USA

Gabriel R. Fries, PhD
Assistant Professor
Department of Psychiatry and Behavioral
Sciences
The University of Texas Health
Science Center
Houston, TX, USA

Adrian Furnham, DPHIL, DSC
Professor
Leadership and Organisation
Norwegian Business School
Nydalsveien, Oslo, Norway

Hermann Garden, PhD
Policy Analyst
Directorate for Science, Technology and
Innovation
OECD
Paris, France

Wayne K. Goodman, MD
Professor & Chair
Department of Psychiatry
Baylor College of Medicine
Houston, TX, USA

David Gratzer, MD
Psychiatry
Department of General Adult Psychiatry
and Health Systems
The Centre for Addiction and
Mental Health
Toronto, ON, Canada

Adrienne Grzenda, MD, PhD
Assistant Clinical Professor
Department of Psychiatry and
Biobehavioral Sciences
David Geffen School of Medicine
University of California
Los Angeles, CA, USA

Laura M. Hack, MD, PhD
Postdoctoral Fellow, VA Advanced
Fellowship in Mental Illness Research
and Treatment, Palo Alto VA; Clinical
Instructor
Department of Psychiatry
and Behavioral Sciences
Stanford University School
of Medicine
Stanford, CA, USA

Reid Hoffman, MSt
Patron, BrainMind
Founder, LinkedIn
Partner, Greylock Partners
Board Member, Microsoft
Menlo Park, CA, USA

Malcolm Hopwood, MD, FRANZCP
Ramsay Health Care Professor of
Psychiatry
Department of Psychiatry
University of Melbourne
Parkville, VIC, Australia

Felipe A. Jain, MD
Director of Healthy Aging Studies and
Assistant Professor, Depression Clinical
and Research Program
Department of Psychiatry
Massachusetts General Hospital and
Harvard Medical School
Boston, MA, USA

Dilip V. Jeste, MD
Senior Associate Dean for Healthy Aging
and Senior Care, Estelle and Edgar Levi
Memorial Chair in Aging, Distinguished
Professor, Director of Sam and Rose Stein
Institute for Research on Aging
Department of Psychiatry and
Neurosciences
University of California San Diego
La Jolla, CA, USA

Patrick J. Hunt, BS
MD-PhD Student
Medical Scientist Training Program
Baylor College of Medicine
Houston, TX, USA

**Rahul Khanna, MBBS, BA, MPsychiatry,
FRANZCP**
Psychiatrist & Fellow
Department of Psychiatry
University of Melbourne
Parkville, VIC, Australia

Kelsey T. Laird, PhD
Adjunct Professor
Master of Arts in Counseling Psychology
Program
California Institute of Integral Studies
San Francisco, CA, USA

Raymond W. Lam, MD
Professor
Department of Psychiatry
University of British Columbia
Vancouver, BC, Canada

Helen Lavretsky, MD, MS
Professor
Department of Psychiatry and
Biobehavioral Sciences
University of California
Los Angeles, CA, USA

Ellen E. Lee, MD
Assistant Professor
Department of Psychiatry
University of California San Diego
La Jolla, CA, USA

Grace Lethlean, BS
VP Program Design and Delivery
University of Melbourne
Melbourne, VIC, Australia

Victor Li, MD, PhD
Medical Resident
Department of Psychiatry
UBC
Vancouver, BC, Canada

Julio Licinio, MD, PhD, MBA, MS
SUNY Distinguished Professor
Department of Psychiatry; Pharmacology;
Medicine; and Neuroscience & Physiology
SUNY Upstate Medical University
Syracuse, NY, USA

Gary Liu, PhD
Medical Student
Department of Medicine
Baylor College of Medicine
Houston, TX, USA

Georgia Lockwood Estrin, PhD, MSc, BSc
Research Fellow
Department of Psychological Sciences
Birkbeck College, University of London
Bloomsbury, London, UK

Ian MacRae, BA, MSc, MBPsS
Managing Director
High Potential Psychology
London, Greater London, UK

Michael McCullough, MD, MSc
Founder, BrainMind, Entrepreneur in
Residence, Greylock Partners,
Assistant Clinical Professor of
Emergency Medicine, UCSF,
Founder, QuestBridge
Department of Emergency Medicine
University of California
San Francisco, CA, USA

Louise J. I. McWhinnie, PhD
Dean and Professor
Faculty of Transdisciplinary
Innovation
University of Technology Sydney (UTS)
Sydney, Australia

Arlen Meyers, MD, MBA
Professor Emeritus of Otolaryngology,
Dentistry, and Engineering
Schools of Medicine and Public Health
University of Colorado
Denver, CO, USA

Bruce L. Miller, MD
Professor of Neurology, Director of the
UCSF Memory and Aging Center
Department of Neurology
University of California
San Francisco, CA, USA

Nidal J. Moukaddam, MD, PhD
Associate Professor
Department of Psychiatry and Behavioral
Sciences
Baylor College of Medicine
Houston, TX, USA

Debarati Mukherjee, PhD
INSPIRE Faculty
Centre for Chronic Conditions and
Injuries
Indian Institute of Public Health—
Bengaluru, Public Health Foundation
of India
Bengaluru, KA, India

Chee H. Ng, MBBS, MD, FRANZCP
Professor
Department of Psychiatry
University of Melbourne
Parkville, VIC, Australia

Calvin Nguyen, BBA
Co-Founder and COO, BrainMind
Woodside, CA, USA

Amruta Pai, MS
PhD Student
Department of Electrical and Computer
Engineering
Rice University
Houston, TX, USA

Vikram Patel, MBBS, PhD, FMedSci
The Pershing Square Professor of
Global Health
Department of Global Health and Social
Medicine
Harvard Medical School
Boston, MA, USA

Seth W. Perry, PhD
Associate Professor
Department of Psychiatry, and
Neuroscience & Physiology
SUNY Upstate Medical University
Syracuse, NY, USA

James A. Randall, MPH
Associate
Center for Strategic Philanthropy
Milken Institute; Loyola University
Chicago Stritch School of Medicine
Maywood, IL, USA

**Thomas Rego, MBBS, BMedSci, MPM,
FRANZCP**
Consultant Psychiatrist, NorthWestern
Mental Health, Melbourne Academic Unit
of Psychiatry of Old Age
Department of Psychiatry
University of Melbourne
Melbourne, VIC, Australia

Charles F. Reynolds III, MD
Emeritus and Distinguished Professor of
Psychiatry
University of Pittsburgh
Pittsburgh, PA, USA

Edmund M. Ricci, PhD
Professor
Behavioral and Community Health
Sciences
University of Pittsburgh
Pittsburgh, PA, USA

**Laura Roberts, MD, MA,
DLFAPA, FACLP**
Chairman, Katharine Dexter McCormick
and Stanley McCormick Memorial
Professor
Department of Psychiatry and Behavioral
Sciences
Stanford University School of Medicine
Stanford, CA, USA

Benjamin Rosner, MD, PhD
Associate Professor
Division of Hospital Medicine, Center for
Clinical Informatics and Improvement
Research
University of California
San Francisco, CA, USA

Ashutosh Sabharwal, PhD
Professor
Department of Electrical and Computer
Engineering
Rice University
Houston, TX, USA

Diana Saville, BA
Co-founder and CCO
BrainMind
Boston, MA, USA

Sophie C. Schneider, PhD
Assistant Professor
Menninger Department of Psychiatry and
Behavioral Sciences
Baylor College of Medicine
Houston, TX, USA

Bo Shao, MBA
Co-Founder and Chairman
Evolve Ventures and Foundation
San Rafael, CA, USA

Amy Sheon, PhD, MPH
Research Scientist
School of Medicine
Case Western Reserve University
Cleveland, OH, USA

**Erin Smith, BS (undergraduate BS degree
in progress)**
Department of Neurology & Neurological
Sciences
Stanford University
Lenexa, KS, USA

Kunmi Sobowale, MD
Child and Adolescent Psychiatry Fellow
Department of Psychiatry and
Biobehavioral Sciences
University of California Los Angeles Semel
Institute
Los Angeles, CA, USA

Garen K. Staglin, BS, MBA
Chairman & Co-Founder, One Mind
Rutherford, CA, USA

Eric A. Storch, PhD
Professor and Vice Chair
Department of Psychiatry and Behavioral
Sciences
Baylor College of Medicine
Houston, TX, USA

Kylie Ternes, MD
Medical Resident
Department of Neurology
UCLA
Los Angeles, CA, USA

Emily B. H. Treichler, PhD
Research Psychologist & Assistant
Professor Mental Illness Research,
Education & Clinical Center (MIRECC),
VA San Diego Psychiatry
University of California, San Diego
La Jolla, CA, USA

Marion T. Turnbull, PhD
Assistant Professor
Department of Neurology
Mayo Clinic
Jacksonville, FL, USA

Brian Van Winkle, MBA
Executive Director
C-Suite
NODE.Health
Denver, CO, USA

Nina Vasan, MD, MBA
Founder and Executive Director,
Brainstorm: The Stanford Lab for Mental
Health Innovation
Department of Psychiatry and Behavioral
Sciences
Stanford University School of Medicine
Stanford, CA, USA

Leanne M. Williams, PhD
Professor
Psychiatry and Behavioral Sciences
Stanford University School of Medicine
Director
Center for Precision Mental Health and
Wellness
Stanford University School of Medicine
Director
Precision Psychiatry and Translational
Neuroscience Lab
Stanford School of Medicine and MIRECC
VA Palo Alto
Director
Education and Precision Medicine,
MIRECC, VA Palo Alto
Stanford, CA, USA

Niki Wilson, BSc, MEDes
Science Journalist

David E. Winickoff, JD, MA
Senior Policy Analyst
Directorate for Science, Technology and
Innovation
OECD
Paris, France

Ma-Li Wong, MD, PhD
Professor
Department of Psychiatry, and
Neuroscience & Physiology
SUNY Upstate Medical University
Syracuse, NY, USA

Sharon Wulfovich, BA
Medical Student
UCSD School of Medicine
San Diego, CA, USA

Wei Zhang, PhD
Postdoctoral Research Fellow
Faillace Department of Psychiatry and
Behavioral Sciences
University of Texas Health
Science Center
Houston, TX, USA

1

Framing Definitions

Accelerator: Accelerator programs typically support early-stage, growth-driven companies through education, mentorship, and financing. *See Chapter 29.*

Affective computing: The study and development of systems and devices that can recognize, interpret, process and simulate emotion or other affective phenomena. Also referred to as artificial emotion intelligence or emotion artificial intelligence. *See Chapter 21.*

Blockchain: Blockchain is an innovative data management technology using distributed ledgers that has potential to achieve efficiency in data processing and greater control over healthcare record access. *See Chapter 23.*

Brain health: Brain health focusses on neurodegenerative disorders such as dementia and other cognitive disorders. *See Chapter 27.*

Clinical neurosciences: The branch of neuroscience focused on understanding the fundamental mechanisms that underly brain and mental health challenges; developing new ways of conceptually understanding, diagnosing, and ultimately developing novel treatments is especially important. *See Chapter 19.*

Consumer participation: A critical component to successfully develop and implement personalized psychiatry that enables greater involvement of patients at every level, ranging from during research to novel solution development to clinical care to policy. Greater partnership between researchers and patient communities is critical to address gaps in translating research, improve quality of life and outcomes, and adapt treatments for marginalized communities. *See Chapter 32.*

Convergence mental health: A convergence science approach applied to solving global mental health challenges. *See Chapters 2 and 37.*

Convergence neuroscience: An approach to study of the mechanisms that underly brain and mental health challenges that integrates ideas and approaches from an array of disparate disciplines to promote novel conceptual frameworks, understanding and innovations that can advance the field of neuroscience. *See Chapter 5.*

Convergence science: An approach that integrates knowledge, tools, and thought strategies from various fields and is the point where novel insights arise. *See Chapter 4.*

Deep technology: Technology that is characterized by substantial scientific advances and extensive engineering innovation. Often requires extensive research and development and a lengthy amount of time to reach commercial application and the large amounts of investment necessary for commercial success.

Fourth Industrial Revolution: An upcoming era that will be characterized by the disintegration of boundaries among the physical, digital, and biological worlds. It signifies the merging of robotics, 3D printing, artificial intelligence, the internet of things, genetic engineering, quantum computing, and other deep technologies. *See Chapter 2.*

Global mental health: The area of study, research, and practice that places a priority on improving mental health and achieving equity in mental health for all people worldwide. *See Chapter 10.*

High potential personality: Six traits (conscientiousness, adjustment, ambiguity acceptance, curiosity, risk approach, and competitiveness) that at optimal levels may correlate with greater success and work and provide a critical backbone for transformative leadership. *See Chapter 30.*

Interdisciplinarity: Involves the blending of diverse perspectives that offers more than the sum of its parts. *See Chapter 2.*

Mental health: The confluence of mind, brain, and behavior that constitutes a broad spectrum of health with implications across individual well-being, population health, economic prosperity, etc.

Microbiomics: The scientific study of the microbiome. Microbiota are ecological communities of commensal, symbiotic, and pathogenic microorganisms. *See Chapter 22.*

Mind–body therapies: Mind–body practices are techniques designed to enhance the mind's positive impact on the body. These techniques practices include behavioral, psychological, social, expressive, and spiritual approaches. *See Chapter 16.*

Multidisciplinarity: Draws on knowledge from two or more disciplines, but the disciplines remain distinct and existing knowledge is not questioned. *See Chapter 2.*

Pharmacogenetics: Pharmacogenomics is the study of the role of the genome in drug response. Its name reflects its combining of pharmacology and genomics. *See Chapter 20.*

Pharmacomicrobiomics: Defined as the effect of microbiome variations on drug disposition, action, and toxicity. Pharmacomicrobiomics is concerned with the interaction between xenobiotics, or foreign compounds, and the gut microbiome. *See Chapter 22.*

Philanthropy: Generous donations and investments that can be strategically deployed to create a better world. A potential creative funding vehicle to help address the most pressing global problems. *See Chapter 35.*

Positive psychiatry: Positive psychiatry may be defined as the science and practice of psychiatry that seeks to understand and promote well-being through assessment and interventions involving positive psychosocial characteristics in people who suffer from or are at high risk of developing mental or physical illnesses. *See Chapter 13.*

Precision psychiatry: An emerging approach for treatment and prevention that takes each person's variability in genes, environment, and lifestyle into account. *See Chapter 12.*

Psychiatry: The branch of medicine focused on the study and treatment of mental health conditions and overall psychological well-being.

Social impact investing: Impact investing refers to investments made into companies, organizations, and funds with the intention to generate a measurable, beneficial social or environmental impact alongside a financial return. Impact investments provide capital to address social and/or environmental issues. *See Chapter 34.*

Transdisciplinary: A comprehensive intellectual and social integration of paradigms, systems, and theories from many different disciplines that enables novel conceptualizations, methodologic approaches and innovations to be produced, moving beyond discipline-specific approaches to address a common problem. *See Chapter 2.*

Transdisciplinary orientation: The guiding principle behind convergence science that aims to foster innovative collaborations and integration of many diverse disciplines. *See Chapter 2.*

Translational psychiatry: Aims to bridge the gap between advancements of knowledge in neuroscience and novel treatments for patients. Especially focused on the pathway from discovery to clinical applications, healthcare, and global health. *See Chapter 9.*

Unidisciplinarlity: Relating to a single discipline. *See Chapter 2.*

SECTION I

INTRODUCING THE CONVERGENCE AGENDA

2

Leveraging Convergence Science to Address Global Mental Health Challenges

Erin Smith, Helen Lavretsky, Charles F. Reynolds III, Michael Berk,
and Harris A. Eyre

Introduction

"I believe the children are our future." Decades after this brazen tautology graced the opening line of Whitney Houston's 1986 hit song, her words continue to reverberate across the world. What do we owe our children? What world are we building for future generations to inhabit? Who is speaking for our youth, and are we listening?

Today, mental health problems kill more young people than any other cause in the world [1, 2]. Suicide rates among youth aged 10 to 24 in the U.S. have increased by over 56% in the last two decades [3]. Especially alarming, the suicide rate among young teen girls has nearly tripled during this time. Half of all mental disorders begin by age 14 and three-quarters by age 24 [4]. Across the entire age spectrum, "deaths of despair" by suicide, drugs, or alcohol are reversing decades of longer life expectancy within the U.S. [5]. The rise in the U.S. mortality rate is a symptom of larger, unfolding health trends. Developing and developed country alike, every country in the world is facing and failing to tackle a mental health epidemic, ranging from anxiety and depression to conditions caused by violence and trauma [6].

The world is in the throes of a global mental health crisis with severe physical, social, and economic ramifications. According to a recent World Health Organization (WHO) report, around 450 million people currently suffer from mental health conditions, marking brain disorders among the leading causes of ill health and disability worldwide [7]. Further, one in four people in the world will be affected by brain disorders at some point in their lives. Although treatments are available, nearly two-thirds of people with a known mental health disorder never seek help from a health professional [2]. Surveys in India and China, which have a third of the global population, have suggested that this number is even higher, with more than 80% of people with any mental health or substance use disorder not seeking treatment [2]. When individuals do seek help, treatment quality is often poor. According to a recent report from a team of 28 global experts assembled by *Lancet*, the world's failure to respond to the mental health crisis has resulted in a "monumental loss of human capabilities and avoidable suffering" [8]. The commission estimates that more than 13 million lives could be saved every year if mental illness was treated properly—or at all. Beyond the profound costs of human lives and avoidable suffering, there are colossal financial ramifications. Indeed, epidemiological modeling suggests the rising cost of mental illness will hit $16 trillion by 2030 [8]. A multitude of other issues are outlined in Box 2.1.

A historic opportunity exists to reframe mental health as a sustainable development goal at a global, institutional level and to promote good mental health as key to "sustainable socioeconomic development, improved general health, and a more equitable world" [8, 9]. Opportunities to reframe and address the global burden of brain disorders arise from three main areas: global mental health, neuroscience advances, and technological innovation.

The field of global mental health has comprehensively articulated the key issues and potential solutions needed to reduce the treatment gap, alleviate the global burden, and improve outcomes of mental health disorders of whole populations at a global level. Addressing gaps in prevention and quality of care is especially critical. *The Lancet* has progressed several major projects in this area such as "The Lancet Commission on Global Mental Health and Sustainable Development" [8] and "The Lancet–World Psychiatric Association Commission on the Global Burden of Depression" [10]. The proposed Partnership for Global Mental Health also provides a useful model for raising and dispersing large-scale funds from diverse stakeholders (e.g., donors, countries, civil society) [11].

Box 2.1. Major Issues in Global Mental health

- High and rising burden of disease
- Poor reliability of current diagnostic methods
- Trial-and-error treatment approaches
- Inadequate utilization of prevention methods
- Inadequacies of current screening approaches
- Global population aging
- Lack of adequate caregiver support
- High rates of comorbidity with other mental and physical disorders
- Lack of investment in novel therapeutics by pharmaceutical companies
- Insufficient global health care resources devoted to mental health
- Mental health issues arising from COVID-19 pandemic social and physical distancing
- Lack of translation of evidence-based data from randomized controlled trials into pragmatic, real-world care and caring
- Need for greater dissemination and implementation science
- Need for integration and innovation of social sciences
- Loss of novel innovations progressing through the "valley of death" (solution development period after the discovery phase and before the commercialization phase)

The field of neuroscience has a range of burgeoning findings. Indeed, it has been proposed that the future of mental health is best grounded in the clinical neurosciences because "advances in the assessment, treatment, and prevention of brain disorders are likely to originate from studies of etiology and pathophysiology based in clinical and translational neurosciences" (p. 1) [12].

With increasing rates of technological ubiquity, decreasing costs, and rapidity of innovation, the impact of technology on society is more visible than ever—and this is increasingly seen in technological innovation in mental health. The World Economic Forum has conceptualized a Fourth Industrial Revolution as a model for articulating the disintegration of boundaries among the physical, digital, and biological worlds [13]. It signifies the merging of robotics, 3D printing, artificial intelligence (AI), the internet of things, genetic engineering, quantum computing, and other deep technologies. In the mental health sector, there are numerous reports highlighting the rapid growth in early-stage company formation and venture capital funding of such companies [14–16].

Despite the enormous individual advances of disciplines such as global mental health, neuroscience studies, and technology innovation in the past decades, these disciplines may not individually have the required capacity to resolve the previously stated global challenges [14]. Modern mental health problems are characterized by their complexity, multisystemic nature, and broad societal impact, hence making them poorly suited to siloed approaches of thinking and innovation. Mental health involves the integration of insights from the mind, the brain, and behavior. To solve the unprecedented complexities and challenges associated with the current global mental health crisis, a paradigm shift is needed. Indeed, scientific progress can be seen as "a series of peaceful interludes punctuated by intellectually violent revolutions" [17]. We propose that a convergence science approach is needed to address the global mental health crisis, bringing about an urgently needed revolution.

Convergence (from the Latin, *convergere*, meaning to "incline together") encompasses the juncture between diverse industries, cultures, departments, and disciplines [18]. It is the node where traditional concepts meld, intersect, clash, and cross-pollinate. Convergence is the point where novel insights arise—termed the Medici Effect for its role in catalyzing the Renaissance [19].

Convergence science was recently defined and promoted in three large reports [20–22] as "an approach to problem solving that cuts across disciplinary boundaries. It integrates knowledge, tools, and thought strategies from various fields for tackling challenges that exist at the interfaces of multiple fields" (p. 1) [20]. In the context of medical science, convergence involves integration of computer science, physics, mathematics, engineering, medicine, the arts, chemistry, and biology; synergy between government, academia, and industry is also vital. Convergence, or transdisciplinary science, offers more comprehensive integration and distinctive benefits over multidisciplinary and interdisciplinary approaches [18]. Multidisciplinarity juxtaposes two or more disciplines focused on a question, problem, topic, or theme; however, the disciplines remain distinct and existing knowledge is not questioned. Interdisciplinarity involves a blend of diverse perspectives that offers more than the sum of its parts, yet it remains hindered. Ongoing debates remain around the differentiation between inter- and transdisciplinary approaches to science and medical innovation [23]. However, transdisciplinarity offers a more comprehensive intellectual and social integration of paradigms, systems, and theories for disciplines with problem-oriented research and development [20]. Convergence aims to foster transdisciplinary language and knowledge integration to solve specific problems, as well as to foster mutual learning and innovative collaborations [20]. Convergence is uniquely characterized by the creation of these novel conceptualizations and methodologic approaches, providing a backbone for innovation and growth.

Arguably, if oncology is so complex to require a convergent approach, then the study of mental health (mind, brain, and behavior) is complexity on a whole different level. Therefore, promoting the importation of convergence science into mental health is important for several reasons. It could further assist the psychiatric profession in developing research and clinical and public health innovations that can more optimally tackle complex challenges. These complex challenges include rising rates of chronic physical and mental disorders resulting from population aging and suboptimal health behaviors, inefficient health systems, low rates of treatment success with current approaches, and the mental health effects of rapid urbanization and social inequality. These problems share diverse and multifactorial etiologies, manifestations, and consequences extending across often unconnected sectors. Convergence science insights can enhance the engagement of the psychiatric profession with nonclinical innovations that include molecular biology discoveries, neuroimaging advances, a reduction in the cost of genomic and proteomic profiling, increased computing power, increased uptake of electronic health records, increased uptake of Internet and smartphone use, and an improved understanding of the social determinants of mental health.

In this opening chapter, we introduce the model of convergence mental health and put forth example projects and training approaches that are currently operating.

Introducing and Defining Convergence Mental Health

Convergence science in mental health involves leveraging a transdisciplinary approach to achieve improved outcomes for patients and healthcare systems. This means robust integration of scientists, clinicians, bioinformaticists, global health experts, engineers, technology entrepreneurs, medical educators, caregivers, and patients [14]. Convergence mental health will be realized when there is an abundance of clinical tools in use leveraging convergence science and many examples demonstrating the progression toward it. Figure 2.1 provides a graphical overview of convergence mental health and the building blocks required to achieve an abundant utilization of convergence science-based solutions globally.

Predicate Examples of Convergence Science in Adjacent Fields to Mental Health

It is helpful as we develop the convergence mental health model to explore examples of convergence science in adjacent fields such as neurology and biomedicine. The following discussion provides predicate examples of convergence science projects.

Convergence Mental Health

A field aiming to improve mental health outcomes via the wide-spread deployment of convergence science-based clinical tools.

Foundational convergence science disciplines	Computer science	Physics	Engineering	Chemistry	Biology

Elements of a "transdisciplinary orientation"	Values	Beliefs	Attitudes	Behaviors	Conceptual skills and knowledge

Applied disciplines core to convergence mental health		Social sciences		Neuroscience	
	Public health (*global health, management, epidemiology*)	Biomedical engineering	Entrepreneurship (*social, for profit, intrapreneurship*)		Big Data (*artificial intelligence etc*)

Efforts to enrich convergence mental health	Continue to build the case for novel convergence approaches	Bolster networks and communities of practice	Refine structures that support and incentivize convergence	Refine criteria for success reflective o convergence

Operational approaches	**Public**	**Not for profit**	**Academia**	**Private**	**Blended**
	• Local government • State government • National government • Bilateral • Multinational • Transnational • Departments of Social Sciences, Health, Science, Innovation, Industry	• Advocacy organizations • Foundations	• Basic sciences • Clinical sciences • Translational sciences • Educational and workforce development • National • International	• Small and medium sized enterprises • Large corporations (health insurance, tech, pharma, biotech, health providers) • Angel investors • VCs, private equity investors • Philanthropists • Social impact investing	• Public-private partnerships

Example Convergent Projects	Healthy Brains Financing Initiative, OneMind, WorldBank, National Academy of Medicine		Global Brain Health Institute, UCSF & Trinity College Dublin
APEC Digital Mental Health Hub	BRAIN Initiative	WEF Future Council on Neurotechnologies
Brainstorm Lab, Stanford University	Brain Mind	ORCATECH, OHSU
	Harvard McLean Institute for Technology in Psychiatry	Translational Research Institute for Space Health, BCM

Figure 2.1 Convergence mental health overview.

The Global Brain Health Institute (GBHI) [71] is funded by Atlantic Philanthropies and based between the University of California, San Francisco, and Trinity College Dublin. The GBHI works to reduce the scale and impact of dementia around the world by training and supporting a new generation of leaders to translate research evidence into effective policy and practice. Atlantic fellows hail from across the world and comprise a diverse array of professions including medicine, law, business, social science, journalism, and the arts. Atlantic fellows include everyone from an American ethnomusicologist designing and implementing interdisciplinary education models for dementia education within university arts and humanities departments [24] to a journalist and writer from Brazil who is leveraging social networks and media to demystify dementia and empower aging [25] to a health economist from Sweden who seeks to provide research on the cost-effectiveness of different interventions to facilitate evidence-based policy decision-making [26]. Atlantic fellows' unique insights and professional backgrounds help connect the missing dots in dementia.

Neuroscape [27] is a translational neuroscience center at University of California, San Francisco, involved in research and development of cutting-edge technologies to improve brain assessment and optimization. The center provides state-of-the-art development studios and research facilities to transform neuroscience research into real-world solutions. Their mission is to use modern technology and a wide range of industry partners to harness the brain's plasticity to ultimately enhance cognition and improve brain function. Neuroscape believes that partnerships with private companies serve as bridges between academia and industry, with the goal of more rapidly accelerating advances in science, education, and medicine. Neuroscape is specifically focused on six main pillars of research: cognitive neuroscience, healthy aging, video game training, noninvasive brain stimulation, cognitive brain computer interface, and mobile assessments. Neuroscape is especially at the forefront of developing video games as assessment tools and neurotherapeutics. A large host of projects centered around the potential of video games have been developed at Neuroscape. Some prior video game projects include Engage, a mobile game to develop delayed gratification and sustained attention skills, and Body Brain Trainer, a full-body motion capture video game that integrates cognitive and physical training with adaptive algorithms. Beyond video game technologies, other technologies that have been built and researched at Neuroscape include novel cognitive paradigms coupled with neural recordings to better understand the neural mechanisms of cognitive control and Glass Brain, a 3D brain visualization that displays real-time, personalized brain activity and connectivity between brain areas via neuroimaging technologies of magnetic resonance imaging and electroencephalography.

The Oregon Center for Aging and Technology (ORCATECH) [28], based at Oregon Health and Science University, is a multidisciplinary organization that is transforming clinical research by developing and implementing leading-edge technologies that measure life's data in real time. ORCATECH specializes in the following: medical technology consultation, design, and development; technology-based medical trial consultation and coordination, from focus groups to field-testing; and high-resolution data handling and analysis. A central focus of ORCATECH is their Life Lab. The Life Lab consists of a network of homes whose residents go about their daily lives while researchers measure and observe their interactions with technology. The ORTECH technology platform, including a variety of sensors and smart devices, is installed within homes of the Life Lab. These technologies measure and provide insights into home-based daily activities and behavioral markers such as walking speed, sleeping patterns, and the number of times someone left their home. Researchers can leverage this comprehensive profile to assess changes in daily routine that could mark changes in schedule or even the onset of disease. Some of the other studies ORCATECH has spearheaded include the SHARP Study, which uses smartphone technology coupled with neighborhood history to create engaging walking groups for the elderly population, especially among the African American population in northern Oregon. The E-Find Study is another focus area, which studies how financial behaviors change with age, especially in relation to cognitive health.

Francis Crick Institute in London [29] opened in 2010. "The Crick" is novel for a number of reasons. The internal structure is not arranged along disciplinary lines; instead, the bottom–up development of "interest groups" that bring together researchers from across the organization to share insights and plan activities in areas of common scientific interest is encouraged. The building was constructed to encourage mixing among all scientific staff (i.e., break-out spaces, transparent partitions, open spaces). Postgraduate students and researchers are intentionally drawn from a diverse array of scientific and industry fields. The Crick has become a hub for biomedical innovation applicable across the UK and at a global level. The Crick seeks to discover the biology underlying human health; improve the treatment, diagnosis, and prevention of human disease; and generate economic opportunities for the UK. A primary aim is gaining understanding on why diseases develop and new ways to diagnose, prevent, and treat a wide spectrum of illnesses such as cancer, heart disease, stroke, infections, and neurodegenerative diseases. To achieve this focus, the Crick brings scientists from all disciplines and career stages to carry out research. The unique structure, convergent mentality, and diverse approaches the Crick embraces keep it at the forefront of medical innovation.

Examples of Convergence Mental Health in Action

When considering convergence mental health in action, we can look to several areas. These include early-stage growth companies, neuroscience initiatives, public health projects, and unconventional funding mechanisms.

Early-Stage Growth Companies

Akili Interactive Labs (Palo Alto, CA) [30] builds clinically validated cognitive therapeutics, assessments, and diagnostics that look and feel like video games (aka video game therapeutics). It has submitted prescription video game for people with attention deficit/hyperactivity disorder for U.S. Food and Drug Administration approval. Select clinical trials include NCT02265718, NCT02828644, and NCT03310281. Akili has raised $72.9 million from Amgen Ventures, Merck Ventures, Jazz Venture Partners, Canepa Advanced Healthcare Fund, and PureTech Health.

Mindstrong (Palo Alto, CA) [31] utilizes digital phenotyping and an AI-powered platform to monitor patterns of interaction on smartphone devices and relate them to objective measures of brain function. The platform aims to provide continuous digital biomarkers of mood and cognition to support diagnosis, prognosis, and treatment monitoring. As one example of their convergent work, Mindstrong has entered a partnership with Takeda Pharmaceutical Company Limited to explore the development of digital biomarkers for selected mental health conditions—in particular, schizophrenia and treatment-resistant depression. The clinical trial is NCT03429361. Mindstrong raised $29 million from ARCH Venture Partners, Berggruen Holdings, Bezos Expeditions, Decheng Capital, Foresite Capital, and One Mind Brain Health Impact Fund.

MindX Sciences (Indianapolis, IN) [32] seeks to leverage advancements in psychiatric genomics and precision medicine to develop the first objective test to measure pain, suicide risk, posttraumatic stress disorder, depression, and other indications using novel blood biomarkers. MindX Sciences leverages a three-pronged approach. First, the company's proprietary app enables doctors to assess risk of mental health issues and track symptoms. Then, at-risk patients undergo the relevant blood tests to objectively assess disease state and risk of future events. The blood tests for chronic pain and mental health issues utilize novel biomarker findings [33]. Lastly, repeated testing monitors response to treatment and can help doctors adjust their treatment going forward, including a combination of pharmaceutical, nutraceutical, and behavioral solutions. The findings from the blood test may also help develop new treatments.

Pragmatic Innovation Models

Affective Computing

Affective computing (also referred to as artificial emotion intelligence or emotion AI) is the study and development of systems and devices that can recognize, interpret, process, and simulate emotion or other affective phenomena [34, 35]. It is an interdisciplinary field that combines engineering and computer science with psychology, cognitive science, neuroscience, sociology, education, psychophysiology, value-centered design, ethics, and more [36]. Although core ideas can be traced back to early philosophical inquiries into emotion [37, 38], the modern branch of computer science originated with Rosalind Picard's 1995 seminal paper on affective computing [35] and her subsequent book [38]. This accumulated in the creation of the Affective Computing group at MIT Media Lab, which has been a pioneer in the space. Affectiva [39], which develops software to recognize human emotions based on facial cues or physiological responses, and Empatica [40], which created an U.S. Food and Drug Administration–cleared watch to detect seizures using physiological and behavioral biomarkers coupled with AI systems, are both spin-offs from the MIT Media Lab group. Other notable organizations progressing affective computing include the University of Southern California's Institute for Creative Technology [41] and Jeffrey Cohn's research at University of Pittsburgh and Carnegie Mellon University [42]. Although applications for affective computing span a broad array of fields, healthcare may especially benefit, such as using emotion detection technology for posttraumatic stress disorder and depression screening and monitoring [43, 44]. Affective computing embraces a convergence science approach to bring together the technical, artistic, and human abilities necessary to push the boundaries of what can be achieved to improve human affective experience with technology and improve humanity [36].

Convergent Functional Genomics

Convergent functional genomics (CFG) is an approach for identifying and prioritizing candidate genes and biomarkers for complex psychiatric disorders. This approach integrates evidence from gene expression and genetic data from human and animal model studies. Working akin to the Google PageRank algorithm, the more lines of evidence for a gene, the higher it comes up on the CFG prioritization list. Large CFG-curated data sets have demonstrated the genetic, neurobiological, and phenotypic levels of complexity, heterogeneity, overlap, and interdependence of major psychiatric disorders [45]. For example, previous studies using this methodology have demonstrated significant molecular overlap between bipolar disorder and schizophrenia [46]. Other studies using CFG have led to the theory that the vulnerability or resilience to disease may be the result of cumulative combinatorics of common (normal) genetic variants, in lieu of or in addition to rare (abnormal) mutations [47]. This would reframe psychiatric disorders as a combinatorial modular Lego game-like model [45]. As a result, it is likely that panels of markers (SNPs, biomarkers) rather than single markers will enable useful profiling tools for precision medicine approaches [45].

Brain Health Innovation Diplomacy

Global mental health diplomacy refers to the conventional approach of improving global brain health via diplomacy, as well as a focus on strengthening health systems and leveraging both public and not-for-profit sectors. Brain health innovation diplomacy (BIND) extends this and aims to improve global brain health outcomes by leveraging technological innovation, entrepreneurship, and innovation diplomacy [48, 49]. It is an acknowledgment of the key role that technology, entrepreneurship, and digitization play and will increasingly play in the future of brain health for individuals and societies alike. It strengthens the positive role of novel solutions and recognizes and works to manage both real and potential risks of digital platforms. It is a recognition of the political, ethical, cultural, and economic influences that mental health technological innovation and entrepreneurship can have in the 21st century.

BIND also helps highlight and create a framework for the ethical considerations that must be taken with convergence science, especially in the way patients and colleagues are treated. Trust and good faith are essential to the progress of convergence science and BIND. It is an inherently human (i.e., social) undertaking, for which the predicate is trust and respect. Sustainable progress will not be achieved unless ethical considerations are continuously integrated.

Social Determinants of Mental Health and Integration of Social Sciences

Recent advancements have been made in understanding the social determinants of mental health. According to a recent report by the WHO Commission for Social Determinants entitled "Social Determinants of Mental Health," many common mental health disorders and challenges are greatly shaped by the social, economic, and physical environments in which people live [50]. Social inequalities are associated with increased risk of many common mental health disorders. The report helps build a framework for shaping individual and collective levels of mental health and well-being by addressing social determinants of health, especially during early childhood and formative stages of life. Innovative methodologies for shifting from institutional to community-based mental healthcare are included.

Further, the world's immense cultural diversity is importantly intertwined with the social determinants of health. Médecins Sans Frontières (also referred to as Doctors Without Borders) has a research arm finely attuned to cultural adaption of science-based practices, including mental health [51]. Médecins Sans Frontières works to ensure specialists are available to provide technical expertise and consultation to national staff on the development, implementation, and evaluation of culturally and socially approach psychosocial interventions. Further, locally hired mental health workers help adapt tools to local cultural needs and contexts and to changing circumstances in the field.

Addressing the social determinants of mental health is a complex task that will require rethinking our concept of disease and integration among health systems, local community partners, and coordination at a national or international level. However, addressing the social determinants of mental health provides unprecedented opportunity to prevent mental health disorders, improve mental health at a population level, and reduce social and health inequalities. Ensuring that there is a place for social science is critical to achieve a convergence science approach to mental health.

Translational Psychiatry
There have been calls for many years to innovate psychiatric research and clinical care through translational psychiatry [52]. Translational skills are believed to be important given that therapies based on the old monoamine model still form the basis of current depression treatment and given the significant gap between the expansion of neuroscience knowledge and translation into novel treatments [52]. The working steps of translational psychiatry as outlined by Licinio [52] include, in a one-way direction (T0) discovery (via preclinical, clinical, and epidemiological science), (T1) bench to bedside, (T2) bedside to clinical applications (clinical trials), (T3) translation to policy and healthcare guidelines, (T4) assessment of health policy and usage, and (T5) global health applications. Many areas of medical research contribute to this area, including molecular biology, genetics, pharmacology, neuroimaging, epidemiology, and immunology.

Responsible Innovation in Mental Health
Responsible innovation in mental health (RIMH) entails a set of principles and practices in the development of technical solutions for complex mental health problems [53]. It encapsulates collaborative endeavors, wherein stakeholders commit to identifying and meeting a set of ethical and social principles, by designing products and services to identify and manage risks to sustainably address the needs and challenges of users.

Responsible innovation is an increasingly prominent initiative. The recent Organization for Economic Cooperation and Development Recommendation on

Responsible Innovation in Neurotechnology [54] proposes the first international standard in this domain. It

aims to guide governments and innovators to anticipate and address the ethical, legal and social challenges raised by novel neurotechnologies while promoting innovation in the field'. It articulates 'the importance of (1) high-level values such as stewardship, trust, safety, and privacy in this technological context, (2) building the capacity of key institutions like foresight, oversight and advice bodies, and (3) processes of societal deliberation, inclusive innovation, and collaboration.

As per the RIMH model, these principles can be usefully adapted to guide the development and implementation of novel technologies for mental health problems.

Global Mental Health Projects

The Asia-Pacific Economic Cooperation (APEC) Digital Mental Health Hub [55] is a digital platform serving as the administrative hub for APEC mental health initiatives to strengthen the mental health and well-being across the Asia-Pacific region in support of sustainable economic growth [56]. With the APEC Digital Hub, we suggest potential outcomes to track may include the impact of tools and projects on suicide rates and the burden of depression, academic outputs, number of multinational projects completed, the adoption of clinical tools generated by the Hub, and funding contributions of foreign governments and foreign owned nonprofits and for-profit corporations. APEC members have identified seven priority focus areas with the greatest potential for critical impact where innovative projects and partnerships have been developed. These mental health focus areas include workplace wellness and resilience, integration with primary care and community settings, advocacy and public awareness, vulnerable communities and children, mental wellness of indigenous communities, disaster resilience and trauma, and data collection and standardization.

World Economic Forum's Global Future Council on Technology for Mental Health [57] convened the Global Future Council on Technology for Mental Health to help advance an ethical framework for neurotechnology development and widespread adoption [58–60]. The increasing ubiquity of technology, such as social media, chatbots, and digital assistants, affects mental health positively and negatively. The Global Future Council on Technology for Mental Health seeks to address the potential and the pitfalls of technology on mental health and create a roadmap to move forward. Further, the Council urges governments, policymakers, business leaders, and practitioners to address barriers to accessibility for effective treatments to those who need them. These barriers include ethical considerations and lack of better, evidence-based research. The Council is especially concerned with the implications that greater use of new and existing technology in mental health will have in the areas of data privacy and individuals' rights. The Council also highlights how technology has vast potential to improve—and even save—millions of life via mental healthcare innovations, solutions, and resources. To achieve a future where this potential is possible, the Council provides frameworks to advance technology development, ethical considerations, and widespread adoption.

The Mental Health Innovation Network [61] is a community of mental health innovators—researchers, clinicians, policymakers, service user advocates, donors from around the world, etc.—sharing innovative resources and ideas to promote mental health and improve the lives of people with mental, neurological, and substance use disorders. The Mental Health Innovation Network aims to facilitate the development and uptake of effective mental health interventions by enabling learning, building partnerships, synthesizing and disseminating knowledge, and leveraging resources.

Neuroscience Projects

The Brain Research Through Advancing Innovative Neurotechnologies (BRAIN) Initiative [62] aims to develop new tools and technologies that will enable the research community to obtain a dynamic picture of the brain in action. With nearly 100 billion cells making 100 trillion connections, this is no small aim and will simply not be achievable with current tools and disciplinary approaches. One of the express themes of action for the BRAIN initiative is to "cross boundaries in interdisciplinary collaborations." The BRAIN initiative consists of teams of engineers, nanotechnologists, computational scientists, materials scientists, and neuroscientists to create the next generation of imaging tools or probes for brain activity. It is funded by public agencies, private companies, and foundations.

The Psychiatric Cell Map Initiative (PCMI) [63, 64] aims to bridge the gap between the genome and clinic in the field of neuropsychiatric disorder research by systematically mapping the physical and genetic interaction networks underlying these disorders and then using these maps to connect the genomic data to neurobiology and ultimately the clinic, which will be a critical resource for precision medicine. PCMI is especially focused on autism spectrum disorders, Tourette disorder, epilepsy, intellectual disability, and schizophrenia. PCMI is the confluence of efforts of a team of geneticists, structural biologists, neurobiologists, systems biologists, and clinicians, leveraging a wide array of experimental approaches and creating a collaborative infrastructure necessary for long-term investigation across a broad range of diseases, such as parallel studies on the significant overlap with genes implicated in cancer, infectious disease, and congenital heart defects.

The Psychiatric Genomics Consortium (PGC) [65] unites investigators worldwide to conduct meta- and mega-analyses of genome-wide genomic data for psychiatric disorders. The PGC began in early 2007 and has rapidly become a collaborative confederation of most investigators in the field. The PGC includes over 800 investigators from 38 countries. There are samples from more than 900,000 individuals currently in analysis, and this number is growing rapidly.

Mental Health Technology Advancement Organizations

The Harvard McLean Institute for Technology in Psychiatry (ITP) [66] aims to advance psychiatric research and practice through innovations in digital health technology and informatics. Working with global leaders in academia, industry, and healthcare, ITP seeks to accomplish the following goals: innovate new technology-based methods for diagnosing, monitoring, and treating psychiatric disorders; support technology-based solutions in research and clinical care; and optimize new and existing technology to meet the needs of clinicians, patients, and the scientific community. McLean Hospital provides a unique environment for optimizing treatments and supporting a wide range of research initiatives. The MultiSense Project and Beiwe are two examples of research projects taking place at or in collaboration with ITP [67]. The MultiSense Project captures naturalistic, face-to-face clinical interviews and uses machine learning to analyze these videos to improve efficiency and robustness of mental health assessment through automatic sensing. Beiwe addresses smartphone-based treatment interventions via a fully encrypted smartphone platform for continuous monitoring coupled with world-class classifiers. The ITP also hosts the annual Technology in Psychiatry Summit, which brings together top leaders in healthcare, academic research, data science, technology, entrepreneurship, policymaking, investing, and patient advocacy to build on the promise of technology in the diagnosis and delivery of mental healthcare.

The Translational Research Institute for Space Health (TRISH), Baylor College of Medicine [68], supported by the NASA Human Research Program and based at the Baylor College of Medicine, provides a range of convergent mechanisms to develop novel solutions for mental health. One mechanism is their Launch Pad [69]. The TRISH Launch Pad aims to prepare early-stage companies and precompanies to meet the needs of the space medicine industry. Launch Pad provides a 10-week intensive program. Sessions are led by industry veterans who help teams create a viable commercialization pathway to Earth's health technology market and a secondary space market. Launch Pad provides companies and precompanies with (1) access to experts working in space health and at NASA, (2) rapid technology maturation and derisking, (3) preparation for commercial success in U.S. healthcare markets, and (4) pathways to government sales in the emerging space market. TRISH also held a conference in 2019 with the MIT Media Lab Space Exploration Initiative focused on "optimizing behavioural health and cognitive performance in confined environments" [70]. TRISH also co-convened the 2019 Space Health Innovation Conference in San Francisco with the University of California, San Francisco [71]. The goal was to "convene a diverse audience of Space experts and Health Tech Innovation stakeholders with a goal to inform, inspire and invite participation in the exciting challenge of optimizing health and medical management in Space environments" [72].

Unconventional Funding Mechanisms

The Healthy Brains Global Initiative (HBGI) is a real-world example of the aforementioned Partnership for Global Mental Health [11, 73]. It is a globally focused effort led by One Mind and the National Academy of Medicine with support from the World Bank, WHO, and the Organization for Economic Development that is developing a plan for a $10 billion social impact bond to fund accelerated global research on mental health [73, 74]. New science and new financing methods are being developed by a coalition of global leaders in neuroscience, finance, policy, and advocacy. Independently verified metrics will prove the reduction in the annual burden of mental illness sufficient to retire the bond [74]. Four separate working groups have been formed involving more than 100 participants. This global collaboration is unprecedented in neuroscience and holds the potential of other chronic illness to follow this lead [74].

BrainMind [75] is a platform and private community of brain scientists, entrepreneurs, philanthropists, investors, and academic institutions dedicated to impactful innovation of brain science. It seeks to coordinate talent from the entrepreneurial community with capital from the philanthropic community to deliver stewardship of neuroscience to impact focused stakeholders. By using the principles of "gather, curate, cultivate," it brings together a powerful community of diverse and motivated leaders interested in changing brain science to establish a roadmap for an effective way forward. The platform recognizes areas in brain science research that are undersupported relative to their impact and provides high consciousness capital and leadership to grow and scale these innovations to ultimately benefit society. BrainMind also convenes a series of private, action-oriented gatherings in collaboration with the world's top brain research institutions. These gatherings create an ecosystem to educate participants on emerging neuroscience; develop intellectual, entrepreneurial, and ethical frameworks for brain endeavors; and accelerate impactful findings in mind and brain science, from basic research to company creation.

A CB Insights report examining venture capital-backed deals into mental health and wellness start-ups since 2012 shows funding to mental health tech start-ups has risen annually and reached nearly $200 million in 2016 [14]. Highlighted companies include Quartet Health, Lyra Health, and AbleTo. Many mental health tech start-ups raising funds today are purportedly working to increase access to mental healthcare. Strategies include telemedicine platforms that enable remote access to care, interactive apps that track fluctuations in emotional states, daily motivational text messaging services, chat bots, and augmented and virtual reality tools.

A CB Insights report [76] found that the major investors in mental health, including hospital systems such as Cedars-Sinai, tech giants like Google, and health insurers like Aetna and BlueCross BlueShield, have been involved in mental health start-ups. Further, many of these corporations are now partnering with early-stage start-ups, such as Aetna with AbleTo. The most active investors are tech accelerators such as Y Combinator or 500 Startups.

Reflections on Mental Health Innovation and COVID-19

Society's psychological reactions to a crisis can be predicted according to disaster response frameworks and COVID-19 is a pandemic-driven disaster [77]. Mental health innovators can use these frameworks to understand *what* to build during this evolving crisis and *when* those innovations will prove most vital. In Figure 2.2 we provide an overview of the phases of a disaster and relevant technologies.

Over the course of March 2020, our world traversed the heroic phase of the disaster response. This phase is characterized by high levels of activity, low levels of

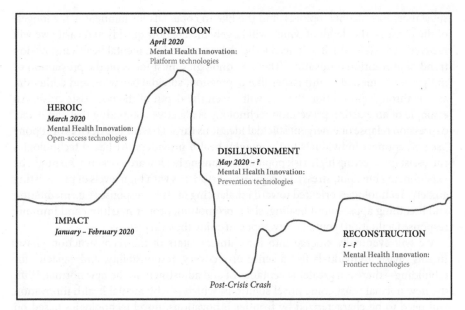

HONEYMOON
April 2020
Mental Health Innovation:
Platform technologies

HEROIC
March 2020
Mental Health Innovation:
Open-access technologies

DISILLUSIONMENT
May 2020 – ?
Mental Health Innovation:
Prevention technologies

IMPACT
January – February 2020

RECONSTRUCTION
? – ?
Mental Health Innovation:
Frontier technologies

Post-Crisis Crash

Figure 2.2 Emotional response to disaster meets mental health innovation.
Source: Carson, Eyre, and Lavretsky [77].

productivity, and a surge in altruistic, adrenaline-induced rescue behavior. In this phase, the mental health innovation trend was that of open-access innovations. A multitude of companies, from meditation apps to teleconferencing technologies, offered free or discounted access to their platforms in this time of limited resources and millions out of work.

As April 2020 progressed, we entered the honeymoon phase. In this phase, disaster assistance was available, community bonding was more prevalent than ever (albeit virtual), and there was a sense of collective optimism. The honeymoon phase seemed to be characterized by the mental health innovation trend of platform innovations—the use of existing technologies (apps, websites, etc.) upon which new products and services can be offered.

Around May 2020, we entered a less hospitable phase—the disillusionment phase. In this phase, the public recognized the limits of the governments in being able to control viral spread, develop vaccines, or provide disaster assistance; felt a heightened sense of discouragement and distress; and began experiencing clinical manifestations of reactions to stress including affective and emotional symptoms (anxiety, phobias, depression, irritability, apathy, and withdrawal), physiological disorders, sleep disorders and dreaming disturbances, memory disorders, behaviors that reinforce and maintain the trauma in the conscience, and repercussions on the basic beliefs of oneself and the world. Experts referred to this phase as the "mental health tsunami"—if the virus outbreak was the earthquake, then mental illness will be the storm surge that comes in its wake. In the disillusionment phase, realities like unemployment, debt, and death begin to sink in, and individuals may rely more heavily on substances like alcohol, opioids, and the like to cope. Disillusionment is the longest of the phases—the depth of which will largely dictate how quickly and easily we will recover—which is why it will need to be characterized by a mental health innovation trend of prevention innovation. These technologies must focus on the prevention or mitigation of mental health issues like depression, suicidal behavior, and addiction, as it is through prevention that we will lessen the depth of the postcrisis crash. An example of an existing prevention technology is affective computing that can detect depression relapse or emergent suicidal ideations through wearable devices or iPhone use and connect individuals to the mental health providers. AI-based technologies can assist in detecting high-risk populations among healthcare workers who might be experiencing burnout, stressed caregivers, or students with high levels of pre-existing anxiety. Technologies oriented toward rebalancing of stress response (e.g., meditation and breathing apps, sound healing, sleep promotion, proper nutrition, and immune response facilitation) could be developed to guide those in distress.

We will eventually emerge into the calmer waters of the reconstruction phase. In this phase, individuals feel a sense of recovery, responsibility, and capacity for rebuilding—there is a greater acceptance of and adjustment to the new normal. With the new normal must come novel solutions, which is why mental health innovation will need to be characterized by frontier innovations, novel technologies based on significant scientific advances and engineering innovation. Examples of frontier technologies include innovations like AI, sensors, -omics, imaging, synthetic biology, smart devices, digital therapeutics, and the like. While this is not to suggest that frontier technologies should not be built throughout the crisis, it is also useful for mental health innovators to consider *what* tools are most crucial and *when* they are most needed. For instance, frontier technologies may not be readily adopted during the disillusionment phase if they are too costly or complex to employ in a time of great uncertainty.

Although these listed stages of response to disasters are true for the population at large, patients with mental disorders are more vulnerable to profound levels of depression, anxiety, and distress and may not reach recovery without additional help from the mental health innovators.

Conclusion

The complexity and multisystemic nature of the global mental health crisis makes it poorly suited to siloed approaches of thinking and innovation. To deal with the unprecedented challenges, a paradigm shift is needed. Convergence science is the Ariadne thread necessary to navigate the intricate labyrinth of global mental health problems. Convergence science integrates knowledge, tools, and thought strategies from various fields and is the point where novel insights arise. There are predicate examples of convergence science in adjacent fields to mental health, such as neurology and biomedicine, that provide a roadmap for the way forward. Further, examples of convergence mental health in action currently include early-stage growth companies, neuroscience initiatives, public health projects, and unconventional funding mechanisms. The world has a historic opportunity to leverage convergence science to lead to a new era of innovation and progress in global mental health.

Disclosures

HE reports ownership of shares in CNSdose LLC. HL has a research grant from Allergan. MB reports personal fees from Servier, Lundbeck, Grunbiotics, Controversias Barcelona, HealthEd, ANZOS, Livanova, Janssen, Catalyst, Norwegian Psych Assocation, Otsuka, allergan, Bioconcepts, and RANZCP, outside the submitted work. MB has a patent modulation of physiological processes and agents useful for the same, issued, and a patent modulation of diseases of the central nervous system and related disorders pending. ES reports ownership of shares in Prodrome Labs Inc. ES has a research grant from the Michael J. Fox Foundation and a patent detection system and methods for neurological diseases pending. There are no other disclosures to report.

Grant Support

HL reports grant support by NIH grant AT009198. MB reports grants from NHMRC Principal Research Fellowship (APP1059660 and APP1156072). No other authors report relevant grant support.

References

1. Patel, V., et al., *Mental health of young people: a global public-health challenge.* Lancet, 2007. **369**(9569): p. 1302–1313 https://doi.org/10.1016/s0140-6736(07)60368-7.
2. Bosely, S., *World in mental health crisis of "monumental suffering," say experts.* The Guardian. October 9, 2018.
3. Curtin, S.C. and M. Heron, *Death rates due to suicide and homicide among persons aged 10–24: United States, 2000–2017.* NCHS Data Brief, **2019**(352): p. 1–8.
4. 5 surprising mental health statistics, 2019. Available from https://www.mentalhealthfirstaid.org/2019/02/5-surprising-mental-health-statistics/.
5. Woolf, S.H., and H. Schoomaker, *Life expectancy and mortality rates in the United States, 1959-2017.* JAMA, 2019. **322**(20): p. 1996–2016 https://doi.org/10.1001/jama.2019.16932.
6. Vigo, D., G. Thornicroft, and R. Atun, *Estimating the true global burden of mental illness.* The Lancet Psychiatry, 2016. **3**(2): p. 171–178 https://doi.org/10.1016/s2215-0366(15)00505-2.
7. Organization, W.H., *The world health report 2001: Mental health: new understanding, new hope.* 2001: World Health Organization.
8. Patel, V., et al., *The Lancet Commission on global mental health and sustainable development.* Lancet, 2018. **392**(10157): p. 1553–1598 https://doi.org/10.1016/s0140-6736(18)32270-0.
9. Timsit, A. *Experts say there are six ways to tackle the world's "monumental" mental health crisis.* 2018. https://qz.com/1419126/world-mental-health-day-a-new-report-calls-the-crisis-monumental/

10. Herrman, H., et al., *Reducing the global burden of depression: a Lancet-World Psychiatric Association Commission.* Lancet, 2019. **393**(10189): p. e42–e43 https://doi.org/10.1016/s0140-6736(18)32408-5.

11. Vigo, D.V., et al., *A partnership for transforming mental health globally.* Lancet Psychiatry, 2019. **6**(4): p. 350–356 https://doi.org/10.1016/s2215-0366(18)30434-6.

12. Reynolds III, C.F., et al., *The future of psychiatry as clinical neuroscience.* Academic Medicine, 2009. **84**(4): p. 446–450 https://doi.org/10.1097/acm.0b013e31819a8052.

13. Stephan, P.E., and R.G. Ehrenberg, *Science and the University.* 2007: Univ of Wisconsin Press.

14. Eyre, H.A., et al., *Convergence science arrives: How does it relate to psychiatry?* Acad Psychiatry, 2017. **41**(1): p. 91–99 https://doi.org/10.1007/s40596-016-0496-0.

15. *Timeline: VC investment in mental health & wellness tech on the rise.* 2017: CB Insights.

16. Fernandez, A. *The digital brain health market 2012–2020: Web-based, mobile and biometrics-based technology to assess, monitor, and enhance cognition and brain functioning;* 2013. SharpBrains. Available from http://sharpbrains.com/market-report.

17. Kuhn, T.S. *The structure of scientific revolutions.* 1962: Chicago.

18. Kemp, S.P., and P.S. Nurius, *Preparing emerging doctoral scholars for transdisciplinary research: A developmental approach.* Journal of Teaching in Social Work, 2015. **35**(1–2): p. 131–150 https://doi.org/10.1080/08841233.2014.980929.

19. Johansson, F., *The Medici effect: Breakthrough insights at the intersection of ideas.* Concepts, and Cultures. 2004: Harvard Business School Press\

20. Council, N.R., *Convergence: Facilitating transdisciplinary integration of life sciences, physical sciences, engineering, and beyond.* 2014: National Academies Press.

21. Roco, M., et al., *Converging knowledge, technology, and society: Beyond convergence of nano-bio-info-cognitive technologies.* 2013: Springer.

22. Arnold, A., and K. Bowman, *Fostering the culture of convergence in research: Proceedings of a workshop.* 2019: National Academies Press.

23. Hall, K.L., et al., *The collaboration readiness of transdisciplinary research teams and centers: findings from the National Cancer Institute's TREC year-one evaluation study.* American Journal of Preventive Medicine, 2008. **35**(2): p. S161–S172 https://doi.org/10.1016/j.amepre.2008.03.035.

24. World Health Organization, *Global health diplomacy, in trade, foreign policy, diplomacy and health.* 2018: World Health Organization.

25. Fernando Aguzzoli-Peres, 2019. Available from https://www.gbhi.org/fernando-aguzzoli-peres.

26. *What is computerized cognitive behavioral therapy?* 2019: Nanalyze.

27. Patel, V. and M. Prince, *Global mental health: A new global health field comes of age.* JAMA, 2010. **303**(19): p. 1976–1977 https://doi.org/10.1001/jama.2010.616.

28. Kohrt, B.A., et al., *Global mental health: Five areas for value-driven training innovation.* Academic Psychiatry, 2016. **40**(4): p. 650–658 https://doi.org/10.1007/s40596-016-0504-4.

29. Miremadi, T., *A model for science and technology diplomacy: How to align the rationales of foreign policy and science.* 2016: SSRN.

30. Leijten, J., *Exploring the future of innovation diplomacy.* European Journal of Futures Research, 2017. **5**: 20 https://doi.org/10.1007/s40309-017-0122-8.

31. Bound, K., and T. Saunders, 2018, November 14. *Innovation policy toolkit: Tradecraft for innovation diplomats.* Available from https://www.nesta.org.uk/toolkit/innovation-policy-toolkit-tradecraft-for-innovation-diplomats/.

32. Fernandes, B.S., et al., *The new field of "precision psychiatry."* BMC Medicine, 2017. **15**(1): p. 80 https://doi.org/10.1186/s12916-017-0849-x.

33. Levey, D.F., et al., *Towards understanding and predicting suicidality in women: biomarkers and clinical risk assessment*. Molecular Psychiatry, 2016. **21**(6): p. 768 https://doi.org/10.1038/mp.2016.31.

34. el Kaliouby, R., *We need computers with empathy*. 2017: MIT Technology Review.

35. Picard, R.W., *Affective computing*. 2000: MIT press.

36. Weiner, S., *Addressing the escalating psychiatrist shortage*. AAMCNews, February 13, 2018.

37. JAMES, W., *II.—What is an emotion?* Mind, 1884. **9**(34): p. 188–205 https://doi.org/10.1093/mind/os-ix.34.188.

38. Picard, R.W., *Affective computing: MIT Media Laboratory Perceptual Computing Section Technical Report No. 321*. 1995: MIT.

39. Affectiva, 2019. Available from https://www.affectiva.com/.

40. Empatica, 2019. Available from https://www.empatica.com/.

41. Jha, A., A. Ilif, and A. Chaoui, *A crisis in health care: a call to action on physician burnout*. 2019: Massachusetts Medical Society.

42. Jeffrey Cohn, 2019. Available from http://psychology.pitt.edu/people/jeffrey-cohn-phd.

43. Gratch, J., et al. *User-state sensing for virtual health agents and telehealth applications*. Studies in Health Technology and Informatics, 2013. **184**: p. 151–157.

44. Dibeklioğlu, H., Z. Hammal, and J.F. Cohn, *Dynamic multimodal measurement of depression severity using deep autoencoding*. IEEE Journal of Biomedical and Health Informatics, 2017. **22**(2): p. 525–536.

45. Niculescu, A.B., and H. Le-Niculescu, *Convergent functional genomics: what we have learned and can learn about genes, pathways, and mechanisms*. Neuropsychopharmacology, 2010. **35**(1): p. 355 https://doi.org/10.1038/npp.2009.107.

46. Le-Niculescu, H., et al., *Towards understanding the schizophrenia code: an expanded convergent functional genomics approach*. American Journal of Medical Genetics Part B: Neuropsychiatric Genetics, 2007. **144**(2): p. 129–158 https://doi.org/10.1002/ajmg.b.30481.

47. Niculescu, A.B., et al., *PhenoChipping of psychotic disorders: a novel approach for deconstructing and quantitating psychiatric phenotypes*. American Journal of Medical Genetics Part B: Neuropsychiatric Genetics, 2006. **141**(6): p. 653–662 https://doi.org/10.1002/ajmg.b.30404.

48. Eyre, H.A., et al., *Mental health innovation diplomacy: An under-recognised soft power*. Australian and New Zealand Journal of Psychiatry, 2019. **53**(5): p. 474–475 https://doi.org/10.1177/0004867419828488.

49. Ternes, K. *Brain health innovation diplomacy (BIND): A model binding diverse disciplines to manage the promise and perils of technological innovation*. 2020: International Psychogeriatrics. https://doi.org/10.1017/S1041610219002266/.

50. World Health Organization and the Calouste Gulbenkian Foundation. *Social determinants of mental health*. 2014. Available from https://www.who.int/mental_health/publications/gulbenkian_paper_social_determinants_of_mental_health/en/.

51. *Mental Health Specialists*, accessed January 15, 2020; Available from https://www.doctorswithoutborders.org/careers/work-overseas/find-role/mental-health-specialists.

52. Licinio, J. and M.L. Wong, *Launching the "war on mental illness."* Molecular Psychiatry, 2014. **19**(1): p. 1–5 https://doi.org/10.1038/mp.2013.180.

53. Eyre, H.A., et al., *Leveraging responsible innovation to steward mental health technology development*. Lancet Psychiatry, 2020. Manuscript accepted for publication.

54. OECD, 2020. *Recommendation of the Council on Responsible Innovation in Neurotechnology*. Available from https://www.oecd.org/science/recommendation-on-responsible-innovation-in-neurotechnology.htm.

55. Staruch, R.M., et al., *Calling for the next WHO Global Health Initiative: The use of disruptive innovation to meet the health care needs of displaced populations.* Journal of Global Health, 2018. **8**(1): p. 010303 https://doi.org/10.7189/jogh.08.010303.

56. Ng, C., et al., *APEC digital hub for mental health.* The Lancet Psychiatry, 2017. **4**(3): p. e3–e4 https://doi.org/10.1016/s2215-0366(17)30034-2.

57. U.S. Department of Health and Human Services, 2019, June 4. *What does "suicide contagion" mean, and what can be done to prevent it?* Available from https://www.hhs.gov/answers/mental-health-and-substance-abuse/what-does-suicide-contagion-mean/index.html#.

58. Doraiswamy, P.M., et al., 2019. *Empowering 8 billion minds: Enabling better mental health for all via the ethical adoption of technologies.* Available from https://nam.edu/empowering-8-billion-minds-enabling-better-mental-health-for-all-via-the-ethical-adoption-of-technologies/.

59. Global Future Council on Technology for Mental Health, 2019. [Home page]. Available from https://www.weforum.org/communities/the-future-of-neurotechnologies-and-brain-science. https://doi.org/10.1016/j.pestbp.2019.12.010.

60. Rommelfanger, K., and A. Fernandez. *We need to rethink neuroscience. And you can help us.* 2018. https://www.weforum.org/agenda/2018/11/rethink-neuroscience-you-can-help/

61. O'Neil, A., et al., *A shared framework for the common mental disorders and non-communicable disease: key considerations for disease prevention and control.* BMC Psychiatry, 2015. **15**: p. 15 https://doi.org/10.1186/s12888-015-0394-0.

62. APC, 2011. *Standards relating to suicide.* Available from https://www.presscouncil.org.au/document-search/standard-suicide-reporting/.

63. Willsey, A.J., et al., *The psychiatric cell map initiative: a convergent systems biological approach to illuminating key molecular pathways in neuropsychiatric disorders.* Cell, 2018. **174**(3): p. 505–520 https://doi.org/10.1016/j.cell.2018.06.016.

64. World Health Organization, 2019. Risk reduction of cognitive decline and dementia: WHO guidelines. Available from https://www.who.int/mental_health/neurology/dementia/guidelines_risk_reduction/en/.

65. Stanford University. Explore courses: PSYC 240: Leadership and Innovation in Mental Healthcare. Available from https://explorecourses.stanford.edu/search?view=catalog&filter-coursestatus-Active=on&q=PSYC%20240:%20Leadership%20and%20Innovation%20in%20Mental%20Healthcare&academicYear=20162017.

66. Tufts University, 2019. *Science diplomacy dialogue series.* Available from https://sites.tufts.edu/sciencediplomacy/2018/09/11/science-diplomacy-dialogue-series/.

67. Zuckerberg, M., 2019. *Four ideas to regulate the Internet.* Available from https://newsroom.fb.com/news/2019/03/four-ideas-regulate-internet/.

68. Alzheimer's Disease International, 2018. *World Alzheimer report 2018: The state of the art of dementia research: New frontiers.* Available from https://www.alz.co.uk/research/WorldAlzheimerReport2018.pdf.

69. Landi, H., *Venture capital investment in AI and mental health startups surges in Q2: report.* 2019: FierceHealthcare.

70. Baum, S., *Payers, large employers are pushing to integrate behavioral health services into member plans.* 2017. https://medcitynews.com/2017/02/payers-large-employers-are-pushing-to-integrate-behavioral-health-services-into-member-plans/

71. Global Brain Health Institute, 2019. [Home page]. Available from www.gbhi.org.

72. Space Health Innovation Conference, 2019. Accessed December 26, 2019; Available from https://shic.swoogo.com/shic19/248306.

73. The World Bank, *Healthy brain bonds: Is this a feasible option.* 2018, World Bank.

74. Staglin, G., *Collaborative research: The path to "Healthy brains for all."* 2019.
75. Norton, S., et al., *Potential for primary prevention of Alzheimer's disease: an analysis of population-based data.* The Lancet Neurology, 2014. 13(8): p. 788–794 https://doi.org/10.1016/s1474-4422(14)70136-x.
76. *Psych 101: The most active investors in mental health tech.* 2017: CB Insights.
77. Carson, J., H.A. Eyre, and H. Lavretsky, *Dear mental health innovators: The COVID-19 honeymoon is almost over.* Psychiatric Times, 2020. Manuscript accepted for publication.

3

On the Road to Convergence Research

Scientists Reaching Across Disciplines
to Tackle Tough Problems

Niki Wilson

Reprinted with permission from *BioScience*, Volume 69, Issue 8, August 2019, pp. 587–593, https://doi.org/10.1093/biosci/biz066

Utqiagvik (previously known as Barrow) is the northernmost city of Alaska. Few of the 5000 people there debate the reality of climate change. Permafrost bluffs are thawing and eroding into the Arctic Ocean. Increasingly, more frequent and intense storms hurl water inland, threatening to swamp the community and destroy homes and infrastructure. Sea ice is disappearing, which, in addition to removing some protection from storms, is also taking out important ocean platforms from which the Iñupiat community there and others across the Arctic hunt for traditional whale, seal, and walrus. These foods are directly tied to the culture and well-being of many communities. Climate change is transforming a way of life.

Finding solutions and adaptations for the people living with this rapid socioecological change in the Arctic is critical and urgent and will require innovation from multiple sectors. It is the kind of complex problem solving that the National Science Foundation (NSF) hopes can be facilitated through convergence research, a way of bringing people together from various disciplines and backgrounds in what the NSF describes as "a deeper, more intentional approach to accelerating discovery." Navigating the New Arctic is a program area that the NSF funds through its convergence research awards—one of its Ten Big Ideas for Future Investment.

The concept of convergence research (also referred to as *convergence science*) is relatively new, having only really come to the fore in the past decade. It is the next stop on a continuum used to describe approaches whereby scientists learn from each other and collaborate across disciplines. One such approach, *multidisciplinarity*, draws on knowledge from different disciplines while staying within the boundaries of those disciplines, as explained in a 2006 paper in *Clinical and Investigative Medicine* by Bernhard Choi and Anita Pak, while *interdisciplinarity* "analyzes, synthesizes and harmonizes links between disciplines into a coordinated and coherent whole." Convergence research teams aim to be *transdisciplinary*—integrating the natural, social, and health sciences in a humanities context and transcending the fields' traditional boundaries.

Definitions of convergence are evolving. On its website dedicated to convergence research (www.convergencerevolution.net), the Massachusetts Institute of Technology (MIT) defines it as "the integration of engineering, physical sciences, computation, and life sciences—with profound benefits for medicine and health, energy and environment." Regardless of the definition, there is general agreement that convergence is not simply a set of experts coming together. Over time, team members absorb knowledge from one another and think with a different mindset, rather than just coming from the perspective of their own training and conditioning. "There is an increasing need to merge expertise that goes beyond the interdisciplinary intersection of fields to the emergence of new disciplines," says MIT's Phillip Sharp and Robert Langer in their 2011 article for *Science* titled "Promoting Convergence in Biomedical Science" (doi:10.1126/science.1205008). Convergence is not something that happens with a snap of the fingers. It requires time—and a paradigm shift from traditional, siloed research approaches.

The science community is on the road to convergence research, but the concept is far from mainstream, and barriers linger. A better understanding of its emergence may shed some light on the journey so far and what to expect next.

Getting Started: Building Convergence Research Networks

The NSF defines convergence research as "being driven by a specific and compelling problem ... whether it arises from deep scientific questions or pressing social need." Once the problem or need has been identified, the first step is to find the right teams to address the problem, and come up with specific research questions. To help facilitate this, convergence science and research networks are popping up around the globe. For example, Australia's Convergence Science Network brings scientists together online and through events around biomedical discovery. The Europe-based Convergence Science Network of Biomimetics and Neurotechnology aims to establish strategic collaborations with key researchers and research communities in the United States and Japan through outreach, workshops, and conferences.

In the United States, the NSF funds research coordination networks (RCNs). Through the aforementioned Navigating the New Arctic Program, in 2016, a team of researchers at the University of Colorado Boulder and the University of Arizona were awarded four years of funding for their RCN, called the Indigenous Foods Knowledges Network (IFKN). Led by cultural anthropologist Noor Johnson, the RCN's goal is to combine indigenous knowledge and perspectives with scientific knowledge across the biological, geological, geographic, anthropological, and information sciences to figure out how to approach issues of food security and resilience.

Indigenous peoples are facing many challenges in maintaining traditional food systems in the Arctic, says Johnson. Rapid environmental change is affecting how food is harvested. In the past, local and traditional knowledge collected over many generations guided communities in the hunt by indicating how animals migrate with the seasons, what time of year to hunt certain species, and when it is safe to travel on sea ice to access and harvest animals. But as the Arctic warms, many of these historic patterns are changing. For example, the formation of sea ice has been important for hunting seal and walrus in the spring, but Johnson says now that the sea ice is less reliable, "It can make it difficult or impossible to access the harvesting territories that are really important to them."

Layered on the environmental problems are challenges around interactions with Western culture that can make it difficult to practice indigenous food knowledge and traditions, says Johnson. For example, one member of the IFKN wants to integrate more traditional foods (such as seal oil) into the cafeteria at a senior center in Nome, Alaska, but it has been difficult to get the US Department of Agriculture to approve foods that are not processed and have not been subject to safety requirements. The complexity of these issues is reflected in other indigenous communities outside of the Arctic that have also experienced rapid environmental and social change. This is why, in addition to bringing together communities from the Arctic and scientists from different disciplines, Johnson and her team wanted to include indigenous communities from the US Southwest, where changes in precipitation are creating significant challenges for agriculture. "The thought was that we could bring communities together to share both some of the challenges they are having around ensuring their food systems are secure, but also some of the solutions and innovations that are emerging from the grassroots in these communities," she says.

The IFKN meets twice a year, alternating between communities in Alaska and communities in the Southwest, where they visit with farmers and learn traditional harvesting techniques through hands-on demonstrations. From these exchanges, participants develop new ideas for convergence research based on the interests and information needs of indigenous communities. Already, a couple of initiatives are taking shape, says Johnson, such as a project to document information about growing and harvesting traditional foods using methods based in digital storytelling. In the meantime, researchers are working to understand how best to share knowledge from their various disciplines. As the team explains in their proposal, "exploring how to merge ideas from diverse groups will contribute to the advancement of both convergence science, and the coproduction of knowledge with Indigenous communities."

Of course, food security is only one of many complex problems Northern communities are facing. Thomas Ravens, professor of civil engineering at the University of Alaska, heads up the Arctic Network for Coastal Community Hazards, Observations, and Integrated Research (ANCHOR), another RCN that is funded through the NSF convergence research grants. ANCHOR aims to integrate social science, the natural sciences, and engineering to address the imminent challenges that coastal communities.in the Arctic face from melting permafrost and rapid erosion. "In the community of Utqiagvik, you have these permafrost bluffs that are thawing and oozing into the ocean," says Ravens. As the ground liquefies and shifts below them, houses can collapse. "You have huge storms happening in August, which didn't really happen in the past," he says, adding that the disappearance of sea ice means less shielding of communities against the battering storm waves of the Chukchi Sea. "During storms, [some community members] are out with their front end loaders [maintaining] a berm to keep the water from flooding the community."

Figuring out exactly how quickly the environment is shifting and understanding how much adaptation is possible will be key in finding solutions. Through ANCHOR, there is already better integration of disciplines. Ravens says that collaboration among engineers, computer scientists, and social scientists, for example, has led to more meaningful data collection in communities and is contributing to the development of coastal hazard forecasting models. "With those models, we'll be forecasting scenarios of flooding, erosion, and permafrost thaw decades into the future," he says. On the basis of modeling, ANCHOR can look at the cost communities face with increased exposure to flooding, erosion, and loss of infrastructure. "The development of these risk scenarios really is a convergence of the physical sciences and engineering, as well as the social science and economic sciences," says Ravens.

Working with social scientists on his team, Ravens is learning how to better interface with community members about the future of their towns and cities. It is difficult to deliver the news that, if things continue the way they are, communities may not be able to stay where they are in 20 to 40 years, he says. He hopes that as they continue to grow ANCHOR, it becomes a bridge between researchers wanting to work in the North, and Northern communities that need the right research questions to be asked and answered to build maximum resilience to the challenges to come.

Convergence Research Institutes

Convergence research institutes are emerging around the globe in an attempt to accelerate discovery around core scientific questions. For example, the French National Research Agency is investing in several large-scale multidisciplinary scientific sites to address key issues at the intersection between societal and economic challenges. As a result, 9 million euros have been given to the Université de Lyon to fund two convergence institutes over 10 years: the François Rabelais Institute for Multi-Disciplinary Cancer Research and the Lyon Urban School examining issues associated with the world's increasing trend toward urbanization.

The Frances Crick Institute in London focuses on biomedical discovery and better understanding the biology underlying human health. Housed in a state-of-the-art building with laboratories designed to physically adapt to change as new scientific opportunities arise, the institute brings together 1500 scientists and support staff collaborating across disciplines. Singularity University in San Francisco is another convergence-focused organization aimed at using rapidly accelerating technology—including artificial intelligence, data science, nanotech, and robotics—to prepare global leaders and organizations to solve what they call "The World's Biggest Problems." This includes ensuring basic needs are met for all and fostering good quality of life. MIT has numerous convergence initiatives, such as the Koch Institute for Integrative Cancer Research and the Precision Medicine Institute.

In Canada, the McGill Centre for the Convergence of Health and Economics (MCCHE) aims "to fundamentally transform individual and community diets, lifestyles, markets, and health systems through better health and economic convergence." At the helm is chair and scientific director Laurette Dubé, also the chair of consumer and lifestyle psychology and marketing.

Dubé works with convergence research teams at the intersection of multiple life sciences, behavioral disciplines such as marketing and management, and digital technologies to "harness the power of both human and artificial intelligence for a better society," she says. As an example of how convergence research gleans novel results, she points to a 2016 study she coauthored examining the connection between genetics and socioeconomic status as it relates to childhood obesity (doi:10.1001/jamapediatrics.2015.4253). It has long been known that certain genes make children more vulnerable to conditions such as obesity, explains Dubé, but her team was able to show that in a different socioeconomic environment, the same gene is an advantage: It makes children eat better. The research team consisted of specialists in pediatrics, mental health, neuroinformatics, psychology, evolutionary biology, and psychiatry. "We were among the first to highlight the neurobehavioral base of obesity, and these results open new horizons for more impactful and better targeted solutions," says Dubé. It is a novel result that comes from understanding data on human behavior in the context of the complex systems around it.

Working with this scientific complexity is one of the things that attracts Dubé to convergence research. Often, our view of systems is simplistic, she explains. For example, though she says society's singular focus on wealth creation has been an important driver of technological innovation since the Industrial Revolution, the model needs to be tweaked to create supply and demand for better social and environmental outcomes. At the MCCHE, Dubé and her colleagues are trying to figure out how the behavioral change that is so well understood and used on the commercial side can be leveraged for more optimal health outcomes. "We can and must have wealth creation that better serves society," she says.

The Importance of Entrepreneurship in Convergence

Harris Eyre is on a mission to end what he calls a "one size fits all" approach to mental healthcare, and he is a proponent of the power of convergence research teams to do it. Eyre is himself an embodiment of convergence: He is a medical doctor with training in psychiatry and neuroscience, and he holds a PhD in the field of precision medicine for mental health. He also maintains advisory or adjunct roles with various industry and academic organizations including the Texas Medical Center Innovation Institute, Brainstorm: The Stanford Lab for Brain Health Innovation and Entrepreneurship, American Psychiatric Association's Innovation Committee, and the University of Melbourne's Department of Psychiatry. However, his primary role is as the chief medical officer of CNSdose, a personalized medicine company that aims to use the information collected from patients' individual genetic profiles to get them the right mental health medications more quickly.

"I got into entrepreneurship because I wanted to make the biggest difference I could in the mental health field, and I figured that I can do that by developing technologies that are scalable, that can help more people," he says. To demonstrate the need for these kinds of solutions, Eyre points to the problem of how medications are prescribed for depression on a trial and error basis. "We know that patients don't like it, because it only works around 50% of the time. They feel like guinea pigs, and it's very demoralizing for them when the medication fails and they have to go to the next line of medication, and the next," he says. When patients do not get the medication they need, it is frustrating for their families and the clinicians trying to help them. "We know that insurers don't like it because it's expensive when people don't get better and you have to pay out more claims."

Eyre says the field of pharmacogenetics—the genetic guidance of medications—is an example of how convergence in research can help get people the medications that work best for them. The field brings together geneticists, psychiatrists, pharmacologists, and primary care doctors (who prescribe most antidepressant medication). By harnessing the discoveries coming out of this field, Eyre's company CNSdose has created a diagnostic tool, Amplis, that, in conjunction with a cheek swab to collect a patient's DNA, can be used by doctors to more precisely prescribe mental health medications. In patients with depression, a trial of this tool compared to trial and error demonstrated the novel approach was able to double rates of remission. It is a product born not just of the convergence found in pharmacogenetics but also of convergence with data science and technical engineering.

Eyre says that there are increasing opportunities to solve mental health issues through convergent research and technologies, and investors are keen to fund related technological innovations. It is a field that is growing rapidly but one that he stresses needs to remain evidence based. Done well, entrepreneurship may play an important role in moving society towards solutions for pressing, healthcare-related issues.

Speed Bumps on the Road to Convergence

There are many steps to be taken on the road to systemically adopt the concept of convergence research and science. Although the goal may be to develop teams that go beyond their silos to embody knowledge across disciplines and adopt new ways of thinking, for many the journey still begins by getting people from different disciplines to sit down together (either physically or remotely). This is not always easy—which is why the NSF and other organizations fund research coordination networks. There are multiple challenges. For example, many scientists spend a lot of time searching for grants and funding for their own work, and may not have the time, desire, or means to participate on con- vergence research teams, especially if they are not convinced it will be of benefit. Ravens recognizes that being closer to the end of his career has allowed him some freedom to let go of "being research competitive" and to instead serve in a facilitation role between researchers and the communities he works with at ANCHOR.

Although convergence research institutes are increasing around the globe, most universities are not designed for convergence education. Eyre thinks the concept needs to be embedded from the level of undergraduate degree, up the academic chain. The education system "needs to be steeped in this kind of thinking ... so that students are deeply immersed in the environment of different disciplines, and picking things up over time to become truly transdisciplinary," he says.

Breaking down silos on convergence teams can also have its challenges. "You need to develop a mutual language, which is interesting, and very humbling," says Eyre. But it takes time. For Johnson, even more challenging is "transcending the boundaries between indigenous knowledge systems and those of us that were trained and continue to work in a western science tradition." These challenges are likely more difficult in groups with greater diversity of disciplines and viewpoints. However, there is also evidence for increased creativity in more diverse teams. It is worth developing governance and operational frameworks that foster a culture of openness and inclusiveness to maximize return on convergence efforts, say proponents.

Getting buy-in to the concept of convergence can also be challenging. Even for established institutes such as the MCCHE, Dubé says she is still fighting to keep the center in existence. "Some people think we're a business school," she says, highlighting a general lack of familiarity with what convergence research is, even among academic peers. Fostering the development of convergence research hubs requires continual outreach to build support.

Despite these and other challenges, convergence research is taking hold and growing. The next few years will see the publication of several books and papers and enhanced education and training to help scientists move toward convergence research teams and, ultimately, convergence mindsets. Proponents ask us to imagine a world in which there is no poverty or malnutrition, a world in which climate change and plastics pollution are not discussed as a daily threat, in which more people get the help needed for mental illness and effective treatment for cancer. Convergence research cannot singlehandedly solve all of these problems, but it could play a key role in accelerating progress. It takes us to the intersection of different fields we have never seen merged before, says Eyre. It is crucial that we bring these fields together, he adds, because, "there will be unexpected findings."

4

Convergence and the Changing Nature of Innovation

Amanda Arnold and Katherine Bowman

Introduction

Convergence has the potential to shape cultures of innovation in health and medicine by providing a framework integrating perspectives from multiple disciplines and sectors to tackle complex challenges. Although multiple definitions are available (see Table 4.1), the convergence concept was described in a 2014 report from the National Academies of Sciences, Engineering, and Medicine as

> an approach to problem solving that cuts across disciplinary boundaries. It integrates knowledge, tools, and ways of thinking from life and health sciences, physical, mathematical, and computational sciences, engineering disciplines, and beyond to form a comprehensive synthetic framework for tackling scientific and societal challenges that exist at the interfaces of multiple fields. By merging these diverse areas of expertise in a network of partnerships, convergence stimulates innovation from basic science discovery to translational application. (p. 1)

The National Academies are not the only institutions discussing the promise of convergence for goal-oriented and curiosity-driven research. Over the past decade, for example, the Massachusetts Institute of Technology, the American Association for the Advancement of Science, the National Science Foundation (NSF), the Science Philanthropy Alliance, and others have held influential meetings and published perspectives on the importance of integration across disciplines and communities. These concepts have been called by several names with sometimes overlapping and complementary definitions. For example, the emphasis on synthesizing knowledge that is a core component of transdisciplinary science (American Academy of Arts and Sciences 2013), is clearly also an important aim of convergence. And because an integral part of the scientific enterprise rests on contributions made by interdependent teams of individuals, evidence on how teams function effectively (the science of team

Table 4.1 Selected Definitions of Convergence

Publication	Convergence as Defined
Sharp and Langer 2011, p. 527	"Convergence of fields represents a third revolution where multidisciplinary thinking and analysis will permit the emergence of new scientific c principles and where engineers and physical scientists are equal partners with biologists and clinicians in addressing many of the new medical challenges. . . . There is an increasing need to merge expertise that goes beyond the interdisciplinary intersection of fields to the emergence of new disciplines. In recent decades there have been two biomedical revolutions: molecular biology and genomics. We believe the convergence of fields represents a third revolution."
Roco, Bainbridge, Tonn, and Whitesides 2013	"Convergence of knowledge and technology for the benefit of society (CKTS) is defined as the escalating and transformative interactions among seemingly different disciplines, technologies, communities, and domains of human activity to achieve mutual compatibility, synergism, and integration, and through this process to create added value and branch out to meet human needs and shared goals. It allows society to answer questions and resolve problems that isolated capabilities cannot, as well as to create new competencies, knowledge, and technologies on this basis. Convergence has been progressing by stages over the past several decades, beginning with nanotechnology for the material world, followed by convergence of nanotechnology, biotechnology, information technology, and cognitive science (NBIC) for emerging technologies. CKTS is the third level of convergence."
National Research Council 2014	"Convergence is an approach to problem solving that integrates expertise from life science white physical, mathematical, and computational sciences, medicine, and engineering, to form comprehensive synthetic frameworks that merge areas of knowledge from multiple fields to address specific challenges."
Government-University-Industry Research Roundtable 2014	"Convergence—the coming together of insights and approaches from originally distinct fields—will make fundamental contributions in our drive to provide creative solutions to the most difficult problems facing us as a society."
Arnold and Greer 2015	"Convergence—an integration of the knowledge, tools, and ways of thinking from the life and health sciences; physical, mathematical, and computational sciences; the engineering disciplines; the social and behavioral sciences; and the humanities to form a comprehensive framework for tackling scientific and societal challenges that exist at the interfaces of multiple fields."

Table 4.1 Continued

Publication	Convergence as Defined
Massachusetts Institute of Technology 2016	"Convergence as applied to health is an approach to problem solving that integrates expertise from life sciences with physical, mathematical, and computational sciences, as well as engineering, to form comprehensive frameworks that merge areas of knowledge from multiple fields to address specific challenges."
Sharp and Hockfield 2017, p. 589	"The integration of the life sciences, physical sciences, mathematics, engineering, and information technology— often referred to as Convergence—has emerged in recent years as a powerful approach to research with the potential to lead to medical and technological breakthroughs."
National Science Foundation 2018	"Convergence is a deeper, more intentional approach to the integration of knowledge, techniques, and expertise from multiple disciplines in order to address the most compelling scientific and societal challenges."

science) can inform the design of strategies to foster convergence (National Research Council [NRC] 2015). This chapter does not attempt to parse this definitional landscape in detail and instead focuses on examples of strategies to establish cultures that support the integrative approaches to research and innovation reflected by the term *convergence*.

Making major progress to enhance the culture of innovation in mental health is one challenge for which a convergence approach may increasingly be welcome. Understanding and addressing the complex biological, social, and behavioral dimensions involved in mental well-being will require bringing together the expertise of diverse research communities and diverse sectors. In fact, the application to psychiatry is already underway: "Convergence science insights can enhance the engagement of the psychiatric profession with non-clinical innovations that include making discoveries in molecular biology, advancing neuroimaging, reducing cost of genomic and proteomic profiling, raising computing power, increasing uptake of electronic health records, increasing uptake of Internet and smartphone use, and improving understanding of the social determinants of mental health" (Eyre et al. 2017, p. 98). The ultimate challenge in this space is the "integration of biological, psychological, socio-cultural, and environmental data into a more comprehensive, individualized portrayal of diagnosis" (Eyre et al. 2017, p. 98). However, the work to create convergence mental health will require a realignment of cross-sectoral cultures, players, and institutions. As the 2014 NRC report noted, without a systematic focus on identifying and overcoming barriers, efforts to establish cultures that support convergence will continued to be "a patchwork of isolated efforts" (NRC 2014, p. 95).

This chapter draws on selected prior work by the National Academies on approaches to convergence and lessons learned from efforts to foster it in academia, industry, foundations, and government agencies. In addition to the 2014 report, it draws on a workshop held in 2018 that highlighted examples of recent efforts undertaken by organizations engaged in convergent science (National Academies of Sciences, Engineering, and Medicine [NASEM] 2019). The chapter concludes with lessons learned in the past to assist future applications.

Convergence and the Changing Culture of Innovation

The nature of innovation emerges from a dynamic ecosystem of diverse stakeholders working together across a cycle of discovery and translation that includes advancing early-stage fundamental research and seeking commercial deployment. Stakeholders include networks of universities and non-profit research institutions, private industry from start-ups to large corporations, and philanthropic supporters, federal agencies, venture capitalists, and other public and private partners.

What is becoming clear is that the nature of innovation is changing—both increasing in speed and requiring more intense interdisciplinarity than ever before. "A dramatically more interconnected, turbulent and transforming world—driven by the convergence of the digital, the atomic and the genetic—places the American innovation enterprise at a distinctive inflection point in history" (Council on Competitiveness 2019, p. 3). Accordingly, "researchers, venture capital investors, start-up companies, large corporations, and others now increasingly engage with each other across the multiple stages of innovation, including in basic research. This requires the integration of a broad spectrum of skill sets and new kinds of partnerships" (NASEM 2019, p. 18).

Convergence can serve as a framework for alignment within this dynamic ecosystem that requires integration across disciplinary boundaries as well as sector boundaries. Discussions of critical elements and lessons learned in fostering successful convergence may help transform institutional cultures in ways that can promote innovation and build momentum toward creating new communities of interest and supportive practices and structures.

Convergence and Innovation: Academic, Corporate, Philanthropic, and Government Sectors

Various public and private institutions within the research and innovation enterprise are embracing the concept of convergence. In some cases, the goals of convergence align smoothly with existing structures and practices. In other cases, barriers to establishing and supporting cultures of convergence arise when approaches that rely on convergence challenge existing research and funding structures and incentives. The following selected examples illustrate some of these efforts across multiple sectors.

Academia

A number of research universities and non-profit research institutes are actively facilitating convergence to aid faculty and students in conducting innovative research drawing on multiple disciplinary fields. What is clear is that there is no one-size-fits-all solution, and universities are adopting convergence in different ways. Academia is traditionally organized along disciplinary lines and fostering convergence can require restructuring systems to create physical and virtual spaces for interaction. It frequently also entails new forms of catalytic administrative and financial support. Identifying metrics for the success of convergent science and designing ways for investigators to receive appropriate credit for convergent science remains an active area of interest and challenge.

Creating Venues for Convergence
The development of cutting-edge convergent science within academia can be fostered by providing opportunities for those with diverse disciplinary expertise to interact. Approaches taken by universities to facilitate such connections include designing new physical facilities and workspaces for convergent science, as well as fostering opportunities for colleagues to interact formally and informally. One commonly employed strategy is to create more nimble, convergence-focused centers or institutes with the larger university organization. For example, the Koch Institute for Integrative Cancer Research at Massachusetts Institute of Technology, opened in 2010, co-localizes faculty from biological and physical sciences, engineering, and medicine on mixed-discipline floors and provides shared access to a number of advanced biotechnology core facilities (NASEM 2014). For many universities, such centers are organized around one or more transdisciplinary themes and faculty members affiliated with the center maintain appointments in disciplinary departments. One new strategy being tested by the California Institute for Quantitative Biosciences (QB3), an innovation hub at the University of California Berkeley, University of California San Francisco, and University of California Santa Cruz is the creation of "pop-up institutes." These seek to more quickly and flexibly bring together faculty from the universities to address a specific topic, such as diseases of aging, rather than creating a more formalized physical institute (Leuty 2018). Other universities such as University of Texas at Austin are trying similar ideas (Dawson 2018).

Offering Financial Support to Catalyze Convergent Science
A number of institutions have established seed funding programs that aim to support initial development of cutting-edge, convergent science and new project collaborations. In addition to providing an incentive for researchers to develop proposals that integrate knowledge across fields, such programs can help mitigate challenges with obtaining initial funding through traditional grant channels. The University of Michigan "Mcubed" program, for example, encourages faculty from different units to partner to receive up to $60,000 of support. Now Mcubed 3.0, the program has so far supported 263 faculty-led "cubes."[1] The Stanford Bio-X Interdisciplinary Initiatives

---

[1] See https://mcubed.umich.edu/about (accessed December 18, 2019).

Seed Grants Program provides two-year, $200,000 support to "high-risk, high re-ward" proposals that advance the mission of human health. Since the program's outset in 2000, the supported projects have reportedly reaped a 10-fold return through subsequent external funding and patent development.[2] Bio-X also supports a NeuroVentures program that provides more substantial support to catalyze target areas.[3]

Providing Additional Forms of Administrative Support

Several examples illustrate the types of additional support universities are deploying to foster convergence. For example, the University of California Irvine offers a team science experts group to provide advice and tools to investigators seeking to design effective collaborative projects (NASEM 2019). A number of convergence centers and institutes also provide resources to aid entrepreneurship and the commercial trans-lation of academic research. The Pritzker School of Molecular Engineering at the University of Chicago involves partnerships not only with nearby Argonne National Laboratory, but also with the University's Institute for Translational Medicine and the Booth School of Business. These connections help participating faculty develop rele-vant skills that have so far resulted in multiple invention disclosures and the founding of a number of startup companies ("$100 Million Commitment" 2019). Providing ex-pertise and support in areas such as program management, business development, and technology translation is an important strategy used by a variety of centers and institutes focused on convergence. In the approach used by the Wyss Institute for Biologically Inspired Engineering at Harvard University, for example, "[t]echnologies conceived in our research laboratories are refined and de-risked technically and com-mercially by our Advanced Technology and Business Development teams," helping to make new technologies available to industry.[4] The Complex Adaptive Systems Institute at Arizona State University has reportedly also found that "combining skilled project managers and research faculty has been critical in progress and successful ef-forts to date" (NASEM 2019).

Supporting Commercialization

Several convergence programs make efforts to engage directly with industry to accel-erate progress. For example, the independent Donald Danforth Plant Science Center holds "Venture Cafes" to successfully build engagement with the start-up community in St. Louis (NASEM 2019). QB3 in the University of California system has devel-oped a number of programs to both advance convergent science and connect aca-demic, start-up, and industry communities. In addition to renting incubator space to life sciences startups, it offers programs including "startup in a box" to new entrepre-neurs and helps to connect QB3 startups with potential partners from larger, estab-lished companies (NASEM 2014 and QB3 website). The Massachusetts Institute of Technology (MIT) is also active in this space, establishing The Engine, an incubator

---

[2] See https://biox.stanford.edu/research/seed-grants (accessed December 18, 2019).
[3] See https://biox.stanford.edu/research/venture/neuroventures (accessed December 18, 2019).
[4] See https://wyss.harvard.edu/team/business-development-team/ (accessed December 18, 2019).

supporting "transformative technology" that may not yet attract venture capital but that can enable innovations across energy, food and agriculture, and biotech.[5]

Industry

Participants from a number of private sector companies present in NASEM discussions and workshops on convergence include Verily Life Sciences, Proctor & Gamble, Microsoft, Johnson and Johnson, DuPont, Intel, and others (NASEM 2014, 2018; Government-University-Industry Research Roundtable 2014; AAAS 2016). The concept of convergence is already a natural fit for many companies whose approaches emphasize flexible teams tackling specific, time-limited missions. Industry speakers consistently emphasize that convergence provides a framework to integrate perspectives from multiple disciples within their company, and to enhance interactions with academia and other partnerships to create new products. The potential for convergence applications to help address anticipated future workforce needs is also a common theme.

For example, the founder and chief science officer of Zymergen, a six-year-old startup company, offered a perspective on the benefits of convergence to his company. The Zymergen business model is based on an automated, technical, and data-strong propriety strain optimization approach to identify or enhance microbes for bio-based chemicals and agricultural products. Although comparatively new, the company, which takes a synthetic biology, or engineering biology, approach, closed the largest aggrotech investment to date in 2018 at $400 million with investors ranging from Goldman Sachs to Two Sigma Ventures (Stine 2018; Feldman 2019). The company's workforce strategy includes hiring a mix of investigators with in-depth expertise in strategic areas of science and technology, as well as ones who can creatively span multiple areas. "A major goal is to seed the system with a sufficient number of transdisciplinary thinkers who can promote teaming and bridge across the work of disciplinary thinkers to access what would have otherwise been lost in the intersections of bounded knowledge" (NASEM 2019, p. 29).

At the opposite end of the spectrum, Lockheed Martin Corporation is a global aerospace and advanced technology company that hires significant numbers of American engineering graduates each year. The company aims to ensure that its future workforce is prepared to help it maintain economic competitiveness across advanced R & D sectors. Characteristics such as learning agility and having a collaborative orientation are seen as valuable skills. "Just as the Convergence approach offers an organizing framework for academia and government institutions to better understand how to enable solutions to our greatest challenges, Convergence offers industry a view inside the university machine and enables a better understanding of the feedback loops necessary to ensure complete training for the 2020 workforce" (Arnold and Greer 2015, p. 62).

[5] See https://www.engine.xyz/ (accessed December 20, 2019).

Box 4.1 The Raymond and Beverly Sackler Prize in Convergence Research

From 2015 to 2018, the prize "recognized significant advances in convergence research—the integration of two or more of the following disciplines: mathematics, physics, chemistry, biomedicine, biology, astronomy, earth sciences, engineering, and computational science—for achievements possible only through such integration." The award is currently inactive.

Recipients and their citations included:

2018 Joseph M. DeSimone: "For integrating chemistry, physics, and engineering disciplines to invent platform technologies that have transformed aspects of nanomedicine and 3D-printing."

2017 Frances H. Arnold: "For her pioneering directed molecular evolution strategies, used worldwide to optimize the functions of enzymes and to engineer cells to produce biofuels and chemicals from renewable resources."

2016 Stephen R. Quake: "For innovative technological advances in microfluidics and genomics that made possible new non-invasive diagnostic procedures to detect at the single cell and single molecule levels a variety of disease conditions, such as brain tumors and the rejection of transplanted organs, as well as the prenatal diagnosis of genetic diseases."

2015 Chad A. Mirkin: "For impressively integrating chemistry, materials science, molecular biology, and biomedicine in the development of spherical nucleic acids and new types of nanostructures that are widely used in the rapid and automated diagnosis of infectious diseases and many other human diseases—including cancers and cardiac disease—and in the detection of drug-resistant bacteria."

Source: http://www.nasonline.org/programs/awards/sackler-prize-convergence.html

---

Foundations

Philanthropic support has provided a proving ground for convergence in several ways. Foundations supported efforts ranging from meetings and awards (see Box 4.1) to centers, institutes, and initiatives. Examples of foundations and philanthropic associations that have taken part in convergence discussions at NASEM and in related fora include the Kavli Foundation, W. M. Keck Foundation, Bill and Melinda Gates Foundation, Raymond and Beverly Sackler Foundation, Burroughs Wellcome Fund, Research Corporation for Science Advancement, Health Research Alliance, and Science Philanthropy Alliance (NASEM 2014, 2019; MIT 2016).

Although philanthropic funding in a particular area may be time-limited, foundations can play valuable roles catalyzing the further development of new areas of knowledge that rely on convergence. One example is the role the Kavli Foundation played in convening initial discussions to articulate what became the Brain Research through Advancing Innovative Neurotechnologies (BRAIN) Initiative. The Kavli Foundation continues to participate in and support the initiative in a variety of ways, including as simple as convening "Kavli BRAIN Coffee Hours" at universities nationwide to facilitate new transdisciplinary connections.[6] Within the National Academies, a philanthropy-funded convergence prize, which ran from 2015 to 2018, offered additional support for senior researchers running convergence style labs (see Box 4.1).

Federal Agencies

Government agencies provide significant sources of funding for fundamental discovery, and exert important influence on research cultures through significant portions of federal programmatic funding. While maintaining important support for disciplinary scholarship, a number of other U.S. federal agencies have developed or take part in programs embodying convergence. A few examples include:

- The Precision Medicine Initiative, which draws on advanced biomedical technology and big data to better tailor treatment to a patient's characteristics, with a federal investment of over $250 million:
- The National Cancer Moonshot Initiative, intended to revolutionize cancer treatment, and prevention, with an investment of $1 billion:
- Programs undertaken by the Defense Advanced Research Projects Agency (DARPA) of the Department of Defense, including through its Biological Technologies Office, which often rely on bringing together multiple areas of expertise to make transformational advances in support of national security: and
- Convergence-style centers at the National Institutes of Health, such as the Physical Sciences—Oncology Network and the NCI Clinical Proteomics Tumor Analysis Consortium (CPTAC), an investment of $150 million since 2006, which extends The Cancer Genome Atlas.[7]

It has been noted in prior discussions that convergent proposals can be more challenging to fully and fairly evaluate (NASEM 2019), and it has also been suggested that "delivering on the full promise of Convergence is hindered by federal research funding practices that often reflect a classical, disciplinary based structure" (MIT 2016, p. 8). Perhaps for these reasons, the NSF was the first federal agency to formally initiate significant funding in the name of convergence as recently as 2016. The NSF included "Growing Convergence Research" in its Ten Big Ideas, identified as "merging ideas, approaches, tools, and technologies from widely diverse fields of science and engineering to stimulate discovery and innovation."[8] NSF also commissioned the National Academy of Engineering to issue a report on the future if its Engineering Research Centers program that recommended an emphasis on convergence approaches (NASEM 2017), a position the Foundation has since adopted by embedding

---

[6] See https://www.braininitiative.org/alliance/the-kavli-foundation/ (accessed December 19, 2019).
[7] For more on these and related programs evoking convergence approaches, see MIT 2016.
[8] See https://www.nsf.gov/news/special_reports/big_ideas (accessed June 10, 2019).

convergence in explanatory and preparatory materials for its Gen-4 ERC RFPs submissions (NSF 2019b).

NSF's Fiscal Year 2020 budget request to Congress includes $76 million for the agency's work on convergence, which includes $16 million for the Growing Convergence Research portfolio and $30 million for Convergence Accelerators (NSF 2019a). The language identifies three areas of a growing portfolio, including capacity-building activities, exploratory grants, and identification of reviewers for convergent grant proposals. An additional $40 million in external funds are expected to push the full convergence effort initiated by NSF over $100 million (Mervis 2019).

Fostering a Convergence Culture to Support Innovation in Mental Health

Diverse efforts are underway to foster convergence cultures and support innovation in academia and industry, as well as among philanthropic and government funders. Mental health is an example of how this approach can be applied to catalyze collaborations and incentivize development and translation of goal-oriented and curiosity-driven research. "Modern psychiatric research problems are characterized by their complexity, multi-systemic nature, and broad societal impact, hence making them poorly suited to siloed approaches of thinking and innovation" (Eyre et al. 2017, p. 91). In addition to integration across disciplines, innovation in mental health and well-being will require input from across research and development sectors, as well as the critical participation of additional stakeholders including potential patient communities. "[A] desire to make progress toward solutions to modern grand challenges is driving change across the research spectrum and provides a catalyst toward convergence" (NASEM 2019, p. 41).

A number of lessons learned arising from the 2018 National Academies workshop discussion are included in Table 4.2. Collectively, these reflect potential opportunities to develop and share best practices.

Suggestions that might have particular relevance to the mental health community include the need to create and sustain communities of practice who can share insights and foster the role of convergence in tackling complex mental health challenges. Creating a network of interested faculty, clinicians, technical staff, trainees, and patient communities across institutions might be especially valuable. One complementary project at the National Academies that may provide community-building opportunities is the newly-launched Forum on Mental Health and Substance Use Disorders, which aims to "provide a structured environment and neutral venue to discuss data, policies, practices, and systems that affect the diagnosis and provision of care" for these issues.[9] In addition, the convergence mental health community may need to consider whether proposal review criteria and processes at major federal and philanthropic funders need to be calibrated to fully evaluate submissions reflective of

---

[9] See Forum on Mental Health and Substance Use Disorders, Institute of Medicine, http://www.nationalacademies.org/hmd/Activities/MentalHealth/MentalHealthSubstanceUseDisorderForum.aspx (accessed November 14, 2019).

Table 4.2 Suggestions for Future Efforts Arising From Workshop Discussions

Potential Opportunity	Future Actions
Build the case for convergence	• Convene focused workshops on case topics to assemble the missing pieces that could support convergence in those specific scientific areas • Build agreement on what is meant by "convergence," including how transdisciplinary research and team science contribute to it, as well as where it differs from or extends beyond these concepts • Develop and collate stories to help internal and external audiences understand what convergence enables
Create networks and communities of practice among those interested in convergence	• Establish a "convergence acceleration forum" across universities, institutes, national laboratories, and industry to convene periodic discussions that share ongoing challenges and identify effective practices and transferable elements • Create a peer community of university provosts or senior research officers to address challenges unique to university structures • Create a peer community or association of convergence center and institute directors to compare cross-sectoral strategies and identify transferable elements that foster convergence • Connect interested faculty, technical staff, and trainees within a university
Design structures that support and incentivize convergence	• Establish "incubators" to provide momentum for the development of convergence centers. Services and support could include creation of "advisory teams" to help researchers launch effective convergent projects. The teams might draw on expertise in areas such as team science, transdisciplinary research, innovation studies, and organizational change • Establish research instrumentation hubs with expert staff scientists, supported through novel funding mechanisms • Consider the advantages and disadvantages of various financial support models
Develop criteria for success reflective of convergence	• Articulate promising proposal review processes and criteria for evaluating convergent funding submissions • Identify outcome metrics of success for the results of convergent research • Explore strategies to address challenges in publication of convergent manuscripts • Collate effective practices and criteria for researcher advancement, including academic promotion and tenure and parallel career paths beyond the traditional tenure track • Discuss expanded metrics of success for departments and institutions that will recognize both disciplinary scholarship and convergence

Source: Reprinted with permission from National Academies of Sciences, Engineering, and Medicine. 2019. *Fostering the Culture of Convergence in Research: Proceedings of a Workshop.* Washington, DC: National Academies Press.

convergence as it applies to the relevant science. Related questions the convergence mental health community may need to consider include challenges associated with multiple authors on convergence manuscripts and pathways for researcher advancement such as promotion and tenure.

Convergence has the potential to shape cultures of innovation by providing a framework to integrate perspectives across disciplines and sectors to tackle major challenges. Shaping the culture of innovation in mental health through convergence may make a valuable contribution to enabling new advances in mental health and well-being.

References

$100 million commitment launches Pritzker School of Molecular Engineering. 2019, May 28. *UChicago News*. Retrieved from https://news.uchicago.edu/story/100-million-commitment-launches-pritzker-school-molecular-engineering

AAAS. 2016. Session: The Impact of Convergence on Innovation Across Sectoral and Global Boundaries (2016 AAAS Annual Meeting, February 11–15, 2016). Retrieved from https://aaas.confex.com/aaas/2016/webprogram/Session12106.html

American Academy of Arts and Sciences. 2013. *ARISE 2: Unleashing American's Research and Innovation Enterprise*. Cambridge, MA: American Academy of Arts and Sciences.

Arnold, A., and M. Greer. 2015. Convergence: A transformative approach to advanced research at the intersection of life, physical sciences and engineering and enhanced university-industry partnerships. *J Transl Sci*. 1(3):61–64.

Council on Competitiveness. 2019. National Commission on Innovation and Competitiveness Frontiers: A council plan to redefine 21st century productivity, prosperity, and security. https://www.compete.org/storage/reports/Commission__Launch.pdf (accessed October 5, 2020).

Dawson, A. (2018, April 13). Pop-up institutes tackle big research questions—quickly. *Office of the Executive Vice President and Provost, University of Texas at Austin*. Retrieved from https://provost.utexas.edu/news/pop-up-institutes-tackle-big-research-questions

Eyre, H. A., H. Lavretsky, M. Forbes, C. Raji, G. Small, P. McGorry, B. T. Baune, and C. Reynolds III. 2017. Convergence science arrives: How does it relate to psychiatry. *Acad Psychiatry*. 41:91–99.

Feldman, A. 2019, August 5. The life factory: Synthetic organisms from this $1.4 billion startup will revolutionize manufacturing. *Forbes*. Retrieved from https://www.forbes.com/sites/amyfeldman/2019/08/05/the-life-factory-synthetic-organisms-from-startup-ginkgo-bioworks-unicorn-will-revolutionize-manufacturing/#51803848145e

Government-University-Industry Research Roundtable. 2014. Convergence: Optimizing cross-sector and interdisciplinary partnerships [Meeting summary]. *The National Academies*. Retrieved from http://sites.nationalacademies.org/cs/groups/pgasite/documents/webpage/pga_152280.pdf

Leuty, R. 2018, February 28. Can "pop-ups" help UCSF move faster, cheaper with medical research? *San Francisco Business Times*. Retrieved from https://www.bizjournals.com/sanfrancisco/news/2018/02/28/pop-up-institutes-ucsf-aging-fibrosis-qb3-calico.html

Massachusetts Institute of Technology. 2016. *Convergence: The Future of Health*. Cambridge, MA: Author.

Mervis, J. 2019, April 9. Novel NSF initiative seeks nimble scientists to create better tools to tackle societal problems. But act now. *Science*. Retrieved from https://www.sciencemag.org/news/ 2019/04/novel-nsf-initiative-seeks-nimble-scientists-create-better-tools-tackle-societal

National Academies of Sciences, Engineering, and Medicine. 2017. *A New Vision for Center-Based Engineering Research*. Washington, DC: The National Academies Press. https://doi. org/10.17226/24767

National Academies of Sciences, Engineering, and Medicine. 2019. *Fostering the Culture of Convergence in Research: Proceedings of a Workshop*. Washington, DC: The National Academies Press.

National Research Council. 2014. *Convergence: Facilitating Transdisciplinary Integration of Life Sciences, Physical Sciences, Engineering, and Beyond*. Washington, DC: National Academies Press.

National Research Council. 2015. *Enhancing the Effectiveness of Team Science*. Washington, DC: National Academies Press.

National Science Foundation. 2018. NSF's 10 big ideas (News release 17082). https://www.nsf. gov/news/special_reports/big_ideas/

National Science Foundation. 2019a. Summary tables: Convergence accelerators and NSF 10 big ideas funding FY2020 budget request to congress. Retrieved from https://www.nsf.gov/ about/budget/fy2020/pdf/07_fy2020.pdf

National Science Foundation. 2019b. Planning grants for engineering research centers (ERC) (Nsf19562. Retrieved from https://www.nsf.gov/pubs/2019/nsf19562/nsf19562.htm

Roco, M., W. Bainbridge, B. Tonn, and G. Whitesides, eds. 2013. *Convergence of Knowledge, Technology and Society: Beyond Convergence of Nano-Bio-Info-Cognitive Technologies*. New York: Springer.

Sharp. P., and R. Langer. 2011. Promoting convergence in biomedical science. *Science*. 333(6042):527.

Sharp, P., and S. Hockfield. 2017. Convergence: The future of health. *Science*. 355(6325): 589.

Stine, L. 2018, December 13. Zymergen Raises $400m Series C in Largest Ever Upstream AgriFood Tech Deal in US. *AgFunder News*. Retrieved from https://agfundernews.com/ breaking-zymergen-raises-400m-series-c-in-largest-ever-upstream-agrifood-tech-deal-in-us.html

5

Developing Convergence Neuroscience as a Model

Marion T. Turnbull and William D. Freeman

Introduction

Nobel Laureate Phillip Sharp, an author on the white paper on convergence,[1] articulated the importance and opportunities that would come from convergence at the American Association for the Advancement of Science (AAAS): "Convergence is a broad rethinking of how all scientific research can be conducted, so that we capitalize on a range of knowledge bases, from microbiology to computer science to engineering design... This merging of technologies, processes, and devices into a unified whole will create new pathways and opportunities for scientific and technological advancement."[2]

The future of the biomedical and life science innovation depends on its ability to integrate and cross-collaborate with other data-hungry and fast-progressing research domains such as bioinformatics, computer science, engineering, and the physical sciences. In the context of this chapter, convergence is the joining of forces between neuro-based life sciences with engineering and the physical sciences, in a trans-directional exchange—or intellectual cross-pollination.[3] This can be represented schematically as a simple quadrant similar to Pasteur's Quadrant,[4] where the vertical axis represents continued progress in neuroscience-based life sciences, and the horizontal axis represents the development of engineering and the physical sciences. True neuroscience convergence occurs when these two fields overlap (top right quadrant; Figure 5.1).

This synergistic progress requires an open, innovative, and collaborative workforce that possesses deep knowledge and understanding of their respective field, combined with the ability to share their expertise and effectively communicate it among other subject matter experts from other fields. To build a diverse biomedical scientific workforce and to continue evolving using a convergence model, we must center on three core objectives:

1. *Focus* on a common theme or scientific/medical problem or challenge.
2. *Encourage* convergence through structural change.
3. *Expand* educational and training programs that teach convergence methodology alongside traditional opportunities for formal and informal discussion and collaborations.

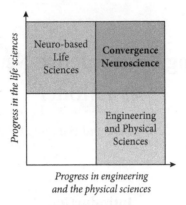

Figure 5.1 Quadrant model of convergence neuroscience as an intersection between neuroscience-based life sciences and engineering and the physical sciences.

The ultimate aim of the convergence initiative is to spur innovative thinking that underlies the advancement of life sciences in basic, translational, and clinical arenas and should arguably be in everything we do to improve healthcare and advance science. Without innovative thinking, progress in science will only continue to advance through slow, incremental steps. Like convergence, true innovation occurs at the interface of disciplines and leads away from the rigid subspecializations of today. Capitalizing on these strategies would foster the advancements necessary to solve current biomedical challenges and meet the growing demand for accessible and affordable healthcare. This chapter aims to expand on each of these three themes in an effort to summarize the bottlenecks facing the convergence initiative and strategize on measures required to progress the field.

Focus Around a Common Theme or Scientific/Medical Challenge

In the 21st century, it is highly unlikely that a single investigator will make another "quantum jump" of scientific discovery in isolation as did Louis Pasteur or Marie Curie. More likely, future breakthroughs will come from "convergence teams." Just like the National Aeronautics Space Administration (NASA) missions that were comprised of many mathematicians, engineers, and physical scientists and required the development of much of the technology and mathematics that was eventually used, convergence science benefits from a focused, goal-oriented approach. Therefore, the strategy to focus or "converge" around a common theme or challenge is aimed at stimulating and supporting cross-collaboration between teams and disciplines.

Nowadays, there is no shortage of challenges that humankind faces in the fields of neuroscience and healthcare, such as curing brain disorders and addressing issues in access to healthcare. The hope that convergence methodology can single-handedly solve these challenges is overly optimistic, yet a convergence approach to these challenges is likely essential to accelerate progress among science teams to ultimately translate treatments back to the patient in need.[5] Convergence strategies have extraordinary potential for many brain-related health challenges: in prevention, in earlier and more accurate diagnoses, in neurotherapeutics, and in drug delivery mechanisms. The overlapping of technology to better monitor and understand biology will bring about a rise in modern artificial intelligences-based sensors, wearables, and smart devices, which will allow for remote monitoring and quantification of biological processes. Novel screening tools will aid in the identification of at-risk populations to prevent, diagnose, or intervene across a broad range of conditions. Non- or minimally invasive methods of brain stimulation and visualization will result in improved control of neurological symptoms and accelerate endogenous healing processes, as well as promote a deeper understanding of neural circuitry and degenerative processes.

To emphasize the extraordinary potential of transdisciplinary collaboration on common themes and challenges in the world of neuroscience, we will focus on two "need-based" convergence initiatives, which represent convergence on a basic research challenge (the Brain Research Through Advancing Innovative Neurotechnologies [BRAIN] initiative), and the other a focus on a clinical challenge (the Neuroscience Intensive Care Unit [NSICU]).

Brain Research Through Advancing Innovative Neurotechnologies Initiative

A convergence neuroscience approach to building tools, analyzing information, has already—and will continue—to create opportunities for investigating one of the greatest challenges in science: the brain. With its nearly 100 billion neurons and 100 trillion connections, the human brain remains one of the greatest mysteries in science and one of the greatest challenges in medicine. Dysfunction of the brain, either acutely or chronically, gives rise to neurological and psychiatric disorders that are devastating for the patient and require tremendous strength and support from family, friends, and society. Despite hundreds of years of investigation into these conditions, and giant leaps forward in recent years, the underlying biology for many of these neurological conditions are still undefined, and there remains a dearth of neurotherapeutics. Recent breakthroughs in tools and technology have allowed us to examine and manipulate the brain with a level of precision that we have never seen before. Tools such as optogenetics and chemogenetics allow us to manipulate the function of cells at the single cell level through manipulation of circuitry and then be measured through behavioral readouts. Imaging technologies allow us to track the movement of individual molecules, measure their binding to other molecules, or allow us to visualize the internal components of single cells with incredible resolution. Relatedly, sequencing the human genome was just the first step toward creating the technology that allows us to sequence the transcriptome of individual neurons or glia through single-cell RNA sequencing. Overall, these technologies and methods have allowed scientists unprecedented access and understanding to the functioning of the brain, and this would not have been possible without convergence of scientific disciplines and collaboration across the life, physical and engineering sciences.

The national goal to create a comprehensive understanding of the brain is a practical example of converging on a theme or challenge to bring together innovative neuroscientists with engineering and technology solutions to accelerate discovery in neuroscience. It was launched by then President Barack Obama in 2013 to "accelerate the development and application of new technologies that will enable researchers to produce dynamic pictures of the brain that show how individual brain cells and complex neural circuits interact at the speed of thought."[6] The BRAIN initiative is a multiyear scientific goal with cross collaboration across 10 different National Institutes of Health (NIH) institutes, and funding opportunities for priority areas.[7] The BRAIN initiative is developed through two phases, the first five years would emphasize rapid advancement of novel and existing perturbation techniques and technology, followed by a phase emphasizing integration of this technology into the nervous system to drive discovery neuroscience.[6] The NIH BRAIN initiative also builds upon the 1990s' "Decade of the Brain," which was rooted in neuroscience and the BRAIN initiative builds upon the science learned in that decade.

The convergence approach of the BRAIN initiative bypasses the classic, discipline-based structures of funding and brings neuroscientists together with engineering and technology experts to accelerate discovery and innovation in neuroscience. The prospects for this funding methodology are endless and have the potential to deliver the full promise of the convergence initiative.

The Neuroscience Intensive Care Unit

The NSICU is a prime example of a clinical convergence unit arising in response to the need for intensive, focused care, and specialized knowledge for life-threatening neurological problems. In essence the patient is at the epicenter of the convergence problem or challenge to solve, but the unmet needs are individualized to the patient and are unique to the patient circumstances (e.g., age and comorbidities) and type of neurological injury (e.g., stroke, traumatic brain injury, or amyotrophic lateral sclerosis). Neurointensive care requires specialized knowledge of neurobiological mechanics, neurological conditions, and the use of dedicated neurological tools and techniques. The NSICU is comprised of multiple professions and specialties with a singular purpose: the health of the patient (Figure 5.2). The NSICU model has evolved over time and functions through collaborative interfacing between different staff such as physicians, nurses, pharmacists, social workers, and rehabilitation specialists. Moreover, this transdisciplinary approach to patient care is guided by those that normally fit within separate, siloed departments—neurologists, neurosurgeons, and intensivists. A NSICU is also a big-data repository with each patient accumulating gigabytes, if not terabytes, of data per day depending on the level and intensity of brain monitoring, physiologic signal processing, imaging, and laboratory biomarkers. This makes the NSICU setting ripe for neuro-injury–based convergence research benefiting the patient by combining this data with machine learning approaches and making predictive assessments of impending deterioration and even outcomes.[8-10]

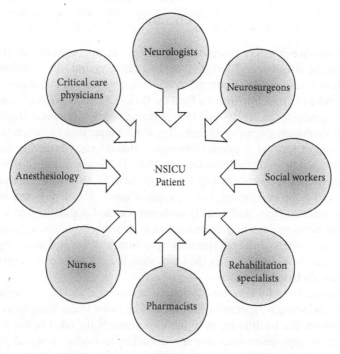

Figure 5.2 Multidisciplinary care centering on the needs of the neurointensive care patient.

In addition to transdisciplinary care, the NSICU fosters a convergence approach to patient health by holding multidisciplinary rounds and informal discussions with the aim of enhancing patient care and improving the quality of healthcare. Multidisciplinary rounds involve multiple medical specialties and stakeholders discussing daily the needs of the patient and what can be improved upon to improve their care and their outcomes. This "need-based" approach to patient care is at the forefront of collaborative, transdisciplinary thinking and ultimately benefits those who need it most: the patients and their families.

Encourage Convergence Through Structural Change

The convergence initiative can be encouraged by careful and thoughtful changes to the current structures of sciences. These adjustments can be made at the individual level, such as encouraging the next generations of scientists, or at the institutional levels, where alterations to infrastructure can help foster transdisciplinary collaborations. Moreover, the overarching funding system is currently set up to emphasize discipline-restricted grants and needs to be rethought to advocate and nurture the convergence initiative.

Personnel

For a convergence model to succeed, the workforce must consist of a diverse and inclusive team of researchers. Therefore, tackling diversity and equity problems in the pipeline is essential. Access to education is just one obstacle to overcome. Over two-thirds of children from low-income families (below $25,000 per year) aim to complete undergraduate studies, yet just 19% of young people from these families obtain a community college degree or higher. This is in comparison to 76% from families with incomes of $76,000 or greater per year.[11] This disparity is further exacerbated and complicated by factors such as race. In 2006, 23.7% of white 20- to 29-year-olds had obtained a four-year college degree, in contrast to 12.2% of individuals of African descents, and 6.7% of Hispanics of equivalent age.[11] Identifying and supporting promising students from traditionally underrepresented populations in science and engineering programs can be achieved through structured mentoring programs and targeted scholarships and opportunities. The future of biomedicine requires this workforce and their ideas to foster the innovation to necessary solve the growing demand for neuro-based healthcare.

The need for diversity in teams is critical—across races and ethnicities and across the gender and sexuality spectrum. Diverse and inclusive teams bring more creativity and innovation due to differences in life experience.[12] Included in the term *diversity*, sources of experience, such like age, disability, neurodiversity, and personality, are often overlooked. Bringing together a diverse team starts with recruitment but is maintained through acknowledging and supporting what makes people different. Listening and learning about their life experiences not only makes a team more successful, but also allows those individuals to reach their full potential, benefiting both the team and the advancement of ideas.

Diverse and inclusive teams make sense from a business perspective. A recent report demonstrated that public companies with gender, ethnic, and racial diversity in management were more likely to have financial returns above the industry mean.[13] Highlighting that commitment to diversity often translate to success in business. In another study, increased cultural diversity was correlated with innovativeness and development of new products.[14] Ultimately, homogeneity in teams—individuals who look, talk, and think alike—discourages innovative thinking, with diverse teams often being smarter and more successful.[15] This is not restricted to the business world; scientific and medical teams also need to think more broadly and innovatively, starting with a commitment to expand diversity in these teams.

Infrastructure

Discipline-based departments are the current standard in academic institutions, designed to foster intradisciplinary support among colleagues and deepen the knowledge of a specific field. However, this traditional set up will be at odds with a convergence innovation approach if this paradigm is to succeed. Some large organizations focus heavily on *process* rather than true technical insights or creativity to make discoveries. While process can be useful once a particular method is established, it cannot invent something new or create an entirely new technology that make tackle a scientific challenge no one has solved before. Conventional hiring practices emphasize long-established preferences for faculty who fit the traditional "subject matter expert" criteria and discourage individuals who approach science with a more transdisciplinary or convergence-oriented research methodology. These "outside the box" thinkers may not fit conveniently into traditional departmental delineations. A transdisciplinary approach to science may also be reflected negatively as fewer traditional lead or senior author journal article qualifications and more middle author or collaborative authorship positions. However this may simply be a reflection of an outdated mechanism to rank or quantify achievement based on authorship, instead of a more holistic measurement of academic productivity.[16,17] Ultimately, moving away from strict, process-driven, and discipline-demarcated departments may help spark more cross-collaborations between fields, and this in itself may make it necessary to revisit methods that truly quantify success within academia.

A realignment or rethinking of academic structures may therefore be required to enhance and facilitate the convergence of disparate specialties and expertise.[18] A recent growth in research centers or science "incubators" located on or near to research campuses is a step in the right direction and begin to encourage a more convergent approach to conducting science. There are already a number of well-known and successful models of this including the Clark Center, which houses the Bio-X program at Stanford University, and the Koch Institute at MIT, as well as the Wyss Institute at Harvard University, the Molecular Engineering Institute at the University of Chicago, and the Petit Institute for Bioengineering and Bioscience at Georgia Tech.[18,19] Essentially what these incubators do is facilitate rapid collaboration, networking, and ideation among different disciplines. Additionally, conventional institutes are beginning to include more open concept spaces meant to catalyze collaboration, powered by access to coffee, sugar, and whiteboards. Newer electronic methods of cross-discipline scientific networking such as Google Hangouts, Skype, and Zoom meetings now exist that allow truly global interconnectedness among diverse groups and world experts to foster innovation. Whether these structural changes are sufficient to fuel more permanent paradigm change has yet to be seen, but perhaps alongside other organizational restructuring, it may help change the culture of innovation and collaboration.[2]

Funding

Traditionally, the challenges facing convergence funding include continuously diminished federal research support alongside structured siloed agencies with discipline-restricted grants and review mechanisms.[5] Despite this, there have been historically successful exceptions to this, with convergence or transdisciplinary approaches to funding a challenge-driven goal. One of the most recognized convergence funding projects is the Human Genome Project by the U.S. Department of Energy and the NIH, which resulted in huge, and largely unanticipated, payoffs.[20,21] Thus, the model already exists for exceptional cases, and perhaps the future of convergence funding just requires fine-tuning of the existing system. Alternatively, it has been argued that a convergence approach may require the dismantling of the existing organization of scientific fields with traditional funding structures.[3] Ultimately, research project driven grants and training grants are needed to encourage convergence directed research and the development of courses and programs that prepare students, postdoctoral researchers, and fellows to think and collaborate across disciplines.

While several governmental agencies including the NIH, National Science Foundation, and the Department of Defense are now involved in the support of this initiative, funding support is still small.[5] The NIH Common Fund is one example of NIH programs aimed at addressing emerging scientific opportunities and current challenges in biomedical research that are outside the scope of a single NIH institute or center—but have been recognized as being high priority for the NIH and scientific community.[22] The Common Fund is managed by the Office of Strategic Coordination/Division of Program Coordination, Planning, and Strategic Coordination/Office of the NIH Director and is unique in that it functions similar to venture capital, where high-risk, high-reward projects are sought. Innovative and creative solutions to pressing challenges are encouraged, with short-term, goal-driven strategic investments driving this transdisciplinary approach to advancing biomedical research.[22]

Similarly, specific institutes may have specific funding programs that fund collaboration between disciplines, but fall short of true convergence. One example is the National Institute of General Medical Sciences,[23] which has a Collaborative Program Grant for Multidisciplinary Teams that supports multiple principal investigators under one grant mechanism that could not be accomplished through a normal grant channel (i.e. multiple principal investigator R01s).[24] The lead investigators must have a unified goal and complementary expertise, and can be at a single institution or spread across multiple institutions. However, there is little emphasis on bringing together disparate disciplines such engineering, computer sciences, and physical sciences.

In parallel, several NIH institutes have begun to embrace convergence initiatives. The National Institute of Biomedical Imaging and Bioengineering mission is to improve health outcomes by developing and accelerating biomedical technologies. To achieve this, it encourages research and development in multidisciplinary, convergence-related areas,[25] and it is "committed to integrating the physical and engineering sciences with the life sciences to advance basic research and medical care."[25] Similarly, the National Center for Advancing Translational Sciences (NCATS) has the goal of catalyzing translational science through a "team sport" approach. In essence, the NCATS strategic principles are centered on innovative and collaborative efforts to bring "more treatments to more patients more quickly."[26] It aims to encompass many disciplines including the life sciences, informatics, engineering, and public health—embodying a convergence approach.[27] These cross-disciplinary structures, unattached to specific disease states, are unlike the traditional knowledge silos and divisions within the NIH. Moreover, the NCATS acknowledge that the future of translational science requires the convergence of disciplines and an emphasis on transdisciplinary training to develop and foster a skilled and diverse translational science workforce.[27] NCATS helped redefine the concept of a "translational scientist" or one who works across disciplines to solve unmet needs of patients and help bridge the gap between various basic scientists and the bedside physician-scientists.

Building and developing a convergence neuroscience workforce will need to model National Institute of Biomedical Imaging and Bioengineering and NCATS priorities and strategic goals. At a national level, funding institutions will need to continue to encourage challenge-driven, multicollaborative projects, as well as expand the funding for infrastructure required for new research centers and the development of the future convergence workforce. Similarly, foundations and institutions should provide seed funding that encourages the convergence initiative and fund the building of transdisciplinary teams.

Expand Educational and Training Programs Alongside Opportunities for Formal and Informal Discussion and Collaborations

Education and Training

To grow a successful convergence-oriented biomedical workforce, there must be greater emphasis placed on development of educational and training programs focused on nontraditional knowledge and skills such as entrepreneurship, cross-disciplinary communication, critical and scientific method thinking, and project management. Moreover, future convergence scientists need to think across disciplines and value the skill sets of other collaborators for their expertise and areas, which ultimately help drive science forward. The ideal convergence scientist or physician has deep expertise in their field, alongside literacy and understanding of a broad range of disciplines.[3] This recognizes that many of today's global problems are too complex to be addressed by a single, specialized discipline and specifically trains and educates the future workforce for cross-disciplinary translation of ideas and concepts. Educational and training programs can be approached from an institution-led angle or prompted and supported by federal funding programs highlighting this methodology. Moreover, continuing education should be targeted at all levels of training, from STEM-based undergraduate students, to graduate and medical students, as well as postdoctoral fellows, residents, and faculty for lifelong learning.

Alongside these training opportunities, collaborative partnerships can be explored with biotechnology companies, pharmaceutical teams, and venture capital communities to learn from their experience and knowledge. To achieve the ultimate goal of helping the patient at the bedside, biomedical research must learn to navigate and make the most of the expertise that these nongovernmental organizations can provide. Specifically, the pharmaceutical industry has a wealth of knowledge in the translational sciences that academia and medicine could effectively leverage and partner with to achieve complementary goals. Moreover joint ventures in therapeutic drug development and clinical trials between academia and industry can benefit patients and advance the science. The business community, including biotechnology companies and venture capital, has an abundance of experience with developing and commercializing technology and clinical/scientific products. The platforms and tools that they have cultivated would be immensely beneficial for the advancement of biomedical research and creation of "exchange" or mini-fellowships between industry and academia could provide opportunities for researchers and scientists to expand their horizons and see different cultures and styles of operations within organization. Such collaboration can also help address gaps in knowledge or technology first-hand, as well as seeing how fast industry moves to most NIH and academic efforts.

The goal of training for a convergence model is to create the ideal convergence workforce that can bring deep understanding of their own field with the capacity to converse in, and value, a broad range of disciplines. The ensuing workforce will not only represent a group of experts coming together, but consequently will merge their expertise and address challenges with a convergence mindset—essentially transcending the traditional boundaries of scientific fields.[28]

Conferences

One approach used to accelerate convergence thinking and provide opportunities for discussion and collaboration is at dedicated conferences meant to engage diverse groups of individuals and stimulate thoughtful discussion, and ultimately, interdisciplinary collaboration. Conferences allow various forms of learning and idea exchange such as didactics question and answer sessions, workshops that teach skills. Conferences also allow some critical time for brainstorming and learning from others outside of one's own discipline. Conferences also are often the place key networking and relationships are made that can lead to future scientific collaboration. We are beginning to see many conferences along this theme—including Exponential Medicine coming out of Singularity University,[29] and Mayo Clinics' Neuroscience Convergence conference.[30]

The Mayo Clinic Neuroscience Convergence Approach

Mayo Clinic is a not-for-profit organization and academic medical center built around the values inspired by the Mayo family: "The best interest of the patient is the only interest to be considered, and in order that the sick may have the benefit of advancing knowledge, union of forces is necessary" (William J. Mayo, M.D., 1910).[31]

This call to action and the "union of forces" inspired the annual Neuroscience Convergence Conference, which calls for groups within the neuroscience-based biomedical and life sciences, as well as engineers and physical scientists, to come together to solve unmet health needs.[30] The conference aims to bring together various scientists, clinicians, biostatisticians, and engineers for creative collaboration and shared problem solving. The conference covers three days and is broken up by panel discussions with the aim of discussing and highlighting pertinent themes or challenges.[30] Talks are presented in a TED-like talk format to promote understanding across all disciplines, and special emphasis is placed on speakers and participants "speaking" the same language and having common reference points. Speakers from governmental and non-governmental research organizations are also invited to discuss future funding opportunities, developmental pipelines, and collaborative strategies (government and industry, philanthropic and government).

Interactions between participants are encouraged throughout the conference, and introductions and networking is stimulated through wearing of special visual pins worn alongside a name tag to indicate which field of origin (science, medical, or industry), and interests such as biology, technology, clinical research, or artificial intelligence. Such visual networking at least allows a "conversation starter" during coffee or food breaks to facilitate networking. At Mayo Clinic's Neuroscience Convergence conference, exchange of traditional business cards and academic emails occur in addition to sharing of newer forms of social media information such as Twitter, Facebook, Instagram, and Google Scholar profiles. These newer social media modes of communication are more powerful for idea exchange since they connect researchers as well as share online curriculum vitae, highly cited papers, personal or work group websites, and social media feeds.

How Could Convergence Mental Health Benefit From Advances in Convergence Neuroscience?

Although still in its infancy, dedicated funding and the rise of convergence-based conferences hints to a bright future for convergence neuroscience. Similarly, the convergence mental health effort can be thought of as fitting under the umbrella of convergence neuroscience, and thus benefits from the development and advancement of convergence neuroscience. Irrespective of this, structural changes in infrastructure, personnel, and the development of specialized, convergence-based education and training would likewise expand and boost the convergence mental health initiative. Additionally, funding structures centered on a common mental health challenge or theme would be immensely beneficial. Similar to what the BRAIN initiative has done for the convergence of neuroscience and technology, an analogous strategy would support and advance the convergence mental health model and this would ultimately benefit the mental health scientific, clinical, and patient community.

References

1. Sharp PA, Cooney CL, Kastner MA, et al. *The Third Revolution: The Convergence of the Life Sciences, Physical Sciences, and Engineering.* Cambridge, MA: Massachusetts Institute of Technology; 2011.
2. Gentile JM. Is "convergence" the Next revolution in science? Published October 11, 2013; Updated December 11, 2013; https://www.huffpost.com/entry/convergence-science-research_b_4078211.
3. Berrett D. The rise of "convergence" science. *Inside Higher Ed.* Published January 5, 2011; https://www.insidehighered.com/news/2011/01/05/rise-convergence-science.
4. Stokes DE. *Pasteur's Quadrant: Basic Science and Technological Innovation.* Washington, DC: Brookings Institution Press; 2011.

5. Sharp P, Hockfield S, Jacks T. Convergence: the future of health. *Science*. 2017;*355*(6325):589. https://doi.org/10.1126/science.aam8563.

6. Bargmann C, Newsome W, Anderson A, et al. BRAIN 2025 report: Brain Research Through Advancing Innovative Neurotechnologies (BRAIN) working group report to the advisory committee to the director. National Institutes of Health. Published June 5, 2014; https://braininitiative.nih.gov/strategic-planning/brain-2025-report.

7. National Institutes of Health. The BRAIN Initiative Overview. Accessed June 20, 2019; https://braininitiative.nih.gov/about/overview.

8. Al-Mufti F, Dodson V, Lee J, et al. Artificial intelligence in neurocritical care. *J Neurol Sci*. 2019;*404*:1–4. https://doi.org/10.1016/j.jns.2019.06.024.

9. Claassen J, Doyle K, Matory A, et al. Detection of brain activation in unresponsive patients with acute brain injury. *N Engl J Med*. 2019;*380*(26):2497–2505. https://doi.org/10.1056/nejmoa1812757.

10. Donald R, Howells T, Piper I, et al. Forewarning of hypotensive events using a Bayesian artificial neural network in neurocritical care. *J Clin Monit Comput*. 2019;*33*(1):39–51.

11. Osterman P. *College for All? The Labor Market for College-Educated Workers*. Washington, DC: Center for American Progress; 2008.

12. Rampton J. Why you need diversity on your team, and 8 ways to build it. *Entrepreneur*. Published September 6, 2019; https://www.entrepreneur.com/article/338663.

13. Hunt V, Layton D, Prince S. Diversity matters. *McKinsey & Company*. Published February 2, 2015; https://www.mckinsey.com/insights/organization/~/media/2497d4ae4b534ee89d929cc6e3aea485.ashx

14. Nathan M, Lee N. Cultural diversity, innovation and entrepreneurship: firm-level evidence from London. *Econ Geogr*. 2013;*84*(4):367–394. https://doi.org/10.1111/ecge.12016.

15. Rock D, and Grant H. Why diverse teams are smarter. *Harvard Business Review*. Published November 4, 2016; https://hbr.org/2016/11/why-diverse-teams-are-smarter.

16. Rawat S, Meena S. Publish or perish: where are we heading? *J Res Med Sci*. 2014;*19*(2):87–89.

17. Enago Academy. Publish or perish: what are its consequences? Last updated July 20, 2019; https://www.enago.com/academy/publish-or-perish-consequences/.

18. Sharp P, Jacks T, Hockfield S. Biomedical engineering: capitalizing on convergence for health care. *Science*. 2016;*352*(6293):1522–1523 https://doi.org/10.1126/science.aag2350.

19. Sharp PA, Langer R. Promoting convergence in biomedical science. *Science*. 2011;*333*(6042):527; https://doi.org/10.1126/science.1205008.

20. Battelle Technology Partnership Practice. Economic impact of the human genome project. *Battelle Memorial Institute*. Published May 2011; https://web.ornl.gov/sci/techresources/Human_Genome/publicat/BattelleReport2011.pdf

21. Jones M. Report suggests big payoff from human genome project. *GenomeWeb*. Published May 11, 2011; https://www.genomeweb.com/report-suggests-big-payoff-human-genome-project.

22. National Institutes of Health. Office of Strategic Coordination—The Common Fund. Last reviewed July 29, 2020; https://commonfund.nih.gov/.

23. National Institute of General Medical Sciences. Overview of NIGMS. Last reviewed November 20, 2019; https://www.nigms.nih.gov/about/overview/pages/default.aspx.

24. National Institute of General Medical Sciences. Collaborative Program Grant for Multidisciplinary Teams (RM1). Last reviewed April 28, 2020; https://www.nigms.nih.gov/grants/RM1/Pages/Collaborative-Program-Grant-for-Multidisciplinary-Teams-(RM1).aspx.

25. National Institute of Biomedical Imaging and Bioengineering. Mission & History. Accessed June 20, 2019; https://www.nibib.nih.gov/about-nibib/mission.

26. National Institutes of Health. National Center for Advancing Translational Sciences. Last updated July 31, 2020; https://ncats.nih.gov/index.php.
27. National Center for Advancing Translational Sciences. NCATS strategic plan 2016. Published Fall 2016; https://ncats.nih.gov/files/NCATS_strategic_plan.pdf.
28. Wilson N. On the road to convergence research. *BioScience.* 2019;69(8):587–593 https://doi.org/10.1093/biosci/biz066.
29. Singularity Education Group. Exponential medicine. Accessed June 20, 2019; https://exponential.singularityu.org/medicine/.
30. Mayo Clinic School of Continuous Professional Development. Neuroscience Convergence 2019. Accessed June 20, 2019; https://ce.mayo.edu/neurology-and-neurologic-surgery/content/neuroscience-convergence-2019#group-tabs-node-course-default1.
31. Mayo Foundation for Medical Education and Research. Quotations from the Doctors Mayo. Accessed June 20, 2019; http://history.mayoclinic.org/toolkit/quotations/the-doctors-mayo.php.

6

Establishing Transdisciplinarity Within a University

Learning From the Experience of the University of Technology Sydney

Louise J. I. McWhinnie

Introduction

It can be challenging to talk conceptually and theoretically about transdisciplinarity, or to conceive of and articulate its scope and application through often emergent research and practice. So how does one practically create capacity for transdisciplinarity and build its application at scale if we recognize the need for it in our complex working and research environments, and what is the role of our educational institutions in preparing graduates for such new and active thinking and practical collaboration?

In a book with a primary focus on convergence, mental health, and a proposed movement toward transdisciplinary innovation, this chapter may reside as an outlier, for it presents an example of its educational application without reference to mental health. Instead, it examines the building of transdisciplinarity at scale within the formal educational structures of a university. This chapter therefore presents the necessity for and challenges of transdisciplinarity through a case study of its feasibility and implementation within a higher educational institution, examining how it is challenging but also possible for such thinking to become core to a university's mission and forward momentum.

The field of mental health (within which this book is placed) resides within a grouping of disciplines that often synthesize their collaboration through what is termed *convergence science*. Yet, according to the American National Science Foundation (n.d.) convergence science is driven by the need to solve "vexing research problems, in particular, complex problems focusing on societal needs" and is thus "research driven by a specific and compelling problem" through "deep integration across disciplines." These definitions could though be as easily be applied to "transdisciplinarity" as "convergence science"; however, the term *convergence* is applied with a specific focus upon the integration of STEM and related disciplines and their application. Transdisciplinarity in its broadest form is often presented as some form of unobtainable nirvana, "historically viewed as the pinnacle of evolutionary integration across disciplines" (National Science Foundation, n.d.). However, does it need to continue to be so perceived, if there is a willingness to commit to and enter into an exploratory space, which is often theorized about, but not so often actively explored?

I have been invited to write this chapter due to my role as the inaugural Dean of the Faculty of Transdisciplinary Innovation at the University of Technology Sydney (UTS) in Australia. Probably unlike the majority of contributors to this book, I am not a scientist, or a medical or health practitioner, or associated with the life sciences. I am a designer. A designer leading a transdisciplinary faculty within a university can sometimes cause surprise, but it shouldn't. For whichever discipline an individual brings to such practice, is just one more component of collaboration. Indeed, the faculty is presently composed of academic staff contributing their depth of disciplinary knowledge from a breadth of specialisms and subspecialisms. In this chapter I will therefore present the reasons for transdisciplinarity, as well as through the examples of its implementation, challenge the perception of it as unobtainable. Through the example of its integration within one university, I will examine not only the challenges transdisciplinarity faces and presents, but also the benefits to be gained. I will not be attempting to theorize it, but primarily use its placement within a single university as an example of its potential.

"A" Not "The" Definition of Transdisciplinarity

Transdisciplinarity as a term is often misapplied and repeatedly confused with multi-, inter-, and cross-disciplinarity. As an emergent academic field, I have learnt to define it as much by what it is, as much as by what it isn't—see Figure 6.1 for further details:

1. Multidisciplinarity simply refers to the obtaining of information from two or more disciplines, without either being altered by this interaction.
2. Cross-disciplinarity is when the aspects of one discipline are imposed upon another discipline, (such as design-thinking being applied to business), which might alter business, but does not alter necessarily design.
3. Interdisciplinarity is where several subdisciplines within a broader disciplinary field cooperate, with no permanent change to any of them.

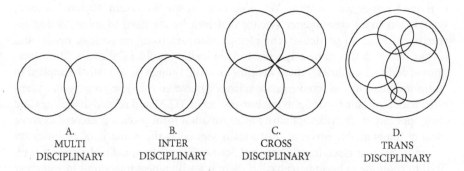

A.	B.	C.	D.
MULTI	INTER	CROSS	TRANS
DISCIPLINARY	DISCIPLINARY	DISCIPLINARY	DISCIPLINARY

Figure 6.1 The differences between multi-, cross-, inter-, and transdisciplinarity.

4. Transdisciplinarity, however takes this both further and broader with a more holistic approach. It is not simply about the joining up of individual outcomes in the interactions between disciplines, but about integrating these interactions into new systems of thinking, resulting in new outcomes that singular or traditionally conjoined disciplines could not create.

In this, the benefit and potential advancement of transdisciplinarity is that unlike disciplinary or inter-, cross-, or multidisciplinary approaches, transdisciplinary outcomes present the potential for new paradigms and methodological approaches for original/innovative outcomes through such new interactions. In other words, transdisciplinary interaction has the potential to create a new whole, greater than the sum of its disciplinary parts. Whilst it is always simplistic to consider that transdisciplinary thinking and collaboration simply required the joining up of disciplines, it is the way in which they collaborate in identifying or addressing a problem that is vital. A simple way to view this might be if one considers individual disciplines as colored lenses. It is when and where they overlap that new colors and vision is formed. Another metaphor might be to consider transdisciplinarity as a palmiped (webbed) structure, for "webbed feet have more surface area to push water backwards and thus propelling the animal forward" (Mooby Di, 2016). Thus, palmipeds generate greater traction through the use of connecting structures. Likewise transdisciplinarity is not simply about the combination of the structured elements, but the way in which the way in which the combination is formed that enables outcomes that the individual or nonconnected components could not.

The Need for Transdisciplinarity

The educational scope of transdisciplinarity is generally acknowledged to have originated during the early 1970s, through a critique of the existing "configuration of knowledge in disciplines in the curriculum" (Bernstein, 2015). However, the debate that surrounds it is now more pertinent than ever before. Whether you regard the time we are now in as the Fourth Industrial Revolution or the second Renaissance, or even just as a time of immense change, it is the acceleration in this change combined with its increasing complexity, and the "wicked" (Brown, Harris, & Russell, 2010) and dynamic nature of the problems that we face and their networked nature (Dorst, 2018) that demands different types of thinking and practice.

The linear nature of the disciplines in addressing complexity causes fragmentation rather than holistic solutions. In educational terms, for students undertaking disciplinary degrees this means that in the passing on of the existing knowledge that the disciplines hold, students engage with instructions and the acquisition of knowledge for entry into that discipline. The transdisciplinary space however is more akin to a sandpit than a designed classroom, where students are provided with ways in which to see, know, and be, and where the education is more akin to a self- and group-navigated journey with no instructional definitions about the required path to be taken.

I do not argue for disciplinary thinking to be superseded, but supplemented, for the necessity for transdisciplinary collaboration is greater now than ever. The speed with which technology is advancing; the complexity of the problems and their networked nature; the ways in which technology, data, and ideas are connecting; and the rapid adoption of changes by industry and the impact upon society have resulted in complex tangled relationships that are often beyond the boundaries of singular disciplines.

Approaching complex problem through the singular vision of a disciplinary lens can limit or even impede the understanding of the complexity of the problem and result in the application of methods and solutions that fit the problem, rather than a free examination of the problem itself, that so that a solution is fundamentally flawed by the linear misunderstanding of the problem itself. It is through transdisciplinary practices that problems can be framed in new ways. Yet if this is required, how is industry to be populated by those who have learnt to think in such new ways, if universities continue to only produce graduates with singular disciplinary education?

Transdisciplinary Formation at UTS

Formed in late 2016, the Faculty of Transdisciplinary Innovation resides within a youthful university. The nature of UTS as well as its relative youth were both significant factors in not only its decision, but also its ability to enter into the transdisciplinary space. While UTS is not a sandstone (Australia), red brick (UK) or Ivy League (US) institution, at the time of writing, it is ranked as the 11th highest performing university in the world under 50 years old (QS World University Rankings, 2020), and as Australia's highest performing young university (Times Higher Education Young University Rankings, 2019; Times Higher Education World University Rankings, 2019). It is also ranked in 2020 by the QS World University Rankings in the top 150 universities in the world and within the top 200 global universities by the Times Higher Education rankings.

Established in its current form in 1988, by 2013 (the year in which the first transdisciplinary course was conceived and designed) UTS was commencing on a significant trajectory in the international educational rankings, and thus the establishment of its own academic confidence. The university was not simply replicating leading national universities, but recognizing its inherent strengths. In other words, in establishing belief in its own abilities and its confidence to not be the same as more long-standing educational institutions, its ability to differentiate itself was formed from its actual difference. University leadership with vision and agility were also factors in its understanding that graduates would increasingly have to develop new ways of thinking and working as a particular form of agility. Another instigator was the university's close relationship with industry, which increasingly articulated their desire for different types of graduates. While they didn't articulate what these students should be, these conversations contributed to fast conceptualization and action, and thus was born a transdisciplinary movement within the university.

The need for students to be prepared for a vastly changed and changing world was becoming clearer, as was the recognition that graduates would require mobility, through the ability to move not just across jobs, but also across careers in a problem-solving world where multidisciplinarity and transdisciplinarity would abound. This was understood as a world of in which skills and knowledge would be built upon and expanded: a time where a university degree is not the final body of learning, but the start of a lifetime of learning.

The articulation of the need for educational change utilizes the prediction that jobs that presently exist will change or no longer exists, or that "in many industries and countries, the most in-demand occupations or specialties did not exist 10 or even five years ago, and the pace of change is set to accelerate" (World Economic Forum, 2016). Within the UTS transdisciplinary model this has proven to be not only true but also possibly conservative, with our students graduating into jobs with job titles that did not exist when they entered their degree study four years previously. Perhaps an unexpected outcome however has been that these students, while highly sought after by industry, enter employment to discover that industry is not always as innovative as it desires to be and that the graduates' knowledge of how to transcend the linear approach to challenges exceeds that for which that industry is presently capable.

The impact of transdisciplinarity upon UTS is that students have been attracted to the university that might have previously considered other local universities. The impact upon core degrees of the Bachelor of Creative Intelligence and Innovation (BCII) combined degree students, has also been noted by the core degree teaching staff, through the distinctive capabilities that the BCII students also bring to their disciplinary degree study. The integration of a transdisciplinary degree with a core degree impact significantly upon students' original core degree career pathways. Students select a core degree with a particular professional pathway in mind. But in combination with a transdisciplinary degree, this results in the creation of greater flexibility in thinking, with different possibilities becoming apparent and open to them through their curiosity, collaboration, and the development of a willingness to fail, that develops skills in students as problem-identifiers and problem-solvers. This generates agility, flexibility, and the ability to pursue a nondefined path, but also the ability to pivot ideas and to seek out new career options.

The impact has also expanded to the formation of industry, government, and social (not-for-profit) sectors, over 700 of whom who have committed to becoming active industry partners. It is often assumed that such partnerships provide excellent opportunities for students, but the importance of such collaboration for industry is not always recognized. In collaboration with the faculty, academics, and students, industry partners gain access to their potential future employees and consumers, as well as this generation's ability to think in new ways across new problem spaces. They thus gain access to thinking and challenges to their problems through the minds of the upcoming generation that as industry they are not yet always able to achieve themselves.

The UTS Faculty of Transdisciplinary Innovation now has 10 programs spanning innovation, creative intelligence, emergent technology, data science, and new forms of visualization and animation, from diploma, degree, masters, and PhD. These programs forefront critical and creative thinking, problem-posing and problem-solving, innovation and invention, complexity, and entrepreneurship, engaging students in not only future-focused learning, but also building in them flexibility and capabilities to be able to adapt to, frame and lead future change. The faculty is one of eight across the university, and the only one formed beyond the model of singular or conjoined disciplines that exist within most other universities. Unlike disciplinary faculties, the faculty's role is to work across, between, and beyond the silos of single disciplines.

The first and still largest transdisciplinary program in the faculty was launched three years prior to the conception of a faculty, with a whole of university approach integrating students from undergraduate degree programs from across all seven of the university's disciplinary faculties of business, arts and social sciences, design, architecture and building, engineering and IT, health, law and science. The BCII was conceived to enable students from, at that time, eighteen of the university's most successful disciplinary undergraduate degrees to undertake double degrees.

Of primary importance was the need to transcend the time commitment of double-degree study, resulting in an accelerated and integrated double-degree program enabling students to undertake two degrees in only one year longer than a single degree. Seven years on, it now encompasses students from twenty-five specialist undergraduate bachelor degrees in information technology, engineering, science, advanced science, forensic science, biomedical physics, medicinal chemistry, sport and exercise science, midwifery, nursing, business, management, architecture, visual communication, fashion and textile design, product design, animation, product design, creative writing, digital and social media, journalism, media arts and production, public communication, social and political sciences and law.

The BCII was created at the intersection of industry desiring more from universities, and a particular new generation of students seeking more from their university experience. With the first degree launched at speed and limited marketing, it received unprecedented applications in that first year alone. That, of course, has since been eclipsed for, within three years, the BCII became the second most applied-for undergraduate degree at the university, with a mark of its popularity being its generation of some of the highest entry scores it was possible for students to achieve. It is often asked why, as the precursor to a faculty with the name 'Transdisciplinary Innovation', this first transdisciplinary program was not formed as a single stand-alone (non-conjoined) degree. The reasoning for this was formed through the understanding that educational innovation across disciplines requires concurrent acquisition, so breadth of transdisciplinarity application could be achieved concurrently with disciplinary depth, as innovation is rarely formed just for its own sake or as the sole but uninformed driver.

At this stage of development, a challenge existed in that transdisciplinary study in Australia was unique to UTS and unfamiliar to many. This meant that prior to the graduation of the first cohort, it was not possible to articulate proven employment outcomes, despite industry's clear articulation to the university of the necessity for graduates with the agility to think across disciplines.

In designing the BCII, a small academic team was formed to undertake the conceptual and pedagogical design with representatives of disciplines from across all seven faculties, and thus a deep dive was undertaken into the potential of transdisciplinarity. Unlike more traditional degree pedagogy, which builds upon historical as well as contemporary disciplinary practices, precedents for a transdisciplinarity degree design and study did not exist. The identification of faculty-specific academic staff champions were vital to its formation. Identified through their genuine curiosity and willingness to engage in such an educational challenge, the co-creation resulted in a final educational outcome described by its designers as the degree that "we all wished we could have studied." In the formation of its first degree program and the subsequent faculty, such curiosity was vital within the university structures, where depth of specialism is highly regarded, and generating research, publication, and the historical hierarchy of academic position (to the pinnacle of a tenured professor) as well as entering into a new academic space without precedent or recognition, demanded not just curiosity, but also academic career bravery. These are academic staff who were willing not only to be risk-takers in the trajectory of their career choice (UTS is still the only Australian faculty of this kind) within still historically formed although shifting institutions, but also to explore new academic spaces. Of course the navigation between and across fields does not simply occur because we wish it to do so; it requires depth of thinking. This understanding of shared ways of knowing also resulted in one of the most important initial forms of engaging others (academic staff and students) in transdisciplinary methodologies.

In establishing a degree program with a student cohort comprised of participants from multiple disciplinary degrees, ways needed to be identified in which these disciplines and the spaces they inhabited could be not simply straddled, but also explored. Thus ways needed to be developed in which transdisciplinary thinking could be successfully facilitated. This is one of the greatest misunderstandings of transdisciplinarity—that simply creating a place for disciplines to collaborate will create successful outcomes. So here resides the other misunderstanding: that the knowledge of disciplines alone will naturally form transdisciplinarity, which leads to the perception that transdisciplinarity as an academic field does not exist. So much of the work that the academics have developed since that initial launch has been without precedent.

One of the fundamental elements in such design required the academic team to achieve a primary understanding of the similarity and difference of individual disciplines. This was achieved through understanding how disciplinary specialists explained their disciplines to those not so affiliated, and to recognize that elements of commonality existed, and that different methodologies of knowing, seeing and articulating, could inform others. A vital component in the creation of the BCII was the set of "method cards." As a result of these discussions, the academic staff from across the university developed a set of methods to be provided to all incoming students as a pack of cards, to enable them to possess potential approaches across disciplines that transcended the dysfunctionality that could have existed in individuals speaking the "language" of their discipline. These enabled students to not retreat into their familiar practices or to see solutions to problems that were often misdiagnosed as a problem due to the singular vision of a disciplinary lens. The new approaches that these method card facilitated (and which have been added to over the years) do not provide a comprehensive answer to transdisciplinary practice, but rather a new way of viewing and developing new methods of transdisciplinary practice to transcend singular practice.

Upon its launch, the BCII immediately drew unprecedented numbers of high-performing applicants, who were attracted based on their desire to not simply confine their curiosity to a single professional path at the age of eighteen. It was easy for some to dismissively assume that this was simply a millennial lack of decisiveness on their part, but it wasn't: it was genuine curiosity and a desire for a different type of nonsingular education and educational experience that their school curriculums in seeking high entry scores for their students had often been restrained from being able to offer. Prospective students clearly indicated a desire for not only depth of single disciplinary study, but also breadth in their university learning experience. Such decisiveness was also often supported by professional parents who themselves were recognizing the speed of change within their professions and acting as advocates for the program to their offspring.

As much as the pedagogical design was born from the academic staffs' curiosity, it also immediately attracted genuinely curious students, seeking more than just a university education. Instead, they were seeking a different university experience that would also provide differentiation for them in a competitive but too often disciplinary generic world. For such students, the education they sought was one that was about the journey, not simply a known end result or a named profession, instead an educational engagement that was about ways of thinking that opened up possibilities.

Professional degrees and professionally recognized disciplinary qualifications have traditionally led to predictably defined and predetermined employment pathways. By introducing the BCII as a double degree, it therefore provided a vital safety net for students (and their parents) by providing a familiar professional qualification with a transdisciplinary qualification. This also meant that if students discovered that they were unsuited to such study, that they could easily withdraw from the double to the single disciplinary degree without risk to their university education. This was vital in the initial stages in reassuring parents for whom the traditional qualification and employment outcomes of a university education were familiar, for in the early stages of delivery, we could not yet provide examples of employment outcomes for graduates, a fact that has now been assessed.

Seven years hence, with a demonstrated concept and with proof of outcome, the necessity for transdisciplinary thinking and study is ever more vital, in addition to now being easier to articulate. This does not however mean it is always easier to persuade traditional disciplinarians. One of the core persuaders however exists in the evidence of the high level of industry, government, and social sector engagement with the faculty's courses, with over 700 industry partners now actively engaged with the faculty, with 95% of the faculty subjects delivered through co-designed delivery with industry partners.

In establishing the BCII, the creation of means by which students could be introduced to forms of navigation required new forms of development. This challenge to the disciplinary traditions could only be solved by the identification of potential academic champions from across the university, whose genuine curiosity, collaborative capabilities, and pedagogical leadership made them open to seeing beyond their long-held disciplinary traditions.

During the development of the degree program, it became obvious that methodologies across disciplines shared certain commonalties, but that these were often submerged in the fragmentation that the university's disciplines inhabited, as well as the language of their disciplinary rhetoric. With academic staff required to explain these methodologies to academics of differing and disparate disciplines, the mantle of rhetoric in the telling shifted and adjusted, and levels of commonality were revealed and so too was the potential applicability of individual practices to new practices.

The Necessity for Transdisciplinarity in Not Only the Complexity, but also the Networked Nature of Problems

At this point it is necessary to step aside from the educational development, to articulate the vital role of transdisciplinarity in addressing the networked nature of problems, in addition to their complexity. The complexity inherent in the creation of new technology creates substantial challenges to, as well as the connectivity of, thinking. Kees Dorst (2018) refers to this as the "networked" nature of today's problems, in that "the networked nature of today's problem situations means that they potentially influence each other constantly. . . . What other people are doing in seemingly unrelated fields might cause an effect that seriously influences your problem field and options for actions" (p. 11).

Let me provide a simple example that is so often in the news as we discuss technological advances and their impact upon society. What is all too often ignored in this era of rapid technological change is not simply the complexity of thinking, but also the complexity of the interconnected layers of thought required. Engineers, technicians, and software developers and designers are some of the primary disciplines engaged in the advancement of our capacity to create autonomous cars. Yet while fundamental to the creation and advances of the technology, these named disciplines are not necessarily sufficient to contribute to the understanding and social adaptation of the new forms of ethical decisions integral in such change.

If a group of children step out in front of an autonomous vehicle, is the car programmed to make the decision to hit the children, swerve one way into the oncoming traffic, or the other way into a solid structure? Does the car make the decision based on children being deserving of saving first or based on the greater number of people that can be saved and therefore the lower number that can be sacrificed? What if there are five people in the car and five people have stepped out into the road in front of the vehicle? Is the car programmed to value children or the number of children before the adult car owner? In fact, in terms of human behavior, do we wish to own a car that in an accident might make the decision to sacrifice us (the driver) first, or does the purchase of the car grant us the moral expectation that the car has loyalty to us as the owner? It is therefore simple here to understand that engineering and IT disciplines are not solely sufficient to address such ethical considerations in the programming of such technological advances and that transdisciplinary collaboration is a requirement of such change.

In creating autonomous cars we are essentially removing the high risk of human failure that results in accidents. One of the results of accidents, apart from injury, is also unfortunately death, so with reduced risk comes altered requirements of insurance and hence the insurance industry. If autonomous vehicles become widely accepted, many things will change, including fuel consumption patterns, the oil industry, service stations and their use for other purchases, and the types of public transportation we use, to name but a few. Also, if we reduce the potential for human error in driving, we will reduce the number of automobile fatalities. If fatalities are reduced, we will also therefore decrease the number of human organs available for transplantation that accidents yield, because at this point, one of the largest sources of organs for transplantation is from automobile fatalities.

In the United States alone, one-fifth of annual organ donations are derived from otherwise healthy people. So from the implementation of autonomous vehicles, we now have to consider the impact of this new technology on our ability to source organs for an ever-growing population that is increasingly lives longer. So with extended life and reduced automobile fatalities, some estimates (Lafrance, 2015) suggest that autonomous cars could save 300,000 lives over a decade in the United States alone. This immediately raises the question of the greater need for organs from alternative sources. So if we are increasing safety, we are reducing automobile fatalities, but at the same time reducing a primary resource for saving other lives. If autonomous cars really do become adopted, will this result in fewer organs being available for transplantation that will result in new ways in which the medical professions ethically and practically have to manage organ donation.

So here is the connectivity, or the networked nature of problems in thinking and where transdisciplinary collaboration is required. With the speed with which we are advancing and the fail fast mentality, there is a risk that we are not considering the connectedness of cause and effect, so we are forced to be reactive to the emergence of unforeseen issues, rather than proactive by predicting them first. It could of course be claimed that technological advance has always caused unforeseen repercussions. But with transdisciplinarity and the potential in connected thinking to transcend the singular disciplinary outcome of the technological advance, are we presented with the ability to connect previously unforeseen dots? I have presented only one example here, and this could as easily be applied to multiple examples, big data being another.

Institutional and Institutionalized Challenges

In addressing challenges, it should be noted that while educational institutions have the potential to bring so many answers to the transdisciplinary space, often they can be regarded as establishments determined by their own past and imbued with the central premise of the "purity of knowledge," both in its application and transfer, through research and education. These two facts alone can be a challenge to the development of transdisciplinary engagement within the institution. Yet so too is the unspoken element of organizational subdivision. Being identified as independent groups can make university divisions competitive, rather than collaborative. Yet unlike most corporations, universities contain all of the component elements for transdisciplinary collaboration, and universities are about new knowledge. So surely this is not be the case?

One of the primary challenges however within universities is that their division and subdivision (through faculties, schools, and departments) has often occurred through the historical determination and formation of now entrenched singular or conjoined disciplines. While universities are also often large institutions, even when subdivided (e.g., through faculties), these still form large groupings of staff and students, but now clustered by singular or conjoined disciplines and thus ways of thinking. Such defining divisions have extraordinary potential but are also limited unless synthesis is also formed. As Matthew Syed (2019) identifies, the larger the institution, the less likelihood there is of interaction between differing schools of thought (178).

The basis upon which educational divisions and subdivisions have been formed, inhabits as Pierre Bourdieu would identify, its own "doxa," whereby cultural norms (the determination of disciplinary groupings) have become established and perpetuated as "truths." This alone presents a challenge when it results in the perception of "pure" and defined disciplines, with resultant siloed perpetuation through application of knowledge. So do university structures primarily inhibit depth of thinking, when in fact they have the capacity to expand upon this, especially at this point in time?

Of course with such a step forward, there are also challenges that institutions presents that are institutionalized. With educational thinking and education generally organized by professional fields, specialisms, and disciplines, over recent years increasing specialist areas of knowledge have been formed, each of which drives a depth of research. But in their subdivision, does this further compartmentalize fields and professions into confined subprofessions and thus hinder collaboration? In the medical profession in the United States alone, specialisms and subspecialisms have increased over the last decade. Certainly these provide highly valuable depth of knowledge, but with increasingly defined specialism, does this constriction limit the connection of symptoms and hinder diagnosis?

Specialisms create depth of knowledge, but as they progress, how do they transcend that singular and often linear depth and fragmented application? Certainly disciplinary specialisms do and can collaborate, but in increasing subdivision, does this further confine disciplines ability to expand through synthesis? Transdisciplinarity requires flexibility in thinking across, between, and beyond the traditional boundaries of disciplines, enabling outcomes to be formed that single disciplines alone cannot generate. Certainly during the initial development of this at UTS, we referred to as "stepping on the cracks in the pavement," probably due to our placement within a university structure in which the paths we tread are traditionally formed from predictably defined patterns of division.

Since the faculty's formation four year ago, the persistent questions by observers have always been, how will success be judged, and can success (in which disciplines recognize, interact and collaborate through transdisciplinary practices) only truly be measured by full adoption university-wide and hence the faculty's redundancy?

Success at a university level is judged in terms of teaching and learning, engagement, research, and impact. Thus far, the first two have been achieved and measured through student feedback (student feedback surveys) and reputationally through elevated application levels, high levels of alumni employment and feedback, unprecedented levels of industry engagement, and a high levels of engagement by schools wishing to integrate such practices into often results-driven high school curriculums.

Transdisciplinary collaboration within a university and its disciplines, and new forms of engagement with industry and resultant research with measurable outcomes, requires more than a few years to engage and persuade as well as form. This therefore is an important point. Within an environment constructed of disciplinary measures, instigating new practices demands not only the conceptual and structural investment in one faculty, but investment in a whole of institutional commitment. Within institutional environments, transdisciplinary forms will always be different to disciplinary structures simply because their outcomes are driven by the act of collaboration in working across, between, and beyond disciplines and by the creation of new methodologies formed as much by the problem space as by the solution.

To be judged through new forms of collaboration at a time of accelerated change and innovation will take time, as well as the willingness to create new measures and view outcomes through new lenses. Within a university environment, transdisciplinarity will need to be judged as possessing a different alternative remit—not simply constructing its own defined boundaries, but collaboratively forming new practices and acting as a persuader/engager/broker in what can be at times still be initially perceived as a space of ambiguity, even within even a relatively new and agile university's environment of traditional boundaries, measures, and expectations.

Conclusion

This chapter did not set out to define transdisciplinarity and its potential, as I am sure many other chapters will have done so. Rather its intent was step aside from theoretical explorations and examples of industry and research practice to instead reveal an example of its introduction within an educational institution. If we recognize the necessity for transdisciplinary practice, then we need to consider the vital role of education in its conceptualization and formation for a new generation and utilize such examples to build and scale, by learning from each other. Work is being undertaken to explore the potential of transdisciplinarity, but development of such work in isolation and without collaboration will only limit its expansion for industry, research, and education to work more holistically together.

Transdisciplinary practice if formed from a place of curiosity, and in a space that facilitates exploration, navigation, and creativity, needs to occur where the confines of traditional practice can be challenged by the problem space. This is as true for education as it is for practice. While radical departures from the norm often receive push back from established interests, those push-backs can be a challenge to forward momentum but also be used to stimulate and refine the development of new paradigms. Every educational reform is not necessarily right first time, but if we don't try, we don't learn. If we are still at the stage that transdisciplinary programs and curriculum are merely emergent and disconnected, we will be unable to produce the compelling evidence that is required to drive forward momentum.

Transdisciplinarity stands on the shoulders of all that has gone before and provides a radical new perspective of how we view the educational process and our ability to address the complexity of where we are now and where we might go. If we stay static as institutions, thinkers, and practitioners, and are unwilling to enter uncharted and often ambiguous space, will single disciplines increasingly be limited in their ability to address the speed and interconnectedness of our increasingly complexity? Transdisciplinarity can be challenging to multiple disciplines within a traditional university structure due to its perceived ambiguity. To move forward however requires that we understand that individual disciplines will continue to remain siloed if they each consider that they possess the answer and recognize instead that the answer lies within the totality of all of them.

Note

While this chapter has predominantly focused on the evolution of its first program, The Faculty of Transdisciplinary Innovation presently delivers the following programs: Bachelor of Creative Intelligence and Innovation (combined with twenty-five of UTS's undergraduate degrees), Bachelor of Creative Intelligence and Innovation (Honors), Diploma in Innovation (combined with all of the university's undergraduate degrees), Bachelor of Technology and Innovation, Graduate Certificate in Transdisciplinary Innovation in Higher Education, Masters of Data Science and Innovation, Masters of Animation and Visualisation (The UTS Animal Logic Academy), Masters of Creative Intelligence and Strategic Innovation, Masters by Research and PhD, in addition to elective subjects available across the university.

References

Bernstein, J. H. (2015). Transdisciplinarity: a review of its origins, development, and current issues. *Journal of Research Practice, 11*(1), R1.

Brown, V. A., Harris, J. A., & Russell, J. Y. (2010). *Tackling wicked problems through the transdisciplinary Imagination*. London: Earthscan.

Dorst, K. (2018). Mixing practices to create transdisciplinary innovation: A design-based approach. *Technology Innovation Management Review, 8*(8), 9–13 https://doi.org/10.22215/timreview/1179

Lafrance, A. (2015, September 29). Self-driving cars could save 300,000 lives per decade in America. *The Atlantic*. https://www.theatlantic.com/technology/archive/2015/09/self-driving-cars-could-save-300000-lives-per-decade-in-america/407956/

Mooby Di. (2016, March 16). Why do some animals have webbed feet? What is their function? *Quora.com*. https://www.quora.com/Why-do-some-animals-have-webbed-feet-What-is-their-function

National Science Foundation. (n.d.). Convergence research at NSF. Accessed October 5, 2019; https://www.nsf.gov/od/oia/convergence/index.jsp

Times Higher Education World University Rankings. (2019). https://www.timeshighereducation.com/world-university-rankings/2020/world-ranking#!/page/0/length/-1/sort_by/rank/sort_order/asc/cols/scores

Times Higher Education Young University Rankings. (2019). https://www.timeshighereducation.com/world-university-rankings/2019/young-university-rankings#!/page/0/length/25/sort_by/rank/sort_order/asc/cols/stats

QS World University Rankings. (2020). https://www.topuniversities.com/university-rankings/world-university-rankings/2020

World Economic Forum. (2016). The future of jobs report. http://www3.weforum.org/docs/WEF_Future_of_Jobs.pdf

7

The OECD Approach to Responsible Innovation

David E. Winickoff and Hermann Garden

Introduction

As other contributions in this volume argue, convergent neurotechnologies targeting mental health could deliver far-reaching benefits, but some pose risks and social questions. In particular, concerns have been raised around privacy, human enhancement, the regulation and marketing of direct-to-consumer devices, and equality of access. Thirty-six member countries of the Organisation for Economic Co-operation and Development (OECD) have recently enacted the Council Recommendation on Responsible Innovation in Neurotechnology (the "Recommendation"), adopted on December 11, 2019 (1). Committed to the idea that we must not just innovate more but innovate *well*, the Recommendation advances a "responsible innovation" approach that could serve as a model for technology governance both in neurotechnology and beyond.

The Recommendation

The Recommendation is the first international instrument in its field. It is soft law, non-binding from a legal matter but enforced through moral suasion and regular monitoring across countries. The Recommendation aims to help public and private actors address the ethical, legal and social challenges of neurotechnology while encouraging innovation. The Recommendation is made up for nine principles (Box 7.1), each principle being specified with more detailed recommendations that are not included here.

Responsible Innovation Approach

The "responsible innovation" approach finds inspiration in the field of Science and Technology Studies (2,3) and recent work funded by the European Union (4) under the Horizon 2020 program. The responsible innovation approach seeks to cope with the so-called Collingridge Dilemma at the heart of technology governance: regulating too early can stifle innovation but regulating further downstream may be too late to

---

Box 7.1. OECD Recommendation on Responsible Innovation in Neurotechnology

---

1. Promote responsible innovation.
2. Prioritize safety assessment.
3. Promote inclusivity.
4. Foster scientific collaboration.
5. Enable societal deliberation.
6. Enable capacity of oversight and advisory bodies.
7. Safeguard personal brain data and other information.
8. Promote cultures of stewardship and trust across the public and private sector.
9. Anticipate and monitor potential unintended use and/or misuse.

---

influence how technology operates in society (5,6). It seeks to anticipate problems in the course of innovation and steer technology to best outcomes and include many stakeholders in the innovation process (7).

Good governance actually can enable, not constrain, technology. This insight—focused on governance from the perspective of innovation—sets the Recommendation apart from other international instruments dealing with technology in society (8). The principles just described are already contributing to the realization of responsible innovation in neurotechnology (9); however at least five overarching elements stand out and make this instrument unique among related statements:

1. *Setting goals and missions for innovation.* The Recommendation responds to societal calls to better align research and commercialization with societal (rather than pure market) needs (10), that is, promotes "mission-oriented" and "purposive" technological transformation to better connect innovation to mental health.
2. *Inclusivity of the innovation process.* When talking about justice and innovation, attention usually focuses on technological divides and access inequality (11). These are worthy considerations. However, the Recommendation emphasizes the need to engage other actors (e.g., citizens, publics, civil society) within the innovation process itself. This is a matter not only of justice, but also of driving innovation. Crowdsourcing health data is only one mechanism for this; another is to create physical and virtual spaces for co-creation (12).
3. *Anticipatory governance.* An end-of-pipe-approach to regulation and governance can be inflexible, inadequate, and even stifling. In the realm of technology governance, the Recommendation encourages governments and policymakers to experiment with collective forms of technology assessment and foresight (7), and forward-looking governance mechanisms like scaled-up test-beds and "living laboratories" (13).
4. *Enabling societal deliberation.* Public engagement is a common refrain in current policy communities. Deliberation is more demanding than "public

engagement" as it implies an iterative exchange of views in hopes of finding reasoned discourse and even common ground (14). The approach demands the enhancement societal capacities to understand, communicate on, and shape technology through the course of development so that technology might advance under conditions of trust and trustworthiness.

5. *Institutional approach and the role of the private sector.* Whereas many technology ethics codes place duties on scientists and clinicians, the Recommendation advances an institutional approach, targeting guidance to policymakers, funding agencies, oversight bodies, and companies. The latter have a critical role to play in governance as they are on the front lines of product development, translation, diffusion and marketing (8). Effective governance of neurotechnology must involve the private sector as a central actor early on—before trajectories are locked in.

The responsible innovation approach can help facilitate pathways for neurotechnology and other converging technologies. Ultimately, technology will be useless unless it can be diffused and built into society in ways that are socially robust—trustworthy, debated, accessible, and acceptable.

References

1. OECD. Recommendation of the Council on Responsible Innovation in Neurotechnology (OECD/LEGAL/0457). Adopted October 12, 2019. https://legalinstruments.oecd.org/en/instruments/OECD-LEGAL-0457
2. Stilgoe J., R. Owen, P. Macnaghten. Developing a framework for responsible innovation. *Res Policy.* 2013;*42*:1568–1580.
3. Owen R., J. Stilgoe, P. Macnaghten, M. Gorman, E. Fisher, D. Guston. A framework for responsible innovation. In: R. Owen, J. Bessant, M. Heintz (Eds.), *Responsible Innovation: Managing the Responsible Emergence of Science and Innovation in Society,* London: Wiley; 2013:27-50.
4. European Commission. Rome Declaration on Responsible Research and Innovation in Europe. Published November 21, 2014. https://ec.europa.eu/research/swafs/pdf/rome_declaration_RRI_final_21_November.pdf
5. Collingridge D. *The Social Control of Technology.* London: Pinter; 1980.
6. Genus A., A. Stirling. Collingridge and the dilemma of control: Towards responsible and accountable innovation, *Res Policy.* 2018;*47*:61–69. https://doi.org/10.1016/j.respol.2017.09.012
7. Guston, D. Understanding "anticipatory governance." *Social Studies of Science.* 2014;*44*(2):218–242. https://doi.org/10.1177/0306312713508669
8. Garden H., D. E. Winickoff, N. M. Frahm, S. Pfotenhauer. *Responsible innovation in neurotechnology enterprises.* OECD Science, Technology and Industry Working Papers. 2019;5.
9. Eyre, H. A., W. Ellsworth, E. Fu, H. K. Manji, M. Berk. Responsible innovation in technology for mental health care. *Lancet Psychiatry.* 2020;*7*(9):728–730. September 01, 2020. https://doi.org/10.1016/S2215-0366(20)30192-9
10. Mazzucato M. *Mission-Oriented Research & Innovation in the European Union: A Problem-Solving Approach to Fuel Innovation-Led Growth.* Brussels: European Commission; 2018.

11. OECD. Making innovation benefit all: policies for inclusive growth. Published March 16, 2017. http://www.innovationpolicyplatform.org/www.innovationpolicyplatform.org/system/files/Inclusive%20Growth%20publication%20FULL%20for%20web/index.pdf.

12. Winickoff D., S. Pfotenhauer. Technology governance and the innovation process. In: OECD, ed. *OECD Science, Technology and Innovation Outlook 2018: Adapting to Technological and Societal Disruption.* Paris: OECD Publishing; 2018:221–240.

13. Engels F., A. Wentland, S. M. Pfotenhauer. Testing future societies? Developing a framework for test beds and living labs as instruments of innovation governance. *Res Policy.* 2019;48:102826

14. Gutmann, A., D. F. Thompson. *Democracy and Disagreement.* Cambridge MA: Belknap Press; 2008.

SECTION II
EXPERT COMMENTARIES ON CONVERGENCE MENTAL HEALTH

8

The Therapeutic Centaur

Training the Half-Human, Half-Computer Clinician of 2040

Rahul Khanna, Juliet B. Edgcomb, and Malcolm Hopwood

Introduction

At the turn of the century, psychiatry was only beginning to reconcile the profound impact that technology would have on clinical practice. Twenty years ago, a person seeking or providing mental healthcare did not have access to an electronic health record (EHR), a smartphone, social media, or many popular websites for disseminating information such as YouTube or Wikipedia. The renaissance of technology of the early 2000s has been coupled with a stark need for advances in mental healthcare—in the United States, suicide rates are the highest recorded in 29 years,[1] the life expectancy gap between those with mental illness and the general population continues to widen,[2] and mental health and addictive disorders affect more than one billion people globally.[3]

In the next two decades, technology, and the convergence of fields that impact and generate technology, including medicine, engineering, physics, computer science, biology, chemistry, and the arts, will continue to transform how mental healthcare is sought, provided, administered, and regulated. As this book describes, convergence, or transdisciplinary, science is a translational field poised to transform mental healthcare. Convergence psychiatry embeds the integrative, innovative, and interactive principles of convergence science into psychiatric clinical practice and research.

In this chapter, we describe how the workflow of contemporary psychiatrists will change over the next two decades as convergence science becomes embedded in clinical practice and discuss how core competencies should evolve. We also provide a framework of new knowledge and skills relevant to future convergent psychiatrists as leaders of mental healthcare teams. Given that the average lag between research and widespread adoption in healthcare is seventeen years,[4] this chapter focuses on near-term technologies that are already in research application. We also reject the alarmist portrayals of humans and machines as direct competitors. Instead, we advocate for a division of labor by aptitude: technology for tasks reducible to data processing and humans to combine technology with tasks centering on human connection. Although this chapter focuses on psychiatrists, many considerations will be applicable to other mental health providers.

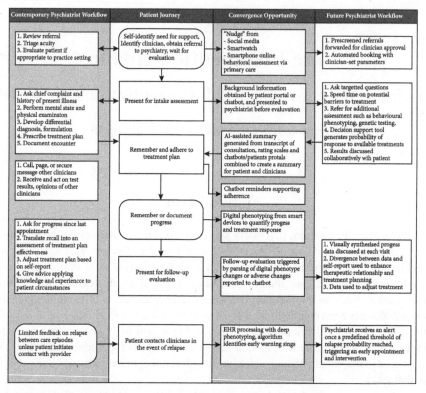

Figure 8.1. Opportunities of convergence science and their impact on clinical workflows. The figure presents the contemporary psychiatrist's workflow (first column) in response to the needs of the patient (second column). Convergence science (third column) provides opportunities to intervene at each step of the patient's journey and transform the psychiatrist's workflow (fourth column).

Psychiatry Pre- and Postconvergence

Contemporary psychiatrists use a range of skills to respond to the needs of each patient, expressed below as the contemporary patient journey. Convergence science can transform the way clinicians provide care at each step. Figure 8.1 summarizes several such opportunities.

Clinical Tasks: Today and Tomorrow

Initial Assessments

Contemporary psychiatrists assess patients through clinical interview, sometimes supplemented by structured questionnaires. In many treatment settings, contemporary psychiatrists work together with psychologists, social workers, primary care providers, and mid-level clinicians to gather clinical data and ascertain a diagnosis. Blood tests and imaging are used in narrow circumstances to exclude organic pathologies but diagnoses and treatment selection remain largely based on self-report data. The clinician elicits the patient's experience of the presenting issue, past medical and psychiatric history, as well as family, social and personal history. A mental state examination is also conducted whereby the clinician incorporates observations of the patient's cross-sectional appearance, mood, affect, speech, thought patterns and behavior.

Many of these details, although important, are collected inefficiently. A patient may have told their story to a primary care provider or therapist and then repeated it to a trainee or an intake clinician before seeing the psychiatrist. Expectations of a structured data flow, where clinical data from medical records could be collected once yet used across multiple relevant encounters have been unrealized due to usability issues.[5] Limited interoperability of EHRs often leaves gaps between data collected by referring providers and psychiatrists.

In the future, we anticipate an increase in technologies to collect and transmit patient data prior to the initial visit. Standardized questionnaires are increasingly administered in in waiting rooms[6] and modern EHR systems strive to increase communication between providers with improved facility of record sharing. More ambitiously, in the future, data could be captured prior to the first appointment using an artificial intelligence (AI) chatbot like the Ada Health Assistant (www.ada.com), which already boasts of conducting a health assessment every three seconds. Patient portals allow consumer-led data checking, preventing the copy-and-paste risks that are commonplace today[7] and incentivizing sensitively worded documentation by all members of the care team.

Parsed appropriately, this information can reduce the duration of assessment appointments and reduce redundant work between providers, while providing a more comprehensive understanding of the patient. Patients may even give a more truthful history to a chatbot compared to a human.[8] Sophisticated virtual humans like SimSensei can interpret facial expressions and body gestures to support rapport building, eliciting a more accurate psychiatric history in military personnel than human assessors.[9]

Ongoing Appointments

A follow-up appointment typically begins by reviewing the progress since the last appointment, covering symptoms, and functional, medical, and psychosocial changes relevant to treatment.

Currently, the treatment orientation of the psychiatrist often dictates the next phase of a consult, where treatment options are discussed. Many psychiatrists work in teams with other mental health clinicians, particularly in the inpatient and intensive outpatient settings. At this stage, the psychiatrist often becomes the team leader for psychotropic medication-related decisions. Psychotherapeutically inclined clinicians may pose questions designed to enlist behavioral, cognitive, or emotional change. Links may be drawn between current problems and the patient's history. Other clinicians use the therapeutic relationship to interpret a patient's current and past relationships and behaviors. A psychopharmacologist may instead spend this time altering dosing or medication choice, simultaneously educating the patients on available options. Final decisions are made collaboratively between the clinical team and patient.

This process is overdue for an update. As Kahneman and Riis describe, our experiencing and evaluative self are distinct.[10] For example, we may be miserable at work daily but when asked to evaluate our job happiness we give a positive account. This is because our evaluative self may be distracted by tangential ideas like perceived prestige. Other cognitive biases like the primacy effect and confirmation bias can skew judgment. As a result, patient responses early in a consult have an outsized influence on diagnosis and treatment compared to later responses. This leads to premature closure, where doctors make decisions before receiving all the relevant information.[11] These tendencies casts doubt on the ritualized progress report that occurs at each appointment. Indeed, more accurate reports of our experiencing self are likely to be collated *between*, rather than *during*, clinical visits. Even a team of health providers who meet with the patient regularly will form a clinical impression based on the patient seeking care when ill, rather than holistically evaluating the patient outside of a health setting, including during periods of wellness. Quantified passively collected data such as GPS activity or social media data, such as posts, direct messaging frequency, and social network size could provide more reliable longitudinal indications of progress compared with cross-sectional self-report. The information, parsed, summarized, and, when appropriate, anonymized, could be available to clinician and patient on any device.

Further, the tendency of treatment to be driven by clinician orientation rather than data requires resolution. Contemporary approaches to this problem using evidence-based yet consensus-framed treatment guidelines have had mixed results. New approaches like the Cochrane Collaboration's Living Evidence initiative seek to create systematic reviews that are constantly updated with new evidence through digital tools. The outputs of such efforts could be paired with EHR decision support tools to improve quality and safety. Ready access to evidence-based decision-making support could also facilitate communication between care providers with diverse backgrounds and expertise working in mental health teams.

Between Appointments

Between appointments, contemporary psychiatrists have little contact with the patient outside emergencies. In a strict sense, this is likely to remain the case, but new AI-based systems may allow interim interactions with clinician avatars. These could perform triage functions or deliver reminders about appointments, medication changes, or homework given during sessions. Such systems are a natural progression of patient-managed health records and ecological momentary assessment methods already proposed for a participatory iHealth era.[12] Similarly, smart assistants such as Amazon's Alexa may assist patients implement behavior change between appointments (e.g., the unofficial Alcoholics Anonymous Alexa app). Administrative tasks such as obtaining prior authorizations for specific pharmaceuticals are also ripe for automation. These technologies raise questions regarding how ecological data will be monitored and evaluated by different members of a treatment team, such as a psychiatrist and therapist or a primary care collaborative mental care team.

Between Patients

Between patients, psychiatrists regularly document previous appointments and exchange clinical information with other treatment providers, increasingly through synchronous secure messaging systems rather than asynchronous methods such as voicemail or fax. Synchronous secure messaging platforms increase facility of communication between providers working within a single system of care (e.g., the U.S. Veterans Affairs use of Skype for Business). However, interoperability and usability issues have still limit communication between providers working in different systems, for which clinicians still frequently turn to fax or even postal mail to health transmit information. In addition to clinician-facing technologies like Skype, patient-centered innovations may also transform communication. Noting that 40% to 80% of healthcare information is forgotten immediately by patients after a consult,[13] Barr et al. reported on a pilot project wherein medical consultations are recorded and summarized, using natural-language processing to highlight key points of interest.[14] The patient can then take the summary home to remember the encounter. Such systems could eliminate or substantially reduce these time-intensive communication tasks in consenting patients, especially when combined with secure transmission to other care providers.

What Will Remain of Contemporary Practice?

As previously discussed, several time-consuming tasks such as clinical data collection, communication, and documentation can be digitally transformed or eliminated by 2040. Britain's Institute of Public Policy Research estimated that a health system that maximized contemporary automation potential would free up 23% of physician time and 31% of general practitioner time.[15]

Without any other change in practice, this extra time alone could make a marked difference in outcomes. A recent study examining home health visits found that each additional minute above the average visit duration decreased re-admission risk by 8%.[16] The finding that antipsychotic prescribing rates are inversely related to the size of the mental health workforce is another intriguing clue of what increased clinician time might mean for patient care.[17] Further, insufficient appointment duration is the most common complaint on physician review sites.[18] The additional time garnered from automation of nonessential tasks would allow psychiatrists to focus on the more uniquely human aspects of their role, although even these are likely to be transformed in form if not in principle. Moreover, reduction in rote tasks enables clinicians to spend more time acting collaboratively within mental healthcare teams. In the following section, we describe clinical duties and skills that will likely remain to core to the work.

The Therapeutic Relationship

The ability to empathically connect with patients and build a therapeutic relationship will remain central. The therapeutic relationship refers to the ability for a patient and clinician to form a collaborative working relationship toward shared goals. Relevant to all health disciplines, this ability is particularly important in mental health. Indeed, meta-analysis suggests the quality of the therapeutic relationship reliably accounts for a substantial portion of the therapeutic benefit of psychotherapy.[19] Therapists skilled in developing such relationships are described as attentive, interested, and understanding—properties that can be enhanced by the judicious use of technology.

By outsourcing the rote aspects of clinical work, psychiatrists can focus on behaviors that are known to enhance the therapeutic relationship, such as accurate expressions of empathy, interpretations, and attunement to nonverbal cues. Contemporary EHRs are frequently experienced as an intruder between patient and clinician,[20] which slows workflow. However, emerging technologies are less intrusive and may even enhance the therapeutic relationship. For example, EHR-based and smartphone-integrated clinical decision support systems could engage providers and patient in mutual discussions regarding clinical progress and treatment. Moreover, technology provides opportunities to quantify and study subtle human experiences; for example, recent research used thermal cameras to detect the autonomic signature of mother–child empathy.[21] These technologies may be applied to better understand how empathic connections between patients and providers are fostered and maintained.

Guidance, Accountability, and Hope

Despite the profusion of advanced e-health interventions for mental illness, research consistently shows improved outcomes with human guidance.[22] Poor physician-patient communication, relationship quality, and trust, as well as infrequent follow-up are all strongly associated with treatment nonadherence.[23] Humans therefore remain crucial to instilling hope and providing accountability and practical guidance.

Accordingly, the personalized therapeutics discussed in this book can only be realized if practitioners continue to hone this ability to promote adherence and change. It is, and will remain, insufficient to merely demand patient action because evidence says the action will help. Maintaining mental well-being requires complex behavior change, needing commitment at a time of vulnerability. By instilling hope and providing practical support and coaching, clinicians provide a crucial scaffold for individual recovery.

Supported Decision-Making

Patient autonomy remains a foundational ethical principal in medicine. Further, patient involvement in decision-making can enhance adherence and outcomes and are therefore important aims for clinicians.[24] As treatment options increase in number and complexity, decision-making becomes increasingly challenging. Clinicians are often asked to support patients in exercising autonomy by providing accurate yet accessible information and actively bolstering self-efficacy. This requires an understanding of the patient's capabilities and value systems—an understanding that would be challenging to automate.

Doing this effectively in 2040 will require psychiatrists to translate algorithms into meaningful guidance for patients. Algorithms do not output a decision but rather a probabilistic statement. For example, an algorithm may suggest a 72% chance that a medication will work or a 40% chance of certain side effects. The role of the psychiatrist will be to provide and translate this information into meaningful clinical guidance, empowering the patient to make informed decisions in the context of this knowledge.

Negotiation and De-escalation

Sadly, some psychiatric conditions are associated with a loss of insight (i.e., an inability to know that one is unwell or with aggression). In these cases, clinicians must negotiate with patients about the need for treatment or de-escalate those at risk of hurting themselves or others. This is task requires a fundamentally "human" touch, and the need for this skill will remain.

Technology is already affecting this process, with telepsychiatry becoming commonplace for emergency psychiatry consults. Other technologies could enable earlier intervention, such as the use of cameras to remotely detect psychophysiological states.[25] Such tools would also provide objective metrics of success, allowing de-escalation skills to be formally studied and improved.

Statutory Responsibility

Contemporary psychiatrists hold considerable statutory responsibility and are informally expected to embody societal values in their practice. They balance competing ethical and legal demands, expressing societal mores around risk tolerance, the value of autonomy, and the definition of justice. Psychiatrists are often invested with significant powers of detention and coercive treatment, with the commensurate legal responsibilities and liabilities ensuring their judicious use. Predictive modeling will add to the complexity of such powers.

For example, if an algorithm predicts with 0.98 accuracy that a patient will attempt suicide, should the psychiatrist automatically put the patient on a hold? If the psychiatrist's judgment differs from the algorithm, who should arbitrate? This is particularly perilous in the current liminal phase of contemporary convergence psychiatry, where promising in vivo algorithms show poor real-world results. A recent review examining 64 suicide prediction models with ≥ 0.80 classification accuracy resulted in huge false-positive rates on simulated patient data sets.[26] The authors found 58 true positives and 49,942 false positives when one million patients were screened, hardly an encouraging statistic to justify detention. Even if the performance was better, the evidence is insufficient to recommend an intervention for such a scenario.

The Convergence Care Team

Mental healthcare will remain a team endeavor, requiring a range of skills for optimal outcomes. The ability to work well with, and at times lead, these diverse teams will remain a core skill. As physicians, psychiatrists have often been the de facto leader of such teams within organizations. However, we anticipate care teams of the future to be more fluid, incorporating nontraditional members such as patients and families with lived experience, mental health coaches or even software designers and data scientists. Stepped care models such as that used by Ginger (www.ginger.io) are likely to be commonplace. Their mobile app-based service allows customers to chat with a behavioral health coach within minutes with care escalated to qualified clinicians if required in a longer timeframe. These novel care team members are unlikely to sit within the same formal hierarchies within institutions and a continued leadership role will require convergent psychiatrists to have more nuanced leadership skills and a broad understanding of how to leverage such diverse teams.

The growing demand for mental health services mean all clinicians must work past turf wars that have constrained some prior attempts at clinical task sharing.[27] Orientating such teams around the patient and their needs, in a manner shown in Figure 8.1, is one way of avoiding such conflicts and illuminating opportunities for all members to contribute helpfully. Further, as high-quality and sensitively managed data underpin convergence mental health, these future teams must develop common understandings and processes for data collection, management, and security. These policies will be particularly important when these novel behavioral health teams interface with other clinician and social service providers. Inappropriate data sharing at such interfaces jeopardizes the whole enterprise of convergence mental health, risking patients and their future willingness to leverage the emerging tools we outline here.

New Skills and Knowledge

In 1940, psychiatry was facing a challenge—the emerging field of applied psychology, with laboratory-based quantitative skills and expertise in research design, was acquiring most available government funding, leaving psychoanalysts with a paltry 5% of federal dollars.[28] Psychiatry had to quickly evolve, marrying psychological theory and research methods to traditional analytic approaches. Coupled with deinstitutionalization and the emergence of psychopharmacology in the mid-1950s, psychiatrists had to again shift the locus of practice, developing outpatient and pharmacological expertise.

In 2020, psychiatry again faces a challenge—the ubiquitous arrival of technology into every sector of life. At a minimum, a smartphone and an EHR system are now in almost every physician–patient encounter. Social media platforms are used by one in three people globally[29] and five billion people have mobile devices, over half of which are smart phones.[30] One hundred years after applied psychology pressed psychiatrists to acquire skills in quantitative and research methods, psychiatry in 2040 is again challenged to improve itself by a new competitor—computers. This time, the path forward may include merging psychiatric practice with new skills and knowledge in informatics and data science.

Convergence Psychiatry as a Translational Field

Translational medicine is an interdisciplinary branch of the biomedical field that connects benchside, bedside, and community.[31] Translational research aims to translate findings in fundamental research into clinical practice and meaningful patient outcomes. Convergence psychiatry is a translational field: translating AI, machine learning, and clinical informatics to understand psychiatric diagnosis, predict patient outcomes, and advance mental health treatment. Convergence mental health expands the scope of translational work, beyond the unidimensional bench-to-bedside, toward a multidisciplinary integration of medical science, engineering, physics, and mathematics.[32]

Psychiatrists cannot become experts in all these fields. Rather, similar to other translational and convergent domains, such as translational neuroscience, the busy clinician is not expected to understand the intricacies of specialized research. However, a foundation in convergence skills will be necessary to interpret the literature, comprehend headline research, and be an informed prescriber and clinician. Similar efforts have been paralleled in the neurosciences, for example, through the National Neuroscience Curriculum Initiative (nncionline.org). Calls to action have also been raised to train new psychiatrists in the principles of clinical informatics.[33] However, in 2020, few psychiatry training programs actively incorporate curricula in informatics. By 2040, we expect this to change.

One challenge in designing curricula and considering how to train psychiatrists in the fundamentals of convergence psychiatry is the breath of the included fields. One framework is to consider convergence psychiatry as a continuum. On one end of the spectrum are forward-facing, point-of-care tools designed to supplement or aid clinical practice. Examples of this include the EHRs, patient portals, apps, and websites. Psychiatrists will increasingly have a role in creating, evaluating, adapting, and adopting these tools in clinical practice. Psychiatrists do not need to know how to design their own EHR or develop a smartphone app. However, psychiatrists will need to understand the fundamentals of these technologies and their appropriate clinical use.

At the other end of the spectrum of convergence psychiatry is data science: the study of scientific methods, processes, algorithms, and systems to extract knowledge from structured and unstructured data.[34] The surge of point-of-care clinical tools has brought an even larger surge of complex data. By 2025, there will be an expected 175 zettabytes of information—that is, enough data that, if stored on BluRay discs and stacked, there would be enough discs to get to the moon 23 times. Psychiatrists still learn the quantitative methods of the early 1900s, such as the t-test (1908), P-value

(1925), and correlation coefficient (1880s). They are not expected to be experts in the development of data mining tools or implementation of machine learning algorithms; however, the psychiatrist of 2040 will need to understand how complex data can be leveraged to diagnose mental illness and evaluate treatments.

In the following sections, we move through the continuum of convergence psychiatry, describing the new skills and knowledge that the psychiatrist of 2040 will require to be an informed clinician. First, we discuss clinical informatics at point of care and then understanding and leveraging data.

The Psychiatrist as an Informatician

In 2020, EHRs are ubiquitous in medical practice. By 2040, we expect even reticent adopters of EHRs to be using electronic systems to document medical information, prescribe, and communicate with other clinicians. Medical and surgical specialties have recognized clinical informatics as a key area of growth and competency among trainees. Perhaps driven by research on the propensity of the EHR to compromise physician–patient relationships and therapeutic rapport,[35] psychiatry has been relatively slow to the game. Psychiatry trainees have limited exposure to clinical informatics and implementation, and many only hear their supervisors' complaints that the EHR interferes with the physician–patient dynamic. But psychiatrists' dissatisfaction with EHRs is recursive—physicians who are involved in designing and customizing the EHR to meet their needs are more likely to be satisfied users.[36]

Already, we are beginning to train experts in mental health informatics. Clinical informatics is now recognized by the American Board of Medical Specialties: fourth-year psychiatry residents and board-certified psychiatrists are eligible to apply for the two-year fellowship. Other countries are yet to implement formal pathways for clinician-informaticians.

In 2020 Australia, for example, has certification courses but no formal physician qualification. As mental health hospitals are anticipated to ubiquitously use EHRs, providers must either outsource leadership roles in health information technology (e.g., chief medical informatics officer) or take on the roles themselves. Leaders in mental health informatics must understand how computers and information systems impact care delivery, clinical decision-making, management of teams, and professionalism.[37] Psychiatry could take a passive stance, reacting to technology only when it is imposed on our practice. However, we argue that by 2040, the profession must establish a clear vision for the use of health information technology in psychiatric practice; share that vision with allied mental health professionals; provide information, knowledge, and methods; and coordinate the conflicting interests of key stakeholders.

Co-existing content (psychiatry) and process (informatics) expertise, enables adaptation of EHR systems for mental health. Across medical and surgical specialties, most specialists are dissatisfied with EHRs compared with primary care,[36] as specialty-specific care requires thoughtful modification of documentation, decision support, and workflows. A psychiatrist who understands informatics can effect positive change in EHRs that advance the practice of mental healthcare. Examples include implementation of a clinical decision support system to flag patients at high cardiometabolic risk or enhanced workflow efficiency in psychiatric emergency department evaluations. In the next two decades, we anticipate EHRs will become more complex, more integrated with diverse sources of patient-generated data, and more intelligent (i.e., with increased capacity for predictive analytics). Without clinical experts guiding this process, EHRs will likely become increasingly onerous and not useful to the busy clinician.

While a subset of psychiatrists will become leaders in the field, the greater workforce will be expected to have a foundational understanding of informatics. Torous[33] proposed core areas of clinical informatics training: patient care (e.g., use of EHRs, electronic diagnostics, digital literacy, patient-generated data), communication (e.g., barriers to technology, telepresence, communication platforms), education (e.g. evaluating information on the web, population health, data science, equipment), and practice management (e.g., digital professionalism, documentation, privacy, confidentiality). We urge medical educators to teach these core skills with intention through formal curricula or designated clinical experience rather than relying on passive absorption. This will ensure future psychiatrists enter the workforce as thoughtful consumers of information technology.

The Psychiatrist as a Data Scientist

The last decade has brought big data in healthcare to the forefront of research and clinical practice. Beyond electronic health and claims records, abundant complex data are now extracted from genomic sequencing, neuroimaging, wearables and patient-generated sources, pharmaceutical research, and medical devices. The psychiatrist of 2040 will need skills and knowledge to incorporate the extraordinarily high-volume, high-velocity, and expansive output from the healthcare industry's digital universe into clinical practice. Big healthcare data has tremendous promise, but also many challenges, including privacy of health information, data security, infrastructure expense, and diversity of format, type, and quality. Two trends will foreseeably increase the importance of big data in mental healthcare. The first is a move from a pay-for-service model to value-based care model. In the latter, physicians are rewarded based on the health of their patient populations, wherein health is operationalized by markers evident in healthcare data, such as psychiatric hospitalizations and re-admissions. The second trend involves using predictive analytics to identify at-risk populations, such as individuals at high risk of suicide, and assess the efficacy of interventions specific to those populations. In this context, the field of psychiatry must train leaders who understand data science while instilling foundational competencies in all mental health trainees.

Despite widespread popular interest in data mining, machine learning, deep learning and other forms of data science within psychiatry, most contemporary psychiatrists could not even define these terms. Without clear definitions, an appreciation of the limitations of these methods also lags, and science quickly becomes hype. In simple terms, data science is the study of data, that is, developing methods of capturing, maintaining, and processing data to extract useful information. Data scientists need to have a strong quantitative background, programming knowledge focusing on data warehousing, mining, and modeling, as well as content expertise. To realize the potential of large-scale data to advance mental healthcare, the field of psychiatry needs an increasing number of physician-scientists versed in data science, with the clinical wherewithal to ask the right questions and with the statistics, mathematics, and programming skills to look for answers in the data. A busy clinician cannot be expected become a statistician but should know how to interpret a P-value. Similarly, we do not expect clinicians to learn the nuances of support vector machines or Hadoop cluster architecture. However, in the next two decades, we anticipate that data will transform mental healthcare so quickly and profoundly that all psychiatrists will need to be able to understand the essential aspects and limitations of data science.

A long-standing adage in research circles has been "garbage in, garbage out," highlighting the fact that feeding flawed data into an algorithm will result in flawed conclusions. Although problematic even in traditional studies, the problem is magnified when developing predictive models from big data in healthcare. Whether from payer records, smart phones, public records, or wearable devices, most large-scale healthcare data was initially recorded for a different purpose. A realistic view of the quality and reliability of the data is key. For example, EHR data collected in the routine course of clinical care are prone to missingness, inaccuracies, and biases.[38] Some researchers have described EHR data, in the statistical taxonomy of missingness, as "nearly completely missing."[39] When a text mining algorithm is used to extract medical terminology from EHR documentation with the purpose of identifying a cohort of interest (e.g., psychotic disorders), the researcher must use clinical judgment in selecting which terms are important to defining the cohort (e.g., hallucinations). The psychiatrist of 2040 must be savvy in evaluating research conclusions from big data. Moreover, clinical research in psychiatry should incorporate rigorous standards for evaluating data quality. An awareness of the internal and external validity of the data will be as important as the methodological details of a novel drug trial are today. Standards of quality research must be upheld, including predefined inclusion and exclusion criteria, time frames for each variable, defined episodes of care, and consistent, generalizable definitions.

Attempts to derive predictive models for rare outcomes in psychiatry have made clear that the clinical judgment of an experienced psychiatrist supported by measurement-based practices is not replaceable by a machine.[26] Here, the promising new field of data science needs the human expert: the most accurate algorithm is ill-informed if the predictors or outcome variables are not reflected in clinical practice. Psychiatrists can play a key role in guiding feature selection, that is, selecting a subset of relevant features (variables or predictors) for use in model construction. While feature selection is performed by the machine learning or statistical algorithm, many aspects of defining variables are left to the discretion of the researcher. For example, a model including medical comorbidity as a predictor may include all individual International Classification of Disease (ICD) codes, parse ICD codes into categories (e.g., presence or absence of a cardiac disorder) or a use a global comorbidity score (e.g., the van

Walraven score[40]). Combining clinical experience, knowledge of the medical literature, and an understanding of machine learning, clinicians would be well-placed to evaluate the degree to which features capture clinically salient phenomena.

Software Advocacy

Given the importance of informatics tools and large-scale healthcare data in the future of convergent psychiatry, the psychiatrist of 2040 has a role in advocating for quality, transparency, accessibility, and interoperability of software used to develop these tools and process data. We are in an age where "big tech" is increasingly scrutinized for infringement on privacy, ill-defined ethical standards, partiality, and bias, while also wielding some of the most powerful tools to harness healthcare data for advancing medical care. Free-to-use software libraries are often controlled by corporations (e.g., TensorFlow, a popular deep learning library, is free-to-use, partially open source, and controlled by Google), and completely open source software is frequently unregulated. In this environment, point-of-care tools, code, and data are often not shared between institutions due to concerns over privacy, security, and economic value. Clinicians have an important role as advocates for the judicious use of software in medical care. Clinicians can witness the benefits of information access to advance mental healthcare as well as the potentially devastating human costs of such data being used for personal or financial gain.

Access and Equity

Given this complex mix of opportunity and risks, clinicians have a further responsibility to advocate for policies that enable equitable access to this convergence future. This includes policies that affect access to patient-facing tools, such as broadband equity, as well as solve clinician barriers like appropriate renumeration for the use of emerging technologies commensurate with their benefits and cost.

Although clinicians and organizations such as the American Medical Association and the Royal Australia and New Zealand College of Psychiatrists have long played advocacy roles on issues pertinent to health, these new technology equity issues demand engagement with a broader range of stakeholders. Policy-setting on broadband access in the United States, for example, falls to the Federal Communications Commission, which clinician organizations would not know to lobby for health outcomes. Despite this, given the multiple social disadvantages faced by the psychologically unwell, such novel lobbying is exactly what is needed. In Australia, despite having the 10th highest GDP per capita globally, one study of schizophrenia suffers published in 2020 revealed only 58% owned a smartphone and 30% had never accessed the internet from any device.[41] A large segment of those in need therefore may miss out on the fruits of the convergence future. Indeed, even with access, certain subpopulations may be particularly susceptible to the risks of our increasingly networked world. The aged, for example, have been shown both to have lower rates of technology adoption but also to be substantially less vigilant of risks around privacy and fake news.[42]

Moreover, some patients may wish to abstain from data sharing or e-tools due to concerns about privacy and data security, cultural values, or personal preference. Psychotic symptoms, particularly paranoia, may also affect willingness to use these tools. We therefore suggest convergent clinicians be mindful of three goals regarding access (i) to ensure that all patients can access the digital tools optimal care demands, (ii) to encourage structures that renumerate and monitor clinical uses of these tools, and (iii) to advocate for tools that are modular enough to suit individual variations in digital engagement.

Conclusion

We live in an age of convergence, where traditionally disparate disciplines are coming together to meet modern challenges. Like the neuroscientific, cognitive and quantitative revolutions of the past, convergence science has begun and will continue to transform psychiatry. Convergent opportunities are likely to change provider workflows by streamlining clinical tasks. Social media screening, chatbots, natural-language processing and living literature reviews will increasingly impact psychiatric practice. Technology will reshape and bring new challenges to enduring skills, including the development of therapeutic relationships, supported decision-making, and de-escalation.

A foundational understanding of the convergence spectrum, ranging from point-of-care informatics tools to large-scale healthcare data, will help psychiatrists develop a wireframe to consider the role of new technologies and research findings. Suitably empowered, practicing clinicians and mental healthcare teams are well placed to maximize the societal benefits of emerging health technologies. At minimum, psychiatrists must effectively use and, when necessary adapt, point-of-care tools such as EHRs, communication technologies and clinical resources like apps and websites. On the data-science side, psychiatrists must understand broadly the opportunities and limits of these investigative methods. Predictive modelling is only as good as the data the model is built on and the human choices made regarding collection and use. Probabilistic outputs require informed clinicians to convey information on risks and benefits accurately to patients. Clinicians must also be aware of new digital divides, identifying and advocating for populations potentially marginalized by new health technologies.

This new era demands convergent psychiatrists, who can maintain humanism, clinical judgment, and rapport, while being flexible to learning new skills and modes of practice. We do not expect psychiatrists to master every contributing discipline, but to be savvy consumers and collaborators in the fields that increasingly intersect with clinical practice. With these reflections in mind, we anticipate that psychiatrists can and must take an active role in leading our bright convergent future.

References

1. Hedegaard H, Warner M, Curtin SC. Increase in suicide in the United States, 1999–2014. *NCHS Data Brief*. 2016;241:1–8.
2. Wahlbeck K, Westman J, Nordentoft M, Gissler M, Laursen TM. Outcomes of Nordic mental health systems: life expectancy of patients with mental disorders. *Br J Psychiatry*. 2011;199(6):453–458. doi:10.1192/bjp.bp.110.085100
3. Rehm J, Shield KD. Global burden of disease and the impact of mental and addictive disorders. *Curr Psychiatry Rep*. 2019;21(2):10. doi:10.1007/s11920-019-0997-0
4. Morris ZS, Wooding S, Grant J. The answer is 17 years, what is the question: understanding time lags in translational research. *J R Soc Med*. 2011;104(12):510–520. doi:10.1258/jrsm.2011.110180
5. Joukes E, Cornet R, De Keizer N, De Bruijne M. Collect once, use many times: end-users don't practice what they preach. *Stud Health Technol Inform*. 2017;228:252–256. doi:10.3233/978-1-61499-678-1-252
6. Jeffrey J, Hajal NJ, Klomhaus A, Marlotte L. The use of behavioral health rating scales for primary care providers why use behavioral health rating scales? 2019;15:884–892.
7. Siegler EL, Adelman R. Copy and paste: a remediable hazard of electronic health records. *Am J Med*. 2009;122(6):495–496. doi:10.1016/j.amjmed.2009.02.010
8. Lucas GM, Gratch J, King A, Morency LP. It's only a computer: virtual humans increase willingness to disclose. *Comput Human Behav*. 2014;37:94–100. doi:10.1016/j.chb.2014.04.043
9. Rizzo AA, Lucas GM, Gratch J, et al. Automatic behavior analysis during a clinical interview with a virtual human. In: Westwood J, ed. *Medicine Meets Virtual Reality* (Vol. 220). Amsterdam: IOS Press; 2016:316–322. doi:10.3233/9781614996255316
10. Kahneman D, Riis J. Living, and thinking about it: two perspectives on life. *Sci Well-Being*. 2005;37:285–304 doi:10.1016/j.chb.2014.04.043
11. Klein JG. Five pitfalls in decisions about diagnosis and prescribing. *Br Med J*. 2005;330(7494):781–783. doi:10.1136/bmj.330.7494.781
12. Berrouiguet S, Perez-Rodriguez MM, Larsen M, Baca-García E, Courtet P, Oquendo M. From eHealth to iHealth: transition to participatory and personalized medicine in mental health. *J Med Internet Res*. 2018;20(1):e2. doi:10.2196/jmir.7412
13. Kessels RP. Patients' memory for medical information. *JRSM*. 2003;96(5):219–222. doi:10.1258/jrsm.96.10.520
14. Barr PJ, Hassanpour S, Haslett W, et al. The development of a personal audio health library (Audio PaHL)—preliminary usability testing & annotation guide development. In: *AMIA Summit 2019*; 2019:6–7.
15. Institute for Public Policy Research. Better health and care for all: a 10-point plan for the 2020s: the Lord Darzi review of health and care (final report). Published 2018. https://www.ippr.org/research/publications/better-health-and-care-for-all
16. Andreyeva E, David G, Song H. The effects of home health visit length on hospital readmission. *NBER Work Pap Ser*. 2018:35. http://www.nber.org/papers/w24566
17. Starace F, Mungai F, Barbui C. Does mental health staffing level affect antipsychotic prescribing? Analysis of Italian national statistics. *PLoS One*. 2018;13(2):1–8. doi:10.1371/journal.pone.0193216
18. Zhang W, Deng Z, Hong Z, Evans R, Ma J, Zhang H. Unhappy patients are not alike: content analysis of the negative comments from China's Good Doctor website. *J Med Internet Res*. 2018;20(1):e35. doi:10.2196/jmir.8223
19. Horvath AO, Del Re AC, Flückiger C, Symonds D. Alliance in individual psychotherapy. *Psychotherapy*. 2011;48(1):9–16. doi:10.1037/a0022186

20. Pearce C, Trumble S, Arnold M, Dwan K, Phillips C. Computers in the new consultation: within the first minute. *Fam Pract.* 2008;25(3):202–208. doi:10.1093/fampra/cmn018

21. Ebisch SJ, Aureli T, Bafunno D, Cardone D, Romani GL, Merla A. Mother and child in synchrony: thermal facial imprints of autonomic contagion. *Biol Psychol.* 2012;89(1):123–129. doi:10.1016/j.biopsycho.2011.09.018

22. Bennett SD, Cuijpers P, Ebert DD, et al. Practitioner review: unguided and guided self-help interventions for common mental health disorders in children and adolescents: a systematic review and meta-analysis. *J Child Psychol Psychiatry Allied Discip.* 2019;60(8):828–847. doi:10.1111/jcpp.13010

23. Kardas P, Lewek P, Matyjaszczyk M. Determinants of patient adherence: a review of systematic reviews. *Front Pharmacol.* 2013;4:1–16. doi:10.3389/fphar.2013.00091

24. Hopwood M. The shared decision-making process in the pharmacological management of depression. *Patient-Patient-Centered Outcomes Res.* 2019;13(1):23–30. doi:10.1007/s40271-019-00383-w

25. Adams ZW, McClure EA, Gray KM, Danielson CK, Treiber FA, Ruggiero KJ. Mobile devices for the remote acquisition of physiological and behavioral biomarkers in psychiatric clinical research. *J Psychiatr Res.* 2017;85:1–14. doi:10.1016/j.jpsychires.2016.10.019

26. Belsher BE, Smolenski DJ, Pruitt LD, et al. Prediction models for suicide attempts and deaths: a systematic review and simulation. *JAMA Psychiatry.* 2019;76(6):642–651. doi:10.1001/jamapsychiatry.2019.0174

27. Waitzkin H, Getrich C, Heying S, et al. Promotoras as mental health practitioners in primary care: a multi-method study of an intervention to address contextual sources of depression. *J Community Health.* 2011;36(2):316–331. doi:10.1007/s10900-010-9313-y

28. Scull A. Contested jurisdictions: psychiatry, psychoanalysis, and clinical psychology in the United States, 1940–2010. *Med Hist.* 2011;55(3):401–406. doi:10.1017/S0025727300005470

29. Ortiz-Ospina E. The rise of social media: our world in data. Published September 18, 2019. https://ourworldindata.org/rise-of-social-media

30. Silver L. Smartphone ownership is growing rapidly around the world, but not always equally. *Pew Research Center: Global Attitudes and Trends.* Published February 5, 2019. https://www.pewresearch.org/global/2019/02/05/smartphone-ownership-is-growing-rapidly-around-the-world-but-not-always-equally/

31. Cohrs RJ, Martin T, Ghahramani P, Bidaut L, Higgins PJ, Shahzad A. Translational medicine definition by the European society for translational medicine. *New Horizons Transl Med.* 2015;2:86–88. doi:10.1016/j.nhtm.2014.12.002

32. Eyre HA, Lavretsky H, Forbes M, et al. Convergence science arrives: how does it relate to psychiatry? *Acad Psychiatry.* 2017;41(1):91–99. doi:10.1007/s40596-016-0496-0

33. Torous J, Chan S, Luo J, Boland R, Hilty D. Clinical informatics in psychiatric training: preparing today's trainees for the already present future. *Acad Psychiatry.* 2018;42(5):694–697. doi:10.1007/s40596-017-0811-4

34. Hayashi C. What is data science ? Fundamental concepts and a heuristic example. In: *Data Science, Classification, and Related Methods: Proceedings of the Fifth Conference of the International Federation of Classification Societies (IFCS-96), Kobe, Japan, March 27–30 1996.* Tokyo: Springer Japan; 1998. doi:10.1007/978-4-431-65950-1_3

35. Kazmi Z. Effects of exam room EHR use on doctor-patient communication: a systematic literature review. *Inform Prim Care.* 2013;21(1):30–39. doi:10.14236/jhi.v21i1.37

36. Redd TK, Doberne JW, Lattin D, et al. Variability in electronic health record usage and perceptions among specialty vs. primary care physicians. *AMIA Annu Symp Proc.* 2015;2015:2053–2062.

37. Finnell J, Dixon B, eds. *Clinical informatics study guide.* Cham, Switzerland: Springer International; 2016. doi:10.1007/978-3-319-22753-5

38. Pathak J, Kho AN, Denny JC. Electronic health records-driven phenotyping: challenges, recent advances, and perspectives. *J Am Med Inform Assoc*. 2013;20(e2):e206–e211. doi:10.1136/amiajnl-2013-002428

39. Hripcsak G, Albers DJ. Next-generation phenotyping of electronic health records. *J Am Med Informatics Assoc*. 2013;20(1):117–1121. doi:10.1136/amiajnl-2012-001145

40. Van Walraven C, Austin PC, Jennings A, Quan H, Forster AJ. A modification of the Elixhauser comorbidity measures into a point system for hospital death using administrative data. *Med Care*. 2009;47(6):626–633. doi:10.1097/MLR.0b013e31819432e5

41. Wong KTG, Liu D, Balzan R, King D, Galletly C. Smartphone and Internet access and utilization by people with schizophrenia in South Australia: quantitative survey study. *JMIR Ment Heal*. 2020;7(1):e11551. doi:10.2196/11551

42. Guess A, Nagler J, Tucker J. Less than you think: prevalence and predictors of fake news dissemination on Facebook. *Sci Adv*. 2019;5(1):eaau4586. doi:10.1126/sciadv.aau4586

9

Update on the War on Mental Illness

Perspectives on Translational Psychiatry

Seth W. Perry, Ma-Li Wong, and Julio Licinio

Copyright Notice and Acknowledgment

Introduction

On December 23, 1971, then US President Richard Nixon signed the National Cancer Act of 1971, a US federal law. The act, as originally stated, was intended "[t]o amend the Public Health Service Act so as to strengthen the National Cancer Institute of Health in order more effectively to carry out the national effort against cancer."[2] This has been widely perceived as the official launch of the colloquially termed "War on Cancer." Looking back, we were arguably technologically unprepared to launch such a war then. At that time, medical research was severely limited by insufficient technology—there was no magnetic resonance imaging, no positron emission tomography, very rudimentary molecular biology, no genetically modified animals, no automated DNA or human genome sequencing, no personal computers, no databases, and far more rudimentary (mostly paper!) means of archiving and accessing scientific and medical literature. Scientific manuscripts were handwritten and then typed with typewriters, and revisions had to be retyped in their entirety. All our current "omics" platforms, such as genomics, proteomics, metabolomics, and lipidomics, were futuristic fantasies. And yet, the enormity of task, the audacity of the goal, and the technical limitations of the era did not prevent the launch of that ambitious and immensely successful effort. While some cancers, such as pancreatic carcinoma and glioblastoma multiforme, are presently understood to be invariably fatal, others have been, for the vast majority of patients, either cured or transformed from a near-term death sentence into a more manageable, longer-term chronic illnesses.

In like fashion, we proposed in 2013 and renew our call here, that now is the time for a "War on Mental Illness" to be launched with renewed vigor, as both intranational and international efforts. The goal of these synergistic efforts will be improved translation of science into mental health care and improved delivery of mental health care, resulting in more rapid, accessible, and efficacious treatments than are available today.

The Need for the "War On Mental Illness"

Mental health disorders represent a substantial burden to the world. They are, by many or most metrics, the leading cause of disease burden in the US,[3] and in the world.[4,5] Major depressive disorder (MDD) is but one excellent case example, as on average it is the second-leading cause of disability in developed countries, undeveloped countries, and in the US (as measured by years lived with disability).[6] (Back pain ranks first in all the aforementioned regional categories.) In many countries, MDD is the leading cause of disability.[6] Between 1999 and 2013, major depression moved from the third to the second leading cause of global disability by years lived with disability,[6] underscoring the pressing need for a comprehensive and united effort to combat mental health disorders worldwide. In the US, depression represents the largest nonfatal disease burden.[7] Depression is also the leading risk factor for suicide: approximately 60% of suicides occur among those with mood disorders.[8,9] In the US in 2017, suicide was the second leading cause of death for ages 10 to 34, the fourth leading cause for ages 35 to 54, and the eighth leading cause of death for ages 55 to 64.[8,10]

Notably, depression may also precipitate or is frequently comorbid with numerous other physical and mental health conditions in both children and adults, leading to reinforcing vicious-cycles between MDD and the comorbid disease(s). Approximately 17% and 18% of individuals with lifetime MDD had an alcohol or drug use disorder, respectively.[11] These numbers were even higher for bipolar disorder: 56% of those with bipolar disorder had a lifetime substance use disorder.[11] In many cases, depression may be the first to occur, thereby leading to alcoholism, and/or alcoholism may precipitate or worsen depression. The presence of either major depression or alcohol use disorder doubles the risk of the other[12] (and see related discussion[13,14]). Research shows that children with depression are more prone to develop alcohol problems once they reach adolescence. Teenagers who have had an episode of major depression are twice as likely as those who are not depressed to start drinking alcohol. Alcohol abuse in adolescence and adulthood is a cause of physical illness as well as traffic accidents. Finally, those who have ever experienced mental illness consume roughly 69% of all alcohol, 84% of all cocaine, and 68% of all cigarettes.[15] Those are staggering figures demonstrating the devastating interrelationships between substance abuse and mental illness.

Furthermore, depression also intertwines closely with and likely contributes to obesity, cardiovascular disease, diabetes, and related conditions, likely leading to mutual reinforcement and exacerbation of these comorbid diseases.[16,17] Depressed patients gain weight during the course of the disorder[18] and also as a result of antidepressant treatment.[19] Having depression makes treatment of obesity particularly challenging, as the symptoms of depression preclude adherence to diet and exercise guidelines and are a major obstacle to healthy lifestyles. Depression by itself also significantly increases the risk of type 2 diabetes and cardiovascular disease.[16,17,20,21] Recent studies have documented that by shortening telomeres, depression has a negative effect on the aging process.[22,23] If one adds to the burden of depression also those of bipolar disorder, schizophrenia, autism, eating disorders, and many other psychiatric disorders, it is easy to see that the cumulative impact of these disorders in the world is truly staggering.

The Time Is Right for the "War on Mental Illness"

One could make the case that psychiatric disorders are more complex to study than cancer and many other diseases, which are perhaps more readily and faithfully reproduced in cell and animal models. While that may be right, it is also true that the infinitely better tools that we have today, compared with what was available for the "War on Cancer" in 1971, give us a stunning advantage that our oncology colleagues of the early 1970s did not have. In some ways, the higher complexity and inaccessibility of psychiatric disorders should arguably be more than offset by the astoundingly superior tools available to us, now in 2020. Therefore, at present, we are far better positioned to launch a "War on Mental Illness" than were our oncology colleagues when they first launched their exceptionally successful "War on Cancer" in 1971.

Moreover, the US in particular,[24-26] as well as some other countries around the world,[27] are experiencing an unprecedented decline in life expectancies among some populations, due in large part to mental-health related ailments such as suicide, drug overdoses and addiction, and even obesity and comorbid diseases, as well as the socioeconomic and related disparities and health inequities that often drive these conditions[8,16,17,25,28-35]—all of which can and should be targeted in this "War on Mental Illness." Gun violence is also another significant contributor, especially for suicide, and we have covered this topic in detail elsewhere.[8]

Early, preventive interventions are critical to combat these trends and must be tightly integrated into this "war," since there is now considerable and robust evidence that early prophylactic interventions are key to ameliorating, delaying, and/or preventing the often crippling downstream sequelae of mental illness, including dementia, amplification of disability secondary to co-occurring medical disorders, erosion of health related quality of life, and foreshortening of life expectancy. Thus, there is now abundant evidence underscoring the importance of early intervention for the sake of brain and mental health, cognitive fitness, and prevention or amelioration of psychiatric disease.

For these reasons, in our view a "War on Mental Illness" is unquestionably necessary, timely, and technically feasible. That being the case, how can we best maintain and accelerate previous and ongoing progress, and most effectively launch bold new initiatives, in this endeavor? In our opinion, this "war" needs to be fought along all fronts of translational medicine. Therefore, it is worthwhile to define those.

The Six Steps of Translational Science

The process of translation in all areas of medicine, including psychiatry, can be conceptualized as occurring along six steps, from T0 to T5, as follows.

T0: Discovery

Because T1 has already been used by many as a level of translation, we suggest a preceding step T0 (T zero). This refers to the fundamental process of discovery, which is sometimes omitted or forgotten in discussions on translational science. Translation cannot be a pipeline only, or a bridge from nowhere. Many fundamental discoveries that will prove instrumental to curing diseases have not yet occurred. Therefore, if we bring (translate) to the clinic only pre-existing discoveries, many diseases will remain unconquered. Much fundamental discovery work still needs to be done so that effective translation can occur. Hypothetically, one could have the best translation pipeline, but without translatable new fundamental science, such a pipeline becomes meaningless. This step is also critical if we are to distinguish translational science from purely applied research. For these reasons, we suggest this step "T0: Discovery" as critical and integral to the translational process.

T1: First in Humans or Proof of Principle

This refers to the now "classical" step of bench-to-bedside, first-in-human studies.

T2: Clinical Trials

The step of translation from bedside to clinical care: clinical trial studies, for example, are in this domain.

T3: Healthcare Policy and Guidelines

This term has been emerging but needs further definition. We believe this step is best defined as translation of new evidence into healthcare guidelines and health policy.

T4: Long-Term Effectiveness and Safety

We define this step as research on the outcomes assessment of translation. Once translation occurs from T0 to T3, from novel fundamental discovery to health policy, the outcomes of such changes in practice need to be meticulously and critically evaluated, as not all new guidelines and policies will be shown to be effective over time. Careful research is needed to determine what is successful in the long run, and what is not, to guide the health care of the future.

T5: Global Health

This consists of global (worldwide) implementation of new guidelines that emerge, as the translational outcomes of T4-level research are further validated for effectiveness and utility on global-scale health.

Within this framework, there are robust opportunities to transition from more traditional multi- and interdisciplinary approaches, to the transdisciplinary approaches of convergence science, notably in but not limited to the National Institute of Mental Health's (NIMH) Research Domain Criteria initiative, which aims to provide a framework for better understanding and treating mental health disorders (T0–T2), and convergent global public mental health efforts to combat mental illness worldwide (T3–T5).[36]

The Three Gaps in the Pathway of Translation

Within these steps T0 to T5 along the pathway of translation, we have identified four major gaps—at the levels of fundamental knowledge, evidence-based validation, practitioner application, and patient adherence—which we refer to as G1, G2a, G2b, G3, and define next (also see Figure 9.1). Two of these four gaps—gaps G2a and G2b—are subcomponents or different elements of the broader "practice" gap concept, which gives us four substantially different gaps within a broader three-gap structure (Figure 9.1).

Translation: A process with four major gaps

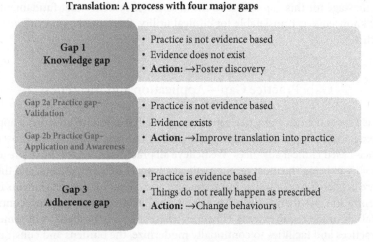

Gap 1 Knowledge gap	• Practice is not evidence based • Evidence does not exist • **Action:** →Foster discovery
Gap 2a Practice gap– Validation Gap 2b Practice Gap– Application and Awareness	• Practice is not evidence based • Evidence exists • **Action:** →Improve translation into practice
Gap 3 Adherence gap	• Practice is evidence based • Things do not really happen as prescribed • **Action:** →Change behaviours

Figure 9.1. Translation: A process with four major gaps. Four major gaps are identified along the pathway of translation, at the levels of fundamental knowledge, evidence-based validation, practitioner application, and patient adherence.

G1: Knowledge Gap

This gap is caused by the lack of discovery, and thus the absence of usable knowledge or data that can ultimately be "translated" into clinical practice. It is remedied by translational step T0. The take-home message for this gap is that in the absence of fundamental scientific knowledge, there can be no translation of knowledge into clinical practice.

G2a: Practice Gap—Validation

Often, existing knowledge is simply not adequately translated into everyday clinical practice. This is also known as translation into practice, or implementation. In many cases, knowledge already exists that may very well be relevant to clinical practice and useful for treating disease, but through nobody's fault, there is simply insufficient awareness, capacity, budget, funding, and/or prioritization among many competing projects and obligations, to further investigate and validate existing knowledge for clinical application. This gap is remedied primarily by translational steps T1 and T2, and to some extent also by steps T3 to T5. The immense challenge of overcoming this gap is illustrated by the fact that it typically takes ~17 years for research evidence to reach clinical practice[37]—if it ever reaches clinical practice at all (i.e. is not forever "lost" in this gap). Overcoming this gap requires multiple "eyes" on the pipeline at all times, to identify new (or old) discoveries that might have clinical utility and efficacy: from researchers, to clinicians, funding bodies/sponsors, and large and small biotechnology and pharmaceutical companies, to name just a few. The take-home message for this gap is that in the absence of evidence that fundamental scientific knowledge is translatable for clinical utility, there can be no evidence-based medicine.

G2b: Practice Gap—Application and Awareness

There is a second kind of practice gap that may result from practitioners not applying, not being able to apply, or perhaps occasionally not being aware of, the most recent evidence-based clinical advances. We believe all practitioners have the desire and innate ability to bring the most recent medical advances to their patients, and these efforts are bolstered by continual infrastructure and technology improvements in (i.e., modernization of) many clinical practices and facilities, and ongoing continuing medical education requirements. However, whether due to the inability of some medical practices and facilities to continually modernize, the burdens and constraints of modern medical practice, and/or the practical limits we all face as humans with multiple competing lives and obligations, many practitioners may simply lack the facilities, infrastructure, resources, capacity, and/or time to be able to do so. Thus while filling this gap is challenging and may require close scrutiny and remedy of some fundamental flaws within the modern medical system and the many burdens placed on practitioners, success will be facilitated by all practitioners' desire to bring the very best care to their patients.

G3: Adherence Gap

It is common that both clinician and patient may appear to agree on a therapeutic course of action, which is then, sooner or later, not followed in the patient's daily life once they leave the provider's office. As an example, a large European study showed that 56% of patients prescribed an antidepressant stopped taking them on their own within four months.[38] This example is particularly concerning given the growing evidence for withdrawal and rebound effects if antidepressants are abruptly discontinued, an area that has only relatively recently gained significant clinical appreciation.[39-48] The critical issue at this level is the modification of patients' (human) behaviors, which is tremendously challenging.

The Necessary Elements for the "War on Mental Illness"

Keeping in mind these six steps and four gaps in the translational process, how can we then proceed to successfully launch a "War on Mental Health?" Our vision for that is summarized in Figure 9.2 and Box 9.1, and described in more detail next.

Investigator-Initiated Research

First, we believe that there is and remains a key role for existing investigator-initiated efforts, which, over many decades if not centuries and often within university or other public sector institutions worldwide, have arguably originated the bulk of translatable knowledge leading to presently available disease therapies. These days, such

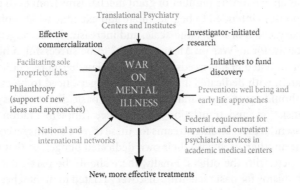

Figure 9.2. A strategy summary for the "War on Mental Illness."

Box 9.1 Components of the "War on Mental Illness"

- Increases in existing investigator-initiated single grants (R01s in the United States, project grants in Australia)
- Increases in center grants (Conte Centers in United States, program grants in Australia)
  - Call for applications with dedicated funding for
  - Basic discovery
  - Psychiatric neuroscience translation
  - Translation into practice(implementation)
- Well-structured and well-funded national consortia
- Well-structured and well-funded international consortia
- Creation or expansion of dedicated translational psychiatry centers and institutes
- Federal requirement for inpatient and outpatient psychiatric services in academic medical centers
- Global treatment efforts: an issue of human dignity
- Promotion of well-being, including positive psychology and resilience building, as well as adoption of health lifestyles
- Philanthropy: support of new hypotheses and approaches
- Infrastructure and seed funding for sole proprietor labs
- Effective commercialization
  - Facilitation and support of start-up/incubators
  - Efficient tech transfer
  - Ethical and appropriate interface with big pharma

---

investigator-initiated research efforts may take the form of single projects (such as the mainstay R01 grants in the US or project grants in many other countries) or increasingly clusters of projects (such as center or program grants in the US and other countries) to promote evermore important collaborative and interdisciplinary science, as well as an expanding number of grant mechanisms from both governmental and private sponsors intended to help facilitate and expedite what is often inter- and transdisciplinary, collaborative, large-scale, and increasingly convergent pipeline research. Obviously, for a "War on Mental Health" to be successful, a higher number of investigator-initiated grants needs to be funded. Furthermore, additional targeted calls for research, with dedicated and sufficient budgets, need to be established. We suggest they should cover, in separate mechanisms, basic discovery, psychiatric neuroscience translation, and translation into practice (implementation). We further suggest it is essential that funding streams for these three domains be completely separate from one another, each with their own dedicated budget, so that one approach does not compete with the others. Finally, there should be particular emphasis on funding mechanisms for basic scientific discovery related to mental health disorders, as fundamental knowledge of the biology underlying many psychiatric diseases remains lacking.

Yet despite the unprecedented successes of this system in producing therapies and even cures for some diseases, in this modern era of stagnating or reduced federal (and thus institutional) budgets for funding basic and translational biomedical research, this traditional system of medical research is beginning to show fissures and stress fractures on many levels, and progress in translational medicine and mental health is suffering as a result. New convergence medicine approaches are needed to help repair or reinvent some of the structural inadequacies and inefficiencies within the current system.

Without getting too far into the weeds of the accounting and logistical details, suffice to say that in many traditional (i.e., university) medical research settings, researchers may be expected or even required, or at the very least strongly encouraged, to maintain 100% self-funded research programs, which are frequently although not exclusively largely unidisciplinary. This long-standing model may soon prove unsustainable for researchers, their funding sponsors, and institutions. That is, researchers are often expected to support (sometimes up to 100% of) their own salaries (plus benefits costs, which may approach 70% or more of the salaries themselves, in some cases); plus the salaries and benefits costs for all personnel in their laboratory; plus all "actual" research costs (i.e., all the supplies and reagents, animals and animal facility costs, core facility fees, and often expensive equipment purchases too, that are required to actually "perform" the research)—with all these costs charged to and paid for in their entirety from the "direct cost" budgets of whatever grant dollars the researcher is able to acquire from external funding sources. In the US, for biomedical research endeavors, this most typically means National Institutes of Health (NIH) grants. Moreover, the institutional infrastructure and facilities are arguably supported not only by researchers' acquired "direct cost" grant dollars in the ways previously described, but also inarguably by substantial supplementary "indirect cost" (aka "facilities and administrative" or "F&A") dollars that institutions receive with every grant that one of their researchers, faculty, or physician-scientists acquire. From federal sponsors, typically an additional 40 to 80 cents in "indirect costs" are awarded to the institution (the exact amount varies with each institutions' negotiated rate), for every dollar of "direct costs" awarded to the researcher's project. For these reasons, it is clear that external grant dollars are the lifeblood of modern medical research institutions, provide tremendous job creation and sustenance to the economy, and are instrumental to translating fundamental knowledge to clinical application.

Despite this seemingly generous federal (and sometimes private) support for the medical research efforts of public sector institutions and their researchers, how then are we still so far away from new or adequate treatments for mental illnesses or other diseases? Perhaps foremost, medical research and discovery simply takes an incredibly long time and vast resources. And that's before any (T0) discoveries even enter translational steps T1 to T5 for direct clinical application—steps that themselves may require equal or greater time and resources than step T0. The problems inherent with these decades-long times scales required to translate knowledge to clinical application are only compounded by continually shrinking (or at best, stagnating) federal budgets for biomedical research. Second, medical and translational research and is inherently and frustratingly unpredictable. Some of the most clinically important discoveries have been or may be entirely serendipitous—that is, not resulting directly from the planned aims and goals of a particular project. Other findings may simply not be recognized or followed-up on as clinically important, a problem that we have previously defined as gap G2a (Practice Gap—Validation). Third, this current system, as worthy as it is and as successful as it has been in many ways, seems to bring about a series of endless catch-22s to the detriment of the researchers, the institutions, and the sponsors that may not be fully sustainable for much longer. Between fully funding their research programs (and not infrequently 100% of their own and their laboratory personnel's salaries and benefits costs) from external grants, writing grants (a full-time occupation in itself, if one is to be successful at it), actually running the research program (i.e., making sure the already funded research gets done), teaching, serving on committees, administrating or performing other forms of university service required for tenure and promotion considerations, and perhaps even performing clinical duties, researchers in academia can easily find themselves working the equivalent of two to three full-time jobs (for the compensation of one job) at great personal cost and sacrifice. And despite the usually well-intentioned efforts of all participants, the current system, like any system, is far from a perfect meritocracy. The sum of these circumstances can drive even the most talented and successful investigators and individuals out of research or academic medicine entirely. The institutions, faced with continual declines in both clinical reimbursement revenues and available external research dollars, and other budgetary strains, may feel they have no choice but to insist that researchers must fully support themselves, all their laboratory personnel, and their research programs often entirely with external funding, lest the institutions be faced with yet more unfunded liabilities, the costs of which must come from somewhere (which, for most academic medical institutions typically means from either clinical revenues, or tuition dollars). Funding sponsors, faced with their own declining budgets and being well-aware, at least in their view, that between direct and indirect costs awarded, they rather than the institutions themselves have long shouldered the substantial majority of costs for university research programs, are increasingly expecting (and sometimes mandating) that institutions have more "skin in the game."

These many inefficiencies and inherent structural and logistical flaws of the current system emphasize the need for a more convergent approach to driving future progress in mental health research, some of which are beginning to evolve as we now describe.

Startups and Similar Research Arrangements (Biohackers)

Perhaps in part as a reaction to what researchers in the traditional academic system may perceive as an exploitative type of structure (as previously described)—in many cases, akin to a form of "self-employment" under the university umbrella—some researchers, also known as biohackers,[49] are becoming de facto sole proprietor businesses, engaged in non-institutional science and technology development. They may lease their own bench space and infrastructure from a university—and ironically and arguably inefficiently for the greater good of scientific progress, in many cases they may also have to pay to license back their own patents from a university, for their own work—thus operating like micro-companies. Many small startups or spin-off companies also begin this way, as well as an increasing number of previously external companies utilizing a growing number of university-linked "incubator" spaces. Often these developing "incubator" infrastructures are designed with an eye toward "open" floor plans and multi/transdisciplinary (convergent) collaboration, both literally and conceptually. There are new funding programs, such as Symbian axlr8r and the Thiel Foundation, that provide early-stage support to high-risk, high-reward independent ventures. SynBio axlr8r is a program that jump starts synthetic biology companies with funding from SOS Ventures, a venture capital firm in Kinsale, Ireland, with a goal of taking an idea through proof of concept to form a company within 90 days. The Thiel Foundation from San Francisco, California, created by Peter Thiel, cofounder of PayPal, supports fellows to "pursue innovative scientific and technical projects, learn entrepreneurship from the ground up, and begin to build the innovative companies of tomorrow."[50] Europe's budding biohacker scene includes La Paillasse in Paris that is growing rapidly and, with public funding and support from the Mayor of Paris, will soon move to a larger building in the city center.

Commercialization

Eventually, new treatment approaches need to be effectively commercialized to reach vast numbers of people and make a difference in their lives. This requires facilitation and support of start-up and incubators and efficient tech transfer, which tend to be a roadblock and source of delayed translation in academic institutions. Given recent conflict of interest scandals in psychiatry, it is also absolutely essential that the "War on Mental Health" not be tainted by such egregious misconduct. Therefore, guidelines and frameworks for interaction with big pharma companies need to be developed to ensure expediency and feasibility in the context of the highest ethical standards. Encouragingly, efforts toward improved and more transparent conflict-of-interest policies and guidelines regulating researchers' interactions with private sector sponsors and other compensated or uncompensated relationships have seen increased focus in recent years from universities, federal granting agencies, and other key stakeholders.

National and International Networks

While investigator-initiated efforts are indispensable, it is highly unlikely that a disease like schizophrenia will be conquered by advances accomplished in one single lab, funded by a single grant or even multiple grants from the same laboratory. All mental illnesses are common and complex disorders of gene–environment interactions. Those are best approached by well-structured and well-funded consortia, which have existed with great success in other areas of medicine, including cancer, heart disease, and endocrine–metabolic diseases. Such consortia should be funded in translational psychiatry both at the national level and internationally. Here we summarize the elements for a proposed International Translational Psychiatry Consortium. This type of international partnership would be structured to fully cover the six steps of translation.

T0—Discovery: to identify and integrate the most promising discovery efforts.

T1—First in humans or proof of principle: partnerships among leading clinical psychiatry research centers.

T2—Clinical trials: to create a rigorous international academic clinical trial network.

T3—Health-care policy and guidelines: Interface with relevant health agencies in various countries.

T4—Long-term effectiveness and safety: is what we are doing working well over time?

T5—Global health: international partnerships and outreach with innovative international clinical and training programs, such as a Global Masters in Translational Psychiatry.

Any opportunities for global transdisciplinary interactions and convergence mental health science should be vigorously explored and incorporated within this framework.

Global Mental Health

The issue of global mental health is very timely. The miserable, inhumane, and appalling conditions faced by the mentally ill in some low- and middle-income countries constitute one of the great human rights scandals of our era.[51] Efforts analogous to those of the Bill & Melinda Gates Foundation, which is doing so much to address infectious diseases, must be created for worldwide mental health, as vital for human dignity. Such global mental health efforts should be an important constitutive element of the "War on Mental Health."

Mental Health in Academic Medical Centers

In developed countries, the stigma of mental health manifests itself in a more insidious way. Groundbreaking advances in treatment tend to occur in academic medical centers. Because psychiatric services do not offer intensive and invasive procedures that can be billed at top dollar, profit-oriented hospital administrators, who may increasingly lack medical background particularly in some systems outside the US model, have in many cases greatly reduced or simply terminated psychiatric services in academic medical centers.[52,53] We suggest a "War on Mental Health" should include a federal requirement for academic medical centers to have inpatient and outpatient psychiatric services in a fixed formula that would be proportional to their size. This way, large academic health sciences centers would have large psychiatric services.

Translational Psychiatry Centers and Institutes

There are very few dedicated translational psychiatry centers and institutes, let alone convergence mental health centers and institutes, in the world. The number of those needs to be increased, both as independent entities and as national intramural research programs, where new ideas can be tested and developed without the long delays caused by the constant and essentially full-time pursuit of extramural funding. Such translational/convergence centers and institutes should be structured to promote integration along both vertical and horizontal axes, as we recently described (see Figure 9.3).[54] Briefly, vertical integration is what we previously presented in steps T0 to T5. Horizontal integration cuts across disease states along either scientific themes, such as inflammation and neuroendocrinology, or along technical domains, exemplified by imaging and the "omics" platforms: genomics, proteomics, metabolomics and lipidomics. Horizontal integration also is, and increasingly needs to be, transdisciplinary in the convergence model, such as the integration of medicine, chemistry, biology, computer science, and economics, at minimum, to develop and distribute new pharmacologic therapies for treating mental illness.

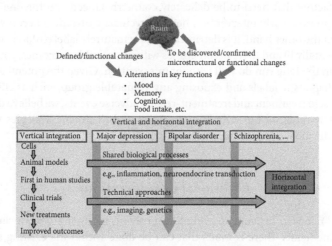

Figure 9.3. A conceptual framework for translational psychiatry. Top panel: In the brain-defined structural changes, such as the plaques and tangles of Alzheimer's disease, or to be discovered or confirmed microstructural or functional changes can lead to key symptoms. Bottom panel: Parallel and simultaneous tracks of integration along both thematic and technical horizontal axes and at the vertical translational level are needed in psychiatry.

Philanthropic Initiatives for New and Untested Ideas

In contrast to cancer and heart disease, philanthropy in psychiatry in still in its infancy. We are grateful for the support of psychiatric research offered by Connie Lieber and the Brain and Behavior Research Foundation (formerly NARSAD), and the Stanley Medical Research Institute, to name a few examples of philanthropy in psychiatric research. Nevertheless, many more similar bodies should be created in our field so that there can be adequate support for new initiatives, innovative approaches, and untested hypotheses, leading to the collection of pilot data and positioning for competitive application to government or private funding.

Prevention: Well-Being, Resilience, and Early-Life Intervention

While a war on established mental illness is very much needed, according to Benjamin Franklin "an ounce of prevention is worth a pound of cure." In that context, efforts to promote wellbeing, such as positive psychology and resilience building,[55,56] as well as adoption of healthy lifestyles including stress reduction, proper nutrition, and exercise, ought to be an integral part of the "War on Mental Illness."

It will likewise be crucial to develop and apply preventive strategies for those who are vulnerable to mental illness in childhood and adolescence, before psychiatric disorders become established chronic conditions. This represents a difficult challenge with two factors that need to be delicately counterbalanced. On the one hand, it is logical to propose early intervention before psychiatric disorders become a chronic burden. On the other hand, it is detrimental to prematurely label children and adolescents as mentally ill and to treat, sometimes with undesirable outcomes, young people who may in the long run do well without intervention. Given the potential pitfalls of applying diagnostic labels and exposing any vulnerable group, such as children and adolescents, to treatment and treatment-related adverse events, we believe that it must be absolutely required for early-life preventive and treatment strategies to be supported by the most rigorous science.

Additional Considerations

This "war" needs to be launched simultaneously on multiple fronts, including convergence medicine. There is much that can be done within the existing structures, and of course more resources are needed to either create or enhance the constitutive elements of the "War on Mental Illness," which are summarized in Figure 9.2 and Box 9.1. Many or most of these elements are highly amenable to convergence science approaches. As the "war" evolves, other elements will undoubtedly emerge. Over time, the "War on Mental Illness" will certainly become bigger and more powerful than the sum of its parts, leading to truly innovative treatments, improved therapeutic approaches, and effective prevention.

It is tempting, but we suggest unwise, to disregard current approaches as having at best reached a plateau and focus resources solely on the search for new treatments.

Many patients with psychiatric disorders achieve full remission with existing interventions, whereas others have only partial or no response. Importantly, some patients may respond very well to some treatments, but not to others. They may also stop responding, for reasons that are unclear at this time. Pharmacogenomics is aimed at unraveling the genetic basis of treatment response. When we discover a priori through genomics, or other types of biomarkers, which patients will respond to which drugs, therapeutics in psychiatry will be much further ahead than it is now.[57] Consequently, efforts to discover new treatments should be complemented by an equally strong emphasis on personalizing and optimizing existing interventions or drugs.

Much emphasis has been placed in recent years on research that is peer reviewed before it is done, as is the case for existing grant mechanisms. In this context, many intramural research institutes have either been reduced in size or dismantled over time.

The US NIMH Intramural Research Program (IRP) has suffered considerable erosion in the last two and a half decades. When we (Licinio and Wong) first joined the IRP in the early 1990s, its budget was 16% of NIMH's budget. In 1994, Cassell and Marks chaired a blue ribbon panel on the NIH's Intramural Research Program, of which the NIMH IRP is part, and specifically recommended that "the total IRP budget for institutes, centers, and divisions (ICDs) should not exceed the current rate of 11.3% of the total NIH budget."[58] In recent years, the NIMH IRP budget has typically remained around 11.3% of that institute's total budget,[59] as recommended by Cassell and Marks in 1994. This represents a relative reduction of ~30% in about 25 years, even before accounting for inflation. Having faced many challenges over the last two and a half decades, we continue to hope the NIMH IRP will see improved budget allocations and achieve new heights in mental health research.

In Australia, the John Curtin School of Medical Research at the Australian National University in Canberra used to be entirely block-funded by a direct allocation from the Australian Commonwealth government. This allowed its scientists to rapidly attain world renown, with milestones such as the awarding of the Nobel Prize in Physiology or Medicine to three individuals who performed their award-winning work there, including neuroscientist Sir John Eccles. However, federal block-funding dedicated directly to John Curtin School of Medical Research has ceased to exist, and that institution's research projects are now entirely supported by competitive grants. At present, Australia does not have a National Institute of Mental Health or any stable, secure, long-term sources of funding for research in psychiatric neuroscience or mental health. Other independent biomedical research institutions in the US and throughout the world, some of which may have used to be 100% supported by direct funding allocations, have also become increasingly grant dependent.

We believe that while there is a key role for research grants, rapid progress at the cutting-edge research can benefit from secure, stable, and dedicated revenue streams. For example, the Manhattan project was launched by President Franklin D. Roosevelt's Executive Order 8807, signed on June 28, 1941, and resulted in the first atomic bomb successfully detonated in New Mexico on July 16, 1945 (Trinity test). While this is indeed an unfortunate example from a humanitarian point of view, and we continue to hope for the day when the world will prioritize healthcare over warfare, the point is simply that such astounding scientific success would not have been achieved as rapidly if instead of an intramural Manhattan project, the US government had relied on the process of investigator-initiated grants that currently exists in medical research.

Under the right conditions, a well-run, solidly funded, and dedicated scientific research program can be more far more efficacious, expeditious, and cost effective than dispersed efforts.

The "War on Mental Illness" needs be fought on many fronts, with a variety of both translational and convergent strategies and mechanisms. For our success, it is vitally important that different approaches do not compete with another. Instead, they should coexist and work cohesively together toward a common target: the generation of new knowledge and its rapid translation to improve mental health.

Launching the "War on Mental Illness"

We have already reached the threshold in which our efforts to launch the "War on Mental Illness" represent medical, scientific, humanitarian and moral imperatives. In concluding this update and renewed call for this effort, we are reminded of the famous statement attributed to Hillel the Elder: "If I am not for myself, who is for me? But if I am for my own self [only], what am I? And if not now, when?"[60]

References

1. Licinio J, Wong ML. Launching the "war on mental illness." *Mol Psychiatry* 2014; **19**(1): 1–5. https://doi.org/10.1038/mp.2013.180.
2. National Cancer Institute. National Cancer Act of 1971. Published February 16, 2016. https://www.cancer.gov/about-nci/overview/history/national-cancer-act-1971
3. Cox C, Sawyer B. What do we know about the burden of disease in the U.S.? Published May 22, 2017. *Peterson-KFF.* https://www.healthsystemtracker.org/chart-collection/know-burden-disease-u-s/
4. Whiteford H, Ferrari A, Degenhardt L. Global burden of disease studies: implications for mental and substance use disorders. *Health Aff (Millwood)* 2016; **35**(6): 1114–1120. https://doi.org/10.1377/hlthaff.2016.0082
5. Vigo D, Thornicroft G, Atun R. Estimating the true global burden of mental illness. *Lancet Psychiatry* 2016; **3**(2): 171–178. https://doi.org/10.1016/s2215-0366(15)00505-2
6. Global Burden of Disease Study C. Global, regional, and national incidence, prevalence, and years lived with disability for 301 acute and chronic diseases and injuries in 188 countries, 1990–2013: a systematic analysis for the Global Burden of Disease Study 2013. *Lancet* 2015; **386**(9995): 743–800.
7. Vos T, Haby MM, Barendregt JJ, Kruijshaar M, Corry J, Andrews G. The burden of major depression avoidable by longer-term treatment strategies. *Arch Gen Psychiatry* 2004; **61**(11): 1097–1103. https://doi.org/10.1001/archpsyc.61.11.1097
8. Perry SW, Allison S, Bastiampillai T, et al. Rising US suicides: Achieving health equity. *OSF Preprints*, 2019:m5q64,
9. Does depression increase the risk for suicide? *HHS.gov.* Last reviewed September 16, 2014. https://www.hhs.gov/answers/mental-health-and-substance-abuse/does-depression-increase-risk-of-suicide/index.html
10. Centers for Disease Control and Prevention. Leading causes of death reports, 1981–2018. Last updated: February 20, 2020. https://webappa.cdc.gov/sasweb/ncipc/leadcause.html

11. Quello SB, Brady KT, Sonne SC. Mood disorders and substance use disorder: a complex comorbidity. *Sci Pract Perspect* 2005; **3**(1): 13–21. https://doi.org/10.1151/spp053113

12. Boden JM, Fergusson DM. Alcohol and depression. *Addiction* 2011; **106**(5): 906–914. https://doi.org/10.1111/j.1360-0443.2010.03351.x

13. Conner KR. Clarifying the relationship between alcohol and depression. *Addiction* 2011; **106**(5): 915–916. https://doi.org/10.1111/j.1360-0443.2011.03385.x

14. Flensborg-Madsen T. Alcohol use disorders and depression--the chicken or the egg? *Addiction* 2011; **106**(5): 916–918. https://doi.org/10.1111/j.1360-0443.2011.03406.x

15. Saffer H, Dave D. Mental Illness and the Demand for Alcohol, Cocaine and Cigarettes. *National Bureau of Economic Research Working Paper Series* 2002; No. 8699. https://www.nber.org/papers/w8699.pdf

16. Perry SW, Licinio J, Wong M-L. The depressed heart. *Heart and Mind* 2019; **3**(2): 35–46. https://doi.org/10.4103/hm.hm_13_19

17. Perry SW, Wong ML, Licinio J. General medical conditions: metabolic disorders. In: Trivedi M, ed. *Primer on Depression*. New York, NY: Oxford University Press; 2020: 136–154.

18. Stunkard AJ, Fernstrom MH, Price A, Frank E, Kupfer DJ. Direction of weight change in recurrent depression. Consistency across episodes. *Arch Gen Psychiatry* 1990; **47**(9): 857–860. https://doi.org/10.1001/archpsyc.1990.01810210065009

19. Mastronardi C, Paz-Filho GJ, Valdez E, Maestre-Mesa J, Licinio J, Wong ML. Long-term body weight outcomes of antidepressant-environment interactions. *Mol Psychiatry* 2011; **16**(3): 265–272. https://doi.org/10.1038/mp.2010.122

20. Engum A. The role of depression and anxiety in onset of diabetes in a large population-based study. *J Psychosom Res* 2007; **62**(1): 31–38. https://doi.org/10.1016/j.jpsychores.2006.07.009

21. Wulsin LR, Singal BM. Do depressive symptoms increase the risk for the onset of coronary disease? A systematic quantitative review. *Psychosom Med* 2003; **65**(2): 201–210. https://doi.org/10.1097/01.psy.0000058371.50240.e3

22. Wolkowitz OM, Mellon SH, Epel ES, et al. Resting leukocyte telomerase activity is elevated in major depression and predicts treatment response. *Mol Psychiatry* 2012; **17**(2): 164–172. https://doi.org/10.1038/mp.2010.133

23. Verhoeven JE, Revesz D, Epel ES, Lin J, Wolkowitz OM, Penninx BW. Major depressive disorder and accelerated cellular aging: results from a large psychiatric cohort study. *Mol Psychiatry* 2014; **19**(8): 895–901. https://doi.org/10.1038/mp.2013.151

24. Bor J, Cohen GH, Galea S. Population health in an era of rising income inequality: USA, 1980-2015. *Lancet* 2017; **389**(10077): 1475–1490. https://doi.org/10.1016/s0140-6736(17)30571-8

25. Case A, Deaton A. Mortality and morbidity in the 21(st) century. *Brookings Pap Econ Act* 2017; **2017**: 397–476.

26. Acciai F, Firebaugh G. Why did life expectancy decline in the United States in 2015? A gender-specific analysis. *Soc Sci Med* 2017; **190**: 174–180. https://doi.org/10.1016/j.socscimed.2017.08.004

27. Mortality GBD, Causes of Death C. Global, regional, and national life expectancy, all-cause mortality, and cause-specific mortality for 249 causes of death, 1980-2015: a systematic analysis for the Global Burden of Disease Study 2015. *Lancet* 2016; **388**(10053): 1459–1544.

28. Brown L, Tucker-Seeley R. Commentary: will "deaths of despair" among Whites change how we talk about racial/ethnic health disparities? *Ethn Dis* 2018; **28**(2): 123–128. https://doi.org/10.18865/ed.28.2.123

29. Case A, Deaton A. Rising morbidity and mortality in midlife among white non-Hispanic Americans in the 21st century. *Proc Natl Acad Sci U S A* 2015; **112**(49): 15078–15083. https://doi.org/10.1073/pnas.1518393112

30. Minton J, Green M, McCartney G, Shaw R, Vanderbloemen L, Pickett K. Two cheers for a small giant? Why we need better ways of seeing data: A commentary on: "Rising morbidity and mortality in midlife among White non-Hispanic Americans in the 21st century." *Int J Epidemiol* 2017; 46(1): 356–361.

31. Stein EM, Gennuso KP, Ugboaja DC, Remington PL. The epidemic of despair among White Americans: trends in the leading causes of premature death, 1999–2015. *Am J Public Health* 2017; 107(10): 1541–1547 https://doi.org/10.2105/ajph.2017.303941.

32. Weinberger AH, Gbedemah M, Martinez AM, Nash D, Galea S, Goodwin RD. Trends in depression prevalence in the USA from 2005 to 2015: widening disparities in vulnerable groups. *Psychol Med* 2018; 48(8): 1308–1315. https://doi.org/10.1017/s0033291717002781

33. Bornstein SR, Ehrhart-Bornstein M, Wong ML, Licinio J. Is the worldwide epidemic of obesity a communicable feature of globalization? *Exp Clin Endocrinol Diabetes* 2008; 116(Suppl 1): S30–S32. https://doi.org/10.1055/s-2008-1081485

34. Dwyer-Lindgren L, Bertozzi-Villa A, Stubbs RW, et al. Inequalities in life expectancy among US counties, 1980 to 2014: temporal trends and key drivers. *JAMA Intern Med* 2017; 177(7): 1003–1011. https://doi.org/10.1001/jamainternmed.2017.0918

35. Chetty R, Stepner M, Abraham S, et al. The association between income and life expectancy in the United States, 2001–2014. *JAMA* 2016; 315(16): 1750–1766. https://doi.org/10.1001/jama.2016.4226

36. Eyre HA, Lavretsky H, Forbes M, et al. Convergence science arrives: how does it relate to psychiatry? *Acad Psychiatry* 2017; 41(1): 91–99. https://doi.org/10.1007/s40596-016-0496-0

37. Balas EA, Boren SA. Managing clinical knowledge for health care improvement. In: Van Bemmel JH, McCray AT, Alexa T, eds. *Yearbook of Medical Informatics 2000: Patient-Centered Systems.* Stuttgart, Germany: Schattauer; 2000: 65–70. https://doi.org/10.1055/s-0038-1637943

38. Serna MC, Cruz I, Real J, Gasco E, Galvan L. Duration and adherence of antidepressant treatment (2003 to 2007) based on prescription database. *Eur Psychiatry* 2010; 25(4): 206–213. https://doi.org/10.1016/j.eurpsy.2009.07.012

39. Davies J, Read J. A systematic review into the incidence, severity and duration of antidepressant withdrawal effects: Are guidelines evidence-based? *Addict Behav* 2019; 97: 111–121. https://doi.org/10.1016/j.addbeh.2018.08.027

40. Schlimme JE. Tapering off is by no means easy. *Dtsch Arztebl Int* 2019; 116(40): 677.

41. Henssler J, Brandt L, Heinz A, Bschor T. In reply. *Dtsch Arztebl Int* 2019; 116(40): 677–678. https://doi.org/10.3238/arztebl.2019.0677b

42. Tomlinson A, Boaden K, Cipriani A. Withdrawal, dependence and adverse events of antidepressants: lessons from patients and data. *Evid Based Ment Health* 2019; 22(4): 137–138. https://doi.org/10.1136/ebmental-2019-300121

43. Fava GA, Cosci F. Understanding and managing withdrawal syndromes after discontinuation of antidepressant drugs. *J Clin Psychiatry* 2019; 80(6). https://doi.org/10.4088/jcp.19com12794

44. Henssler J, Heinz A, Brandt L, Bschor T. Antidepressant withdrawal and rebound phenomena. *Dtsch Arztebl Int* 2019; 116(20): 355-361.

45. Iacobucci G. NICE updates antidepressant guidelines to reflect severity and length of withdrawal symptoms. *BMJ* 2019; 367: l6103.

46. Hengartner MP, Davies J, Read J. Antidepressant withdrawal—the tide is finally turning. *Epidemiol Psychiatr Sci* 2019: 1–3.

47. Horowitz MA, Taylor D. Tapering of SSRI treatment to mitigate withdrawal symptoms. *Lancet Psychiatry* 2019; 6(6): 538–546 https://doi.org/10.1016/s2215-0366(19)30032-x.

48. Jha MK, Rush AJ, Trivedi MH. When discontinuing SSRI antidepressants Is a challenge: management tips. *Am J Psychiatry* 2018; **175**(12): 1176–1184 https://doi.org/10.1176/appi.ajp.2018.18060692.

49. Gewin V. Biotechnology: independent streak. *Nature* 2013; **499**(7459): 509–511 https://doi.org/10.1038/nj7459-509a.

50. Peter Thiel announces 2013 class of "20 Under 20" Thiel fellows. *Business Wire*. Published May 14, 2013. https://www.businesswire.com/news/home/20130509005377/en/Peter-Thiel-Announces-2013-Class-

51. Drew N, Funk M, Tang S, et al. Human rights violations of people with mental and psychosocial disabilities: an unresolved global crisis. *Lancet* 2011; **378**(9803): 1664–1675. https://doi.org/10.1016/s0140-6736(11)61458-x

52. Licinio J. A leadership crisis in American psychiatry. *Mol Psychiatry* 2004; **9**(1): 1. https://doi.org/10.1038/sj.mp.4001467

53. Licinio J. Mental Illness Awareness Week: a leadership crisis in psychiatry [Blog post]. *Nature*. October 8, 2013. http://blogs.nature.com/soapboxscience/2013/10/08/mental-illness-awareness-week-a-leadership-crisis-in-psychiatry

54. Licinio J, Wong ML. A novel conceptual framework for psychiatry: vertically and horizontally integrated approaches to redundancy and pleiotropism that co-exist with a classification of symptom clusters based on DSM-5. *Mol Psychiatry* 2013; **18**(8): 846–848. https://doi.org/10.1038/mp.2013.90

55. Duckworth AL, Steen TA, Seligman ME. Positive psychology in clinical practice. *Annu Rev Clin Psychol* 2005; **1**: 629–651.

56. Seligman ME. Building resilience. *Harv Bus Rev* 2011; **89**(4): 100–106, 138.

57. Licinio J, Wong ML. Pharmacogenomics of antidepressant treatment effects. *Dialogues Clin Neurosci* 2011; **13**(1): 63–71.

58. National Institutes of Health Intramural Research Program. Report of the External Advisory Committee of the Director's Advisory Committee, National Institutes of Health. Published November 17, 1994. https://oir.nih.gov/sites/default/files/uploads/sourcebook/documents/review_science/nih-irp_redbook.pdf

59. National Institute of Mental Health. Budget. https://www.nimh.nih.gov/about/budget/index.shtml

60. Chapters of the Fathers (Pirkei Avot) 1.14, https://www.sefaria.org/Pirkei_Avot.1?lang=bi.

10

Promoting Early Child Development

Using Convergence Science for the Scalable Assessment and Monitoring of Cognitive Development

Supriya Bhavnani, Georgia Lockwood Estrin, Debarati Mukherjee, and Vikram Patel

Introduction

Substantial reductions in infant and under-5 mortality in the past few decades has led to a critical shift in focus from child survival to optimizing developmental potential.[1] The global challenge is enormous with an estimated 200 million children believed to be at risk of suboptimal development, based on proxy measures of poverty and stunting.[2] Even this number is likely to be an underestimate, since they are distal to measures of brain functioning and cognitive development. Using a more direct measure of child development—the Early Childhood Development Index—a study across 35 low- and middle-income countries (LMICs) suggested that over 81 million, or one in every three children aged 3 to 4 years, could be developing suboptimally in cognitive and social-emotional domains.[3] This is because child development is highly sensitive to adversities in early childhood. A recent study from India[4] reported that every additional economic and psychosocial adversity faced in the first year of life negatively impacts growth and development at 18 months of age. Additionally, disadvantaged children not only have poorer development outcomes at an early age, but the impact of adversities continue to accumulate over time, as demonstrated in a large longitudinal study on children and adolescents around the world—the Young Lives Study.[5] For instance, the impact of sociodemographic inequalities is evident in educational outcomes, such as school enrolment rates, in Vietnam, which increasingly amplify as children grow older.[6] Unsurprisingly, Africa and South Asia house a disproportionately large number of the children at risk of developing suboptimally, with India faring the worst at the country level. These disadvantaged children are likely to perform poorly in school, achieve lower grade levels, earn an average of 25% less than their healthy peers, have poorer mental health and higher fertility rates, and thereby continue to propagate the vicious cycle of intergenerational poverty and disadvantage.[7] LMICs also house more than 95% of the children with developmental delays and disorders.[8] A recent population-based study reported the cumulative prevalence of seven common neurodevelopmental disorders in India to be 9.2%,[9] making it the country with the highest number of children with developmental disorders in the world.

Encouragingly though, research has demonstrated that early interventions that promote and protect developmental trajectories can mitigate the impact of early adversities by promoting health and wellness across the life-course and increasing adult productivity and income, thereby reducing inequities arising out of differential early life circumstances.[10] In fact, investing in early childhood is the most cost effective investment a country can make, with up to $17 saved for every dollar spent.[11] In 2015, the United Nations Secretary-General Ban ki-Moon stated, "The Sustainable Development Goals recognize that early childhood development (ECD) can help drive the transformation we hope to achieve over the next 15 years," aptly summarizing the impact that optimizing child development could have in the coming decades.

The foundations and promise of early interventions lie in the dynamic nature of brain development and its capacity for functional and structural changes in response to environmental stimuli, referred to as "plasticity," in the first few years of life. The brain has a unique developmental trajectory compared to the rest of the body. At age 2 years, while the child has only gained about 20% of the adult body weight, the brain is already close to 80% of its adult weight.[12] During this period of rapid growth, emerging functional connectivity is established and strengthened by early experiences and driven by opportunities for learning and relationships with caregivers. Thus, the early years present the best window of opportunity when emerging brain circuits are most receptive to interventions that promote development and likely to result in the best outcomes.

Healthy growth and development of a child is a result not only of their biological constitution, but also of the complex interplay between the individual and their surrounding environment. In the bioecological systems theory, one of the most influential frameworks of development, Bronfenbrenner[13] highlights the critical importance of this environment. This ranges from the proximal immediate surroundings or microsystem, which includes a child's family, school, and neighborhood, which interact with each other to form a mesosystem, to the more distal, like the parents' workplace, and government services such as social welfare and legal services. All these factors constitute the macrosystem and indirectly impact each individual child's life.[13]

To ensure that all children reach their full developmental potential and thrive, we have to design solutions that address all these levels of society as well as their intersections. It is thus critical for experts from a range of disciplines to synergize and work together. Specialists dedicated to the health and well-being of young children, like pediatricians, clinical psychologists, social workers, and teachers, need to work hand in hand with neuroscientists (e.g., assessment of brain structure and function), anthropologists (e.g., societal norms and practices impacting child development), artists and community leaders (e.g., community engagement and advocacy), lawyers (e.g., child protection), economists (e.g., efficient resource utilization and mobilization), public health and implementation scientists (e.g., design of scalable, cost-effective and sustainable programs), and policy experts (e.g., creating roadmaps to achieve national and global goals) to create an ecosystem where children have access to all the opportunities that optimize development.

To this end, the World Health Organization's Nurturing Care Framework[14] provides a roadmap for government, civil society, and families with a holistic approach to promoting ECD. While the framework emphasizes the period from pregnancy to age

3 years, its guiding principles, strategic actions, and recommendations for monitoring progress are applicable to the entire period of early childhood. It divides nurturing care of young children into five essential pillars—adequate nutrition, responsive caregiving, security and safety, opportunities for early learning, and good health.

In the last two decades, strong evidence emerging from LMICs has shown the effectiveness of interventions that target these pillars, implemented during the early years of life.[15] In the early 2000s, a seminal ECD study called Reach Up and Learn was conducted in Jamaica. This study used the principals of the Care for Child Development Package designed by UNICEF in which health workers assist families to adopt play and communication into their caregiving skills. Stunted infants aged 9 to 24 months were provided an intervention comprising either nutritional supplementation or cognitive stimulation or both together. Participants were later followed up at regular intervals till early adulthood. Remarkably, an impact of cognitive stimulation was demonstrated at 7 to 9 and 17 to 18 years as improved performance on developmental tests and, at 22 years, as increased earnings, reduced involvement in fights, reduced violent behavior, and fewer symptoms of depression and social inhibition.[16-19]

Similar results have been obtained by Yousafzai and colleagues in the PEDS (Pakistan Early Child Development Scale Up) study in Pakistan in which the intervention promoting responsive stimulation in parents impacted child cognitive abilities at 2 and 4 years of age.[20,21] Furthermore, the Turkish Early Enrichment Project has demonstrated effectiveness of interventions implemented at a slightly later age, that of 4 to 6 years. This intervention involved training mothers and preschool teachers, which positively impacted school attainment in late childhood and higher occupational status and employment in adulthood.[22,23] Similar interventions implemented in high-income countries have also shown to be effective.[24] These intervention studies strongly support the argument for investing across early childhood.

Barriers to Optimizing ECD

Despite much theory and research having been conducted to highlight the importance of optimizing early child development, and how to best go about achieving this, there are many factors that limit our ability to do so effectively, especially in LMIC contexts. In particular, we aim to highlight the large "detection gap" wherein children in need of interventions fail to be identified. There are two fundamental barriers to their detection: the first is a low demand for services such as assessments to measure and monitor early child development, and the second is a shortage of supply and effective implementation of such services.

Demand Shortages

There is a striking lack of awareness of what optimal child development looks like in the population, which may lead to poor help-seeking behavior. This is illustrated through an example of a qualitative assessment of the universal screening program for child development in Thailand. This highlighted caregiver's low levels of understanding about how to stimulate their child's development, which remained evident even in cases where their child had screened positive for developmental delays.[25] This lack of understanding may have been a key reason that caregivers did not follow the advice provided by health workers to enhance their child's development or return to clinics for follow-up by physicians. Similarly, studies conducted in India and Nepal have demonstrated little explicit awareness of atypical development in children. This is not limited to parents and caregivers, but is also evident in health professionals, school teachers, and educators, as well as members in religious sectors, who are often relied upon for guidance in health matters.[26-29] ·

Socioeconomic factors may be an important influence on whether a child with atypical development receives a diagnosis, such as autism spectrum disorder (ASD), and is therefore able to access interventions and support.[29] This may be related to different patterns of health seeking behaviors due to financial burdens and education as well as misconceptions of health workers. Daley et al. highlighted that in urban India it was a "prevalent belief ... [amongst physicians] that families of lower socioeconomic background and less education are not as sensitive to developmental difficulties."[29] While more recent evidence suggests that awareness by professionals in India may be on the increase, at least in the large cities, staff in government hospitals staff are poorly equipped to identify children with disabilities,[27,2] much less identify those children who are faltering and not reaching their full potential. These studies highlight the urgent need to increase the level of education in the population to create greater awareness of normal growth and development in children.

Supply Shortages

The difficult task of effectively and efficiently measuring child development brings with it multiple limitations. A key limitation is the lack of specialized health professionals for developmental healthcare[30] and their unequal distribution to urban areas. Another key limitation lies in the kind of child development measurement tools that currently exist.[31] Many of them, meant to be used by these skilled professionals, are proprietary, limiting their access in low-resource communities. While a number of tools have been developed for administration by nonspecialists, they mostly rely on direct assessment of standardized activities by a trained assessor, for example Infant and Young Child Development[32] and Guide for Monitoring Child Development.[33] These are dependent on regular and lengthy training sessions and requires extensive time to administer, thereby imposing enormous time and cost barriers for parents and health systems and limiting their scalability. Tools dependent on parent-report present alternatives to these, but they suffer from the disadvantages of recall bias, lack of sensitivity, and poor accuracy because parents' responses tend to differ based on their own knowledge of child development.[34]

The issue of scalability is further called into question by recent evidence demonstrating that there are currently no easily available tools that provide both accurate measures and that are also feasible to administer at scale in low resources community settings.[35] Accessibility, training requirements, clinical relevance, and geographical uptake are particularly poor for most tools. Part of the reason for this is that the majority of tools have been developed in the cultural contexts of high-income settings which are usually not appropriate for LMICs.[31] In some cases, these tools are used with no adaptations for the different settings in which they are being used.[34] Further, the norms created using these tools, which are also used to identify delayed development, have almost entirely been derived in limited populations in high-income countries raising questions about their generalizability across contexts. Development of cross-culturally appropriate tools that are also feasible and affordable and with good psychometric properties in diverse contexts are essential for effective measurement of ECD by nonspecialists in routine LMIC health services.

To address the key issues of scalability, researchers have sought to make use of the unprecedented increase of access to mobile technologies around the world. The wide penetration of mobile devices and internet services across sociodemographic boundaries opens a unique opportunity for newer technologies to address some of these barriers to optimizing ECD and scaling up effective programs in the modern world. The case study described next serves as an example of harnessing the potential of technology to assess ECD in preschool children.

Developing and Validating Scalable Transdiagnostic Assessments for ECD—A Case Study

With an overarching vision of reducing the large detection gap in preschool years,[36] to improve children's health in LMICs, in 2015 we initiated efforts to pull together diverse disciplines through a team of international experts. Acutely aware of the fact that the development of any solution that has this ambition cannot be done by specialists in any single discipline, we ensured that our team converged disciplines of clinical, neuro-, public health, computer, and data sciences (see Figure 10.1). Once we had built our team, a common goal was decided—to develop a suite of digital tools that can holistically assess multiple domains of child development and that can be used at scale. Our first step was ensure that our solution was grounded in the well-founded *theory* of developmental neuroscience, which has been established through decades of research.[37] The neuroscientists on the team also brought the relatively novel perspective of the Research Domain Criteria (RDoC) framework.[38] The RDoC framework is a prime example of a convergence of disciplines in mental health science that arose due to the growing understanding that for mental health, it is unlikely that any one symptom would have a one-on-one and exclusive correspondence with a diagnosis. It is more likely that a set of behaviors, biomarkers and symptoms would cluster in various ways, and this pattern of clustering would determine the most appropriate treatment model for each individual. The advantage of the RDoC approach is its emphasis on dimensional measures, and this encouraged us to go beyond the identification of clinically defined categories of dysfunction and instead design our tools to measure domains of development such as social-communication, attention and cognition, and fine motor, which are integral to a child's healthy mental and physical development.

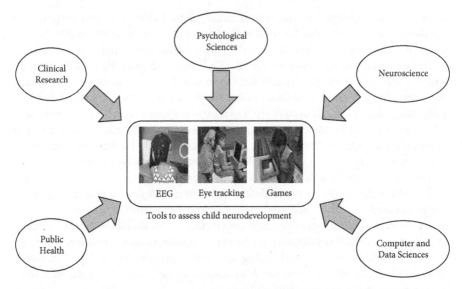

Figure 10.1 Convergence of research disciplines to develop scalable tools for assessment of neurodevelopment in preschool children.

At the same time, the involvement of developmental pediatricians, psychologists, and psychiatrists ensured that the constructs being captured by the tasks on our tools remained clinically relevant and age-appropriate, capturing the dynamic nature of early childhood.

The public health experts on our team advised on the *design* of this solution to ensure that it would not only be acceptable to the end users of children and their families, but also feasible for *delivery* by the implementers. These implementers are nonspecialist workers who are at the frontline of the national public health systems and would, in the long term, be the people administering such digital tools at scale. Finally, through the engagement of computer scientists and digital game designers from conception of this study, we were able to appreciate the vast potential of these technologies and design our solution to harness it. This potential was further enhanced through the expertise of data scientists, who used machine learning methods to design *analytical* models for the novel digital data being generated.

Innovating the Design, Delivery and Analysis of ECD Assessments

Our team chose to integrate technologies that can capture three key modes of assessment of child development: (i) child behavior, through the use of eye-tracking; (ii) child performance, on gamified neuropsychological tasks; and (iii) neurophysiology using electroencephalography. These three elements combine to create a novel solution capable of assessing developmental attainments in the critical preschool years. To truly harness the potential of these technologies, and keeping global applicability as our guiding principle, we ensured that our digital tools would be (i) administered offline on Android tablets, which due to their lower costs, are considerably more prevalent in low resource settings than other counterparts; (ii) administered in the comfort of a child's home; (iii) free of any written instructions for the child; (iv) free of cultural references through the use of globally recognizable images and characters; and (v) feasible for administration by nonspecialist workers. This required us to innovate on the design, delivery, and data analysis of existing technologies, some examples of which are described later in the text.

First, by engaging an agency to *design* this product, our team ensured that this developmental assessment "game" would be greater than the sum of its parts, by being visually attractive, fun, engaging, and exciting for young children on whom it would be administered and a seamless journey for the administrator. Second, to ensure that the *delivery* of these tools could be effectively administered by nonspecialists, the tools were designed to incorporate well-defined "start–stop" rules, such as timers to allow for automatic transition between games. Such rules minimized the requirement of the administrator to exercise judgement on the child's abilities, overcoming the disadvantage of current developmental assessments wherein specialist administrators need to observe and use expert judgement to record child performance, which limits their scalability. The other technology integrated into our solution was electroencephalography, which was ripe to take to scale with relatively low cost, portable devices available on the market.[39] The innovation required to scale this technology has centered around the need to overcome the challenges of the uncontrolled nature of the settings in which the data were being collected (i.e., households instead of laboratories).

Finally, a key example of the innovation of the *analytical methods* applied lies in the use of tablet-based eye-tracking. Eye-tracking was conducted to assess children's preference for social compared to nonsocial stimuli. Such tasks have been shown to have the potential to identify children with social-communication impairments, such as those with ASD.[40] Studies involving the use of eye-tracking are typically conducted in highly controlled settings using expensive laboratory-grade equipment, which had to be replaced to enhance the scalability of this mode of assessment. This was achieved by using the camera at the front end of the tablet to record a video of the child watching videos presented to them on the tablet screen. Subsequently, computer-vision technology was applied to analyze these videos, which involved first identifying the eyes of the child while they watched the video and then capturing the duration for which they looked at a particular part of the screen. This allowed for automated analysis to determine the child's preference, if any, for a particular type of video presented to them.[41]

Our pilot studies in India have demonstrated that the *design* of these digital tools is highly acceptable to children and their families, and their *delivery* is feasible by nonspecialists in rural households.[42] We have also generated preliminary evidence to establish the validity of the novel digital data captured by these tools and *analytical methods* by benchmarking them against gold-standard developmental assessments. For instance, our data indicate the ability of tablet-based eye-tracking to differentiate between typically developing children and those with neurodevelopmental disorders including ASD and intellectual disability based on the amount of time that they look at social compared to non-social dynamic stimuli.[43,44] These groups of children can also be differentiated based on the manner in which they play tablet-based games, for instance, children with neurodevelopmental disorders use greater force to press on the tablet than typically developing ones, a finding that has also been demonstrated by another group.[45] Our pilot data also indicates that, using machine learning, we are able to determine metrics derived from children's performance on tablet-based gamified cognitive tasks that are able to predict their developmental scores based on gold-standard clinical neurodevelopmental assessments.

These results are being replicated in a larger cohort through ongoing studies. Efforts are also underway to establish their global applicability by expanding the diversity of settings in which they are validated. Through longitudinal studies, we also intend to establish the ability of child performance on digital developmental assessment tools and neurophysiology measured at younger ages to predict outcomes such as academic performance in school or emergence of clinical phenotypes at older ages.

Our Vision for Assessment of Early Childhood Development

The vision for these scalable digital tools is to harness the potential of the multiple sources of digital data in our solution to triangulate information from them and determine the combination of metrics that can most accurately identify children who are at risk of developmental disorders or not attaining their full developmental potential and refer them for timely interventions (see Figure 10.2). These tools would eventually allow for large-scale longitudinal developmental surveillance of preschool children by trained nonspecialists from diverse settings to create truly "global" norms characterizing children's attainment in crucial developmental domains (see Figure

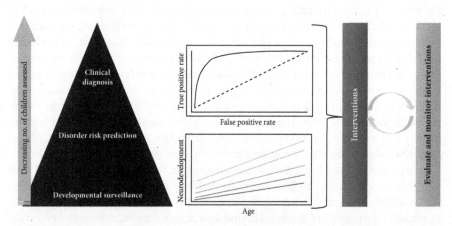

Figure 10.2 The vision for promoting early child development: convergence of sectors, disciplines, and technologies is integral to achieving this vision. True positive rate = proportion of correctly identified positives. False positive rate = proportion of incorrectly identified positives.

10.2) resulting in neurodevelopmental charts analogous to growth charts for anthropometric measures used routinely across the world. These norms would continually be updated and their precision improved as more data becomes available paving the way for the use of cloud computing for data analysis. The nuanced nature of the digital data emerging from these tools also has the potential of being sensitive to improvements brought about through interventions.

Achieving this vision requires the integration of such solutions into existing ECD programs. Child welfare, maternal and child health, and preschool education sectors offer extensive reach to both women and children, from preconception throughout early childhood and are therefore ideally placed to be the starting point to implement services. There needs to be synchrony between all these sectors as well as engagement extending between government, academia, industry, healthcare providers, employers, and patient groups and their families. Interventions that integrate between diverse sectors offer the advantage of providing a more holistic approach to support a child to achieve their optimal development.[7]

One example of a program that is implemented via convergence of governmental departments and aims to address multiple domains of child development, is India's Integrated Child Development Services. This program is implemented through the public preschools (called Anganwadi centers) and a network of 1.4 million workers who form a large part of the public healthcare system in India, and these networks provide basic healthcare within communities, which makes it a potential avenue for integration of scalable developmental assessment services. This program aims to combat high rates of child mortality, malnutrition, and poor learning outcomes in children. It provides multiple health and education services, including medical checks, immunizations, referral services, and health and nutrition education for adolescent girls and mothers, as well as supplementary feeding, for example, the seminal "mid-day meal" scheme, which provides free nutritious meals during lunchtime to every child attending government preschools. The program also provides preschool education and cognitive stimulation during early childhood. However, despite the coherent aims and multiple sectors working to implement this program, the overall impact of this initiative has been mixed. This may be in part due to variable quality of implementation, which highlights the need for successful convergence of sectors relevant to ECD to make such schemes successful.

Ethical and Policy Considerations

Notwithstanding its benefits, it is important to keep in mind the ethical issues related to the use of technology for assessment of neurodevelopment, especially in vulnerable populations such as children. The foremost concerns are the need for improved data protection to maintain privacy, establishing guidelines and regulations on how digital data should be stored, shared, and used to avoid misuse. The identification of developmental delays or disorders in children needs to account for the stigma associated with a positive screen evident in many societies. Therefore, efforts to build awareness about childhood developmental disorders and advocacy to gain access to effective interventions must go hand in hand with developing new technologies directed toward early identification. Ignoring any of the two arms is likely to severely impede the effectiveness of the other.

Finally, for any program to be extensively and effectively implemented at scale, it needs support from policy, cross-sectoral coordination, and financing; as highlighted by Richter et al.: "Laws and policies can improve child development by increasing access and quality of health and other services, as well as money and time for parents to provide nurturing care for their young children."[7] Such policies would include implementation of minimum wage to lift families out of poverty or paid sick leave for parents to provide nurturing care for their infants and children.

Conclusions

In this chapter, we have emphasized the need for convergence across diverse sectors and disciplines to achieve the goal of promoting ECD. We have outlined the barriers that lend to the alarming picture of the state of the children of our world, particularly those residing in low resource settings, and highlighted the potential that the use of technology offers in creating a closed-loop by aiding in both detection and provision of effective intervention services for these children. We illustrate the immense importance of convergence of experts from diverse disciplines to conduct research in this field through a case study on developing and validating assessment tools for preschool children. Finally, we present a reminder of the ethical considerations to bear in mind while harnessing the power of technology to optimize the developmental potential of the next generation.

References

1. Kuruvilla S, Bustreo F, Kuo T, et al. The global strategy for women's, children's and adolescents' health (2016–2030): a roadmap based on evidence and country experience. *Bull World Health Organ*. 2016;94(5):398–400. doi:10.2471/BLT.16.170431
2. Black MM, Walker SP, Fernald LCH, et al. Early childhood development coming of age: science through the life course. *Lancet*. 2017;389(10064):77–90. doi:10.1016/S0140-6736(16)31389-7
3. McCoy DC, Peet ED, Ezzati M, et al. Early childhood developmental status in low- and middle-income countries: national, regional, and global prevalence estimates using predictive modeling. *PLoS Med*. 2016;13(6):e1002034. doi:10.1371/journal.pmed.1002034
4. Bhopal S, Roy R, Verma D, et al. Impact of adversity on early childhood growth & development in rural India: Findings from the early life stress sub-study of the SPRING cluster randomised controlled trial (SPRING-ELS). *PLoS One*. 2019;14(1). doi:10.1371/journal.pone.0209122
5. Young Lives. [Home page]. https://www.younglives.org.uk/. Accessed November 15, 2019.
6. Nguyen HTM. Ethnic gaps in child education outcomes in Vietnam: an investigation using Young Lives data. *Educ Econ*. 2019;27(1):93–111. doi:10.1080/09645292.2018.1444147
7. Richter LM, Daelmans B, Lombardi J, et al. Investing in the foundation of sustainable development: pathways to scale up for early childhood development. *Lancet*. 2017;389(10064):103–118. doi:10.1016/S0140-6736(16)31698-1

8. Olusanya BO, Davis AC, Wertlieb D, et al. Developmental disabilities among children younger than 5 years in 195 countries and territories, 1990–2016: a systematic analysis for the Global Burden of Disease Study 2016. *Lancet Glob Health.* 2018;6(10):e1100–e1121. doi:10.1016/S2214-109X(18)30309-7

9. Arora NK, Nair MKC, Gulati S, et al. Neurodevelopmental disorders in children aged 2–9 years: population-based burden estimates across five regions in India. *PLoS Med.* 2018;15(7):e1002615. doi:10.1371/journal.pmed.1002615

10. Britto PR, Lye SJ, Proulx K, et al. Nurturing care: promoting early childhood development. *The Lancet.* 2017;389(10064):91–102. doi:10.1016/S0140-6736(16)31390-3

11. World Bank. Early childhood development. https://www.worldbank.org/en/topic/earlychildhooddevelopment. Accessed November 15, 2019.

12. Haartsen R, Jones EJ, Johnson MH. Human brain development over the early years. *Curr Opin Behav Sci.* 2016;10:149–154. doi:10.1016/j.cobeha.2016.05.015

13. Bronfenbrenner U. *The Ecology of Human Development.* Cambridge, MA: Harvard University Press; 1979.

14. UNICEF, World Bank, World Health Organization. Nurturing care for early childhood development a framework for helping children survive and thrive to transform health and human potential. *World Health Organization.* https://www.who.int/maternal_child_adolescent/child/nurturing-care-framework/en/. Accessed November 15, 2019.

15. Prado EL, Larson LM, Cox K, Bettencourt K, Kubes JN, Shankar AH. Do effects of early life interventions on linear growth correspond to effects on neurobehavioural development? A systematic review and meta-analysis. *Lancet Glob Health.* 2019;7(10):e1398–e1413. doi:10.1016/S2214-109X(19)30361-4

16. Grantham-McGregor SM, Walker SP, Chang SM, Powell CA. Effects of early childhood supplementation with and without stimulation on later development in stunted Jamaican children. *Am J Clin Nutr.* 1997;66(2):247–253. doi:10.1093/ajcn/66.2.247

17. Walker SP, Chang SM, Powell CA, Grantham-McGregor SM. Effects of early childhood psychosocial stimulation and nutritional supplementation on cognition and education in growth-stunted Jamaican children: prospective cohort study. *Lancet.* 2005;366(9499):1804–1807. doi:10.1016/S0140-6736(05)67574-5

18. Gertler P, Heckman J, Pinto R, et al. Labor market returns to an early childhood stimulation intervention in Jamaica. *Science.* 2014;344(6187):998–1001. doi:10.1126/science.1251178

19. Walker SP, Chang SM, Vera-Hernández M, Grantham-McGregor S. Early childhood stimulation benefits adult competence and reduces violent behavior. *Pediatrics.* 2011;127(5):849–857. doi:10.1542/peds.2010-2231

20. Yousafzai AK, Obradović J, Rasheed MA, et al. Effects of responsive stimulation and nutrition interventions on children's development and growth at age 4 years in a disadvantaged population in Pakistan: a longitudinal follow-up of a cluster-randomised factorial effectiveness trial. *Lancet Glob Health.* 2016;4(8):e548–558. doi:10.1016/S2214-109X(16)30100-0

21. Yousafzai AK, Rasheed MA, Rizvi A, Armstrong R, Bhutta ZA. Effect of integrated responsive stimulation and nutrition interventions in the Lady Health Worker programme in Pakistan on child development, growth, and health outcomes: a cluster-randomised factorial effectiveness trial. *Lancet.* 2014;384(9950):1282–1293. doi:10.1016/S0140-6736(14)60455-4

22. Kagitcibasi C, Sunar D, Bekman S, Baydar N, Cemalcilar Z. Continuing effects of early enrichment in adult life: the Turkish early enrichment project 22 years later. *J Appl Dev Psychol.* 2009;30(6):764–779. doi:10.1016/j.appdev.2009.05.003

23. Kagitcibasi C, Sunar D, Bekman S. Long-term effects of early intervention: Turkish low-income mothers and children. *J Appl Dev Psychol.* 2001;22(4):333–361. doi:10.1016/S0193-3973(01)00071-5

24. Office of Head Start. [Home page]. https://www.acf.hhs.gov/ohs. Accessed November 15, 2019.

25. Morrison J, Chunsuwan I, Bunnag P, Gronholm PC, Estrin GL. Thailand's national universal developmental screening programme for young children: action research for improved follow-up. *BMJ Glob Health*. 2018;3(1). doi:10.1136/bmjgh-2017-000589

26. Heys M, Alexander AE, Medeiros E, et al. Understanding parents' and professionals' knowledge and awareness of autism in Nepal. *Autism Int J Res Pract*. 2017;21(4):436–449. doi:10.1177/1362361316646558

27. Divan G, Vajaratkar V, Desai MU, Strik-Lievers L, Patel V. Challenges, coping strategies, and unmet needs of families with a child with autism spectrum disorder in Goa, India. *Autism Res*. 2012;5(3):190–200. doi:10.1002/aur.1225

28. Krishnamurthy V. A clinical experience of autism in India. *J Dev Behav Pediatr*. 2008;29(4):331–333. doi:10.1097/DBP.0b013e3181829f1f

29. Daley TC. From symptom recognition to diagnosis: children with autism in urban India. *Soc Sci Med*. 2004;58(7):1323–1335. doi:10.1016/S0277-9536(03)00330-7

30. Collins PY, Pringle B, Alexander C, et al. Global services and support for children with developmental delays and disabilities: bridging research and policy gaps. *PLoS Med*. 2017;14(9). doi:10.1371/journal.pmed.1002393

31. Goldfeld S, Yousafzai A. Monitoring tools for child development: an opportunity for action. *Lancet Glob Health*. 2018;6(3):e232–e233. doi:10.1016/S2214-109X(18)30040-8

32. Lancaster GA, McCray G, Kariger P, et al. Creation of the WHO Indicators of Infant and Young Child Development (IYCD): metadata synthesis across 10 countries. *BMJ Glob Health*. 2018;3(5). doi:10.1136/bmjgh-2018-000747

33. Ertem IO, Dogan DG, Gok CG, et al. A guide for monitoring child development in low- and middle-income countries. *Pediatrics*. 2008;121(3):e581–589. doi:10.1542/peds.2007-1771

34. Sabanathan S, Wills B, Gladstone M. Child development assessment tools in low-income and middle-income countries: how can we use them more appropriately? *Arch Dis Child*. 2015;100(5):482. doi:10.1136/archdischild-2014-308114

35. Boggs D, Milner KM, Chandna J, et al. Rating early child development outcome measurement tools for routine health programme use. *Arch Dis Child*. 2019;104(Suppl 1):S22–S33. doi:10.1136/archdischild-2018-315431

36. Dasgupta J, Bhavnani S, Estrin GL, et al. Translating neuroscience to the front lines: point-of-care detection of neuropsychiatric disorders. *Lancet Psychiatry*. 2016;3(10):915–917. doi:10.1016/S2215-0366(16)30186-9

37. Johnson MH. *Developmental Cognitive Neuroscience*. New York: Wiley; 2010.

38. Insel T, Cuthbert B, Garvey M, et al. Research domain criteria (RDoC): toward a new classification framework for research on mental disorders. *Am J Psychiatry*. 2010;167(7):748–751. doi:10.1176/appi.ajp.2010.09091379

39. Lau-Zhu A, Lau MPH, McLoughlin G. Mobile EEG in research on neurodevelopmental disorders: opportunities and challenges. *Dev Cogn Neurosci*. 2019;36. doi:10.1016/j.dcn.2019.100635

40. Falck-Ytter T, Bölte S, Gredebäck G. Eye tracking in early autism research. *J Neurodev Disord*. 2013;5(1):28. doi:10.1186/1866-1955-5-28

41. Bishain R. An open-source, computing platform-agnostic, calibration-free preferential gaze detection approach for social preference assessment. https://insar.confex.com/insar/2019/webprogram/Paper31575.html. Published 2019. Accessed November 15, 2019.

42. Bhavnani S, Mukherjee D, Dasgupta J, et al. Development, feasibility and acceptability of a gamified cognitive developmental assessment on an E-platform (DEEP) in rural Indian pre-schoolers—a pilot study. *Glob Health Action*. 2019;12(1). doi:10.1080/16549716.2018.1548005

43. Chakrabarti B. Mobile computer-mediated assessment of autism risk by non-specialists in home settings: insights from the START Project. https://insar.confex.com/insar/2019/webprogram/Paper31375.html. Published 2019. Accessed November 15, 2019.
44. Dasgupta J. Exploring the acceptability and feasibility of a mobile assessment platform: START (Screening Tools for Autism Risk Using Technology). https://insar.confex.com/insar/2019/webprogram/Paper31383.html. Published 2019. Accessed November 15, 2019.
45. Anzulewicz A, Sobota K, Delafield-Butt JT. Toward the autism motor signature: gesture patterns during smart tablet gameplay identify children with autism. *Sci Rep*. 2016;6:31107. doi:10.1038/srep31107

11

Artificial Intelligence in Mental Health

Adrienne Grzenda

Introduction

Mental health is at a critical impasse. The first big data wave occurred over a decade ago, fueled by the reduced cost of -omics techniques (e.g., genomics, transcriptomics), increased access to neuroimaging equipment, and the transition to electronic medical records (EMRs).[1] Insights from this data, however, have not translated into dramatically improved outcomes for patients. Diagnostic clarity is often elusive and treatment selection remains primarily trial and error. A second wave of big data proliferation is already underway with the increased implementation of mobile applications and wearable devices.[2] Solutions are desperately needed to resolve current bottlenecks in the translational pathway. Factors contributing to delays in discoveries progressing to implementation include:

1. *Nosology conflicts and illness heterogeneity.* Significant overlap exists between the genetic risk factors of most common psychiatric disorders.[3] The *Diagnostic and Statistical Manual of Mental Disorders* and *International Classification of Diseases* (ICD), however, employ strict symptom-based criteria for diagnosis. Illness heterogeneity is thus either underestimated (e.g., missing comorbidities or illness subtypes) or exaggerated (e.g., symptoms represent one rather than multiple diagnoses), chronically confounding reproducibility of research. Dimension-based transdiagnostic frameworks, such as the Research Domain Criteria (RDoC), emphasis the synergism between genomics, neural circuits, and behavior.[4] By aligning symptoms more closely with underlying biological processes, the RDoC dimensions are theorized to increase the homogeneity of study cohorts. Interoperability with *Diagnostic and Statistical Manual of Mental Disorders* and ICD—a pragmatic necessity for treatment reimbursement for the foreseeable future—is lacking and largely predicated on identification of biomarkers that reliably associate to behavioral dimensions.

2. *Reliance on P-values as the primary determinant of study significance.* The de facto standard of a *P*-value of less than 0.05 as the delineation between study success and failure is entirely arbitrary. The measure is prone to "hacking," or the selection of certain data or analysis types to ensure significant results.[5] The current reproducibility crisis in medicine is blamed on the misuse of *P*-values.[6] Sample size is a constant balance between economic resources, time, and projected number of subjects required for statistical significance (power). Low-powered studies may precipitate inflated effects sizes, Type I errors (e.g., false

positives), and Type II errors (e.g., false negatives). Biased results can negatively impact subsequent data synthesis methods such as meta-analysis.

3. *Limitations of traditional statistics with large, multidimensional data sets.* Big data technologies strain traditional statistical analyses as these collect a large number of features (P) in relatively few subjects (n), otherwise known as the "big P, little n" problem, a unique multiple testing challenge. A common example are large-scale -omics data sets, such as microarray and genome-wide association studies, which test thousands of genes in a small number of patients.[7] Given the complexity of gene × gene interactions, simplifying an entire biological system to a short list of "statistically significant" features is problematic. Numerous potentially informative targets are abandoned with heightened risk of lurking false positives receiving undue emphasis. A recent reanalysis of 18 often-studied candidate genes for depression found these were no more associated with a depressive phenotype than noncandidate genes.[8]

4. *Lessening participation in population-based research.* Cohort studies and clinical trials are suffering from dwindling rates of participation and high attrition, exacerbating selection bias.[9] Nonparticipants in mental health research frequently suffer a higher degree of symptoms burden and mortality.[10] As a result, the generalizability of results from population-based studies is increasingly questionable.

5. *Limited utility of EMR data.* EMR data suffers from a pervasive lack of standardization. A large portion of records are comprised of unstructured free text notes of variable depth and quality. The structured portion of the EMR (e.g., inputted variables with finite options such as diagnoses, medications, vitals) is often incorrect or incomplete. These issues present significant barriers to secondary analysis as the data often requires substantial organization and recoding, which may introduce additional errors.[11]

6. *Lack of objective measures for diagnosis and treatment monitoring.* Whereas other specialties possess quantitative measurements to assess illness presence and severity, the mental status exam is entirely subjective and reliant on clinician observation. Rare manifestations of illness may be readily missed in a brief interview, particularly with an inexperienced clinician. Monitoring of treatment response and adherence is largely dependent on patient self-report. Psychometric scales are easily skewed by under- or over-reporting. Where treatment failure is the result of unstated non-adherence, inadequate dosing, or actual inefficacy of a particular medication is never clear.

In addition to the previously onted challenges, delivery of mental health services is fraught by perennial issues of access, stigma, and quality of care. The shortage of mental health providers is only anticipated to grow in the coming years. According to a report from the National Council for Behavioral Health, demand may outstrip supply by 6,090 to 15,600 psychiatrists by 2025.[12] Mental health providers are at a heightened increased risk for emotional exhaustion, hazards that contribute to clinician burnout.[13] The dearth of providers often places matters related to quality and equity of care at a lower priority. Although more individuals are pursuing help than ever before, many of the most vulnerable individuals never seek care prior to an adverse outcome, such as suicide.[14]

Artificial intelligence (AI) holds substantial promise in addressing these and other critical issues within the field. A recent survey of psychiatrists found that only about 50% believe that AI will significantly transform clinical practice, which may reflect a healthy cynicism born of thwarted expectations of past overhyped technologies.[15] As will be discussed at length in the current chapter, AI is less of a singular goal than a framework for facilitating a convergence approach to mental health's most vexing challenges.

Overview of Artificial Intelligence

Humanity's fascination with the promise and peril of autonomous machines possesses ancient roots. Homer originated the term αὐτόματον, or automaton, meaning "acting of one's own will," to describe objects that behave of their own accord by means of an internal force.[16] Automata appear frequently in Greek mythology, such as Talos, the bronze man forged by Hephaistos to defend the shores of Crete against invading pirates attempting to kidnap Europa.[17] Manufactured mechanical automata reached peak popularity in the 17th and 18th centuries and were a favorite subject of the Enlightenment philosophers, including Voltaire and Descartes.[18] Descartes contended that automata could never achieve human-level reasoning. As he noted in *Discours de la méthode*: "Although such machines might execute many things with equal or perhaps greater perfection than any of us, they would, without doubt, fail in certain others from which it could be discovered that they did not act from knowledge, but solely from the disposition of their organs."[19]

History and Theoretical Foundations

The modern foundations of AI trace back to Alan Turing's, "On Computable Numbers, with an Application to the *Entscheidungproblem* (1936)," which proposed the theoretical foundations of a "universal computing machine," or a single computer capable of solving many difference types of calculations.[20] Turing's "bombe," the mechanical device employed to decipher German Enigma-encrypted communications in World War II, required substantial manual input by a human operator, rendering it unsuitable for general computation. However, the bombe's limitations inspired Turing to ponder if machines could eventually "think" and learn from experiences to solve complicated problems.[21] Significant advances in computing, including the advent of the silicon transistor and integrated computing chips as well as the emergence of early programming languages (e.g., COBAL, LISP), occurred over the next 20 years.[22] In 1956, Arthur Samuel, an IBM engineer, unveiled a checkers-playing program for the IBM 701 on national television, providing proof of concept as to the ability for machines to acquire and re-apply knowledge to specific tasks.[23]

Dartmouth convened a two-month workshop in the summer of 1956 to explore the newly named field of "artificial intelligence" or "the conjecture that every aspect of learning or any other feature of intelligence can in principle be so precisely described that a machine can be made to simulate it."[24] In the decade following the Dartmouth workshop, enthusiasm for AI remained high, buoyed by substantial funding from the U.S. Department of Defense, specifically the Defense Advanced Research Projects Agency (DARPA), which hoped to conscript intelligent machines to automate translation of Russian texts to English for an advantage in the Cold War.[25] In 1973, on behalf of the British Science Research Council, Sir James Lighthill published a report criticizing the state of American and British AI. He noted that early successes on relatively "simple" challenges heightened expectations for similar progress on complex projects, but that "in no part of the field have discoveries made so far produced the major impact that was then promised."[26] The report exacerbated existing pessimism within and toward the field. Funding fell drastically from government sources, leading to a stagnation of interest, precipitating the first AI "winter."[27]

In the 1970 and 1980s, commercial successes with "expert systems," or rules-based decision software, prompted renewed interest in AI. The eXpert CONfigurer (or XCON) developed by Carnegie Mellon University in 1978 for the Digital Equipment Corporation inspired widespread emulation.[28] XCON assisted customers by automatically ordering all of the parts associated with their desired computer configurations. Previously, components were ordered separately, resulting in frequent errors and lost profits from customer refunds. XCON saved DEC an estimated $25 million per year by the mid-1980s.[29] Expert systems generated excitement in healthcare as well. Among the first health expert systems was MYCIN, a system constructed of approximately 600 rules to assist clinicians with antibiotic selection.[30]

While able to generate impressive results, expert systems suffered from knowledge acquisition bottlenecks, as capturing specific domain knowledge for rule building necessitated interviews with experts and manual compilation of rules, a time-consuming process.[31] Regardless of red flags, research and industry pursued expert systems with fervor, investing considerable funds to build specialized computers to optimally run the systems. The arrival of the personal computer reduced enthusiasm for expensive proprietary hardware. By the early 1990s, the field entered a second winter with AI a verboten term in funding applications.

In the late-2000s, several shifts in the technological landscape sparked renewed enthusiasm for AI. First, computing capacity increased exponentially. In 1965, Gordon Moore, co-founder of Intel, remarked that the density of silicon transistors appeared to double every year (later amended to every two years) with concurrent reductions in cost.[32] Known as Moore's law, the phenomenon drove advancements in the performance of central processing units (CPUs) at a linear rate until approximately 2010.[33] Parallel processing and distributed computing, the splitting of a task across multiple processors or networked computers, respectively, afforded further performance enhancements.[34] The repurposing of graphics processing units (GPUs), to data science is a more recent milestone.[35] GPUs were originally designed to accelerate rendering of video game graphics and contain thousands of processing cores, whereas even the most powerful and cutting-edge of CPUs contains no more than a few dozen. While more abundant, GPU cores lag behind CPU cores in speed and sophistication.

However, by operating in parallel, GPUs can significantly accelerate tasks that require myriad simultaneous simple calculations, while CPUs remain appropriate for more complex computation. These advances in computing performance enabled the application of more complex algorithms to larger datasets, improving the accuracy and speed of results.

The second major technological shift occurred with the maturation of the Internet. In the past, AI research was largely siloed in computer science and engineering departments as other disciplines lacked the necessary resources and programming expertise to readily adapt this methodology to their investigations. Faster data transfer speeds and lessening service and data storage costs popularized cloud-based storage and computing. Cloud-based infrastructures enabled projects to scale resources to a given project, reducing the overhead associated with maintaining dedicated equipment. Concurrently, increasing availability of open-source tools significantly lowered the technical barriers to entry into the field.[36] The democratization of AI broadened its use in a wider variety of contexts, increasing the community invested in the endurance of the field.

Finally, a plethora of data is now available for training models. Nearly every aspect of daily life is now digitized. New communication tools have also emerged, such as social media. In the biological and health sciences, reduced costs of large-scale data acquisition (e.g., genome sequencing, imaging) and the transition to electronic documentation is further contributing to a virtually unchecked data proliferation. Processors, sensors, and wireless networking components have grown ever smaller, faster, and cheaper, enabling numerous Internet-capable devices, ranging from sophisticated wearables (e.g., Apple watch) to everyday objects (e.g., lightbulbs).[37] Known collectively as the internet of things, these devices continuously capture, store, and disseminate data. The number of internet of things devices is anticipated to exceed 75 billion by 2025.[38]

According to economist Klaus Schwab, we are on the verge of the Fourth Industrial Revolution, which will see a rise in cyber-physical systems that blur "the lines between the physical, digital, and biological spheres."[39] Virtual reality environments, brain-computing interfaces, wearable or implantable devices, and mobile applications will continue to contribute to the current data explosion. Automated, high-throughput analysis is essential to extracting timely and actionable insights from this data. AI is no longer a novelty, but a requisite set of tools for navigating the "digital revolution."

Subtypes

The historical gold standard for intelligence is *human* intelligence. However, many existing intelligent agents have surpassed humans in knowledge capacity, computational ability, and information processing speed. Systems that synthesize copious amounts of data to execute a single or narrow range of tasks, such as pattern or anomaly detection, are known as artificial narrow intelligence (ANI).[40] ANI is already ubiquitous in the background of daily life, from catching fraudulent credit charges to freeing email inboxes from spam. ANI such as Google's AlphaGo and IBM's DeepBlue are considered "reactive machines," lack the ability to form or employ memories. All decision-making is based on the current information available (e.g., configuration of the game pieces). Virtual semi-autonomous assistants such as Siri and Alexa as well as self-driving vehicles are "limited memory" agents, capable of continuously monitoring the environment and employing information about the recent past to make decisions (e.g., positions of other cars, road markings).

Systems capable of the full range of human intelligence, known as artificial general intelligence (AGI), are currently hypothetical.[41] The prominent distinction from ANI is the ability of AGI to generalize or flexibly adapt and apply knowledge from different domains and experiences to complete any task. Among the oldest and most frequently cited tests of AGI is Turing's Imitation Game, otherwise known as the Turing Test.[42] In the game, a human and a machine converse blindly with a human evaluator, who poses questions to each participant. If the machine is able to "pass" as human for the majority of the test, it wins the game. Critics argue the test is invalid as mimicry without genuine intelligence is theoretically sufficient to pass.[43] In 2010, Apple co-founder Steve Wosniak suggested a better test of intelligence would be for an AGI to enter an unknown home and "make me a cup of coffee."[44] He contended that this assesses a broader, if not the full, range of human intelligence tasks.

The necessity—or desirability—of consciousness, sentience, sapience, or emotion in AGI is debated.[45] The technological singularity is a hypothesized point in the future in which AGI develop recursive self-improvement, resulting in an uncontrolled "intelligence explosion" that generates an artificial superintelligence that exceeds humans in every capacity. A 2012 survey of AI experts predicted a 90% chance of the realization of AGI by 2075 with the singularity anticipated to occur no more than 30 years later.[46] AGI and artificial superintelligence remain in the realm of science fiction, in no small part due to Moravec's paradox, an observation described by AI researcher Hans Moravec in his book, *Mind Children*. Per Moravec, tasks that humans find difficult, such as mathematics, are relatively easy to program, while seemingly simple, innate tasks, such as walking, are computationally difficult.[47] He offered the following as explanation: "The deliberate process we call reasoning is, I believe, the thinnest veneer of human thought, effective only because it is supported by this much older and much more powerful, though usually unconscious, sensorimotor knowledge."[47]

Methods

AI integrates knowledge from myriad disciplines, including computer science, data science, mathematics, engineering, physics, statistics, linguistics, signal processing, ethics, and philosophy. The term *AI* is often used interchangeably with its methods and applications, generating confusion. Figure 11.1 illustrates the relationship between contributing disciplines, core methods, and common applications.

Machine Learning

Machine learning (ML) is the ability for a computer to iteratively learn from data to improve its efficiency and accuracy on a problem without explicit instructions.[48] Per ML expert Tom Mitchell, "a computer program is said to learn from experience *E*

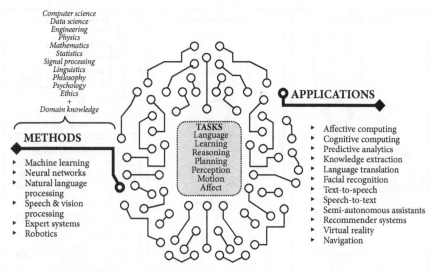

Computer science
Data science
Engineering
Physics
Mathematics
Statistics
Signal processing
Linguistics
Philosophy
Psychology
Ethics
+
Domain knowledge

METHODS

▸ Machine learning
▸ Neural networks
▸ Natural language
  processing
▸ Speech & vision
  processing
▸ Expert systems
▸ Robotics

TASKS
Language
Learning
Reasoning
Planning
Perception
Motion
Affect

APPLICATIONS

▸ Affective computing
▸ Cognitive computing
▸ Predictive analytics
▸ Knowledge extraction
▸ Language translation
▸ Facial recognition
▸ Text-to-speech
▸ Speech-to-text
▸ Semi-autonomous assistants
▸ Recommender systems
▸ Virtual reality
▸ Navigation

Figure 11.1 Artificial intelligence domains, core methods, and applications. Artificial intelligence is comprised of novel methods derived from numerous disciplines to accomplish tasks related to human intelligence.

with respect to some class of tasks T and performance measure P if its performance at tasks in T, as measured by P, improves with experience E."[49] There are three broad categories of ML techniques (Figure 11.2). In supervised learning, the task is prediction, either of a categorical (classification) or continuous outcome (regression). The learning algorithm is supplied with a set of training data in which there are a number of independent predictive features (e.g., age, ethnicity, gender) and the labeled dependent outcome of interest (e.g., responders versus nonresponder) labeled for each observation. The algorithm will then "study" the training data to optimize which combination of features and model parameters yields the highest predictive accuracy. In unsupervised learning, the learning algorithm is supplied with unlabeled data and searches for underlying patterns or trends in the features among the included observations. A common example is clustering, or the subgrouping of observations such that the observations in a subgroup or more similar than those in another. In re-enforcement learning, the algorithm learns by trial and error to maximize a notion of a cumulative reward. The algorithm will take actions toward the indicated goal (e.g., win a game of chess), receiving feedback as to the reward associated with each action. The numerous learning algorithm types (e.g., decision trees, support vector machines) are beyond the scope of this chapter.

ML enables the rapid synthesis of massive quantities of data and identification of subtle patterns that might otherwise elude human detection. The focus of classical inferential statistics is to describe the relationship between predictive factors and a designated outcome within a single set of data. While the resultant equation may be employed for prediction, the accuracy of the prediction is unlikely to be robust when applied to new data. ML seeks to enable repeatable predictions in new, unseen data

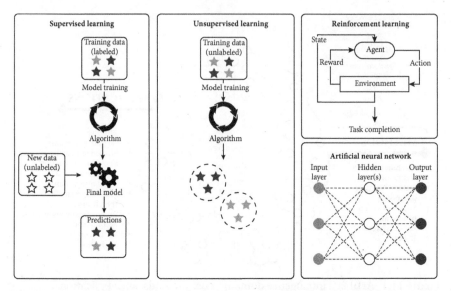

Figure 11.2 Machine learning methods. The core machine learning methods include supervised learning, in which the learning algorithm (e.g., decision tree, support vector machine) is supplied with a set of training data with predictive features and a labeled outcome of interest. The process of model building involves the algorithm mapping the best solution between the features and outcome. The final trained model may then be applied to new, unseen, unlabeled data to make predictions. In unsupervised learning, the algorithms searches for the underlying patterns or trends within the data. A simple example is clustering, in which the algorithm divides observations into subgroups, striving for maximal similarity among the observations within a subgroup. Reinforcement learning enables an algorithm to learn the optimal solution to a designated task by undertaking actions and assessing each action's impact a notion of reward (trial and error). Artificial neural networks are an advanced type of learning technique modeled after the biological neuron. The network learns by mapping the relationships between the inputs and desired output, performing iterative adjustments to internal parameters to maximize accuracy. Deep learning involves the use of neural network with more than one hidden layer of information processing. Neural networks may be used for supervised and unsupervised machine learning tasks.

with less concern regarding the relationship between variables and outcomes; however, some inference is still possible. Whereas traditional predictive modeling restricts the number of predictive features for inclusion to avoid overfitting, in ML, automated feature selection techniques enable all possible features to be considered with the algorithm penalizing or excluding irrelevant features.

Artificial Neural Networks

Artificial neural networks (ANNs) are a ML technique loosely modeled after biological neurons that may be employed for supervised and unsupervised learning tasks.[50] The network is composed of two primary layers—an input layer (features) and an output layer (predictions). A simple ANN will have one hidden layer for additional information processes, where as "deep learning," involves the use of ANNs with multiple hidden layers. Learning involves the mapping of the relationships between the inputs and desired output with iterative adjustment of internal model weights (connected edges between neurons) to improve accuracy. ANNs are well-suited to detecting unseen and nonlinear relationships between a large number of inputs and the outcome of interest. ANNs also tolerate a high degree of heteroskedasticity (volatility and nonconstant variance) in data. Together, these properties make ANN a powerful solution for the irregularity of real-world data and highly complex tasks, such as image classification and voice recognition.[51] However, ANNs are a bit of a "black box," as the precise learning steps occurring in the hidden layers are difficult to interpret.

Natural Language Processing

Natural language processing (NLP) studies how computers comprehend, process, and communicate in human language.[52] NLP models employ ML and deep learning algorithms on the word features extracted from a digested text to learn its underlying formal grammar (syntax) and meaning (semantics). NLP can be employed to quickly extract meaning from volumes of unstructured written texts. Subtasks can include labeling key entities (named entity recognition), determining the predominant themes (topic modeling), or assessing the underlying tone or emotion of the text (sentiment analysis). NLP is among the hardest of AI techniques due to the ambiguity of human language. Applications range from language translation to chatbots. The latter are an excellent example of the complexity and breadth of tasks that NLP seeks to accomplish. When a chatbot receives a question from a user, it must deconstruct the text to deduce the user's meaning, extract the factual information for the response from its knowledge base, and then construct an intelligible reply.

Speech and Vision Processing

Speech and vision processing involves capturing, interpreting, and manipulating auditory and visual digital signals.[53,54] Such signals possess numerous informative features that vary in time and space with impact on interpretation of the content. Examples of speech and vision processing are pervasive in daily life, particularly in interacting with mobile devices. Speech recognition is the manner of input into semiautonomous helper agents such as Siri and Alexa. The agent must capture the spoken signal, deconstruct the analog signal to discrete words, then employ NLP to determine the underlying request content and formulate a sensical response, and finally map the response back into an auditory signal for replying to the user. Facial recognition follows a similarly complex processing pathway that involves multiple ML and NLP subtasks.

Expert Systems

Expert systems are designed to solve problems by mimicking the human decision-making process, which is deductive (Figure 11.2).[55] The systems are composed of two parts—a knowledge base and an inference system. The knowledge base is a collection of factual and heuristic data supplied by domain experts or extracted from reliable sources and organized as "IF-THEN-ELSE" logic. To recommend a solution, the inference engine will evaluate all facts and apply available rules to the question at hand to produce an answer for the user. Expert systems are advantageous in improving efficiency for repeated, clearly defined problems. While the system can be continuously updated with the latest studies and best practices to remain current, this process must be done manually. Additionally, expert systems lack "common sense." As noted by AI expert John McCarthy, "this lack makes them "brittle." ... They are difficult to extend beyond the scope originally contemplated by their designers, and they usually don't recognize their own limitations."[56] When presented with outlier cases, the system will follow its internal logic to a solution, even one that does not make sense.

Fuzzy Logic

Computational logic is typically Boolean, a type of algebraic reasoning that combines data with "AND-OR-NOT" operators."[57] Inputs and outputs are precise, carrying absolute truth or falseness (e.g., 0 or 1). Fuzzy logic, by contrast, better resembles human reasoning as inputs and outputs may take on imprecise or continuous values (i.e., variable degrees of truth or falseness). Fuzzy logic tolerates the noisiness and complexity of real-world data. While relatively simple to construct and interpret, such models are inappropriate for tasks that require high accuracy.

Robotics

Robotics encompasses all of the mechanical, electrical, and software components that enable control of an AI system and dictate its interactions and manipulation of the surrounding environment.[58] For intelligence machines, AI is the "brain" to a "body" supplied by robotics. Of note, not all robots are intelligent. For example, a simple robot may be programmed to transport objects from point A to point B and will continue to do so until interrupted, albeit with variable precision. If equipped with sensors and a learning algorithm, an intelligent robot can "see" and place each object accurately, stopping when it detects that no more objects are present.

Cognitive and Affective Computing

No hard delineation exists between AI methods and applications. Cognitive and affective computing are often considered philosophically distinct from AI due to differences in intent and downstream application. IBM defines cognitive computing as "systems that learn at scale, reason with purpose and interact with humans naturally."[59] Cognitive computing uses AI methods to learn and mimic human reasoning to augment the decision-making process.[60] AI, by contrast, may supersede human capabilities in information synthesis and analysis to pinpoint the best solution to a problem. The best solution as determined by an algorithm, however, may be incorrect or even harmful in practice. Advocates of cognitive computing contend that their approach enables users to leverage the power, speed, and precision of ML without concern for autonomous decision-making. The system provides data-driven guidance, but the final decision is the responsibility of the human user.

Affective computing, often referred to as artificial emotional intelligence, seeks to use AI subsystems to recognize and simulate human affect in order to enrich interactivity between humans and intelligent machines.[61] Cameras, microphones, and sensors passively collect visual, auditory, and physiological data from the user. ML enables extraction of the informative features from this data, enabling classification of the user's emotional state, information that may influence how the system responds to the user. For example, the system may simulate empathy if a user appears or sounds distressed. For an extensive treatment as to the advantages and drawbacks of affective computing, please see the corresponding Chapter 21 in this book.

Benefits of Artificial Intelligence for Mental Health

Improved Data Quality for Exploratory and Predictive Analyses

Harmonization of Disparate Data Sets

Data harmonization involves creating a single consistent macro-data source from multiple, potentially disparate micro datasets. Contributing datasets are structured to remove inconsistencies, creating "harmony," such that the final dataset provides a cohesive view of a subject from many different perspectives. ML enables automatization of this process, permitting integration of clinical, behavioral, -omic, imaging, neurosignals, and other datatypes for data mining and predictive modeling.[62] For example, Squeglia et al. trained a model with demographic, neuropsychological, and magnetic resonance imaging (MRI) data from 12- to 14-year-old subjects to predict development of alcohol abuse by age 18. The model performed with an accuracy of 74% with 34 predictive features, including male gender, higher socioeconomic status, positive alcohol expectancies, worsening executive functioning, thinner cortices, and less observed brain activation.[63] Deep learning in combination with multidimensional biological data (e.g., genomics, proteomics) enables examination of the full portrait of the impact of genetic variation or other system disturbances on transcription, translation, signaling, and resultant phenotypic variation.[64] Such approaches could assist in achieving interoperability between RDoC-based dimensions and practical diagnostic criteria, furthering progression toward the unrealized goal of precision psychiatry.

Automated Organization of Unstructured Data

NLP enables automated data extraction and labeling of unstructured free text, such as clinical notes and social media posts. Manual curation of unstructured data is resource-intensive but also prone to subjectivity, requiring additional individuals to review to minimize interoperator variability. Structured data, such as inputted diagnoses and medications, can be validated against free text. For example, if a patient is diagnosed with bipolar, the free text may be analyzed for confirmatory terms, such as sleep difficulties and prior receipt of mood stabilizers. This workflow can automate selection of potential candidates for research recruitment with improved homogeneity of desired diagnoses or other traits. For example, Geraci et al. generated a set of 861 free-text outpatient clinical notes spanning 366 patients labeled by two psychiatrists to train a deep learning model to phenotype psychiatric diagnoses from note language to identify suitable candidates for a study on depression in youth.[65] NLP is also effective in de-identifying clinical data at scale, a common barrier to access for secondary analysis.[66]

Illness Subtyping

Unsupervised learning tasks, such as clustering, are helpful for identifying potentially important signatures related to a desired phenotype. For instance, Doshi-Velez et al. employed hierarchical clustering on ICD codes extracted from the medical records of subjects with autism spectrum disorder (ASD) to identify the most common medical comorbidities. Four subgroups were identified, the largest of which was characterized by seizures (77.5% subgroup prevalence).[67] Liston et al. employed clustering with functional MRI in patients with depression to define four neurophysiological subtypes distinguished by limbic and frontostriatal network dysfunction.[68]

Improved Biomarker Identification

Biomarker identification is the most prevalent use of ML in neuroscience mental health research.[69] Lin et al. trained a deep learning network using single nucleotide polymorphisms (SNPs) to predict antidepressant response in major depressive disorder. None of the 4,241,701 SNPs were significantly associated with treatment response as assessed by standard statistical analysis. However, deep learning generated a model of approximately two dozen features that together could accurately predict treatment response.[70] Nicodemus et al. investigated genetic interactions between promising candidate susceptibility genes in a schizophrenia case-control study. Using a prediction classifier, the group tested for gene epistasis, finding seven SNPs with four significant interactions. Three of the four interactions were validated by functional MRI and predicted cortical insufficiency in the n-back task, a schizophrenia-linked phenotype.[71]

Less Restrictive Modeling of Large-Scale Data

Classical inferential statistics is limited in the number of features that can be incorporated into the analysis without overfitting. The selection of features for inclusion is often dependent on what the user or the field considers important, creating bias and risking hidden confounders. A recent meta-analysis of suicide studies found that 80% of the risk factors tested were encompassed by five broad categories.[72] ML affords the ability to consider all available factors and automatization of feature selection can remove the user and potential bias from the model building process. For example, Kessler et al. developed an actuarial risk model predicting suicide in the 12 months following inpatient hospitalization in US veterans using five years of administrative data converged from 38 Army/Department of Defense systems across 53,769 hospitalizations and 68 suicides. Investigators included 421 features in the model, employing penalized techniques to exclude those features of low predictive value. The final fitted model included sociodemographic features (male, enlistment at age 27+, Armed Forces Qualification Test score), access to firearms, crime perpetration, prior suicidality, prior psychiatric treatment, and hospitalization reason.[73]

Expanded Repertoire of Monitoring and Intervention Options

New Methods for Public Health Surveillance

Finding more naturalistic ways of monitoring public health can facilitate prevention efforts. The rise of social media and other Internet-based forums has generated massive repositories of unstructured data capturing discussions on the entire spectrum of mental health topics. ML/NLP can facilitate "digital epidemiology." For example, Chary et al. collected 3.6 million publicly available Twitter posts from 2012 to 2014 and used NLP to characterize tweets mentioning prescription opioid misuse. Extracted location data permitted estimation of the location of each tweet. The resultant geographical distribution performed comparably to the 2013–2015 National Surveys on Drug Usage and Health.[74] Nikfarjam et al. used an unsupervised deep learning model to extract language about adverse drug reactions from over one million social media posts (Twitter, DailyStrength). The model learned the context of the drug-related words and mapped these to representative vectors. The clustered vectors were found to contain words of a similar semantic type (e.g., drug names, dosages, symptoms), permitting estimation of the prevalence of known and unknown drug side effects.[75]

Real-Time, Continuous Monitoring and Intervention

Mobile and sensor technologies support ecological momentary assessment, or the repeated sampling of an individual's behaviors and emotional state in real time in his or her own environment.[76] Context-sensitive data may assist in the development of just-in-time interventions for situations otherwise difficult to capture, such as the transition from suicidal ideation to attempt and cravings to substance use relapse. Data generated from mobile applications and wearable sensors contains up to hundreds of features measured continuously, a volume and complexity of data that outpaces traditional analysis. For example, Burns et al. provided depressed subjects with a mobile application that collected 38 sensor features, including GPS, ambient light, and phone usage. The application periodically prompted users to self-report their emotional state and used this as labeled data to train a predictive classifier. Users could access an associated website for tailored didactics and behavioral activation tools. Subjects improved significantly over the course of eight weeks with a remission rate of 85.7%.[77] Wahle et al.'s application collected 120 features, which, in combination with biweekly self-reported PHQ-9 scores, permitted prediction of depression and determined the delivery of a tailored cognitive-behavioral therapy intervention via ML prediction. After eight weeks, depressed subjects demonstrated a significant reduction in PHQ-9 scores.[78] Bae et al. piloted an application that employed 20 sensor datapoints and self-reported alcohol consumption using a random forest classifier to stratify low- to high-risk drinking. High-risk drinking could be predicted with 90.9%

accuracy. The most informative sensor features were time, movement, device usages, and communication.[79]

Automating the Mental Status Exam

Facial and voice recognition models can permit detection of mental state, including intensity. In situations where the patient is not forthcoming as to symptoms or refuses to speak with a clinician, an automated exam could still occur. Bedi et al. treated healthy volunteers with MDMA, methamphetamine, or placebo and asked subjects to speak about a person of importance in their life for approximately 10 minutes. The audio transcripts were analyzed using syntactical and semantic analysis to determine topological structure and topic differences. A classifier trained on these features discriminated between MDMA intoxication and placebo with 88% accuracy as well as MDMA and methamphetamine intoxication with 84% accuracy.[80] ML may also assist in refining current psychometric inventories.[81] Wall et al. used a classifier to predict ASD from healthy controls using the Autism Diagnostic Observation Schedule-Generic (ADOS) and found that only eight of nine items were necessary to achieve 100% accuracy. The final model performed at nearly 100% sensitivity in two independent cohorts.[82]

Improved Access to Care

Resource-Limited Screening

If diagnostic model requires expensive or time-consuming-to-generate biomarkers for accuracy, its feasibility for use across a range of clinical contexts and resource levels is questionable. Developing alternative models that use readily available clinical data or easily obtained on-the-spot measures (e.g., speech analysis), permits portability. This does not obviate the more complex model. Simplified models could be used as fast preliminary screens with borderline cases escalated to more refined measures. Where early diagnosis is critical to treatment outcomes, such as ASD and schizophrenia, widespread screening would be highly beneficial. Bedi et al. assessed 34 youths at risk for the development of psychosis and followed the subjects for 2.5 years. Baseline free speech interviews were transcribed for semantic and syntactic analysis. A classifier trained on the word features outperformed the Structured Interview for Prodromal Syndromes/Scale of Prodromal Symptoms scores in predicting transition to psychosis (100% vs. 33% accuracy).[83] Liu et al. trained a classifier on eye movement data derived during a face recognition task in children to predict ASD to an accuracy of 88.5%.[84]

New Ways to Intervene and Deliver Care

Generating cost-effective alternative avenues to access mental health treatment is essential, particularly for those who would not otherwise seek assistance due to stigma or other factors. Modern life is now intrinsically intertwined with technology and the Internet. Some individuals may feel more comfortable divulging sensitive information to a non-human agent. Darcy et al. reported that college students with self-identified anxiety and depression, who used Woebot, a fully automated conversational agent for the delivery of a two-week program of cognitive behavioral therapy, demonstrated substantial improvements.[85] In similar fashion, some individuals may be more responsive to an anonymized intervention and offer of service, such as when search engines present crisis information to those searching topics related to suicide. Passive surveillance of social media data presents challenges in relation to privacy rights and responsibility for intervention.[86] Passive surveillance raises can also use images or video. For example, Reece et al. analyzed 43,950 Instagram photos from 166 individuals and collected depression data using surveys through Amazon's Mechanical Turk (MTurk), a crowd-sourcing platform. A classifier trained on facial features outperformed human raters in predicting depression.[87]

Improved Treatment Selection

ML models can assist with treatment selection through prediction of response. For instance, Chekroud et al. trained a model using a subset of data from the Sequenced Treatment Alternatives to Relieve Depression (STAR*D) trial to predict antidepressant response.[88] The model included 25 patient-report features and achieved an accuracy of 64.6% in predicting treatment response in unseen cases. Shortreed et al. employed reinforcement learning and Clinical Antipsychotic Trials of Intervention Effectiveness (CATIE) data to build a model to recommend antipsychotic treatment using a low Positive and Negative Syndrome Scale score as the "reward."[89] "Smart" recommender systems, compared to older rules-based expert systems, can continuously update predictive models with new findings. Such systems can assist primary care providers in preliminary treatment selection and prioritize need for referral to specialty care to complex or refractory patients.

Quality Improvement

Reduced Variability in Clinical Documentation

Speech-to-text dictation software already assists clinicians with reducing documentation time. However, in the near future, clinical documentation may be generated in real-time by a virtual assistant that extracts important features from the physician–patient dialogue via NLP. Entity recognition could enable population of the appropriate record fields with the pertinent data, such as current symptoms, past psychiatric history, current medications and side effects.[90] Data included are then no longer in the hands of the time-pressed clinician, and the missingness or irregularity of EMR data improves. Time saved could be used for psychoeducation or addressing patient concerns.

Monitoring of Treatment Quality

Objective measures for assessing the quality of psychotherapy delivery would be beneficial. Training in psychotherapy relies on a supervision model that is resource intensive. Blackwell et al. used a deep learning classifier to analyze therapist language from the transcripts of 90,000 hours of Internet-enabled cognitive-behavioral therapy. The data revealed that increased quantities of change methods language on the part of the therapist resulted in consistent improvements in patient symptoms, whereas a high degree of nontherapy related content demonstrated poor response.[91] AI-based supervision of psychotherapeutic interventions could permit real-time feedback to the providers, enabling skill progression and generate immediate improvement for the patient.

Implicit bias, or associations outside of conscious awareness that negatively impact a clinician's evaluation of a patient based on factors such as gender or race, is a known contributor to disparities in healthcare.[92] Investigating implicit bias in physician behavior is difficult as highly dependent on anonymous surveys or small-scale documentation review. NLP, however, offers an efficient pipeline for digesting and scoring clinical documentation to highlight clinician-level issues. For instance, McCoy et al. performed sentiment analysis on 2,484 free-text discharge notes for 2,010 individuals from a psychiatric inpatient unit, as well as 20,859 hospital discharges for 15,011 individuals from general medical units from a three-year period. Higher positive discharge sentiment was associated with significantly decreased risk for re-admission not explainable by differences in diagnosis. Public insurance additionally associated with diminished positive sentiment in psychiatric but not medical discharge notes.[93] As with psychotherapy monitoring, clinical scoring feedback can assist physicians in continuous learning.

Barriers to Implementation of Artificial Intelligence in Mental Health

Numerous technical and ethical considerations exist in implementing AI/ML in mental health. ML models are reliant upon the quantity and quality of labeled training data, which can be costly and time-consuming to produce. Optimization of a model on poor quality training data may result in a model that fails to generalize to new data sets. Training data may also be inherently biased, yielding biased models.[94] For example, an important step in preprocessing data for ML model building is to examine the amount of missing values for each feature in the training data and consider the reasons for missingness. Values may be missing completely at random or a significant relationship may exist between a feature and its tendency to be missing (e.g., reported income in disadvantaged populations). Removing observations with missing data can thus skew the resultant predictions and bias against an absent population. In NLP, text-based models have shown a tendency to adopt the biases of the text authors that must be controlled to avoid propagation of systematic inequalities.[95]

There is often a sacrifice between model accuracy and interpretability, the latter largely dictates trust in implementation, particularly in clinical decision-making. Each ML learning algorithm confers advantages and disadvantages that dictate an algorithm's sensitivity to outliers and missing data, speed, accuracy, and interpretability. Too often, however, algorithm selection is arbitrary or biased toward the model that produces the highest accuracy. Standards in the reporting and validation of ML models are notably lacking, although under active discussion.[96] For example, external validation of predictive ML models, or application of an ML model to a data set not using in training, is rare. Cross-validation, or the holding back of a subset of the training data set for internal validation is more common, but inconsistently employed. Due to the rise of tools for automating ML model building and optimization, there is a heightened need for multidisciplinary tram to review manuscripts and grants to ensure methodological rigor.

The degree to which AI systems will be permitted to perform autonomously in the future is unclear. Higher degrees of autonomy require thoughtful solutions to problems related to the current insensitivity of ML algorithms to the real-world consequences of solutions.[97] Reinforcement algorithms searching for optimal solutions to a task may engage in "unsafe exploration," in which the algorithm makes dangerous choices to increase its learning. In the case of mobile applications with real-time tailoring of interventions, empowering the algorithm to make an automated decision is critical. How such decisions should be audited is unclear. Furthermore, when and how clinicians overrule the recommendations of a system required consideration. If a clinician fails to overrule an incorrect decision, to what extent is he or she liable for the action or expected to possess competence in the advanced technology at play?[98]

Clinician Training and Workforce Development

Consider the following case scenario. Ms. B, a 25-year-old female with a history of depression, presents for an urgent outpatient follow-up appointment. On examination, she exhibits pressured, hyperverbal speech and elevated affect, reporting new insomnia and impulsive spending. Dr. C suspects bipolar disorder and notes that his medication guide system, PsychotroSelect®, suggests initiation of olanzapine and lithium. Dr. C hesitates due to her known history of unsuccessful suicide attempts on prescribed and over-the-counter medications. However, Dr. C is also cognizant of the substantial literature supporting the use of lithium for suicide risk reduction that he assumes informs PsychotroSelect®'s guidance. However, he is unclear as to precisely what data the system employs to render a recommendation.

Would Dr. C be justified in overruling the algorithm? Would he be liable for prescribing lithium if Ms. B died by overdose? Would he be liable for not prescribing lithium if Ms. B later died by suicide by another means? What if he were to select an alternative mood stabilizer to which she develops a severe adverse reaction?

In considering the ethical and legal implications of AI in clinical practice, excitement tends to drive the discussion to the imagined extreme—virtual or robotic clinicians delivering autonomous care. The more immediate scenario is that of the case above. In 2017, MD Anderson discontinued use of IBM Watson for Oncology, a cognitive computing system for cancer treatment selection, dissatisfied with the poor quality of the system's treatment recommendations. In total, MD Anderson spent three years and upwards of $60 million before declaring the effort exhausted.[99] Watson struggled in reliable extraction of information from the hospital's EMRs. Additionally, the same issue that historically plagued expert systems in business re-emerged—insufficient quantity of training data.

The success of AI/ML in clinical practice is contingent on skilled clinician–system interaction. Incorporation of AI/ML recommendations into informed consent requires that clinicians understand a system's fundamental methodology, its limitations, and how to interpret an output for the patient during the informed consent process. The situation is similar to that posed in recent years by the rising popularity of pharmacogenomic testing. While grounded in familiar biological concepts, full understanding of the limitations of such assays, including assessment of clinical outcomes, requires a breadth of knowledge in genomics, pharmacodynamics, and statistics beyond that acquired during routine medical training. Among the critical barriers to the use of pharmacogenomic testing, advanced genomics education has been cited as a pressing area for remediation.[100] In 2005, the International Society of Pharmacogenomics called for increased coverage of pharmacogenomics in the curricula of medical and pharmaceutical training programs.[101]

Despite increasing reliance on digital tools in clinical practice, educational requirements for medical school have changed little in the last 20 to 30 years. Medical schools typically require a year of college-level mathematics, preferably a semester of calculus and a semester of statistics, although few enforce this as a set requirement. No medical schools require multivariable calculus. The laxity is curious, particularly given the push toward evidence-based medicine over the last 20 years.[102] A study of medicine residents found that while 95% believe that evidence-based clinical practice is important, less than 25% were confident in fully understanding the statistics reported in journals.[103] The level of understanding required to answer standardized test questions on research study design or statistics is static across training levels. The same depth and difficulty of questions may be found on the Medical College Admission Test (MCAT) as the United States Medical Licensing Examinations (USMLE) and specialty-specific board certification exams.[104–106] The current system neither requires nor encourages a progression.

A re-alignment is long overdue between state of practice and the content of corresponding premedical, medical, and residency/fellowship curricula. Longitudinal incorporation of data science principles into the medical curricula are already belated given the widespread implementation of the EMR. Clinicians are simultaneous curators and consumers of EMR data; however, data management is only covered as an afterthought in relation to patient privacy the Health Insurance Portability and Accountability Act. The quality of insights derived from EMR data is directly related to the quality of data.[107] This is also true of classical inferential statistics but is a particular hurdle to AI/ML models. No matter how poor the training data supplied, an ML algorithm will always produce an optimized solution. Understanding the quality of a training data set used by an algorithm as well as the features informing a prediction substantially furthers the ability to interpret a model, even without detailed mathematical knowledge.

The knowledge base to evaluate AI/ML technology does not require substantial expertise in hardware, specific programming languages, or networking infrastructures. However, statistics, and more broadly data science, can no longer be considered optional curricula. Data science is the field focused on the extraction and manipulation of data, which includes data management and manipulation, algorithms, and statistics. The distinction between data science and major areas of data-driven health and medical research is largely semantic and delineated on the basis of content, not methodology. Data science with a biological focus is bioinformatics, with a clinical focus, clinical informatics, and with a population-level focus, epidemiology. Implementing data science as a core component of training along with discussion of related ethical and legal issues provides a solid foundation for navigating modern clinical practice and eases subspecialization, if desired. Currently, if a psychiatry resident wishes to pursue computational research, this may require substantial additional training to remediate in these areas. Increased emphasis on data science fundamentals can reduce the gap and encourages the interested to pursue research at any stage of training. Implementing such a framework necessitates recruitment of faculty from multiple disciplines. Developing the ability to communicate across disciplines is not only inherently important to modern clinical practice, but essential to truly impactful convergence research.

Data science is readily incorporated and assessed within the current longitudinal training framework. The MCAT may include material from introductory statistics, otherwise known as descriptive statistics. Premedical students should be able to readily describe the strengths and flaws of a data set and challenges this may pose on further analysis. The first two years of medical school may then focus on developing skills in inferential statistics, enabling facility in interpreting odds ratios, confidence intervals, and significance testing using real-world data. Prior to a trainee ever touching an EMR, information science principles should be instilled, including an appreciation for how data quality impacts the subsequent extraction of meaningful insights. Rather than contain this training to a single isolated block of teaching, incorporation where relevant in each preclinical course would better solidify these skills. Statistical critique of landmark studies reinforces not only specific clinical knowledge but fosters familiarity with the data science mindset. In the clinical rotation years, priority may transition to hands-on experience with specific AI/ML software packages in practice. In addition to standardized testing on the USMLE Step examinations, completion of a required, longitudinal data-driven research project may additionally help reinforce core principles of data management and analysis. In residency training, in-depth training in specific AI/ML tools in practice may be combined with deeper knowledge acquisition as to methodological considerations inherent to field. The focus should be in developing a systematic, informed approach to the supervision of automated recommendations. Board certification exams may include extended vignette-style, rather than stand-alone questions, to assess the multitude of facets involved in evaluating an ML/AI-based recommendation. For clinicians already in practice, development of online curricula and workshops may assist in closing knowledge gaps with requirements enforced via audit of continuing medical education credits.

The implementation of AI/ML in clinical practice raises concerns as to overreliance resulting in errors of commission (taking the wrong action) or omission (failing to take a necessary action).[108] Automation bias occurs if a human accepts a decision from an autonomous system as correct in deference to its typical pattern of superior performance and ignoring contradictory information, a situation similar to that of the case scenario above. If Ms. B were to present to the emergency department endorsing ongoing suicidal ideation and an autonomous triaging system fails to recommend ordering a lithium level to assess for occult ingestion, this would be considered an error of omission. These scenarios are combated by requiring competent, proactive supervision of AI/ML-based decisions. Future practice may require certification in the use of specific AI/ML-based software in clinical decision-making. Furthermore, clinical documentation may evolve to comparative discussion of the AI/ML-based recommendation versus accepted practice and justification for acceptance or over-rule. Development of standardized assessment metrics accompanying automated recommendations can further assist clinicians in auditing decisions and remaining critically engaged in the decision-making process.

Conclusion

As illustrated in this chapter, AI/ML is advancing mental health research and clinical practice in innumerable ways.[109-111] AI/ML is an especially powerful framework for the integration and analysis of large-scale, multidimensional data. However, AI is not a panacea to every problem in the field. Enthusiasm should be tempered by an appreciation for AI/ML's limitations as well as the technical and ethical complexities of implementation outside of a research environment. Collaboration between AI-associated fields and mental health will be critical to establishing the evidence base necessary for building confidence in AI/ML systems operating in routine clinical care.

References

1. Monteith S, Glenn T, Geddes J, Bauer M. Big data are coming to psychiatry: a general introduction. *International Journal of Bipolar Disorders*. 2015;3(1):21 https://doi.org/10.1186/s40345-015-0038-9.
2. Torous J, Staples P, Onnela J-P. Realizing the potential of mobile mental health: new methods for new data in psychiatry. *Current Psychiatry Reports*. 2015;17(8):61 https://doi.org/10.1007/s11920-015-0602-0.
3. Doherty JL, Owen MJ. Genomic insights into the overlap between psychiatric disorders: implications for research and clinical practice. *Genome Med*. 2014;6(4):29 https://doi.org/10.1186/gm546.
4. Lilienfeld SO, Treadway MT. Clashing diagnostic approaches: DSM–ICD versus RDoC. *Annu Rev Clin Psychol*. 2016;12:435–463 https://doi.org/10.1146/annurev-clinpsy-021815-093122.
5. Head ML, Holman L, Lanfear R, Kahn AT, Jennions MD. The extent and consequences of P-hacking in science. *PloS Biology*. 2015;13(3):e1002106 https://doi.org/10.1371/journal.pbio.1002106.
6. Wasserstein RL, Lazar NA. The ASA statement on P-values: context, process, and purpose. *The American Statistician*. 2016;70(2):129–133 https://doi.org/10.1080/00031305.2016.1154108.
7. Fadista J, Manning AK, Florez JC, Groop L. The (in)famous GWAS P-value threshold revisited and updated for low-frequency variants. *European Journal of Human Genetics*. 2016;24(8):1202–1205 https://doi.org/10.1038/ejhg.2015.269.

8. Border R, Johnson EC, Evans LM, et al. No support for historical candidate gene or candidate gene-by-interaction hypotheses for major depression across multiple large samples. *American Journal of Psychiatry.* 2019;176(5):376–387 https://doi.org/10.1176/appi.ajp.2018.18070881.

9. Arfken CL, Balon R. Declining participation in research studies. *Psychother Psychosom.* 2011;80(6):325–328 https://doi.org/10.1159/000324795.

10. Haapea M, Miettunen J, Veijola J, Lauronen E, Tanskanen P, Isohanni M. Non-participation may bias the results of a psychiatric survey. *Social Psychiatry and Psychiatric Epidemiology.* 2007;42(5):403–409 https://doi.org/10.1007/s00127-007-0178-z.

11. Weiskopf NG, Weng C. Methods and dimensions of electronic health record data quality assessment: enabling reuse for clinical research. *J Am Med Inform Assoc.* 2013;20(1):144–151 https://doi.org/10.1136/amiajnl-2011-000681.

12. Butryn T, Bryant L, Marchionni C, Sholevar F. The shortage of psychiatrists and other mental health providers: Causes, current state, and potential solutions. *Int J Acad Med.* 2017;3(1):5–9.

13. Morse G, Salyers MP, Rollins AL, Monroe-DeVita M, Pfahler C. Burnout in mental health services: a review of the problem and its remediation. *Adm Policy Ment Health.* 2012;39(5):341–352 https://doi.org/10.1007/s10488-011-0352-1.

14. Centers for Disease Control and Prevention. More than a mental health problem. https://www.cdc.gov/vitalsigns/suicide/index.html. Published February 11, 2019. Accessed July 1, 2019.

15. Doraiswamy PM, Blease C, Bodner K. Artificial intelligence and the future of psychiatry: insights from a global physician survey. *Artif Intell Med.* 2020;102:101753 https://doi.org/10.1016/j.artmed.2019.101753.

16. Kalligeropoulos D, Vasileiadou S. The homeric automata and their implementation. In: Paipetis SA, ed. *Science and Technology in Homeric Epics.* Dordrecht, The Netherlands: Springer; 2008:77–84.

17. Mayor A. *Gods and Robots: Myths, Machines, and Ancient Dreams of Technology.* Princeton, NJ: Princeton University Press; 2018.

18. Voskuhl A. *Androids in the Enlightenment: Mechanics, Artisans, and Cultures of the Self.* Chicago: University of Chicago Press; 2013.

19. Descartes R, Veitch J. *Discourse on Method.* New York: Barnes & Noble Books; 2004.

20. Turing AM. On computable numbers, with an application to the Entscheidungsproblem. *Proc London Math Soc.* 1937;s2-42(1):230–265 https://doi.org/10.1112/plms/s2-42.1.230.

21. Turing AM. Computing machinery and intelligence. *Mind.* 1950;59:433–460 https://doi.org/10.1093/mind/lix.236.433.

22. O'Regan G. *A Brief History of Computing.* 2nd ed. London: Springer; 2012.

23. Samuel AL. Some studies in machine learning using the game of checkers. *IBM J Res Dev.* 1959;3(3):210–229 https://doi.org/10.1147/rd.33.0210.

24. John M, Marvin LM, Nathaniel R, Claude ES. A proposal for the Dartmouth summer research project on artificial intelligence, August 31, 1955. *AI Mag.* 2006;27(4).

25. Toma P. Systran as a multilingual machine translation system. Proceedings of the Third European Congress on Information Systems and Networks: Overcoming the Language Barrier; 1977. http://mt-archive.info/CEC-1977-Toma.pdf

26. McCarthy J. Artificial intelligence: a paper symposium: Professor Sir James Lighthill, FRS: artificial intelligence: a general survey. In: Science Research Council, 1973. *Artif Intell.* 1974;5(3):317–322 https://doi.org/10.1016/0004-3702(74)90016-2.

27. Nilsson NJ. *The Quest for Artificial Intelligence: A History of Ideas and Achievements.* Cambridge, UK: Cambridge University Press; 2010.

28. Judith B, John M. R1 revisited: four years in the trenches. *AI Mag.* 1984;5(3).

29. Leonard-Barton D, Sviokla J. Putting Expert Systems to Work. *Harvard Business Review*; March1988. https://hbr.org/1988/03/putting-expert-systems-to-work

30. Buchanan BG, Shortliffe EH. *Rule-Based Expert Systems: The MYCIN Experiments of the Stanford Heuristic Programming Project*. Reading, MA: Addison-Wesley; 1984.

31. Neale IM. First generation expert systems: a review of knowledge acquisition methodologies. *Knowledge Engineering Review*. 1988;3(2):105–145 https://doi.org/10.1017/s0269888900004288.

32. Moore G. Cramming more components onto integrated circuits, Reprinted from Electronics, volume 38, number 8, April 19, 1965, pp.114 ff. *Solid-State Circuits Newsletter, IEEE*. 2006;11:33–35 https://doi.org/10.1109/n-ssc.2006.4785860.

33. Waldrop MM. The chips are down for Moore's law. *Nature*. 2016;530(7589):144–147 https://doi.org/10.1038/530144a.

34. Hwang K, Fox GC, Dongarra JJ. *Distributed and Cloud Computing: From Parallel Processing to the Internet of Things*. Amsterdam: Morgan Kaufmann; 2012.

35. Raina R, Madhavan A, Ng AY. Large-scale deep unsupervised learning using graphics processors. In: *Proceedings of the 26th Annual International Conference on Machine Learning*. New York: ACM; 2009.

36. Fernández A, del Río S, López V, et al. Big data with cloud computing: an insight on the computing environment, MapReduce, and programming frameworks. *WIREs Data Mining and Knowledge Discovery*. 2014;4(5):380–409 https://doi.org/10.1002/widm.1134.

37. Xia F, Yang LT, Wang L, Vinel A. Internet of things. *Int J Commun Syst*. 2012;25(9):1101 https://doi.org/10.1002/dac.2417.

38. Lucero S. IoT platforms: enabling the internet of things. https://cdn.ihs.com/www/pdf/enabling-IOT.pdf. Published March 1, 2016.

39. Schwab K. *The Fourth Industrial Revolution*. New York: Crown; 2017.

40. Miailhe N, Hodes C. The third age of artificial intelligence. *Field Actions Sci Rep*. 2017(Special Iss 17):6–11.

41. Adams S, Arel I, Bach J, et al. Mapping the landscape of human-level artificial general intelligence. *AI Mag*. 2012;33(1):25 https://doi.org/10.1609/aimag.v33i1.2322.

42. Turing AM. I.—Computing machinery and intelligence. *Mind*. 1950;59(236):433–460 https://doi.org/10.1093/mind/lix.236.433.

43. Levesque HJ. On our best behaviour. *Artif Intell*. 2014;212:27–35 https://doi.org/10.1016/j.artint.2014.03.007.

44. *Wozniak: Could a computer make a cup of coffee?*[video file]. https://www.youtube.com/watch?v=MowergwQR5Y. Published March 2, 2010.

45. Hildt E. Artificial intelligence: does consciousness matter? *Front Psychol*. 2019;10:1535.

46. Müller VC, Bostrom N. Future progress in artificial intelligence: a survey of expert opinion. In *Fundamental Issues of Artificial Intelligence*. Cham, Switzerland; 2016:555–572.

47. Moravec H. *Mind Children: The Future of Robot and Human Intelligence*. Cambridge, MA: Harvard University Press; 1988.

48. Shalev-Shwartz S, Ben-David S. *Understanding Machine Learning: From Theory to Algorithms*. New York: Cambridge University Press; 2014.

49. Mitchell TM. *Machine Learning*. New York: McGraw-Hill; 1997.

50. Hagan MT, Demuth HB, Beale MH. *Neural Network Design*. 1st ed. Boston: PWS; 1996.

51. Goodfellow I, Bengio Y, Courville A. *Deep Learning*. Cambridge, MA: MIT Press; 2016.

52. Manning CD, Schütze H. *Foundations of Statistical Natural Language Processing*. Cambridge, MA: MIT Press; 1999.

53. Schwab EC, Nusbaum HC. *Pattern Recognition by Humans and Machines*. Orlando, FL: Academic Press; 1986.

54. Chen CH. *Handbook of Pattern Recognition and Computer Vision*. 5th ed. Hackensack, NJ: World Scientific; 2016.

55. Giarratano JC, Riley G. *Expert Systems: Principles and Programming*. 3rd ed. Boston: PWS; 1998.

56. McCarthy J. Some expert systems need common sense. *Ann N Y Acad Sci*. 1984;426:129–137 https://doi.org/10.1111/j.1749-6632.1984.tb16516.x.

57. Kartalopoulos SV; IEEE Neural Networks Council. *Understanding Neural Networks and Fuzzy Logic: Basic Concepts and Applications*. New York: Institute of Electrical and Electronics Engineers; 1996.

58. Matarić MJ. *The Robotics Primer*. Cambridge, MA: MIT Press; 2007.

59. Schroeer T. Cognitive computing: hello Watson on the shop floor. https://www.ibm.com/blogs/internet-of-things/iot-cognitive-computing-watson/ Published May 9, 2017.

60. Kelly JE, Hamm S. *Smart Machines: IBM's Watson and the Era of Cognitive Computing*. New York: Columbia Business School; 2013.

61. Picard RW. *Affective Computing*. Cambridge, MA: MIT Press; 1997.

62. Lee JS, Kibbe WA, Grossman RL. Data harmonization for a molecularly driven health system. *Cell*. 2018;174(5):1045–1048 https://doi.org/10.1016/j.cell.2018.08.012.

63. Squeglia LM, Ball TM, Jacobus J, et al. Neural predictors of initiating alcohol use during adolescence. *Am J Psychiatry*. 2017;174(2):172–185 https://doi.org/10.1176/appi.ajp.2016.15121587.

64. Ching.T, Himmelstein DS, Beaulieu-Jones BK, et al. Opportunities and obstacles for deep learning in biology and medicine. *J R Soc Interface*. 2018;15(141).

65. Geraci J, Wilansky P, de Luca V, Roy A, Kennedy JL, Strauss J. Applying deep neural networks to unstructured text notes in electronic medical records for phenotyping youth depression. *Evid Based Ment Health*. 2017;20(3):83–87 https://doi.org/10.1136/eb-2017-102688.

66. Szarvas ·G, Farkas R, Busa-Fekete R. State-of-the-art anonymization of medical records using an iterative machine learning framework. *J Am Med Inf Assoc*. 2007;14(5): 574–580.

67. Doshi-Velez F, Ge Y, Kohane I. Comorbidity clusters in autism spectrum disorders: an electronic health record time-series analysis. *Pediatrics*. 2014;133(1):e54–63 https://doi.org/10.1542/peds.2013-0819.

68. Drysdale AT, Grosenick L, Downar J, et al. Resting-state connectivity biomarkers define neurophysiological subtypes of depression. *Nature Medicine*. 2017;23(1):28–38 https://doi.org/10.1038/nm.4246.

69. Orru G, Pettersson-Yeo W, Marquand AF, Sartori G, Mechelli A. Using support vector machine to identify imaging biomarkers of neurological and psychiatric disease: a critical review. *Neurosci Biobehav Rev*. 2012;36(4):1140–1152 https://doi.org/10.1016/j.neubiorev.2012.01.004.

70. Lin E, Kuo PH, Liu YL, Yu YW, Yang AC, Tsai SJ. A deep learning approach for predicting antidepressant response in major depression using clinical and genetic biomarkers. *Front Psychiatry*. 2018;9:290 https://doi.org/10.3389/fpsyt.2018.00290.

71. Nicodemus KK, Callicott JH, Higier RG, et al. Evidence of statistical epistasis between DISC1, CIT and NDEL1 impacting risk for schizophrenia: biological validation with functional neuroimaging. *Hum Genet*. 2010;127(4):441–452 https://doi.org/10.1007/s00439-009-0782-y.

72. Franklin JC, Ribeiro JD, Fox KR, et al. Risk factors for suicidal thoughts and behaviors: a meta-analysis of 50 years of research. *Psychol Bull*. 2017;143(2):187–232 https://doi.org/10.1037/bul0000084.

73. Kessler RC, Warner CH, Ivany C, et al. Predicting suicides after psychiatric hospitalization in US Army soldiers: the Army Study To Assess Risk and rEsilience in Servicemembers (Army STARRS). *JAMA Psychiatry.* 2015;72(1):49–57 https://doi.org/10.1001/jamapsychiatry.2014.1754.

74. Chary M, Genes N, Giraud-Carrier C, Hanson C, Nelson LS, Manini AF. Epidemiology from tweets: estimating misuse of prescription opioids in the USA from social media. *J Med Toxicol.* 2017;13(4):278–286 https://doi.org/10.1007/s13181-017-0625-5.

75. Nikfarjam A, Sarker A, O'Connor K, Ginn R, Gonzalez G. Pharmacovigilance from social media: mining adverse drug reaction mentions using sequence labeling with word embedding cluster features. *J Am Med Inform Assoc.* 2015;22(3):671–681.

76. Nahum-Shani I, Smith SN, Spring BJ, et al. Just-in-time adaptive interventions (JITAIs) in mobile health: key components and design principles for ongoing health behavior support. *Ann Behav Med.* 2018;52(6):446–462 https://doi.org/10.1007/s12160-016-9830-8.

77. Burns MN, Begale M, Duffecy J, et al. Harnessing context sensing to develop a mobile intervention for depression. *J Med Internet Res.* 2011;13(3):e55 https://doi.org/10.2196/jmir.1838.

78. Wahle F, Kowatsch T, Fleisch E, Rufer M, Weidt S. Mobile sensing and support for people with depression: a pilot trial in the wild. *JMIR Mhealth Uhealth.* 2016;4(3):e111 https://doi.org/10.2196/mhealth.5960.

79. Bae S, Chung T, Ferreira D, Dey AK, Suffoletto B. Mobile phone sensors and supervised machine learning to identify alcohol use events in young adults: Implications for just-in-time adaptive interventions. *Addict Behav.* 2018;83:42–47 https://doi.org/10.1016/j.addbeh.2017.11.039.

80. Bedi G, Cecchi GA, Slezak DF, Carrillo F, Sigman M, de Wit H. A window into the intoxicated mind? Speech as an index of psychoactive drug effects. *Neuropsychopharmacology.* 2014;39(10):2340–2348 https://doi.org/10.1038/npp.2014.80.

81. Markowetz A, Blaszkiewicz K, Montag C, Switala C, Schlaepfer TE. Psycho-informatics: big data shaping modern psychometrics. *Med Hypotheses.* 2014;82(4):405–411 https://doi.org/10.1016/j.mehy.2013.11.030.

82. Wall DP, Kosmicki J, Deluca TF, Harstad E, Fusaro VA. Use of machine learning to shorten observation-based screening and diagnosis of autism. *Transl Psychiatr.* 2012;2:e100 https://doi.org/10.1038/tp.2012.10.

83. Bedi G, Carrillo F, Cecchi GA, et al. Automated analysis of free speech predicts psychosis onset in high-risk youths. *NPJ Schizophr.* 2015;1:15030 https://doi.org/10.1038/npjschz.2015.30.

84. Liu W, Li M, Yi L. Identifying children with autism spectrum disorder based on their face processing abnormality: a machine learning framework. *Autism Res.* 2016;9(8):888–898 https://doi.org/10.1002/aur.1615.

85. Fitzpatrick KK, Darcy A, Vierhile M. Delivering cognitive behavior therapy to young adults with symptoms of depression and anxiety using a fully automated conversational agent (Woebot): a randomized controlled trial. *JMIR Ment Health.* 2017;4(2):e19 https://doi.org/10.2196/mental.7785.

86. Coppersmith G, Leary R, Crutchley P, Fine A. Natural language processing of social media as screening for suicide risk. *Biomed Inform Insights.* 2018;10:1178222618792860 https://doi.org/10.1177/1178222618792860.

87. Reece AG, Danforth CM. Instagram photos reveal predictive markers of depression. *EPJ Data Science.* 2017;6(1) https://doi.org/10.1140/epjds/s13688-017-0118-4.

88. Chekroud AM, Zotti RJ, Shehzad Z, et al. Cross-trial prediction of treatment outcome in depression: a machine learning approach. *Lancet Psychiatry.* 2016;3(3):243-250 https://doi.org/10.1016/s2215-0366(15)00471-x.

89. Shortreed SM, Laber E, Lizotte DJ, Stroup TS, Pineau J, Murphy SA. Informing sequential clinical decision-making through reinforcement learning: an empirical study. *Mach Learn*. 2011;84(1-2):109–136 https://doi.org/10.1007/s10994-010-5229-0.

90. Jeblee S, Khan Khattak F, Crampton N, Mamdani M, Rudzicz F. Extracting relevant information from physician–patient dialogues for automated clinical note taking. In: *Proceedings of the Tenth International Workshop on Health Text Mining and Information Analysis*. Hong Kong: Association for Computational Linguistics; 2019.

91. Ewbank MP, Cummins R, Tablan V, et al. Quantifying the association between psychotherapy content and clinical outcomes using deep learning. *JAMA Psychiatry*. 2020;77(1):35–43 https://doi.org/10.1001/jamapsychiatry.2019.2664.

92. Chapman EN, Kaatz A, Carnes M. Physicians and implicit bias: how doctors may unwittingly perpetuate health care disparities. *J Gen Intern Med*. 2013;28(11):1504–1510 https://doi.org/10.1007/s11606-013-2441-1.

93. McCoy TH, Castro VM, Cagan A, Roberson AM, Kohane IS, Perlis RH. Sentiment measured in hospital discharge notes is associated with readmission and mortality risk: an electronic health record study. *PLoS One*. 2015;10(8):e0136341 https://doi.org/10.1371/journal.pone.0136341.

94. Gianfrancesco MA, Tamang S, Yazdany J, Schmajuk G. Potential biases in machine learning algorithms using electronic health record data. *JAMA Intern Med*. 2018;178(11):1544–1547 https://doi.org/10.1001/jamainternmed.2018.3763.

95. Costa-Jussà MR. An analysis of gender bias studies in natural language processing. *Nature Mach Intell*. 2019;1(11):495–496 https://doi.org/10.1038/s42256-019-0105-5.

96. Riley P. Three pitfalls to avoid in machine learning. *Nature*. 2019;572(7767):27–29 https://doi.org/10.1038/d41586-019-02307-y.

97. Challen R, Denny J, Pitt M, Gompels L, Edwards T, Tsaneva-Atanasova K. Artificial intelligence, bias and clinical safety. *BMJ Quality & Safety*. 2019;28(3):231 https://doi.org/10.1136/bmjqs-2018-008370.

98. Price WN, II, Gerke S, Cohen IG. Potential liability for physicians using artificial intelligence. *JAMA*. 2019;322(18):1765–1766 https://doi.org/10.1001/jama.2019.15064.

99. Strickland E. IBM Watson, heal thyself: how IBM overpromised and underdelivered on AI health care. *IEEE Spectrum*. 2019;56(4):24–31 https://doi.org/10.1109/mspec.2019.8678513.

100. McKinnon RA, Ward MB, Sorich MJ. A critical analysis of barriers to the clinical implementation of pharmacogenomics. *Ther Clin Risk Manag*. 2007;3(5):751–759.

101. Gurwitz D, Lunshof JE, Dedoussis G, et al. Pharmacogenomics education: International Society of Pharmacogenomics recommendations for medical, pharmaceutical, and health schools deans of education. *Pharmacogenomics J*. 2005;5(4):221–225 https://doi.org/10.1038/sj.tpj.6500312.

102. Greenhalgh T, Howick J, Maskrey N. Evidence based medicine: a movement in crisis? *BMJ*. 2014;348:g3725.

103. Windish DM, Huot SJ, Green ML. Medicine residents' understanding of the biostatistics and results in the medical literature. *JAMA*. 2007;298(9):1010–1022 https://doi.org/10.1001/jama.298.9.1010.

104. Association of American Medical Colleges. Scientific inquiry & reasoning—Skill 4: database statistical reasoning. https://students-residents.aamc.org/applying-medical-school/article/mcat-2015-sirs-skill4/. Published 2015. Accessed February 24, 2020.

105. Examination USML. Step 1 content description and general information. https://www.usmle.org/pdfs/step-1/content_step1.pdf. Published 2019. Accessed February 24, 2020.

106. American Board of Psychiatry and Neurology. Certification examination in psychiatry. https://www.abpn.com/wp-content/uploads/2019/10/2020_Psychiatry_CERT_Content_Specifications.pdf. Published October 30, 2019. Accessed February 24, 2020.

107. Chang IC, Li Y-C, Wu T-Y, Yen DC. Electronic medical record quality and its impact on user satisfaction—healthcare providers' point of view. *Gov Info Q.* 2012;29(2):235–242 https://doi.org/10.1016/j.giq.2011.07.006.

108. Parasuraman R, Manzey DH. Complacency and bias in human use of automation: an attentional integration. *Hum Factors.* 2010;52(3):381–410 https://doi.org/10.1177/0018720810376055.

109. Shatte ABR, Hutchinson DM, Teague SJ. Machine learning in mental health: a scoping review of methods and applications. *Psychol Med.* 2019;49(9):1426–1448 https://doi.org/10.1017/s0033291719000151.

110. Cho G, Yim J, Choi Y, Ko J, Lee SH. Review of machine learning algorithms for diagnosing mental illness. *Psychiatry Investig.* 2019;16(4):262–269 https://doi.org/10.30773/pi.2018.12.21.2.

111. Dwyer DB, Falkai P, Koutsouleris N. machine learning approaches for clinical psychology and psychiatry. *Annu Rev Clin Psychol.* 2018;14:91–118 https://doi.org/10.1146/annurev-clinpsy-032816-045037.

SECTION III
CONVERGENT FIELDS OF MENTAL HEALTH INNOVATION

12

Precision Mental Health

Focus on Depression

Laura M. Hack and Leanne M. Williams

Envisioning New Models for Precision Psychiatry

Paradigm shifts in the integration of psychiatry and neuroscience are motivated by the search for an innovative model that connects a neurobiological understanding of psychiatric disorders with clinical phenomenology to improve the precision of classification, treatment decisions; and prevention efforts. Thus far, clinicians and clinical researchers have tended to orient toward precision in predictors of treatment outcomes or disease progression independent of mechanism. In contrast, neuroscientists and other basic researchers have been focused on precision in terms of mechanistic understanding, independent of meaningful clinical outcomes. Precision psychiatry requires effective interdisciplinary convergence between these orientations.

The development of non-invasive functional neuroimaging (e.g., positron emission tomography, functional magnetic resonance imaging [fMRI]), has led to more precise methods for quantifying the brain in action and synthesizing multiple sources of complex data over time. A dimensional framework is relevant for implementing neuroimaging within a mechanistically oriented approach. Within a dimensional framework, we may consider psychiatric illnesses as disorders of functional systems and their underlying neural circuits. Variables such as brain activation and connectivity serve a dual function; on the one hand, they contribute to normal variation in brain capacities and, on the other, they also confer vulnerability to mental disorders. Observable discontinuities in behavior, and ultimately psychiatric disorders, occur when neural trait vulnerabilities are coupled with other risk factors, including environmental variables such as stress, and forced to their extreme. In cardiovascular disease, an analogous variable would be blood pressure, which has a fairly wide range of normal distribution, but higher levels of blood pressure confer vulnerability to pathological conditions. Observable discontinuities such as stroke may occur when high blood pressure is coupled with the effects of other risk factors (e.g., stress, diet). Although this analogy does not capture the complexity of brain circuits and their interaction, it serves as an illustration for how extremes of brain activation and connectivity can produce identifiable failures of function and result in psychiatric disorders. To add to the complexity, the source of the extremes in brain circuit activation and connectivity are a result of a complex combination of genetic and environmental inputs, along with the continual plasticity that occurs with each person's experience and learning.

Overall, there has been a tremendous accumulation of evidence about brain circuitry in psychiatric disorders. This has formed the foundation of large biomarker discovery trials using neuroimaging[1-4] and novel classification systems.[5,6] Next we highlight exciting literature on neuroimaging, inflammatory markers, and pharmacogenetic variants and provide examples of their use in tailoring treatment efforts with a focus on depressive disorders.

Precise Classification and Treatment Planning

Neuroimaging

Modern imaging technologies allow us to reconceptualize depression (and other neuropsychiatric conditions) as disorders of functional brain circuits. These advanced technologies enable researchers to see the brain at work, examine differences in how an individual's brain is functioning, and develop a stratified medicine approach for psychiatry. Through identifying more homogenous types of depression, based on brain circuit dysfunctions, we have the opportunity to use these circuit dysfunctions and types to predict what treatments may work best for an individual, and thus advance a personalized approach to treatment choices. Scientists using these technologies have identified an intrinsic neural architecture of large-scale circuits that are responsible for generating our thoughts, emotions, and behaviors.[7,8] The universality of this intrinsic architecture has been demonstrated with meta-analyses of the relationships between neural regions in the brain at rest, termed *functional connectivity* (FC).[8] Additionally, converging evidence exists that these same intrinsic circuits are disrupted in psychiatric disorders.[6,9]

Of particular interest are the default mode, salience, and attention (sometimes called central executive or frontoparietal) circuits. The default mode has core nodes in the anterior medial prefrontal cortex, posterior cingulate cortex, and angular gyrus. It has been implicated in self-reflective thought, and there is evidence that high FC in this network is associated with maladaptive self-reflective thoughts such as rumination and worry.[10] The salience circuit is defined by core nodes in the anterior cingulate cortex, amygdala, and anterior insula and detects salient internal sensations and external changes. Low FC in this circuit occurs in those with social anxiety disorder and may lead to anxious avoidance.[6,11,12] Core nodes in the attention circuit include medial superior frontal cortex, anterior inferior parietal lobe, and precuneus. Low connectivity may partially underlie the inattention symptoms common across depressive and anxious disorders,[6,13]

In addition to this intrinsic architecture, large-scale circuits related to specific processing of threat, reward, and cognitive load have been identified. The extent to which these circuits are engaged by threatening, rewarding, or cognitively challenging tasks varies across individuals and may relate to specific biomarkers of psychopathology. For example, increased activation in the amygdala within the threat circuit to threatening stimuli has been associated with heightened anxiety[14] whereas decreased activation of the ventral striatum, a core node of the reward circuit, has been associated with anhedonia.[15,16]

Several promising examples provide proof-of-concept illustrative examples of subtypes based on specific dysfunctions in brain circuits. Combining findings from the previously described circuits, we have characterized the function and dysfunction of six large-scale brain circuits that may underlie different subtypes ('biotypes') of affective psychopathology.[6,17] Although these biotypes are anchored in brain circuits, we anticipate that they can be refined based on inflammatory, genetic, and other biological and environmental variation, such as early life trauma, as well as specific symptom profiles. The ultimate test of this model will be in its ability to differentially predict treatment outcomes. Data-driven approaches have similarly identified subtypes for depression and other psychiatric disorders based on intrinsic FC and structural imaging data.[5,18,19]

Precise classification based on etiologically relevant biomarkers such as neuroimaging is only valuable to the extent that it can be utilized to ameliorate suffering. Precisely diagnosing a problem allows precise tailoring of treatment choices; for example, identifying which patients may benefit from pharmacotherapy, which patients may not or even may worsen, selecting among types of pharmacotherapy, and limiting side effects. Several biomarker trials in depression have yielded potential predictors relevant to precise treatment planning,[1,3] and more are underway.[2]

The International Study to Predict Optimized Treatment for Depression (iSPOT-D) trial[3] has uncovered several promising environmental, clinical, and neuroimaging-based predictors of treatment response. In this study, over 1000 unmedicated adults with major depressive disorder were randomized to receive escitalopram, sertraline, or venlafaxine for eight weeks. All participants received a comprehensive baseline assessment of clinical variables, cognitive function, electroencephalogram and genotyping for candidate genetic variants, and a subset completed functional neuroimaging prior to initiating treatment. The iSPOT-D trial found that clinical variables such as early life stress[3] and high anxious arousal symptoms[20] predict poorer treatment response to any medication, while higher body mass index predicts better response specifically to venlafaxine.[21] Functional neuroimaging analyses in iSPOT-D suggest that intact cognitive control circuitry[22] and less-responsive threat circuitry[23] are predictive of good antidepressant outcomes in general. Additionally, a single-nucleotide polymorphism in the *ABCB1* gene (which plays a role in controlling antidepressant concentrations in the brain) predicts good response to escitalopram and sertraline for individuals with the common variant and good response to venlafaxine for those with the more rare variant.[24] Hypothalamic–pituitary–adrenal axis and cortisol genes have also been implicated in determining who is likely to experience symptom remission with antidepressants.[25] Furthermore, other analyses in this sample indicate that pretreatment level of FC in cognitive circuitry predicts treatment-specific response such that those with higher FC respond better to sertraline, while those with lower FC responded better to venlafaxine. Importantly, interactions and combinations of predictors are beginning to be examined[26] so that recommendations can be made for patients with more than one predictive marker.

Inflammatory Markers

Researchers have demonstrated a relationship between chronic inflammation and a number of psychiatric disorders, including depression, for which this association has been most studied.[27] Reliable increases in inflammatory response markers, including inflammatory cytokines, acute phase reactants, chemokines, and cellular adhesion molecules, have been observed in depression.[27] Meta-analyses show that the most reproducibly elevated markers in the peripheral blood include the inflammatory cytokines tumor necrosis factor, interleukin-1ß, and interleukin-6, as well as the acute phase reactant C-reactive protein (CRP).[28-30] Depending on the relevant risk factors and sample, about 30% of depressed individuals exhibit increased inflammation.[29] While estimates vary depending on the definition, this is also approximately the prevalence of treatment-resistant depression in the population. Notably, recent research suggests that patients with treatment-resistant depression exhibit increased markers of inflammation.[31,32]

Regarding the effect on large-scale neurocircuits discussed in the previous section of this chapter, inflammation reproducibly decreases ventral striatum-based reward circuitry[33,34] through inhibition of dopamine synthesis.[35] Evidence suggests that inflammatory cytokines decrease tetrahydrobiopterin, an enzyme cofactor necessary for the activity of all major enzymes responsible for the synthesis of monoamines, including dopamine.[35] Acute administration of inflammatory stimuli in healthy volunteers reduces task-evoked ventral striatal activity in response to reward accompanied by behavioral changes including anhedonia, a core feature of depression.[36,37] Such effects align with studies in depressed patients showing that elevated CRP is associated with decreased FC within reward circuitry, including decreased connectivity between the ventral striatum and the ventromedial prefrontal cortex in association with symptoms of anhedonia.[38]

A large extant literature exists exploring the association between response to antidepressant treatment in depressed patients and level of inflammatory biomarkers. Strawbridge and colleagues[39] showed in their meta-analysis of 35 studies of depressed patients that a composite measure of inflammation significantly predicted nonresponse to pharmacotherapy (mostly conventional antidepressants) in depressed outpatients. Consistent with this, post hoc analyses of three clinical trials revealed that level of inflammatory biomarkers, particularly CRP, may be associated with differential response to particular classes of conventional antidepressants.[40-42] Specifically, the trials suggest that CRP (using a cutoff of ≥ 1 mg/L) could help guide treatment selection given that patients with higher inflammation appear to respond less well to selective serotonin reuptake inhibitors and serotonin–norepinephrine reuptake inhibitors and preferentially respond to drugs such as bupropion or nortriptyline.

Pharmacogenetics

While pharmacogenetics is covered more thoroughly in the chapter by Bousman and colleagues (Chapter 20), we discuss it here briefly given that we plan to utilize it in our implementation of a translational precision psychiatry clinic (see section on Stanford Translational Precision Mental Health Clinic). Through identification and tailoring of pharmacotherapy based on an individual's genetic information, pharmacogenetic testing offers a method for addressing variability in drug response. Genetic variants that influence medications used to treat depressive disorders can be parsed into those that code for proteins affecting pharmacokinetic (i.e., metabolism of drugs occurring in the liver and kidneys via enzymes), pharmacodynamic (i.e., therapeutic and toxic effects of drugs via receptors and transporters), and immune-related (i.e., hypersensitivity reactions mediated through human leukocyte antigen [HLA]) processes.

Currently, the most robust evidence exists for the clinical relevance of three genes encoding pharmacokinetic enzymes that are part of the cytochrome P450 (CYP450) system (*CYP2C19, CYP2C9,* and *CYP2D6*) and two genes that are part of the HLA system (*HLA-A* and *HLA-B*). Variants in the CYP450 genes contribute to metabolizer status (i.e., poor, intermediate, normal, rapid, ultrarapid) of multiple drugs for depressive disorders, affecting the length of time an individual is exposed to the drug. In terms of the HLA system, the alleles *HLA-A**31:01 and *HLA-B**15:02 are the most supported in the literature for causing serious cutaneous side effects for those taking carbamazepine.[43,44] Guidelines to assist with the translation of this information into clinical recommendations are freely available,[45-47] and their application in clinical practice has been recommended by multiple professional societies.

Compared to pharmacokinetic and immune-related genes, the evidence base for pharmacodynamic genes is not as strong and no clinical guidelines currently support their use. However, there is some evidence for the involvement of genes encoding receptors and transporters affecting the efficacy of antidepressants in the glutamatergic, dopaminergic, and serotonergic systems.[48] As mentioned previously, the iSPOT-D trial provided evidence for the involvement of variants in the *ABCB1*[24] and *HPA*[25] axis genes in differential response to conventional antidepressants.

Closing the Translational Gap

Despite the progress described in the preceding sections, precision psychiatry is not yet a clinical reality. To escalate progress toward a clinically applicable precision psychiatry model of mental disorders, we need standardized protocols, normative data, multimodal data integration, new computational models, and application of precision psychiatry to optimize existing interventions and develop novel interventions.

Standardized Protocols

Our current understanding of the role that brain circuits play in clinical dysfunction is limited in part by inconsistent findings arising from a lack of standardization across research protocols. While novel imaging protocols are important for new scientific discoveries, standardized protocols will be essential for the future viability of routine scans for mental health assessment. To advance the field of precision psychiatry, it will be necessary to undertake larger, multisite investigations made possible by the use of standardized protocols, integrative analytic models, and databases.[49,50] This approach has been implemented with success in several large interventional and observational imaging studies to date (e.g., Trivedi et al.[2]; Korgaonkar, Grieve, Etkin, Koslow, and Williams[49]; Casey et al.[51]; Marcus et al.[52]).

Norms, Psychometric Properties, and Clinical Thresholds

We must be able to characterize an individual's functioning as normal or abnormal to incorporate pathophysiology into psychiatric diagnoses. This is straightforward for self-report scales and cognitive testing for which population norms are often available. Neuroimaging, however, presents more of a challenge. It will therefore be important to define the normative distribution of neural circuit function in healthy individuals (as in Ball, Goldstein-Piekarski, Gatt, and Williams[53]) and identify thresholds for overt disorder and failures of function. Methods for establishing the psychometric properties, including the reproducibility of imaging data across people, sites, and time, and the reliability of the measures themselves, are also needed.[54]

Integration Across Modalities Within the Same Patients

Our current insights about the biological, behavioral, and experiential characteristics of psychiatric disorders are typically derived from studies that have focused on the individual contributions of these characteristics rather than their combined effects. Correspondingly, within each of these domains of characteristics, the focus has typically been a particular modality (such as functional imaging or structural imaging), rather than on the integration of information across modalities. Of course, this modality-specific focus has been necessary for building the requisite scientific and technological foundations. However, an integrated understanding of a patient across modalities will likely be necessary to obtain the most precise classification and treatment prediction.

Systematic mapping of combinatorial and interactive effects across modalities is a significant challenge and requires purposefully interdisciplinary effort. To refine classifications based on neural circuits, there is a need to consider the relationships among activation, connectivity, and structure within a circuit, as well as the more nuanced interactions between circuits. In parallel, it is necessary to obtain an in-depth understanding of the precise ways that brain circuits relate to behavior and symptoms: which specific symptoms reflect the activation of particular circuits, are there symptoms that reflect a "final common pathway" as the outcome of multiple different types of circuit disruptions, does a change in a brain circuits predict a change in symptoms, and so on. An integrated understanding of how neural circuit dysfunctions are modulated by more distal factors, such as genetic variation, epigenetic influences, inflammation, the microbiome, life events, and their interaction will also be paramount. These multimodal efforts will necessarily accumulate increasingly "big data." In turn, big data requires computational innovation,[55] which is discussed in depth in Chapters 11 and 17 of this book.

Impact on Society and Challenges for Application

Even if the preceding issues are resolved and the scientific grounding of precision psychiatry is accelerated, realizing its promise will rely on a variety of societal- and systems-level factors. When consensus about which evidence is "field ready" has been reached, translating precision models from the laboratory to the clinic will still require the capacity to scale assessment techniques, integrate with existing workflow and reimbursement models, develop new training models, and carefully consider social and ethical issues.

Scale

Scaling neurobiological insights may be aided by their integration with wearable sensing and smartphone sampling technologies that are accessible in each person's natural settings. Scale can also be achieved by combining technologies based on evidence-based risk assessment. For example, in cardiovascular medicine, imaging tools that require intensive on-site testing may be indicated when symptoms are present and function is being disrupted, whereas field-accessible tests akin to blood pressure readings are available for routine screening. Furthermore, sensors track fitness and heart health indicators over time to maintain adherence to treatments or signal changes that may need further assessment. The technology and app revolution has delivered a multitude of opportunities for such real-time monitoring, and rich temporal information about individuals in psychiatry. The challenge is how to tie this information to clinically interpretable data and ultimately to medical records. New research designs that ground scalable technologies with more intensive lab-based neurobiological tests are also needed, to ground both in a common understanding of the mechanisms of psychiatric disorders. Such designs will rely on interdisciplinary communication across clinical, neurobiological, engineering, and data science disciplines to develop scalable systems that are clinical meaningful, valid, and reliable and have the capacity to integrate with interventions and not simply sense signals.

The integration of neuroscience insights with natural world sensors has the added-value capacity for richer temporal information about the trajectory of each patient's risk, recovery, and adherence to interventions. Of course, sensor technology also entails accumulations of massive data sets that will reply on innovative computational approaches, outlined earlier. Furthermore, to scale will not only mean access to populations but also speed of computation, to bridge the translational divide. Clinical viability would rely on close to real time data crunching and delivery (in the form of reports, individualized profiles, etc.), rather than the timeframe of months that is more typical of lab settings.

In terms of scaling inflammatory markers, CRP is already assessed in clinical laboratories throughout the United States under standardized, high-quality conditions. Notably, the measurement of CRP through finger-stick blood sampling is also starting to be utilized in point-of-care testing,[56] suggesting promise for use in primary care settings for rapid assessment and clinical decision-making. Pharmacogenetic testing in psychiatry is further along than both neuroimaging and inflammatory markers. The last 20 years have witnessed an exponential growth in pharmacogenetic testing options[48,57] with psychiatry leading the way in terms of implementation in the clinic.[58-60]

Workflow and Reimbursement Issues

Application of precision psychiatry in practice will require consideration of how testing information and precision measurement-based management is incorporated into the workflow and reimbursement models. One barrier to routine application of imaging is the presumption that it would be too expensive, but the economic case for how such costs might be offset by savings due to reduced utilization and disability has not been tested. Because psychiatric disorders confer significant disability and often involve prolonged periods of trial and error to find effective treatments, it would not be surprising if the cost of introducing precision testing in the short-term was dwarfed by reductions in this toll over the longer term. Furthermore, when imaging can reliably refine diagnosis, help select among treatment options, and monitor treatment progress, imaging is routinely reimbursed without question (e.g., for a broken bone or torn ligament). Integrating imaging and inflammatory, and pharmacogenetic, and markers, as well as other biological data, into clinical workflow will require resolving challenges such as introducing new referral, reimbursement, and reporting systems, as tests for these measures become part of the psychiatric toolkit. CRP testing is covered under the Centers for Medicare and Medicaid Services and many private insurance plans for certain conditions, while particular psychiatric pharmacogenetic decision support tools are fully covered by Centers for Medicare and Medicaid Services with at least partial coverage by several private insurance companies.

Ethical Issues

It is vital for researchers to partner with patients, providers, and key stakeholders at every phase of discovery and translation to ensure that new models are relevant, culturally centered, and effective across populations. Too often innovative new technologies and biomedical advances initially widen disparities in health outcomes such that those with resources are able to take advantage and those without resources are left out. Because serious mental illnesses are often poorly understood by patients and families, many of the treatments involve values-based decision-making, and gathering of personal health information, particularly genetic data, may have unanticipated psychosocial consequences, attention to the distinct ethical issues in personalized psychiatry is essential.

Furthermore, our vision of precision psychiatry requires continuous integration and updating of disease models and treatment planning based on emerging neuroscience and other research findings. A major challenge to this continual updating is that researchers are often hesitant to disseminate findings without an extremely high level of certainty, and providers are often hesitant to adopt new approaches. Caution is certainly warranted; adopting new scientific results into clinical practice too early has the potential for causing harm to patients, particularly if novel and invasive interventions are trialed without adequate safety testing. On the other hand, adopting new scientific results into clinical practice too late also has the potential for causing great harm, as patients miss the opportunity to receive intervention or assessment procedures that could have benefited them.

Training Future Leaders and Translating Research Findings Into the Clinic

Research efforts must be deeply intertwined with educational programs. It is of no use to patients if providers are not competent to incorporate precision psychiatry models into practice. Case-based learning provides a good foundation, as it affords the opportunity to discuss how individual patients' treatment plans can be precisely optimized based on specific patient characteristics. At the national level, the National Neuroscience Curriculum Initiative was established in 2013 to promote the inclusion of a modern neuroscience prospective in psychiatry training through resources that can be integrated into residency programs. As neuroimaging, inflammatory, pharmacogenetic, and other biological markers become incorporated into routine clinical assessments, additional curriculum that more thoroughly addresses the integration of neuroscience and psychiatry will be critical.

The Stanford Center for Precision Mental Health and Wellness

The Stanford Center for Precision Mental Health and Wellness was founded by one of us (LW) in 2018 as an emerging world leader for neuroscience-based mental health research. The Center features a strong integrative team and close interactions among basic neuroscientists, neuroimaging experts, experimental psychologists, behavioral specialists, computational specialists, and clinicians. As part of the Center, we launched a first-in-the-nation "discovery clinic" as a collaboration between researchers, educators, and clinicians in the Stanford Psychiatry Department in 2017. This clinic took place within the context of the year-long third year resident (PGY3) training Continuity Clinic rotation that is required for all Stanford Psychiatry residents. The goals of the discovery clinic included (i) to accelerate the translation of neuroscience into the clinical workflow and (ii) to introduce neuroscience-informed precision psychiatry into a training curriculum.

Patients entering the training clinic were offered a multimodal assessment of symptoms, cognition, and brain circuit functioning. Symptoms of depression, anxiety, rumination, and emotion regulation were assessed by self-report and trained interview-administered questionnaires. Cognition was measured with an online assessment called WebNeuro,[61] in which both general (including executive function, processing speed, attention, and memory) and emotional (including positive and negative emotion identification and bias) cognitive domains were evaluated. We also obtained both resting state and task-based fMRI from which we derived brain circuit profiles for each patient. Each of six biotypes of depression and anxiety[6,17] were summarized using a single score (range: 1–10) representing the extent of dysfunction within each circuit. The large-scale neural circuits mentioned previously, including three intrinsic (default mode, salience, and attention) and three task-based (threat, reward, and cognition) circuits were characterized using anatomical regions based on our theoretical model and defined using a meta-analytic database called NeuroSynth[62] (neurosynth.org). Activation in and connectivity between these regions were combined based on the hypothesized direction of dysfunction in each circuit from our theoretical model.[6]

The treatment team received information from the assessment prior to their first appointment for half of the patients, and the team had the option of incorporating the suggestions of the research team based on interpretation of the multimodal data. The remaining patients received the information 12 weeks later, to allow the research team to test the impact of receiving information from neuroscience-based assessments relative to usual care. The research team also provided advanced training in neuroscience models and their applicability to clinical care to the residents rotating in the clinic. This trial was the first of its kind to integrate assessments for precision psychiatry into routine clinical care and provided valuable insights into the pragmatics and benefits of such integration. The majority of patients agreed that the information provided to them in the reports helped them understand how their brain functioned, provided new insights into their symptoms, and enabled them to feel more committed to treatment. Although the "discovery clinic" spanned one year only, we continue to provide didactics to Stanford Psychiatry residents on our neuroscience-informed model of depression and anxiety, along with additional lectures on neurocognition, active and passive monitoring, inflammatory markers, pharmacogenetics, machine learning, and precision targeting using transcranial magnetic stimulation in the form of a Precision Psychiatry elective.

Stanford Translational Precision Mental Health Clinic

We have launched of the Stanford Translational Precision Mental Health Clinic in 2020, which we hope will serve as a unique exemplar and pave the way for future clinics of its kind. The goal of this consultation clinic will be to offer cutting-edge, multimodal assessment for treatment-resistant patients with mood and/or anxiety disorders to help better match patients with treatments. Similar to our discovery clinic, patients will undergo a comprehensive battery of evaluations assessing symptoms, neurocognition, resting and task-based fMRI, as well as pharmacogenetic markers and CRP. Any patients qualifying for one of our research studies will have the opportunity to learn more about it. All patients will receive a printed summary of their feedback report, along with a thorough explanation of the findings and their implications for treatment recommendations, as well as communication with their primary psychiatrist regarding these findings.

Concluding Thoughts and Future Directions

We are at an exciting moment in history when a new paradigm for precision psychiatry is being realized. We envision that new knowledge about brain circuits and other biological measures along with behavioral, cognitive, and experiential variables will be incorporated into models of assessment, care delivery, and prevention; residency programs will prepare graduates with training in these topics; and clinicians will have access to neuroscience-based tools to inform their decision-making as part of the routine, reimbursable workflow. Findings synthesized in this chapter are encouraging because they indicate that we can use biomarkers to subtype patients and to predict with precision which patients are likely to benefit from which treatment and why. We foresee a future in which the field uses a clinical toolkit that is the psychiatry equivalent of cardiology: multiple imaging modalities and blood-based markers that help differentially diagnose the source of the underlying pathophysiology and guide choice of treatments accordingly across the wide spectrum of options, including lifestyle changes, medications, behavioral therapies, neuromodulation, and their combination. With such a precision approach that translates mechanistic brain insights into clinically actionable tools, we have the opportunity to reduce mortality and morbidity from psychiatric illness and greatly ameliorate suffering.

References

1. Dunlop BW, Binder EB, Cubells JF, et al. Predictors of remission in depression to individual and combined treatments (PReDICT): study protocol for a randomized controlled trial. *Trials.* 2012;13:106 https://doi.org/10.1186/1745-6215-13-106.
2. Trivedi MH, McGrath PJ, Fava M, et al. Establishing moderators and biosignatures of antidepressant response in clinical care (EMBARC): rationale and design. *J Psychiatr Res.* 2016;78:11–23 https://doi.org/10.1016/j.jpsychires.2016.03.001.

3. Williams LM, Rush AJ, Koslow SH, et al. International Study to Predict Optimized Treatment for Depression (iSPOT-D), a randomized clinical trial: rationale and protocol. *Trials*. 2011;12:4 https://doi.org/10.1186/1745-6215-12-4.

4. Tamminga CA, Pearlson G, Keshavan M, Sweeney J, Clementz B, Thaker G. Bipolar and schizophrenia network for intermediate phenotypes: outcomes across the psychosis continuum. *Schizophr Bull*. 2014;40(Suppl 2):S131–S137 https://doi.org/10.1093/schbul/sbt179.

5. Clementz BA, Sweeney JA, Hamm JP, et al. Identification of distinct psychosis biotypes using brain-based biomarkers. *Am J Psychiatry*. 2016;173(4):373–384 https://doi.org/10.1176/appi.ajp.2015.14091200.

6. Williams LM. Precision psychiatry: a neural circuit taxonomy for depression and anxiety. *Lancet Psychiatry*. 2016;3(5):472–480 https://doi.org/10.1016/s2215-0366(15)00579-9.

7. Buckner RL, Krienen FM, Yeo BT. Opportunities and limitations of intrinsic functional connectivity MRI. *Nat Neurosci*. 2013;16(7):832–837 https://doi.org/10.1038/nn.3423.

8. Cole MW, Bassett DS, Power JD, Braver TS, Petersen SE. Intrinsic and task-evoked network architectures of the human brain. *Neuron*. 2014;83(1):238–251 https://doi.org/10.1016/j.neuron.2014.05.014.

9. Whitfield-Gabrieli S, Ford JM. Default mode network activity and connectivity in psychopathology. *Annu Rev Clin Psychol*. 2012;8:49–76 https://doi.org/10.1146/annurev-clinpsy-032511-143049.

10. Hamilton JP, Farmer M, Fogelman P, Gotlib IH. Depressive rumination, the default-mode network, and the dark matter of clinical neuroscience. *Biol Psychiatry*. 2015;78(4):224–230 https://doi.org/10.1016/j.biopsych.2015.02.020.

11. Mulders PC, van Eijndhoven PF, Schene AH, Beckmann CF, Tendolkar I. Resting-state functional connectivity in major depressive disorder: a review. *Neurosci Biobehav Rev*. 2015;56:330–344 https://doi.org/10.1016/j.neubiorev.2015.07.014.

12. Peterson A, Thome J, Frewen P, Lanius RA. Resting-state neuroimaging studies: a new way of identifying differences and similarities among the anxiety disorders? *Can J Psychiatry*. 2014;59(6):294–300 https://doi.org/10.1177/070674371405900602.

13. Keller AS, Ball TM, Williams LM. Deep phenotyping of attention impairments and the "inattention biotype" in major depressive disorder. *Psychol Med*. 2019 Sep 3:1–10 doi:10.1017/S0033291719002290. Online ahead of print.

14. Shin LM, Liberzon I. The neurocircuitry of fear, stress, and anxiety disorders. *Neuropsychopharmacology*. 2010;35(1):169–191 https://doi.org/10.1038/npp.2009.83.

15. Der-Avakian A, Markou A. The neurobiology of anhedonia and other reward-related deficits. *Trends Neurosci*. 2012;35(1):68–77 https://doi.org/10.1016/j.tins.2011.11.005.

16. Greenberg T, Chase HW, Almeida JR, et al. Moderation of the relationship between reward expectancy and prediction error-related ventral striatal reactivity by anhedonia in unmedicated major depressive disorder: findings from the EMBARC Study. *Am J Psychiatry*. 2015;172(9):881–891 https://doi.org/10.1176/appi.ajp.2015.14050594.

17. Goldstein-Piekarski AN, Ball TM, Samara Z, et al. *Mapping neural circuit biotypes to symptoms and behavioral dimensions of depression and anxiety* (4/24/2020). Available at SSRN: https://ssrn.com/abstract=3588580 or http://dx.doi.org/10.2139/ssrn.3588580.

18. Drysdale AT, Grosenick L, Downar J, et al. Resting-state connectivity biomarkers define neurophysiological subtypes of depression. *Nat Med*. 2017;23(1):28–38 https://doi.org/10.1038/nm.4246.

19. Williams LM, Goldstein-Piekarski AN, Chowdhry N, et al. Developing a clinical translational neuroscience taxonomy for anxiety and mood disorder: protocol for the baseline-follow up Research Domain Criteria anxiety and depression ("RAD") project. *BMC Psychiatry*. 2016;16:68 https://doi.org/10.1186/s12888-016-0771-3.

20. Saveanu R, Etkin A, Duchemin AM, et al. The international Study to Predict Optimized Treatment in Depression (iSPOT-D): outcomes from the acute phase of antidepressant treatment. *J Psychiatr Res.* 2015;61:1–12 https://doi.org/10.1016/j.jpsychires.2014.12.018.

21. Green E, Goldstein-Piekarski AN, et al. Personalizing antidepressant choice by sex, body mass index, and symptom profile: an iSPOT-D report. *Pers Med Psychiatry.* 2017;1–2:65–73 https://doi.org/10.1016/j.pmip.2016.12.001.

22. Gyurak A, Patenaude B, Korgaonkar MS, Grieve SM, Williams LM, Etkin A. Frontoparietal activation during response inhibition predicts remission to antidepressants in patients with major depression. *Biol Psychiatry.* 2016;79(4):274–281 https://doi.org/10.1016/j.biopsych.2015.02.037.

23. Williams LM, Korgaonkar MS, Song YC, et al. Amygdala reactivity to emotional faces in the prediction of general and medication-specific responses to antidepressant treatment in the randomized iSPOT-D trial. *Neuropsychopharmacology.* 2015;40(10):2398–2408 https://doi.org/10.1038/npp.2015.89.

24. Schatzberg AF, DeBattista C, Lazzeroni LC, Etkin A, Murphy GM, Williams LM. ABCB1 genetic effects on antidepressant outcomes: a report from the iSPOT-D trial. *Am J Psychiatry.* 2015;172(8):751–759 https://doi.org/10.1176/appi.ajp.2015.14050680.

25. O'Connell CP, Goldstein-Piekarski AN, Nemeroff CB, et al. Antidepressant outcomes predicted by genetic variation in corticotropin-releasing hormone binding protein. *Am J Psychiatry.* 2018;175(3):251–261 https://doi.org/10.1176/appi.ajp.2017.17020172.

26. Goldstein-Piekarski AN, Korgaonkar MS, Green E, et al. Human amygdala engagement moderated by early life stress exposure is a biobehavioral target for predicting recovery on antidepressants. *Proc Natl Acad Sci U S A.* 2016;113(42):11955–11960 https://doi.org/10.1073/pnas.1606671113.

27. Miller AH, Raison CL. The role of inflammation in depression: from evolutionary imperative to modern treatment target. *Nat Rev Immunol.* 2016;16(1):22–34 https://doi.org/10.1038/nri.2015.5.

28. Dowlati Y, Herrmann N, Swardfager W, et al. A meta-analysis of cytokines in major depression. *Biol Psychiatry.* 2010;67(5):446–457 https://doi.org/10.1016/j.biopsych.2009.09.033.

29. Osimo EF, Baxter LJ, Lewis G, Jones PB, Khandaker GM. Prevalence of low-grade inflammation in depression: a systematic review and meta-analysis of CRP levels. *Psychol Med.* 2019;49(12):1958–1970 https://doi.org/10.1017/s0033291719001454.

30. Goldsmith DR, Rapaport MH, Miller BJ. A meta-analysis of blood cytokine network alterations in psychiatric patients: comparisons between schizophrenia, bipolar disorder and depression. *Mol Psychiatry.* 2016;21(12):1696–1709 https://doi.org/10.1038/mp.2016.3.

31. Chamberlain SR, Cavanagh J, de Boer P, et al. Treatment-resistant depression and peripheral C-reactive protein. *Br J Psychiatry.* 2019;214(1):11–19 https://doi.org/10.1192/bjp.2018.66.

32. Haroon E, Daguanno AW, Woolwine BJ, et al. Antidepressant treatment resistance is associated with increased inflammatory markers in patients with major depressive disorder. *Psychoneuroendocrinology.* 2018;95:43–49 https://doi.org/10.1016/j.psyneuen.2018.05.026.

33. Felger JC, Treadway MT. Inflammation effects on motivation and motor activity: role of dopamine. *Neuropsychopharmacology.* 2017;42(1):216–241 https://doi.org/10.1038/npp.2016.143.

34. Treadway MT, Cooper JA, Miller AH. Can't or won't? Immunometabolic constraints on dopaminergic drive. *Trends Cogn Sci.* 2019;23(5):435–448 https://doi.org/10.1016/j.tics.2019.03.003.

35. Haroon E, Raison CL, Miller AH. Psychoneuroimmunology meets neuropsychopharmacology: translational implications of the impact of inflammation

on behavior. *Neuropsychopharmacology.* 2012;37(1):137–162 https://doi.org/10.1038/npp.2011.205.

36. Eisenberger NI, Berkman ET, Inagaki TK, Rameson LT, Mashal NM, Irwin MR. Inflammation-induced anhedonia: endotoxin reduces ventral striatum responses to reward. *Biol Psychiatry.* 2010;68(8):748–754 https://doi.org/10.1016/j.biopsych.2010.06.010.

37. Harrison NA, Voon V, Cercignani M, Cooper EA, Pessiglione M, Critchley HD. A neurocomputational account of how inflammation enhances sensitivity to punishments versus rewards. *Biol Psychiatry.* 2016;80(1):73–81 https://doi.org/10.1016/j.biopsych.2015.07.018.

38. Felger JC, Li Z, Haroon E, et al. Inflammation is associated with decreased functional connectivity within corticostriatal reward circuitry in depression. *Mol Psychiatry.* 2016;21(10):1358–1365 https://doi.org/10.1038/mp.2015.168.

39. Strawbridge R, Arnone D, Danese A, Papadopoulos A, Herane Vives A, Cleare AJ. Inflammation and clinical response to treatment in depression: a meta-analysis. *Eur Neuropsychopharmacol.* 2015;25(10):1532–1543 https://doi.org/10.1016/j.euroneuro.2015.06.007.

40. Jha MK, Minhajuddin A, Gadad BS, et al. Can C-reactive protein inform antidepressant medication selection in depressed outpatients? Findings from the CO-MED trial. *Psychoneuroendocrinology.* 2017;78:105–113 https://doi.org/10.1016/j.psyneuen.2017.01.023.

41. Uher R, Tansey KE, Dew T, et al. An inflammatory biomarker as a differential predictor of outcome of depression treatment with escitalopram and nortriptyline. *Am J Psychiatry.* 2014;171(12):1278–1286 https://doi.org/10.1176/appi.ajp.2014.14010094.

42. Zhang J, Yue Y, Thapa A, et al. Baseline serum C-reactive protein levels may predict antidepressant treatment responses in patients with major depressive disorder. *J Affect Disord.* 2019;250:432–438 https://doi.org/10.1016/j.jad.2019.03.001.

43. Yip VL, Pirmohamed M. The HLA-A*31:01 allele: influence on carbamazepine treatment. *Pharmgenomics Pers Med.* 2017;10:29–38.

44. Tangamornsuksan W, Chaiyakunapruk N, Somkrua R, Lohitnavy M, Tassaneeyakul W. Relationship between the HLA-B*1502 allele and carbamazepine-induced Stevens–Johnson syndrome and toxic epidermal necrolysis: a systematic review and meta-analysis. *JAMA Dermatol.* 2013;149(9):1025–1032 https://doi.org/10.1001/jamadermatol.2013.4114.

45. Caudle KE, Klein TE, Hoffman JM, et al. Incorporation of pharmacogenomics into routine clinical practice: the Clinical Pharmacogenetics Implementation Consortium (CPIC) guideline development process. *Curr Drug Metab.* 2014;15(2):209–217 https://doi.org/10.2174/1389200215666140130124910.

46. Hicks JK, Bishop JR, Sangkuhl K, et al. Clinical Pharmacogenetics Implementation Consortium (CPIC) guideline for CYP2D6 and CYP2C19 genotypes and dosing of selective serotonin reuptake inhibitors. *Clin Pharmacol Ther.* 2015;98(2):127–134 https://doi.org/10.1002/cpt.147.

47. Phillips EJ, Sukasem C, Whirl-Carrillo M, et al. Clinical Pharmacogenetics Implementation Consortium Guideline for HLA genotype and use of carbamazepine and oxcarbazepine: 2017 update. *Clin Pharmacol Ther.* 2018;103(4):574–581.

48. Bousman CA, Hopwood M. Commercial pharmacogenetic-based decision-support tools in psychiatry. *Lancet Psychiatry.* 2016;3(6):585–590 https://doi.org/10.1016/s2215-0366(16)00017-1.

49. Korgaonkar MS, Grieve SM, Etkin A, Koslow SH, Williams LM. Using standardized fMRI protocols to identify patterns of prefrontal circuit dysregulation that are common and specific to cognitive and emotional tasks in major depressive disorder: first wave results

from the iSPOT-D study. *Neuropsychopharmacology*. 2013;38(5):863–871 https://doi.org/10.1038/npp.2012.252.

50. Siegle GJ. Beyond depression commentary: wherefore art thou, depression clinic of tomorrow? *Clin Psychol (New York)*. 2011;18(4):305–310 https://doi.org/10.1111/j.1468-2850.2011.01261.x.

51. Casey BJ, Cannonier T, Conley MI, et al. The Adolescent Brain Cognitive Development (ABCD) study: imaging acquisition across 21 sites. *Dev Cogn Neurosci*. 2018;32:43–54 https://doi.org/10.1016/j.dcn.2018.03.001.

52. Marcus DS, Harms MP, Snyder AZ, et al. Human Connectome Project informatics: quality control, database services, and data visualization. *Neuroimage*. 2013;80:202–219 https://doi.org/10.1016/j.neuroimage.2013.05.077.

53. Ball TM, Goldstein-Piekarski AN, Gatt JM, Williams LM. Quantifying person-level brain network functioning to facilitate clinical translation. *Transl Psychiatry*. 2017;7(10):e1248 https://doi.org/10.1038/tp.2017.204.

54. Biswal BB, Mennes M, Zuo XN, et al. Toward discovery science of human brain function. *Proc Natl Acad Sci U S A*. 2010;107(10):4734–4739.

55. Paulus MP, Huys QJ, Maia TV. A roadmap for the development of applied computational psychiatry. *Biol Psychiatry Cogn Neurosci Neuroimaging*. 2016;1(5):386–392 https://doi.org/10.1016/j.bpsc.2016.05.001.

56. Bukve T, Stavelin A, Sandberg S. Effect of participating in a quality improvement system over time for point-of-care c-reactive protein, glucose, and hemoglobin testing. *Clin Chem*. 2016;62(11):1474–1481 https://doi.org/10.1373/clinchem.2016.259093.

57. Haga SB, Kantor A. Horizon scan of clinical laboratories offering pharmacogenetic testing. *Health Aff (Millwood)*. 2018;37(5):717–723 https://doi.org/10.1377/hlthaff.2017.1564.

58. Ramsey LB, Prows CA, Zhang K, et al. Implementation of pharmacogenetics at Cincinnati Children's Hospital Medical Center: lessons learned over 14 years of personalizing medicine. *Clin Pharmacol Ther*. 2019;105(1):49–52 https://doi.org/10.1002/cpt.1165.

59. Volpi S, Bult CJ, Chisholm RL, et al. Research directions in the clinical implementation of pharmacogenomics: an overview of US programs and projects. *Clin Pharmacol Ther*. 2018;103(5):778–786 https://doi.org/10.1002/cpt.1048.

60. Müller DJ, Kekin I, Kao AC, Brandl EJ. Towards the implementation of CYP2D6 and CYP2C19 genotypes in clinical practice: update and report from a pharmacogenetic service clinic. *Int Rev Psychiatry*. 2013;25(5):554–571 https://doi.org/10.3109/09540261.2013.838944.

61. Silverstein SM, Berten S, Olson P, et al. Development and validation of a World-Wide-Web-based neurocognitive assessment battery: WebNeuro. *Behav Res Methods*. 2007;39(4):940–949 https://doi.org/10.3758/bf03192989.

62. Yarkoni T, Poldrack RA, Nichols TE, Van Essen DC, Wager TD. Large-scale automated synthesis of human functional neuroimaging data. *Nat Methods*. 2011;8(8):665–670 https://doi.org/10.1038/nmeth.1635.

13

Emerging Role for Technology in Positive Psychiatry Interventions

Importance of Convergence Medicine in Improving Mental Well-Being

Emily B. H. Treichler, Ellen E. Lee, and Dilip V. Jeste

Acknowledgment

This study was supported, in part, by the NARSAD Young Investigator grant from the Brain and Behavior Research Foundation (PI: Ellen E. Lee, MD), National Institute of Mental Health [NIMH T32 Geriatric Mental Health Program MH019934 (PI: Dilip V. Jeste), NIMH R01 MH115127-01 (PI: Dilip V. Jeste), and NIMH MH094151-07 (PI: Dilip V. Jeste), and by the Stein Institute for Research on Aging at the University of California San Diego.

> *Happiness is the consequence of personal effort. You fight for it, strive for it, insist upon it, and sometimes even travel around the world looking for it. You have to participate relentlessly in the manifestations of your own blessings. And once you have achieved a state of happiness, you must never become lax about maintaining it.*
>
> —Elizabeth Gilbert (from *Eat, Pray, Love*)

Positive Psychiatry

Traditional psychiatry has focused on assessment and alleviation of specific symptoms and functional impairments (e.g., depressed mood, hallucinations, anxiety, sleep impairment). The psychiatric assessment methods currently in use rate the severity and impairment of targeted symptom and functional domains and focus on how medications and psychotherapies can reduce problematic symptoms and alleviate impairment. However, this model does not consider going beyond symptom reduction and relapse prevention by seeking to increase happiness and greater well-being among people with mental illnesses. In short, traditional psychiatric research and practice are oriented around the traditional medical model, wherein the focus is on identifying and treating disease states and avoiding exacerbations.

Yet, the medical model itself is changing. Patient satisfaction and well-being are increasingly considered the top priority for modern healthcare. In that spirit, our group has been advocating positive psychiatry as the "the science and practice of psychiatry that seeks to understand and promote well-being through assessment and interventions aimed at enhancing behavioral and mental wellness" (Jeste et al., 2015, p. 676). Thus, improvement in positive psychological traits, such as optimism, resilience, wisdom, social engagement, personal mastery, coping self-efficacy, and spirituality are the focus of positive psychiatry (Jeste & Palmer, 2015). Such traits have been closely linked with better well-being, lower perceived stress, greater posttraumatic growth, recovery, and prevention of psychopathology as well as improved physical health and cognitive function along with optimal levels of aging-related biomarkers and decreased mortality (Diener & Chan, 2011; Lee et al., 2018; Rasmussen et al., 2009).

The roots of positive psychiatry can be traced back to the early perspectives of psychologist-physician William James who introduced the concept of a "mind-cure," defined as the healing abilities associated with positive emotions and beliefs (Froh, 2004). Half a century later, James's mind cure concept was expanded and extended by Abraham Maslow and colleagues in the form of humanistic psychology (Maslow, 1971). According to Maslow, clinical outcomes among people with mental disorders were best improved by assessing and enhancing overall health and creativity. In the late 1990s, Martin Seligman and colleagues shepherded the positive psychology movement, aiming to improve wellness in the general population (i.e., people without psychiatric, cognitive, or physical illnesses; Seligman & Csikszentmihalyi, 2000).

Positive psychiatry is an emerging subdiscipline that incorporates the complementary training backgrounds of psychiatrists, psychologists, and other mental health clinicians like nurses, social workers, occupational therapists, etc. to further enhance mental health for people with mental and physical illnesses (Eglit et al., 2018; Jeste & Palmer, 2015; Jeste et al., 2015, 2017). Thus, the purpose of the current chapter is to showcase positive psychiatry interventions and the opportunities for convergence psychiatry—that is, development and use of technology to both assess and promote positive psychological traits and experiences.

One challenge for positive psychiatry, especially in the arena of empirical evidence-based research, is the historically heavy reliance on self-rated assessments of positive psychological traits, common to most studies of personality and well-being. While there is great value in assessing the subjective experience of individuals, there are potential pitfalls of both conscious (e.g., deliberate deception) and unconscious (e.g., impression management) biases in human introspection and subsequent reporting (Chan, 2009). Development of well-validated and psychometrically sound scales for positive psychological traits is warranted for people with and without mental illnesses. Furthermore, there are opportunities to use technology in the form of mobile applications, passive sensors on smartphones, and wearable sensors to assess and promote behaviors that would improve positive psychiatry-related outcomes. For example, ecological momentary assessment (EMA) on smartphones (such as an application that randomly surveys a participant throughout the day about how they are feeling and what they are doing) is one such tool that would more accurately gauge an individual's social engagement and their enjoyment of those activities. Similarly, passive sensors on smartphones could be used to objectively assess a person's online/

social media-related activities to derive "behavioral biomarkers" that reflect traits like social advising, emotional regulation, compassion, or decisiveness. Data from wearable sensors that track sleep, heart rate, physical activity, and GPS location could be analyzed using artificial intelligence (AI) algorithms to track behavioral changes in real-time. Abrupt shifts in sleep or activity, such as a reduction in the number of hours of sleep in a person with bipolar disorder, could herald worsening mood symptoms like mania, depression, or psychosis. In this way, technology can be used to proactively connect patients to their mental health treatment teams to avoid a full-fledged relapse via medication or psychotherapy-driven interventions.

Increasing well-being, resilience, happiness, and related positive psychiatry outcomes is possible via behavioral and psychological interventions. These interventions target populations with a range of levels of baseline well-being; meaning that people who are already doing fairly "well" can benefit from these interventions as well as those who are actively symptomatic. Among some clinicians, there is a misperception that in persons with psychiatric disorders one must focus on remission of symptoms before working on increasing positive outcomes like happiness, meaning, and well-being. This is assuredly not the case. In fact, targeting outcomes like hope, self-determination, and meaning in life can often be the mechanism by which people with psychiatric disorders would find relief (Winsper et al., 2020).

Positive Psychiatry Interventions

Convergence of psychiatry with computer science, engineering, and related disciplines will allow for the impact of these interventions to be personalized, maintained, and augmented in a number of ways. To illustrate these potential impacts, we use an example of a recent trial of a novel psychosocial group intervention in senior housing communities to improve resilience and reduce perceived stress (Treichler et al., 2020). See Table 13.1 for a list of interventions described in this chapter.

Older adults commonly experience stressors related to a decline in physical, cognitive, and functional abilities, loss of purpose and of independence, bereavement, societal ageism, and financial hardships (Almeida et al., 2015). Chronic stressors have cascading effects on physical and mental outcomes, including worse overall well-being, increased depression, and greater physical disability and mobility limitation (Dautovich et al., 2014; Frias & Whyne, 2015; Kulmala et al., 2013). Stressful events increase the likelihood of chronic metabolic, pulmonary, and cardiovascular diseases (Scott et al., 2013). These stressors are often unavoidable in modern Western societies, given the realities of aging, so identifying methods to enhance older adults' ability to manage stressors is essential.

Resilience refers to the trait as well as the process of adapting well in the face of adversity, trauma, loss, and other sources of stress (Ong et al., 2009; Rutter, 2007; Jeste et al., 2013). Resilience is a modestly heritable personality trait and is partially malleable (Chmitorz et al., 2018; Johnston et al., 2015). Resilience is associated with lower levels of anxiety, depression, and general psychological distress and has a mediating effect on physical and mental health in people who have experienced trauma as children

Table 13.1. Interventions described in this chapter

Intervention	Mode	Target Population(s)	Target Outcome(s)	Implementation Considerations	Convergence Potential
Cognitive Behavioral Therapy (CBT)[1]	12–16 individual or group sessions, including at-home practice	Children and adults with a range of psychiatric diagnoses and medical diseases	Depression, anxiety, psychotic symptoms	Effective for many different populations; allows for transdiagnostic training of therapists	Scaling down may increase accessibility; e.g., use of telehealth sessions
Mindfulness-based stress reduction[2]	8 session group based intervention; includes at-home practice	Adults with a range of psychiatric diagnoses; medical diseases; and those without a diagnosis	Quality of life, anxiety, depression, chronic pain	Effective for many different populations; scalable across settings	Machine learning could help identify most successful mindfulness strategies for individuals
CommonGround[3]	In-office web application completed with peer facilitation prior to psychiatry appointments	Adults with serious mental illnesses	Shared decision making, empowerment, appropriate treatment personalization	Increased cost, time, and technology requirements can be a barrier; use of peers can offset some of these concerns	Web application amplifies patient voices and increases patient-provider communication
CBT$_2$go[4]	Single 90-minute CBT session combined with CBT$_2$go app	Adults with schizophrenia or bipolar disorder	Global psychopathology, community functioning, defeatist attitudes	Single session; use of app requires access to smart phone and computer literacy	Connecting in-person session to evidence-based app increases access to care
+Connect[5]	Positive psychiatry app	Young adults with social anxiety disorder, psychosis, and without any psychiatric diagnosis	Loneliness, social confidence	No in-person session required; use of app requires access to smart phone and computer literacy	Using technology may increase engagement of young adults

Intervention	Format	Target population	Outcomes	Implementation considerations	Technology considerations
Savoring Intervention[6]	1 week intervention; 5 minute savoring activity twice/day	Older adults	Resilience, happiness, depression	Short, savoring activity completed independently	Use technology to increase fidelity (e.g., reminders)
Raise Your Resilience (RYR)[7]	3 session group; includes ongoing use of daily diary	Older adults	Resilience, perceived stress, wisdom	Short; delivered by unlicensed residential staff in senior housing communities	Use technology to facilitate daily diary completion or otherwise augment treatment

[1]Beck & Beck, 2011; [2]Gu et al., 2015; [3]Deegan et al., 2007; [4]Depp et al., 2019; [5]Lim et al., 2019b
[6]Smith& Hanni, 2019; [7]Treichler, Glorioso, et al., 2020.

Table summary: These seven interventions are the primary interventions described in this chapter. This table summarizes the key elements of these interventions, including their target population and outcome, along with their congruence with convergence mental health and implementation considerations. Some of these interventions (i.e., CommonGround, CBT2go, +Connect) were developed specifically for convergence purposes, and are therefore described in the chapter as models, while others (i.e., CBT, MBSR) were developed prior to the advent of many of the technologies discussed and are currently undergoing adaptation. The other two interventions (i.e., Savoring, RYR) were included because of their focus on positive psychiatry outcomes and their clear scalability, leaving a number of entry points for convergence to maximize implementation potential.

or adults, and those managing chronic health conditions (Hjemdal et al., 2011; Mujeeb & Zubair, 2013; Stewart & Yuen, 2011; Wingo et al., 2010; Lee et al., 2018). Resilience decreases perceived stress, and people who are less impacted emotionally by daily stressors have lower incidence of mood disorders 10 years later (Charles et al., 2013), indicating the long-term value of pursuing methods of decreasing perceived stress.

Among older adults, high resilience has been shown to be a significant determinant of well-being and is associated with lower levels of perceived stress as well as greater happiness and better quality of life (Jeste et al., 2013; Lavretsky, 2014; MacLeod et al., 2016; Smith & Hollinger-Smith, 2015). Similarly, other constructs characterizing positive psychology and psychiatry (Jeste, 2018), including wisdom, optimism, personal growth, and happiness, positively impact well-being, mental health, and physical functioning among older adults (Depp et al., 2014; Engel et al., 2011; Jeste et al., 2015; Laird, 2019; Reichstadt et al., 2010). Therefore, enhancing these outcomes may promote successful aging (Reichstadt et al., 2010; Depp et al., 2006). However, only about a third of the older adults score high on resilience measures (Jeste et al., 2013; Hildon et al., 2010), indicating that increasing resilience may be a promising strategy to enhance well-being and quality of life among older adults.

Existing literature on methods to improve resilience among older adults is limited. The only published study in this specific arena that we found was a pilot study examining the use of a one-week savoring intervention, which reported that adults over aged 60 who completed the brief intervention with high fidelity (i.e., engaged in the intervention for at least six days; 60% of the sample) showed reduced depression and improved resilience and happiness, unlike the other 40% participants, indicating that consistent engagement was important (Smith & Hanni, 2019). More broadly, a few interventions in older adults targeting related positive psychology/psychiatry domains have found evidence of benefit (Ho et al., 2014; Killen & Macaskill, 2015; Meléndez Moral et al., 2015).

The population of older adults living in senior housing communities is increasing (Jeste et al., 2019; Jeste & Childers, 2017), presenting an important opportunity to improve physical and mental healthcare in these communities (Borson et al., 2019; Guo & Castillo, 2012). Implementing positive prevention strategies in senior housing communities offers a method to assist older adults in maintaining health, well-being, and independence as they age (Guo & Castillo, 2012; Dong, 2017). Our team at the University of California, San Diego, along with the Mather Institute developed a manualized psychological intervention, Raise Your Resilience (RYR), intended to improve resilience and related outcomes among older adults living in senior housing communities.

Development of RYR was driven by empirical literature including consistent findings that experience of positive emotions, savoring of positive experiences, and use of adaptive coping skills are associated with greater resilience among older adults (MacLeod et al., 2016). RYR included savoring, gratitude, and engagement in value-based activities to improve resilience. Group members were taught to savor by recording one event each day that made them feel happy and one accomplishment or activity that made them proud in a daily diary. Gratitude practices were incorporated because they are associated with improved physical and mental health (Jans-Beken et al., 2019; Killen & Macaskill, 2015). Due to past findings that perceived age discrimination negatively impacts well-being and mental health *via* more negative perceptions of aging (Marquet et al., 2018; Martin et al., 2019), RYR incorporated explicit discussion of the impact of age discrimination and associated stereotypes along with methods to fight those stereotypes and improve self-perceptions of aging.

RYR was delivered in three 90-minute sessions at weeks 1, 2, and 4 by an unlicensed but researcher-trained residential facilitator, and focused on three positive psychology-oriented topics: aging as a time of continued growth and enjoyment, making small changes to increase positive emotions, and engagement in values-driven activities. At the beginning of RYR, participants set short-term individualized goals to make life more enjoyable and meaningful. The group facilitator assisted in identifying and encouraging concrete values-driven activities to achieve participants' short-term goals. At the end of the one-month RYR intervention, the participants were encouraged to continue the daily diary and other activities during the three-month follow-up period and beyond.

We designed our trial based on the principles of pragmatic clinical trials (Mdege et al., 2011; Patsopoulos, 2011). These are randomized controlled trials that focus on participants in real world, with few exclusion criteria, randomization at group rather than individual level, and administration of the intervention by unlicensed nonresearch staff. This study used a modified stepped-wedge trial design, which is an alternative method of conducting cluster randomized trials (Copas et al., 2015; Hemming et al., 2015; Woertman et al., 2013). This approach allows for all participants to receive the intervention while still having data from a control period to compare the intervention data to. Unlike a classical stepped-wedge design, start dates were not uniformly staggered; they were chosen based on the availability and readiness of each site. The control period consisted of treatment as usual. Each group underwent baseline assessment at month 0, followed by pre-intervention assessment at month 1, post-intervention assessment at month 2, and follow-up assessment at month 5.

Eighty-nine older adults residing in independent living sector of five senior housing communities across three states (California, Illinois, and Arizona) participated. These individuals were expected to have relatively high resilience at baseline though they still experienced a range of significant stressors. Our primary hypothesis was that older adults who participate in RYR would have higher levels of resilience and well-being and lower level of perceived stress at the end of the one-month intervention. We also examined changes in these parameters at the end of the follow-up period.

We used generalized estimating equations (Tang et al., 2012) and self-report measures of resilience, well-being, perceived stress, and wisdom. Compared to the control period, resilience improved among participants from pre-intervention to three-month follow-up, and perceived stress and wisdom improved from pre-intervention to post-intervention. Among wisdom subscales, emotional regulation and social advising improved significantly while tolerance of divergent values approached significance during the intervention period compared to the control period. Effect sizes for the significant outcomes were small (Cohen's $d = 0.115$–0.221). There were no changes in physical or mental well-being.

Although the effect sizes of the outcomes that changed significantly were small, this may be attributable, in part, to the high baseline resilience of the sample, resulting in a ceiling effect. Still, it is notable that among these highly resilient participants, further significant improvements were detected, consistent with our goal of preventing decline in health and well-being by fostering protective psychological mechanisms. Although scores trended upwards from pre-intervention to post-intervention, changes in resilience were only significant from pre-intervention to three-month follow-up. This indicates the value of continued use of the practices taught in RYR, including use of a daily diary and engagement in value-based behavior.

Our conclusions regarding maintenance of practices taught in RYR lead to the first potential way that technology could help maximize potential impact of positive psychiatry interventions. In many psychosocial and behavioral interventions, clinicians work with patients to learn new behaviors including coping mechanisms and often provide resources like printed handouts for patients to use as they practice. For example, the RYR intervention included use of a daily gratitude diary. During the intervention itself, participants reported remarkably high adherence to the diary: the median number of days completed was 28 out of a possible maximum of 31. However, adherence to at-home practice is often low, despite its importance for treatment outcomes (Decker et al., 2016).

Technology for Positive Psychiatry

Technology can be used to monitor and enhance treatment adherence outside of treatment appointments, for example, via EMA (Moore et al., 2016). Thus, EMA could be used to monitor engagement in previously identified value-based behaviors as they occur, or at n times throughout the day. EMA is most commonly used via apps installed on a smartphone that prompt participant response, although other models use automated or live phone calls (Shiffman et al., 2008). EMA is more sensitive and more accurate than asking participants to estimate their behaviors retrospectively (Ebner-Priemer & Trull, 2009). In addition, clinicians can access EMA data as these are collected to monitor participant treatment engagement, increasing the ability to respond proactively and adjust treatment as needed. Implementation of EMA or other monitoring may itself improve treatment engagement on its own, by creating embedded reminders about at-home practice.

At the end of positive psychiatry interventions, patients are responsible for continuing the use of newly learned behaviors, with few interpersonal or functional supports to do so. It is no surprise, therefore, that many patients struggle to use such coping strategies learned, despite their effectiveness. For example, one small qualitative study of nine people who completed cognitive-behavioral therapy (CBT) noted that in some moments, like times of crisis, it was more difficult to recognize that it was a good time to try a CBT technique and that introducing new behaviors felt too overwhelming or challenging in specific situations like a long-term family conflict (Glasman et al., 2004). Technology offers valuable approaches to provide resources and support after therapy ends to facilitate maintenance of benefits already acquired, as well as continued growth in targeted areas. In the RYR study, we did not monitor continued use of the daily diary post-intervention, but posit that such use is key to continued benefit, given that the theoretical mechanism of change included gratitude and savoring practices, both of which were facilitated by the diary. Technological strategies like EMA can *measure* post-intervention treatment engagement, but more than that, these strategies can *facilitate and promote* treatment engagement.

The ubiquity of smart phones, smart phone apps, and at-home access to the Internet among most adults provides an accessible way for ongoing, free methods to support ongoing engagement in positive psychiatry practices. These methods can be remarkably simple: for example, a reminder to complete the RYR daily diary at each participants' chosen time of day. Equipment that incorporates sensors can be paired with monitoring using reminders—for instance, collecting biological data like heart rate, movement and other activity to identify potentially impactful moments throughout the day to prompt for potential pleasure savoring later. By incorporating technological solutions like these, participants may continue to utilize effective strategies they learned during positive psychiatry interventions, leading to maintenance of benefits. In addition, some research indicates that patients continue to improve following the end of interventions (e.g., Jackson et al., 2007) and facilitating ongoing engagement in helpful therapeutic activities via technological means may increase the number of patients who experience this continued improvement.

However, it is important not to get ahead of the current technology available prematurely. A recent, large-scale review of smart phone apps for mental health noted that although there are thousands of apps, only a few are based on any scientific evidence and even fewer have been studied rigorously (Larsen et al., 2019; Torous et al., 2019). Therefore, although there is considerable promise in this area, there is much research to be done to identify specific, effective technologies. Fortunately, a number of innovative clinical trials are currently underway, and we expect that within five years of this book's publication, the number of evidence-based apps and similar technological methods will have greatly expanded.

Some interventions are already considering more complex and dynamic apps that are responsive to individual needs, including, for example, collecting daily moods and suggesting coping strategies based on past successful strategies for a given mood (Depp et al., 2019). The potential to use technology to improve treatment personalization is particularly promising. Psychiatry broadly has invested in precision medicine (sometimes also called *personalized medicine*), often focusing on the identification of biomarkers, an objectively measurable, dynamic or static indicator of presence or severity of a medical or psychiatric illness. Precision medicine is currently being used for purposes including identification of aberrant neurological, neurocognitive, and associated phenomena indicative of prodromal psychosis (e.g., Clark et al., 2016, Chung et al., 2019, Ramanathan et al., 2017) and indicators that given therapies are likely to be effective (e.g., Hochberger et al., 2019a, 2019b; Perez et al., 2017), using technology related to genetics, electroencephalography, magnetic resonance imaging, machine learning, and artificial intelligence (AI).

A recent review of AI techniques for mental illness detection and treatment highlights its potential and pitfalls (Graham et al., 2019). The authors reviewed 28 studies of AI and mental health that used electronic health records, mood rating scales, brain imaging data, novel monitoring systems (e.g., smartphone, video), and social media platforms to predict, classify, or subgroup mental illnesses including depression, schizophrenia or other psychiatric illnesses, and suicide ideation and attempts. These studies indicated a high level of accuracy overall and provided excellent support for AI's potential in psychiatry. However, most studies were early proof-of-concept works demonstrating the potential for using machine learning algorithms to address mental health-related questions and helping determine which types of algorithms yield the best performance. AI for mental illnesses and their treatments is not ready for broad implementation at clinical level at the present time. As AI techniques continue to be studied and improved, it may be possible to use them in pursuit of more effective mental illness categorization, identify these illnesses at an earlier or prodromal stage when interventions may be more effective, and personalize treatments based on an individual's unique characteristics. Treatment personalization, in particular, may increase positive psychiatry interventions, and although this was outside of the review's scope, we also feel optimistic that AI could incorporate positive psychiatric constructs in its assessment for both prevention and early identification purposes in the future. However, caution is necessary to avoid overinterpreting preliminary results, and more work is required to bridge the gap between AI in mental health research and clinical care.

Person-centered care is highly overlapping with the intentions of precision medicine, although it typically focuses on integrating subjective data like patient perceptions, perceptions, and cultural values into care. Technology can play an important role here too, as it does in CommonGround, a program that uses software to increase the engagement of people with serious mental illness in their recovery (Deegan, 2007, 2010). For example, patients log into CommonGround prior to psychiatric appointments to help them organize their priorities for the appointment and communicate these priorities to their psychiatrists. CommonGround utilizes ideas like "personal medicine," activities that provide meaning and well-being to each patient, like spending time in nature or with family. These principles generalize easily to positive psychiatry, for example, use of similar software to identify individualized value-based behavior (which holds similarities to the principle of "personal medicine") could facilitate RYR sessions.

The strategies currently being deployed to identify, prevent, and improve treatment of psychiatric illnesses, including machine learning and other types of AI, could also be used to identify and increase positive psychiatry outcomes like resilience, happiness, and wisdom. Positive psychiatry research includes a number of studies to identify factors that facilitate these coveted states of being like those targeted in RYR: pleasure savoring, gratitude practice, engagement in value based living, dismantling of self-stigma and other negative self-concepts, and other factors like positive social support, mindfulness, and behavioral activation. Use of machine learning could create a complex model of these factors that is responsive to individuals, enabling personalized well-being seeking. There are a range of positive psychiatry interventions available, and an even larger number of other behaviors, that a given person might find effective in their search for greater happiness and well-being. For example, there are many ways to practice mindfulness, including mindfulness-based stress reduction (Gu et al., 2015; Khoury et al., 2015), an empirically supported therapy; Zen Buddhism; yoga; walks in nature; listening to instrumental music; mindful eating; or even mindful dishwashing. A personalized model created through machine learning or other AI strategies could help individuals cultivate a well-being practice that works best for them.

Perhaps the most exciting way that technology could benefit positive psychiatry research and positive psychiatry interventions is by increasing scalability and expanding accessibility of those interventions. Dissemination and implementation of evidence-based interventions is fundamental to positively impacting public health. However, the research-to-practice gap is large—according to some estimates, it takes an average of 17 years for an evidence-based health intervention to reach the general public (Westfall et al., 2007). Many promising interventions never reach the public at all, due to a lack of research or implementation funding, policy backing, administrative buy-in, provider training, or other essential resources (Aarons et al., 2009; Beidas et al., 2016; Bond et al., 2014; Rapp et al., 2010; Torrey et al., 2001). Psychiatric interventions often face additional obstacles to implementation due to stigma, difficulty with insurance coverage for specialty care, and low mental health literacy among the public, and sometimes among primary care providers responsible for referring patients to specialty care.

In addition, even when behavioral interventions are available, some patients may struggle to engage in them due to the time commitment, difficulties with travel, and accessibility issues. Finding methods to break down these obstacles is key. Scalability looks to find strategies to increase access to through changing resources. For example, RYR is particularly scalable because it (i) involves only three sessions, (ii) is delivered by non-licensed staff already working at retirement communities, and (iii) is offered where older adults live, rather than asking them to come to specialty care clinics. Technology offers a potential way to navigate such issues, especially for new or empirically supported but relatively non-pragmatic interventions. For example, CBT is an empirically supported therapy for a range of psychiatric conditions including major depression disorder, schizophrenia, generalized anxiety disorder, obsessive-compulsive disorder, panic disorder, social anxiety disorder, and insomnia, among others (Burns et al., 2014; Carpenter et al., 2018; Linardon et al., 2017; Ljótsson et al., 2017; van der Zweerde et al., 2019). Traditionally, CBT is delivered in 12 to 16 (or more) in-person, individual, weekly, 50-minute sessions, with at-home practice in between. However, implementation scientists have considered methods of scaling CBT interventions down to increase accessibility, for example, by decreasing the number of sessions required or by combining in-person sessions with telehealth sessions via web, phone, or video connections (Karyotaki et al., 2017; Mohr et al., 2019; Reding et al., 2018). Through this method, technology can augment interventions to increase accessibility and extend resources, ideally increasing the number of patients who access care while maintaining the high impact of care.

Mobile apps offer another method of augmenting CBT and other existing empirically supported interventions. A recent three-armed randomized controlled trial (Depp et al., 2019) evaluated how an app, CBT2go, could augment a single, 90-minute, in-person CBT session among 255 individuals with schizophrenia or bipolar disorder. The CBT2go app includes components to help guide participants through cognitive restructuring exercises that are individualized to specific symptoms and cognitive distortions that participants endorse. It also monitors symptoms, socialization, and medication adherence, and includes personalized adaptive coping prompts. The CBT2go condition was compared with two other interventions: treatment-as-usual (TAU), where participants continued to work with their regular providers and completed study assessments, but nothing else, and self-monitoring (SM), an active control condition where participants engaged in a 90-minute psychoeducational session and then had access to an app that included questions about symptoms, socialization, and medication adherence, but none of the intervention components (e.g., cognitive restructuring) that CBT2go provides. Both the CBT2go and SM groups experienced decreases in symptoms compared to TAU, but only participants in the CBT2go group experienced improvements in community functioning (compared to TAU) and declines in defeatist attitudes (compared to both TAU and SM). These improvements sustained over the 24-week follow-up, indicating the long-term impact of this scalable intervention.

These methods of augmenting intervention with technology offer a promising way forward for positive psychiatry interventions. For example, perhaps the existing RYR intervention could be extended by a CBT2go-style app, or a single in-person session of RYR or other positive psychiatry interventions could be augmented by two or three monthly telehealth sessions. In this way, effective interventions can reach more people more easily, while maintaining or even increasing their effectiveness.

Another approach is online or smart phone–based forums, which many people already use to find likeminded people. Loneliness is a key problem facing older adults, among other populations, and can seriously undermine well-being and happiness (Lee et al., 2019). Online socialization is one way to decrease loneliness and increase social support, particularly for the individuals who struggle to find in-person social support, due to decreased mobility, transportation issues, living in a rural area, or other accessibility difficulties. A clinician- or peer-facilitated forum developed for people following engagement in a single-session of RYR could help older adults continue to engage in coping strategies learned in RYR and increase adherence to the daily diary while also providing an opportunity to make social connections. A peer-facilitated forum, in particular, would provide the peers new opportunities to take leadership roles and develop relationships with other members of the forum, giving them meaning and purpose in life, which is a key element to successful aging (Reichstadt et al., 2010; Aftab et al., 2019).

A recent set of pilots of a positive psychiatry app called +Connect, targeting young adults with social anxiety disorder, with psychosis, and without any psychiatric diagnosis highlights the promise of this approach (Lim et al., 2019a, 2019b). These studies were small pilots that found evidence of initial feasibility, and preliminary evidence that +Connect reduced loneliness and increased social confidence among the young adults with psychosis. This evidence is early, but there is reason to think that not only can technology facilitate positive psychiatry's aims by extending its reach, but it can also provide an innovative way to reach people who may not have been willing or able to engage in standard psychiatric treatments. Young adults with prodromal psychosis, for example, tend to be difficult to engage in traditional treatment programs (Becker et al., 2015). By combining positive psychiatry-related content areas of most interest, like meaning in life, social connection, personal identity development, and empowerment, with technology, using a familiar and comfortable approach, young adults may be more willing to engage in treatment and more likely to benefit from it.

Some scalability efforts seek to use technologically based interventions instead of in-person interventions, rather than solely as augmentation strategies. This can be particularly useful for patients for whom even one in-person session would be diffi-cult to accomplish. For example, mobility can be difficult for many older adults, and asking them to leave their home for every medical and mental health appointment is burdensome and leads to attrition from care. Other people may not have access to personal transportation and live in areas without reliable public transportation or may be caregivers of minor children or family members with disabilities. Transitioning as many appointments as needed, when possible, to in-home appointments using telehealth equipment allows for people who have increased burden due to various reasons to access their appointments.

Beyond the interventions themselves, technology can also be used for other aspects of scalability. For example, the staff who delivered RYR could be primarily trained through teleconferencing rather than in-person. Similarly, staff who deliver inter-ventions can record their work through audio and/or video and have long-distance supervisors provide feedback. This increases the reach of interventions and allows fa-cilities and staff who otherwise could not afford such training opportunities. In the same vein, using technology to connect remote teams to the same training sessions or to prerecorded trainings by experienced providers will improve dissemination of the intervention. High fidelity to the original intervention relies heavily on the uni-formity of the training. Staff should receive standardized training to ensure that they will deliver the intervention similarly in their different sites. Next, successful dissemi-nation of interventions depends upon the adaptability of the intervention to different residential facilities. Again, technology can be used to personalize the intervention to senior housing communities of different sizes, educational backgrounds, primary languages, and economic challenges. Interpreter services, groups led via videocon-ference, or web-based class materials are among the ways in which technology can further the potential reach of interventions.

It is clear that positive psychiatry interventions are feasible, desirable, and effec-tive, leading to outcomes that help improve quality of life across a number of outcome domains for both people with mental illnesses and those without. Investing in the further development and implementation of these interventions, including by scaling up and out, is essential. Across populations, the research literature identifies similar constructs of importance such as well-being, gratitude, resilience, wisdom, hope, meaning, values-based living, social connectedness, and connection to communities and activities relevant to personal, cultural, and spiritual meaning. Therefore, we can expect that the mechanisms by which effective positive psychiatry interventions work might be similar across populations, indicating that existing interventions may be ef-fectively applied to new populations. For example, the previously described +Connect app was tested in three young adult populations, two diagnosed with mental illness and one without.

However, adjustments would be needed to increase accessibility or to personalize treatments to individuals. As we previously described, use of technology can achieve both of these means, increasing the adaptability of a single intervention so it is opti-mally effective for each individual who engages in it. For example, some older adults who engage in RYR may benefit from increased focus on pleasure savoring to increase daily positive emotion, while others may benefit from increased support around age-related stigma to help combat discrimination due to ageism that they are experiencing.

Conclusions

Interdisciplinary approaches, like those supported by convergence science strategies are critical to expanding the field of positive psychiatry and increasing its impact. Continuing to invest in interdisciplinary collaborations with convergence scientists will aid in ongoing efforts to increase targeted outcomes *via* improved accuracy and precision of assessment, personalized behavioral assessment and interventions, improved fidelity and impact of interventions, increased accessibility and scalability of interventions, and broad dissemination and implementation of effective interventions. A marriage of positive psychiatry and convergence psychiatry is likely to help develop a new system of mental healthcare that would promote well-being across the lifespan for those with and without psychiatric diagnoses, leading to improved longevity and more fulfilling lives.

References

Aarons GA, Wells RS, Zagursky K, Fettes DL, Palinkas LA. Implementing evidence-based practice in community mental health agencies: a multiple stakeholder analysis. *Am J Pub Health.* 2009;99(11):2087–2095. doi:10.2105/AJPH.2009.161711

Aftab A, Lee EE, Klaus F, Daly R, Wu T-C, Tu X, Huege S, Jeste DV. Meaning in life and its relationship with physical, mental, and cognitive functioning: a study of 1,042 community-dwelling adults across the lifespan. *J Clin Psychiatry.* 2019;81(1):19m13064. doi:10.4088/jcp.19m13064

Almeida RS de, Bourliataux-Lajoinie S, Martins M. Satisfaction measurement instruments for healthcare service users: a systematic review. *Cad Saúde Pública, Cad saúde pública.* 2015;31:11–25. doi:10.1590/0102-311X00027014

Beidas RS, Stewart RE, Adams DR, et al. A multi-level examination of stakeholder perspectives of implementation of evidence-based practices in a large urban publicly-funded mental health system. *Adm Policy Ment Health.* 2016;43(6):893–908. doi:10.1007/s10488-015-0705-2

Bond GR, Drake RE, McHugo GJ, Peterson AE, Jones AM, Williams J. Long-term sustainability of evidence-based practices in community mental health agencies. *Admin Policy Ment Health.* 2014;41(2):228–236. doi:10.1007/s10488-012-0461-5

Borson S, Korpak A, Carbajal-Madrid P, Likar D, Brown GA, Batra R. Reducing barriers to mental health care: bringing evidence-based psychotherapy home. *J Am Geriatr Soc.* 2019;67(10):2174–2179. doi:10.1111/jgs.16088

Burns AMN, Erickson DH, Brenner CA. Cognitive-behavioral therapy for medication-resistant psychosis: a meta-analytic review. *PS.* 2014;65(7):874–880. doi:10.1176/appi.ps.201300213

Chan, D. *So Why Ask Me? Are Self-Report Data Really That Bad?* New York, NY: Taylor & Francis; 2009. doi:10.1176/appi.ps.201300213

Chmitorz A, Kunzler A, Helmreich I, et al. Intervention studies to foster resilience—A systematic review and proposal for a resilience framework in future intervention studies. *Clin Psych Rev.* 2018;59:78–100. doi:10.1016/j.cpr.2017.11.002

Clark SR, Baune BT, Schubert KO, et al. Prediction of transition from ultra-high risk to first- episode psychosis using a probabilistic model combining history, clinical assessment and fatty-acid biomarkers. *Transl Psychiatry.* 2016;6(9):e897–e897. doi:10.1038/tp.2016.170

Copas AJ, Lewis JJ, Thompson JA, Davey C, Baio G, Hargreaves JR. Designing a stepped wedge trial: three main designs, carry-over effects and randomisation approaches. *Trials*. 2015;16(1):352. doi:10.1186/s13063-015-0842-7

Dautovich ND, Dzierzewski JM, Gum AM. Older adults display concurrent but not delayed associations between life stressors and depressive symptoms: a microlongitudinal study. *Am J Geriatr Psychiatry*. 2014;22(11):1131–1139. doi:10.1016/j.jagp.2013.02.008

Decker SE, Kiluk BD, Frankforter T, Babuscio T, Nich C, Carroll KM. Just showing up is not enough: homework adherence and outcome in cognitive–behavioral therapy for cocaine dependence. *J Consult Clin Psychology*. 2016;84(10):907–912. doi:10.1037/ccp0000126

Deegan PE. The lived experience of using psychiatric medication in the recovery process and a shared decision-making program to support it. *Psychiatr Rehab J*. 2007;31(1):62–69. doi:10.2975/31.1.2007.62.69

Deegan PE. A web application to support recovery and shared decision making in psychiatric medication clinics. *Psychiatr Rehab J*. 2010;34(1):23–28. doi:10.2975/34.1.2010.23.28

Depp CA, Harmell AL, Jeste D. Strategies for successful aging: a research update. *Curr Psychiatry Rep*. 2014;16(10):476. doi:10.1007/s11920-014-0476-6

Depp CA, Jeste DV. Definitions and predictors of successful aging: a comprehensive review of larger quantitative studies. *Am J Geriatr Psychiatry*. 2006;14(1):6–20. doi:10.1097/01.JGP.0000192501.03069.bc

Depp CA, Perivoliotis D, Holden J, Dorr J, Granholm EL. Single-session mobile-augmented intervention in serious mental illness: a three-arm randomized controlled trial. *Schizophr Bull*. 2019;45(4):752–762. doi:10.1093/schbul/sby135

Diener E, Chan MY. Happy people live longer: subjective well-being contributes to health and longevity: health benefits of happiness. *Appl Psychol-Hlth We*. 2011;3(1):1–43. doi:10.1111/j.1758-0854.2010.01045.x

Dong X. Advancing community and health equity: health and wellbeing of U.S. Chinese populations. *J Gerontol A Biol Sci Med Sci*. 2017;72(Suppl 1):S1–S4. doi:10.1093/gerona/glx049

Ebner-Priemer UW, Trull TJ. Ecological momentary assessment of mood disorders and mood dysregulation. *Psychol Assess*. 2009;21(4):463–475. doi:10.1037/a0017075

Eglit GML, Palmer BW, Martin AS, Tu X, Jeste DV. Loneliness in schizophrenia: Construct clarification, measurement, and clinical relevance. *PLOS ONE* 2018;13(3):e0194021.

Engel JH, Siewerdt F, Jackson R, Akobundu U, Wait C, Sahyoun N. Hardiness, depression, and emotional well-being and their association with appetite in older adults. *J Am Geriatr Soc*. 2011;59(3):482–487. doi:10.1111/j.1532-5415.2010.03274.x

Frias CM de, Whyne E. Stress on health-related quality of life in older adults: the protective nature of mindfulness. *Aging Ment Health*. 2015;19(3):201–206. doi:10.1080/13607863.2014.924090

Froh JJ. 2004. The history of positive psychology: truth be told. *NYS Psychologist* 16(3), 18–20.

Glasman D, Finlay WML, Brock D. Becoming a self-therapist: using cognitive-behavioural therapy for recurrent depression and/or dysthymia after completing therapy. *Psychol Psychother-T*. 2004;77(Pt 3):335–351. doi:10.1348/1476083041839385

Gu J, Strauss C, Bond R, Cavanagh K. How do mindfulness-based cognitive therapy and mindfulness-based stress reduction improve mental health and wellbeing? A systematic review and meta-analysis of mediation studies. *Clin Psych Rev*. 2015;37:1–12. doi:10.1016/j.cpr.2015.01.006

Guo K, Castillo R. The U.S. long term care system: development and expansion of naturally occurring retirement communities as an innovative model for aging in place. *Ageing Int*. 2012;37(2):210–227. doi:10.1007/s12126-010-9105-9

Hemming K, Haines TP, Chilton PJ, Girling AJ, Lilford RJ. The stepped wedge cluster randomised trial: rationale, design, analysis, and reporting. *BMJ*. 2015;350(1):h391–h391. doi:10.1136/bmj.h391

Hildon Z, Montgomery SM, Blane D, Wiggins RD, Netuveli G. Examining resilience of quality of life in the face of health-related and psychosocial adversity at older ages: what is "right" about the way we age? *Gerontologist*. 2010;50(1):36–47. doi:10.1093/geront/gnp067

Hjemdal O, Vogel PA, Solem S, Hagen K, Stiles TC. The relationship between resilience and levels of anxiety, depression, and obsessive-compulsive symptoms in adolescents. *Clin Psychology Psychother*. 2011;18(4):314–321. doi:10.1002/cpp.719

Ho HCY, Yeung DY, Kwok SYCL. Development and evaluation of the positive psychology intervention for older adults. *J Posit Psychol*. 2014;9(3):187–197. doi:10.1080/17439760.2014.888577

Hochberger WC, Joshi YB, Thomas ML, et al. Neurophysiologic measures of target engagement predict response to auditory-based cognitive training in treatment refractory schizophrenia. *Neuropsychopharmacology*. 2019. 44(3), 606–612. doi:10.1038/s41386-018-0256-9

Hochberger WC, Thomas ML, Joshi YB, et al. Oscillatory biomarkers of early auditory information processing predict cognitive gains following targeted cognitive training in schizophrenia patients. *Schizophr Res*. 2020;215:97–104. doi:10.1016/j.schres.2019.11.015

Jans-Beken L, Jacobs N, Janssens M, et al. Gratitude and health: an updated review. *J Posit Psychol*. 2019:1–40. doi:10.1080/17439760.2019.1651888

Jeste DV, Childers J. Strategic planning for transformative senior living: developing tomorrow's leadership and workforce. *Seniors Housing Care J*. 2017;25(1):113–126.

Jeste DV, Glorioso D, Lee EE, et al. Study of independent living residents of a continuing care senior housing community: sociodemographic and clinical associations of cognitive, physical, and mental health. *Am J Geriatr Psychiatry*. 2019;27(9):895–907. doi:10.1016/j.jagp.2019.04.002

Jeste D, Palmer, BW. *Positive Psychiatry: A Clinical Handbook*. Washington, DC: American Psychiatric Publishing; 2015. doi:10.1016/j.jagp.2019.04.002

Jeste DV, Palmer BW, Rettew DC, Boardman S. Positive psychiatry: its time has come. *J Clin Psychiatry*. 2015;76(6):675–683. doi:10.4088/JCP.14nr09599

Jeste DV, Palmer BW, Saks ER. Why we need positive psychiatry for schizophrenia and other psychotic disorders. *Schizophr Bull*. 2017;43(2):227–229. doi:10.1093/schbul/sbw184.

Jeste DV, Savla GN, Thompson WK, et al. Association between older age and more successful aging: critical role of resilience and depression. *AJP*. 2013;170(2):188–196. doi:10.1176/appi.ajp.2012.12030386

Johnston MC, Porteous T, Crilly MA, et al. physical disease and resilient outcomes: a systematic review of resilience definitions and study methods. *Psychosomatics*. 2015;56(2):168–180. doi:10.1016/j.psym.2014.10.005

Karyotaki E, Riper H, Twisk J, et al. Efficacy of self-guided Internet-based cognitive behavioral therapy in the treatment of depressive symptoms: a meta-analysis of individual participant data. *JAMA Psychiatry*. 2017;74(4):351. doi:10.1001/jamapsychiatry.2017.0044

Khoury B, Sharma M, Rush SE, Fournier C. Mindfulness-based stress reduction for healthy individuals: a meta-analysis. *J Psychosom Res*. 2015;78(6):519–528. doi:10.1016/j.jpsychores.2015.03.009

Killen A, Macaskill A. Using a gratitude intervention to enhance well-being in older adults. *J Happiness Stud*. 2015;16(4):947–964. doi:10.1007/s10902-014-9542-3

Kulmala J, von Bonsdorff MB, Stenholm S, et al. Perceived stress symptoms in midlife predict disability in old age: a 28-year prospective cohort study. *J Gerontol A Biol Sci MedSci*. 2013;68(8):984–991. doi:10.1093/gerona/gls339

Laird KT, Lavretsky H, Paholpak P, et al. Clinical correlates of resilience factors in geriatric depression. *Int Psychogeriatr.* 2019; 31(2):193–202. doi:10.1017/S1041610217002873

Lavretsky H. *Resilience and Aging: Research and Practice.* 1st ed. Baltimore, MD: Johns Hopkins University Press; 2014.

Larsen ME, Huckvale K, Nicholas J, et al. Using science to sell apps: Evaluation of mental health app store quality claims. *npj Digit Med.* 2019;2:18. doi:10.1038/s41746-019-0093-1.

Lee EE, Lavretsky H, Renn BN, Arean P. Positive psychiatry in geropsychiatric clinical practice: in schizophrenia, cognitive disorders, and affective disorders. *Am J Geriatr Psychiatry.* 2018;26(3):29–30 doi:10.1016/j.jagp.2018.01.047.

Lee EE, Depp C, Palmer BW, et al. High prevalence and adverse health effects of loneliness in community-dwelling adults across the lifespan: role of wisdom as a protective factor. *Int Psychogeriatr.* 2019;31(10):1447–1462. doi:10.1017/S1041610218002120

Lee EE, Martin AS, Tu X, Palmer BW, Jeste DV. Childhood adversity and schizophrenia: the protective role of resilience in mental and physical health and metabolic markers. J Clin Psychiatry. 2019;79(3):17m11776. doi:10.4088/JCP.17m11776

Ljótsson B, Hedman E, Mattsson S, Andersson E. The effects of cognitive–behavioral therapy for depression are not falling: a re-analysis of Johnsen and Friborg (2015). *Psychol Bull.* 2017;143(3):321–325. doi:10.1037/bul0000055

MacLeod S, Musich S, Hawkins K, Alsgaard K, Wicker ER. The impact of resilience among older adults. *Geriatr Nurs.* 2016;37(4):266–272. doi:10.1016/j.gerinurse.2016.02.014

Marquet M, Chasteen AL, Plaks JE, Balasubramaniam L. Understanding the mechanisms underlying the effects of negative age stereotypes and perceived age discrimination on older adults' well-being. *Aging Ment Health.* 2018;0(0):1–8. doi:10.1080/13607863.2018.1514487

Martin AS, Eglit GML, Maldonado Y, et al. Attitude toward own aging among older adults: implications for cancer prevention. *Gerontologist.* 2019;59(Suppl 1):S38–S49. doi:10.1093/geront/gnz039Mdege

Maslow AH. *The Farther Reaches of Human Nature.* New York, NY: Arkana/Penguin Books; 1971. doi:10.1016/j.jclinepi.2010.12.003

Mohr DC, Lattie EG, Tomasino KN, et al. A randomized noninferiority trial evaluating remotely-delivered stepped care for depression using internet cognitive behavioral therapy (CBT) and telephone CBT. *Behaviour Research and Therapy.* 2019;123:103485. doi:10.1016/j.brat.2019.103485

Moral JCM, Terrero FBF, Galán AS, Rodríguez TM. Effect of integrative reminiscence therapy on depression, well-being, integrity, self-esteem, and life satisfaction in older adults. *J Posit Psychol.* 2015;10(3):240–247. doi:10.1080/17439760.2014.936968

Mujeeb A, Zubair A. Stress, anxiety, depression, and resilience among internally IDPs. *Pakistan J Soc Clin Psychol.* 2013;9(3):20–26. doi:10.1080/17439760.2014.936968

Ong AD, Bergeman CS, Boker SM. Resilience comes of age: defining features in later adulthood. *J Pers.* 2009;77(6):1777–1804. doi:10.1111/j.1467-6494.2009.00600.x

Patsopoulos NA. A pragmatic view on pragmatic trials. *Dialogues Clin Neurosci.* 2011;13(2):217–224. doi:10.1111/j.1467-6494.2009.00600.x

Perez VB, Tarasenko M, Miyakoshi M, et al. Mismatch negativity is a sensitive and predictive biomarker of perceptual learning during auditory cognitive training in schizophrenia. *Neuropsychopharmacology.* 2017;42(11):2206–2213. doi:10.1038/npp.2017.25

Ramanathan S, Mattiaccio LM, Coman IL, et al. Longitudinal trajectories of cortical thickness as a biomarker for psychosis in individuals with 22q11.2 deletion syndrome. *Schizophr Res.* 2017;188:35–41. doi:10.1016/j.schres.2016.11.041

Rapp CA, Etzel-Wise D, Marty D, et al. Barriers to evidence-based practice implementation: results of a qualitative study. *Comm Ment Health J.* 2010;46(2):112–118. doi:10.1007/s10597-009-9238-z

Rasmussen HN, Scheier MF, Greenhouse JB. Optimism and physical health: a meta-analytic review. *Ann Behav Med.* 2009;37(3):239–256. doi:10.1007/s12160-009-9111-x

Reding MEJ, Guan K, Regan J, Palinkas LA, Lau AS, Chorpita BF. Implementation in a changing landscape: provider experiences during rapid scaling of use of evidence- based treatments. *Cogn Behav Pract.* 2018;25(2):185–198. doi:10.1016/j.cbpra.2017.05.005

Reichstadt J, Sengupta G, Depp CA, Palinkas LA, Jeste DV. Older adults' perspectives on successful aging: qualitative interviews. *Am J Geriatr Psychiatry.* 2010;18(7):567–575 doi:10.1097/jgp.0b013e3181e040bb.

Rutter M. Resilience, competence, and coping. *Child Abuse Negl.* 2007;31(3):205–209. doi:10.1016/j.chiabu.2007.02.001

Seligman ME, Csikszentmihalyi M. Positive psychology. an introduction. *Am Psychol* 2000;55(1):5–14. doi:10.1037//0003-066x.55.1.5

Scott KM, Koenen KC, Aguilar-Gaxiola S, et al. Associations between lifetime traumatic events and subsequent chronic physical conditions: a cross-national, cross-sectional study. *PLOS ONE.* 2013;8(11):e80573. doi:10.1371/journal.pone.0080573

Shiffman S, Stone AA, Hufford MR. Ecological momentary assessment. *Annu Rev Clin Psychol.* 2008;4(1):1–32. doi:10.1146/annurev.clinpsy.3.022806.091415

Smith JL, Hanni AA. Effects of a savoring intervention on resilience and well-being of older adults. *J Appl Gerontol.* 2019;38(1):137–152. doi:10.1177/0733464817693375

Smith JL, Hollinger-Smith L. Savoring, resilience, and psychological well-being in older adults. *Aging Ment Health.* 2015;19(3):192–200. doi:10.1080/13607863.2014.986647

Stewart DE, Yuen T. A systematic review of resilience in the physically ill. *Psychosomatics.* 2011;52(3):199–209. doi:10.1016/j.psym.2011.01.036

Tang W, He H, Tu XM. *Applied Categorical and Count Data Analysis.* Boca Baton, FL: Chapman & Hall/CRC; 2012. doi:10.1016/j.psym.2011.01.036

Torous J, Andersson G, Bertagnoli A, et al. Towards a consensus around standards for smartphone apps and digital mental health. *World Psychiatr.* 2019;18(1):97–98. doi:10.1002/wps.20592

Torrey WC, Drake RE, Dixon L, et al. Implementing evidence-based practices for persons with severe mental illnesses. *PS.* 2001;52(1):45–50. doi:10.1176/appi.ps.52.1.45

Treichler, EBH, Glorioso, D, Lee, EE, et al. A pragmatic trial of a group intervention to increase resilience in residents of senior housing communities. *Int Psychogeriatr.* (2020). doi:10.1176/appi.ps.52.1.45.

van der Zweerde T, Bisdounis L, Kyle SD, Lancee J, van Straten A. Cognitive behavioral therapy for insomnia: A meta-analysis of long-term effects in controlled studies. *Sleep Med Rev.* 2019;48:101208. doi:10.1016/j.smrv.2019.08.002

Westfall JM, Mold J, Fagnan L. Practice-based research—"blue highways" on the NIH roadmap. *JAMA.* 2007;297(4):403–406. doi:10.1001/jama.297.4.403

Wingo AP, Wrenn G, Pelletier T, Gutman AR, Bradley B, Ressler KJ. Moderating effects of resilience on depression in individuals with a history of childhood abuse or trauma exposure. *J Affect Disord.* 2010;126(3):411–414. doi:10.1016/j.jad.2010.04.009

Winsper C, Docherty AC, Weich S, Fenton S-J, Singh SP. How do recovery-oriented interventions contribute to personal mental health recovery? A systematic review and logic model. *Clin Psychol Rev.* 2020;76:101815. doi:10.1016/j.cpr.2020.101815

Woertman W, de Hoop E, Moerbeek M, Zuidema SU, Gerritsen DL, Teerenstra S. Stepped wedge designs could reduce the required sample size in cluster randomized trials. *J Clin Epidemiol.* 2013;66(7):752–758. doi:10.1016/j.jclinepi.2013.01.009

14

A Social, Behavioral, and Implementation Science Perspective on Convergence Mental Health

Steven M. Albert and Edmund M. Ricci

Introduction

In this chapter we discuss the value of broadening convergence in mental health research to include the social and behavioral sciences. We cast the discussion within a systems framework and suggest that this approach is critical for identifying underlying causes of mental illness as well as evidence-based treatments and implementation strategies.

The social and behavioral sciences are critical to convergence mental health for a number of reasons. First, while mental illness can, in part, be traced to the genetic and cellular components of the connectome and human biological systems, it is also well documented that these fundamental biological factors can be modified through cultural, social, and psychological exposures. There are social/behavioral as well as molecular/biological causes of mental illness.

Second, the social and behavioral sciences have spawned the specialties of health policy, management, evaluation, and, most recently, implementation. These specialties take findings from basic social/behavioral science to determine how changes in one domain (e.g., reducing food insecurity) may affect mental health outcomes (e.g., anxiety disorders concurrent with diabetic complications and asthma exacerbations that appear to be more common when food vouchers are depleted at the end of each month). Finally, the social sciences have also usefully incorporated operations engineering principles for examining dynamics of states and their components. A systems framework is useful for specifying pathways and time scales for influence (including feedback processes) among sets of interrelated factors. Convergence is best approached through a systems science lens because it includes multiple levels of influence and organization and a host of mutually reinforcing parts.

We start with a definition of convergence in mental health science. Following Eyre, Lavretsky, and Insel (2015), the hallmark of convergence mental health science is the integration of "biological, psychological, sociocultural, and environmental data into a more comprehensive, individualized portrayal of diagnosis." They point to examples of convergence currently underway, including the following:

- Continuous assessment of mental state using voice analytics, facial expression monitoring, actigraphy, and engagement of social networks to track depression or mania;
- Interventional psychiatry using implanted devices for the management of hallucinations and obsessive thoughts;
- Use of multiple diagnostic modalities, crossing different brain sciences, to predict risk of first episode psychosis;
- Electronic mental health interventions using personalized smartphone apps to deliver psychosocial treatments; and
- Deployment of socially assistive robotics to promote social interaction that may benefit mental health.

Each of these efforts brings together different disciplines, leverages new technologies to address old problems, and allows us to think about mechanisms for mental illness in a different way and in this sense change our conceptual framework for mental disorders. To take one example, why should a smartphone app be more effective in addressing adolescent depression than traditional therapies? The app interface captures real-time data for tracking mood and function and can provide cognitive behavioral therapy tailored to particular daily challenges. Is its success due to this constant availability linked to challenging moments across the day? This feature would suggest that depression cannot be separated from social triggers and that therapy needs to be delivered on an as-needed basis. Or is the success of the app platform due to its ability to link therapy to other aspects of behavior tracked by the interface, such as an increased heart or breathing rate, which are often physical signs for an impending anxiety episode? This would suggest an alternative mechanism for the condition and other routes for therapy. In either case, the convergent science producing the app, from engineering to psychiatry to human–machine interaction, leads us to recognize that adolescent depression is different in some ways from how we have thought about it historically.

To take this example one step further, consider the social and behavioral implications of using an app-based intervention that has a scalability undreamt of for traditional therapies. For example, the Australian "MoodGYM" has more than 1.2 million users from across the globe, with approximately 40% referred to the program by clinicians (Doraiswamy et al., 2019). Unfortunately, it has been estimated that less than 1% of the approximately 10,000 depression or anxiety self-help apps currently available for download have been subjected to rigorous evaluation (Funnell, 2017). Also, the apps are easily accessible but carry a heavy cost in privacy; almost all gather personal data for commercial purposes. Moreover, users eventually develop fatigue and stop use, lowering benefit. The apps presume people are effective consumers and capable of making effective choices for self-care, but results from research in consumer use in other health domains, such as over-the-counter medications, suggest this assumption may be inappropriate (Albert et al., 2017). Patients may need in-person contact with a therapist to choose an appropriate app and in-person boosters to support effective use. Use of the app and its effectiveness depend on social-behavioral factors. Each of these factors requires behavioral and social science research to ensure that convergence is appropriately anchored in the experience of patients and their communities.

Convergence Behavioral Science in Mental Health: An Example

What is the role of the social and behavioral sciences in the effort to promote convergence in mental health? One way to approach the question is to begin with an example of convergence science in public health. Consider the following situation: In a typical city in the United States, it has been estimated that approximately 15% of the land is vacant or abandoned (Branas, South, Kondo, et al., 2018; South et al., 2018). These vacant plots tend to be concentrated in low-income neighborhoods. Proximity to vacant lots and physical blight has been associated with crime, less outdoor physical activity, and poorer mental health (Kondo, Morrison, Jacoby, et al., 2018; Kondo, Fluehr, McKeon et al., 2018). Vacant lots also increase the risk of environmental hazards, such as lead in soil from demolitions and flooding from storm runoff, which may be mixed with sewage backup. Greening these areas may improve air and water quality as well as community aesthetics. Further, interventions to address physical blight, such as planting trees, removing trash, and working with local organizations to clean and plant vacant lots, have also been shown to strengthen community resilience by supporting mental health and improving neighborhood safety (Branas, South, Kondo, et al., 2018). Efforts to create green areas also encourage community residents to organize to promote environmental justice and other initiatives that have a positive impact on mental health.

U.S. communities as different as Philadelphia, New Orleans, Detroit, and Youngstown, Ohio, have reported benefit from such efforts, both in observational studies and in randomized controlled trials. For example, in Philadelphia, participants living near places receiving a greening intervention experienced significant reductions in depressed mood (from about 20% to 10% of participants). The areas targeted for greening also saw reductions in firearm violence (7%–9%) relative to control areas (Branas, South, Kondo, et al., 2018; Moyer, MacDonald, Ridgeway, and Branas, 2019). In New Orleans, drug crimes per square mile decreased 5.7% from historic levels for residents living near remediated lots (Kondo, Morrison, Jacoby, et al., 2018). In Detroit, census tracts that completed 5+ demolitions of abandoned buildings saw an 11% reduction in firearm assaults, relative to control locations (Kondo, Hohl, Han, and Branas, 2016). An observational study in Australia found that more total green space (tree canopy, in particular) was associated with about a 30% lower incidence of psychological distress (Astell-Burt and Feng 2019). In addition, evidence suggests that greening is associated with increases in outdoor physical activity. Linking jobs programs to greening efforts may augment these benefits because residents gain income and work experience.

Thinking about the public health impact of vacant lots this way, including its diverse effects, suggests many mechanisms for health effects and the benefits of remediation. However, the convergence perspective allows us to go further. Now consider this expanded public health perspective: Urban areas in the United States are burdened with sewer systems that collect rainwater runoff, domestic sewage, and industrial waste together, in one pipe, for wastewater treatment. The volume of wastewater often exceeds system capacity. The result is direct discharge of untreated sewage into streams and rivers, as well as sewer backups into homes. Pathologic microorganisms and industrial contaminants may enter drinking water but also affect residents through air and skin exposure if overflows enter home basements. In Pittsburgh, Pennsylvania, low-income communities are more likely to be located in flood zones or areas that experienced earlier mining extraction. Surveys suggest that 40% of homes in these communities experience a wet basement during flood events and perhaps 20% have sewer backups (Grounded GSI, 2018).

Drilling down further, we find that communities with the highest flood risk also have the highest incidence of gastrointestinal illness involving Centers for Disease Control and Prevention (CDC)-reportable GI pathogens (salmonella, cryptosporidium, campylobacter) in the city, with rates double the average of Pittsburgh as a whole: 2.28 to 2.16/1,000 versus 1.05/1,000 (unpublished data, Allegheny County Health Department, 2016–2018). With this information, a convergence science approach would suggest an expanded outcome for public health impact. First, we include hydrogeologic expertise to map flood areas in communities. Then we include the expertise of environmental engineering to correlate chemical/bacteriologic analysis of water samples with reports of GI symptoms (e.g., days with diarrhea) and community-level GI-related health care (from local hospital electronic health records). We can explore a host of questions otherwise inaccessible without such convergence: (i) Are GI symptoms in flood areas higher than in periphery areas? (ii) Are GI symptoms most prevalent in households with flooding characterized by sewage backup? (iii) Are GI pathogens more prominent in water samples with high levels of sewage backup? Most critically, (iv) Does greening remediation reduce indoor flooding, sewage backup, GI pathogens, and GI symptom burden?

The social and mental health effects of such an intervention, if successful, are likely to be profound. Addressing such an environmental health threat may boost home sale prices, promote neighborhood satisfaction, and boost community social capital and resilience, with corresponding mental health benefit. This broadscale convergence effort is inconceivable without the input of multiple disciplines, a wide range of methodologies (including hydrogeologic mapping, laboratory testing for bacteriology and contaminants, storm water sewage characterization using oxygen and nitrogen isotope ratios, address-based sampling, and community-level analysis of electronic health record data), and the population-based perspective of public health.

Convergence and Implementation Science

The social and behavioral sciences are also central for assessing and shortening the time between the development and translation into practice of a new treatment/program. Implementation science, built on systems thinking, remains the most powerful conceptual tool available to scientists who study complex human behaviors that have multilevel influences. In Figure 14.1 we present a diagram showing the multitude of factors involved when a convergence approach is applied to mental health science to assess evidence-based treatments. The model identifies four domains of activity that could be included in a robust convergence effort.

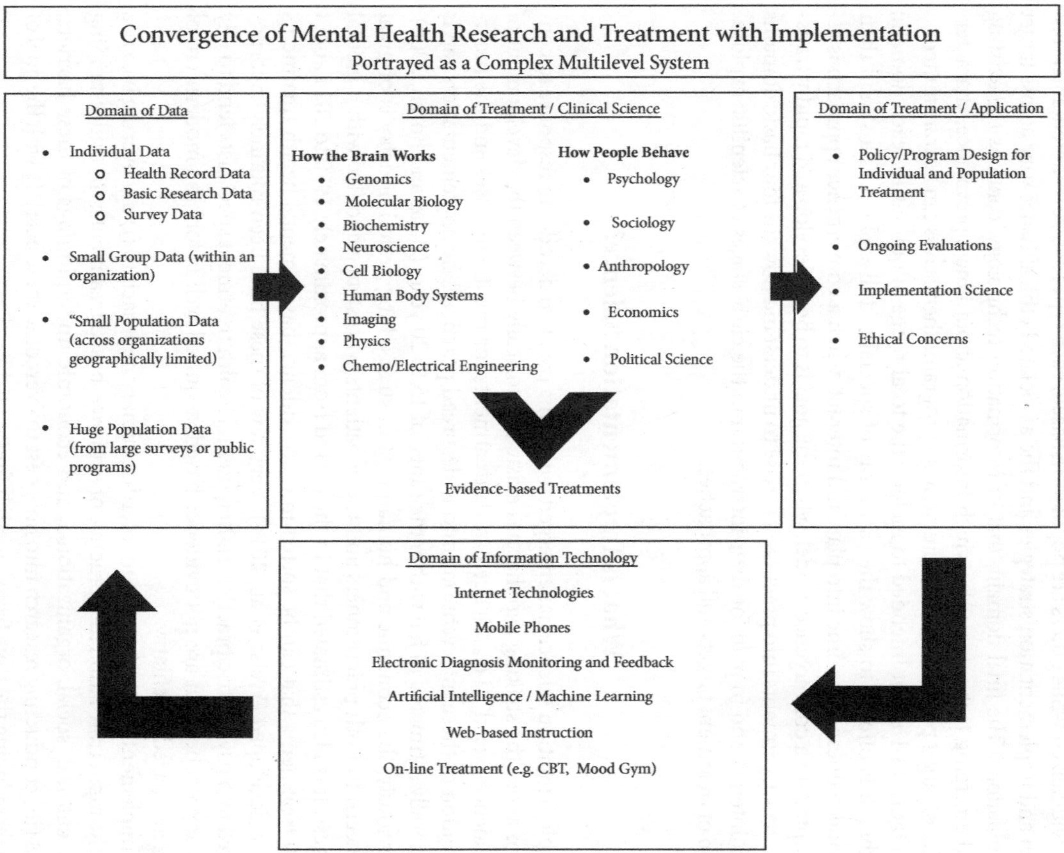

Convergence of Mental Health Research and Treatment with Implementation
Portrayed as a Complex Multilevel System

Domain of Data

- Individual Data
  o Health Record Data
  o Basic Research Data
  o Survey Data

- Small Group Data (within an organization)

- "Small Population Data (across organizations geographically limited)

- Huge Population Data (from large surveys or public programs)

Domain of Treatment / Clinical Science

How the Brain Works
- Genomics
- Molecular Biology
- Biochemistry
- Neuroscience
- Cell Biology
- Human Body Systems
- Imaging
- Physics
- Chemo/Electrical Engineering

How People Behave
- Psychology
- Sociology
- Anthropology
- Economics
- Political Science

Evidence-based Treatments

Domain of Treatment / Application

- Policy/Program Design for Individual and Population Treatment

- Ongoing Evaluations

- Implementation Science

- Ethical Concerns

Domain of Information Technology

Internet Technologies

Mobile Phones

Electronic Diagnosis Monitoring and Feedback

Artificial Intelligence / Machine Learning

Web-based Instruction

On-line Treatment (e.g. CBT; Mood Gym)

Figure 14.1 Mental health research, treatment, and implementation as a complex multilevel system.

The domain of data shows that information about health can derive from numerous sources and can be applied to individuals through small, medium, and large groups. The domain of biological and behavioral science includes all disciplines that study the structure and functioning of the human body from its molecular and cellular organization and functioning to the social and cultural influences upon behavior. The domain of treatment, implementation, and policy addresses the reality that some treatments are individualized while others are population based; each type requires different intervention and implementation strategies and the associated ethical issues vary across target populations. The final domain, that of information technology, contains the existing and emerging technologies by which information about illness prevalence, characteristics of target populations and intervention programs themselves can be transmitted.

Figure 14.1 is not intended to include the total range of options for each domain; rather, it is offered to show the vast array of specialized disciplines (silos) and their connectedness that come into play, and interact, when a convergence approach is attempted. In a convergence model, when the goal is to both develop and rapidly translate new treatments into practice, it is wise to understand how the four basic domains can interact and to plan for their interaction in the early stages of scientific exploration of treatment targets and approaches.

What Is Implementation Science?

Implementation science has emerged within the past two decades in response to concern about the striking gap that has existed historically between the development of "evidence-based" (i.e., science based) treatments for mental illnesses and the incorporation of these interventions into widespread practice. The implementation gap is generally estimated to fall within the range of 15 to 20 years (Balas and Boren, 2000). Obviously, the economic and human cost of such a long period of delay is of great concern to both practitioners and those patients who struggle to live with a mental illness. It is also estimated that in the period from approximately 1970 to 2014 about 500 treatments that can be sorted into 86 evidence-based mental health treatments were developed (Weisz et al., 2014). Very few of these have been routinely incorporated into psychiatric practice; rather, mental health treatment specialists tend to rely on approaches that are not evidence based, acquired well before the modern era of science-based psychiatry.

Implementation science is an interdisciplinary approach to (i) uncovering barriers to the rapid translation into practice of evidence-based treatments; (ii) understanding the cultural, social, organizational, and economic underpinnings of these barriers; and (iii) conducting research into how best to overcome these barriers with the goal of vastly reducing the time from research finding to practice.

As implementation science is a newly emerging field of scientific inquiry one can find numerous definitions of this specialized area of research. The CDC defines implementation research as "the systemic study of how a specific set of activities and designated strategies are used to successfully integrate an evidence- based public health intervention within specific settings" (RFA CD 07-005). One definition that the authors of this chapter find useful delineates the difference between

implementation and dissemination. Dissemination is defined as "the targeted distribution of information and intervention materials to a specific public health or clinical practice audience … with the intent to spread knowledge and the associated
evidence-based interventions." Implementation is defined as "the use of strategies
to introduce … [new] evidence-based health interventions within specific settings"
(Proctor et al., 2009, p. 26). Implementation research is therefore needed to identify
the strategies most likely to lead to uptake of new treatment approaches. Further,

> Implementation research comprises study of processes and strategies that move, or
> integrate, evidence-based effective treatments into routine use in usual care settings.
> Understanding these processes is crucial for improving care, but currently this re-
> search is largely case study or anecdotal report. Systematic, empirical or robust re-
> search on implementation is just beginning to emerge. (Proctor et al., 2009, p. 27)

Several recent reviews of the state of implementation research indicate that it is
in an early stage of development and is based primarily upon single case studies of
unknown internal and external validity. The authors of these reviews conclude that
implementation scientists should (i) design and implement more "experimental" research into the barriers and facilitators of rapid translation into practice; (ii) identify a
core set of implementation outcomes; (iii) specify specific implementation strategies
for varying types and levels of intervention targets (individual/small group/ large
populations/ varying subcultures); and (iv) assess the feasibility and cost effectiveness
of varying implementation strategies in order to provide evidence- based guidance to
policy and program specialists (Williams and Beidas, 2019).

Historically and into the present time period, it has been the belief that implementation scientists and practitioners should be consulted near the time when a new
evidence-based treatment program has been approved; however, recently that assumption is being challenged. Ramsey (2019) has suggested that the early inclusion of implementation scientists into the treatment research process can have several benefits:

- Accelerating the transfer innovations into practice: … by collecting data on implementation perceptions (e.g., attitudes) and resources (e.g., staffing) … will
  bring us to the point of system-ready innovations sooner. …
- Improving the design and packaging of innovations: Attending to feasibility and
  the innovation-organization fit through small scale early stage implementation
  efforts can ensure more useful and usable innovations and inform ongoing and
  necessary adaptions.
- Refining organizational and system processes involved in implementation: Trialing implementation efforts, pilot testing implementation strategies,
  and modifying these approaches as the evidence based for the innovation evolves
  will better prepare the setting for implementation and ensure that the context is
  receptive for timely uptake of the innovation. (Ramsey, 2019, p. 4)

We believe that the early inclusion of an implementation specialist in the intervention development process can, at a minimum, lead to modifications in the treatment
itself that can facilitate and shorten the translation into practice.

An Illustration of Systems Thinking and Simulation in Mental Health Convergence Science

We conclude this chapter with an illustration showing how a simulation, built using a systems design and convergence approach, can be a useful tool in developing a "treatment" for a tragic public health problem, namely, deaths resulting from firearm violence. Consistent with the public health approach described here, including the social-behavioral perspective in convergence science, we can conceptualize mental health as an ecosystem. A rendering of this ecosystem, from the perspective of technological interventions for mental health, is displayed in Figure 14.2.

The person is at the center of this ecosystem but only as a node in a web of interacting factors. Several new technologies (mobile phones, internet, extended

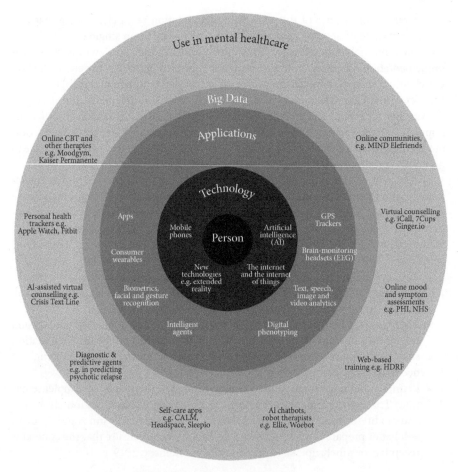

Figure 14.2 The mental healthcare technology ecosystem.

Reprinted with permission from World Economic Forum, *Empowering 8 Billion Minds: Enabling Better Mental Health for All via the Ethical Adoption of Technologies*, 2019. Available at: http://www3.weforum. org/docs/WEF_Future%20Council_Mental_Health_and_Tech_Report.pdf#page=24

reality, artificial intelligence) allow tracking of internal (mood, physiology, "digital phenotypes," and ultimately brain signatures) and external (interactions, situations) states across time and space. A data platform can be designed to capture patterns and dysregulation relative to either population norms or one's own baseline. These signals are parsed, perhaps in a machine-learning algorithm, and used to refer appropriate mental health services, or perhaps to design a personalized mental health intervention. Outcomes from this effort are tracked, again by the same technologies, and used to refine tracking and referral.

This complex human–mental health technology interface is still emerging, and whether it truly benefits vulnerable populations remains to be seen. We must recognize its dystopian potential as well and consider appropriate safeguards. Still, acknowledging this ecosystem is important. The ecosystem's different layers are related over a meaningful time scale. That is, dysregulation captured in data systems is used to tailor interventions, which may in turn affect the internal and external states of our system. This feedback loop indicates dynamics that can be modeled in a systems science framework. A systems science perspective allows us to capture the effects of behavioral and social factors in this dynamic process.

Our ongoing research in community violence prevention shows the value of a systems perspective for mental health convergence science. Using a simulation framework derived from infectious disease modeling, we developed a simple "artificial society" whose population at any given time can be divided into four mutually exclusive states: (i) not owning a firearm; (ii) owning a firearm; (iii) carrying a firearm; and (iv) suffering injury or death from firearm violence. We implemented the model in Netlogo software (Wilensky, 2019), an agent-based modeling framework. Agent (individual)-based models create a population of discrete entities with certain properties, movement patterns, and rules of behavior. These agents move and interact in time. They may change states based on interactions with others. In our simple model, we gave agents different properties, such as the likelihood of changing states (called transition probabilities) per unit of time, and counted the number of agents in each state over time. Figure 14.3 shows output and sample transition properties for the model. This is a "toy model" in that it does not reference any real population and includes only a small number of possible states and relationships. Such models are useful for showing emerging patterns even if they are oversimplified and do not

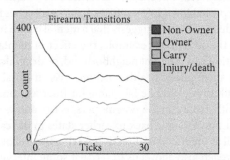

Figure 14.3 Firearm transitions across four states in a "toy model."

capture the full complexity of the social environment and behavior. We allowed plausible transitions between most pairs of states, including feedback relationships, and chose transition probabilities (probability of transitioning from one state to another each step) reported in the research literature, when available. In the simple model, only people carrying guns can transition to injury or death from firearms. Transition probabilities for the baseline model are specified in Figure 14.3.

Model implemented in Netlogo. Transition probabilities as shown in the following table: BehaviorSpace, 10 iterations over 36 timesteps in initial population of 400 agents.

	Transition Probability
Carrier to owner	0.2 [0.4]
Injury to carrier	0.1
Carrier to injury/death	0.05
Non-owner to owner	0.1
Carrier to nonowner	0.1
Injury to non-owner	0.05
Owner to nonowner	0.1
Owner to carrier	0.1
Injury to owner	0.05

The model begins with 400 agents and updates their status at each timestep. These timesteps represent a unit of time in which every agent has an opportunity to change state based on the assigned transition probability. The model reaches equilibrium at about 30 timesteps, and the status of agents at each timestep is plotted in the figure. The output shows that this matrix of transition probabilities yields about 12 injuries/deaths in the initial population of 400 (meant to represent a high incidence neighborhood). This model includes a transition probability of 20% per timestep for people carrying guns to revert to simply owning a gun (i.e., having a gun but not carrying it). In our model these might be considered people using guns for defensive purposes only in their homes. Notably, if we double the rate at which people carrying guns revert to this state of defensive use only (transition from yellow to green in the figure), injuries and deaths decline by about a third, yielding 8 rather than 12 injuries or deaths. These results average stochastic outcomes over 10 different model iterations with each transition probability (20% vs. 40%), holding all other transitions constant.

This systems-modeling exercise suggests that a mental health intervention affecting a single pathway in the system, for example, the effect of mental health counseling, employment, relocation to a different neighborhood, or drug-alcohol treatment, may be enough to affect a key public health outcome, even if distal to that outcome. In fact, any of these pathways would be fair game for interventions designed to reduce firearm injury or death. Note that the systems perspective allows us to assess the effect of interventions that move people back to earlier states in the causal chain (as in the example here) as well as the effects of directly lowering the risk of transition to higher-risk states. This approach also allows us to see that some interventions may not produce desired effects without unrealistic changes in transition probabilities, suggesting low feasibility or return on investment.

Note the limitations of this model. There is no actual geography, no social influences or network effects, no sociodemographic factors, no aging over time, no relocation, guesses on the transition probability for some pairs of states, and limiting the population to only four discrete states. Yet we would argue this approach is still valuable for convergence science. It suggests dynamics and points of intervention and, in this way, uncovers potential putative mechanisms. It also allows additional complexity to be added to the model. For example, we could assess the effect of changes in gun access (transition from nonownship to firearm ownership), greater confidence in neighborhood safety (transition from carrying to defensive use of firearms), and more effective policing (transition from carrying to injury/ death). Systems thinking is an important adjunct to convergence mental health and is essential for incorporating the full range of social and behavioral influences on mental health outcomes.

Conclusion

This overview of the social and behavioral sciences in mental health convergence science suggests the need for broadscale efforts that link mental health to population science to systems thinking, which place mental health within the broader framework of population health and to implementation science for reducing the time from the development of a new treatment to its widespread use. These efforts presume multidisciplinary teamwork, a wide array of research methodology, interventions across different scales, and attention to the various causes of mental illness. The approach has implications for data collection and analysis, in that is entails much larger data sets than we have been used historically and a need for greater computational power. It presumes new technologies for delivering interventions and tracking patient experience. The social and behavioral sciences will be critical to delivering treatments are developed from emerging convergence science.

Is there a downside to convergence thinking? The greatest challenge to convergence science is putting appropriate boundaries on complexity for research and intervention efforts. All models, and all science, require abstraction and simplification. Convergence asks us to add multiple levels to take in a larger and larger context for the phenomena we wish to explain. The danger is that too much complexity and too many factors may ultimately obscure a clear view and clear test of hypothesized disease and treatment mechanisms. The art of convergence science may be knowing when to bring in additional levels of complexity and when to put bounds on each possibly relevant level or factor.

References

Albert SM, Roth T, Toscani M, Vitiello MV, Zee P. Sleep Health and Appropriate Use of OTC Sleep Aids in Older Adults: Recommendations of a Gerontological Society of America Workgroup. Gerontologist. 2017;57(2):163–170 https://doi.org/10.1016/j.jclinepi.2013.01.009.

Astell-Burt T, Feng X. Association of Urban Green Space with Mental Health and General Health Among Adults in Australia. JAMA Netw Open. 2019;2(7):e198209 https://doi.org/10.1001/jamanetworkopen.2019.8209.

Balas EA, Boren S. Managing Clinical Knowledge for Health Care Improvement. Yearb Med Inform. 2000;9(1):65–70. https://doi.org/10.1055/s-0038-1637943.

Branas CC, Kondo MC, Murphy SM, South EC, Polsky D, MacDonald JM. Urban Blight Remediation as a Cost-Beneficial Solution to Firearm Violence. Am J Public Health. 2016;106(12):2158–2164 https://doi.org/10.2105/ajph.2016.303434.

Branas CC, South E, Kondo MC, Hohl BC, Bourgois P, Wiebe DJ, MacDonald JM. Citywide Cluster Randomized Trial to Restore Blighted Vacant Land and Its Effects on Violence, Crime, and Fear. Proc Natl Acad Sci U S A. 2018;115(12):2946–2951 https://doi.org/10.1073/pnas.1718503115.

Doraiswamy P, London E, Canderos V. *Empowering 8 Billion Minds: Enabling Better Mental Health for All Via the Ethical Adoption of Technologies.* World Economic Forum, Geneva, Switzerland; 2019.

Grounded GSI. 2016–2018 grounded strategies for Richard King Mellon Foundation. https://groundedpgh.org/wp-content/uploads/2019/03/20181102_Grounded-GSI-Report_RKM-compressed.pdf

Eyre HA, Lavretsky H, Insel TR. Convergence Science: Shaping 21st Century Psychiatry. *Psychiatric Times*, November 13, 2015. https://www.psychiatrictimes.com/schizophrenia/convergence-science-shaping-21st-century-psychiatry.

Funnell A. Depression and Mental Health Apps: How to Tell the Good From The bad. *ABC New (Australia)*, December 5, 2017. https://www.abc.net.au/news/2017-12-06/depression-mental-health-apps-how-to-tell-the-good-from-the-bad/9228178.

Kondo MC, Fluehr JM, McKeon T, Branas CC. Urban Green Space and Its Impact on Human Health. Int J Environ Res Public Health. 2018;15(3):E445. https://doi.org/10.3390/ijerph15030445.

Kondo MC, Hohl B, Han S, Branas C. Effects of Greening and Community Reuse of Vacant Lots on Crime. Urban Stud. 2016; 53(15): 3279–3295 https://doi.org/10.1177/0042098015608058.

Kondo MC, Morrison C, Jacoby SF, Elliott L, Poche A, Theall KP, Branas CC. Blight Abatement of Vacant Land and Crime in New Orleans. Public Health Rep. 2018;133(6):650–657 https://doi.org/10.1177/0033354918798811.

Moyer R, MacDonald JM, Ridgeway G, Branas CC. Effect of Remediating Blighted Vacant Land on Shootings: A Citywide Cluster Randomized Trial. Am J Public Health. 2019;109(1):140–144.

Proctor EK, Landsverk J, Aarons G, Chambers D, Glisson C, Mittman B. Implementation Research in Mental Health Services: An Emerging Science with Conceptual, Methodological, and Training Challenges. *Adm Policy Ment Health*. 2009;36:24–34 https://doi.org/10.1007/s10488-008-0197-4.

Ramsey A. *More Than Just the Endgame: The Role of Implementation Science for Early Stage Innovations in Behavioral Health. Institute for Public Health.* Washington University, St. Louis; 2019.

South EC, Hohl BC, Kondo MC, MacDonald JM, Branas CC. Effect of Greening Vacant Land on Mental Health of Community-Dwelling Adults: A Cluster Randomized Trial. JAMA Netw Open. 2018 Jul 6;1(3):e180298. https://doi.org/10.1001/jamanetworkopen.2018.0298.

Wilensky, U. *NetLogo.* Center for Connected Learning and Computer-Based Modeling, Northwestern University, Evanston, IL; 2019. http://ccl.northwestern.edu/netlogo/.

Williams NJ, Beidas RS. Annual Research Review: The State of Implementation Science in Child Psychology and Psychiatry: A Review and Suggestions to Advance the Field. J Child Psychiatr Psychol. 2019;60(4):430–450 https://doi.org/10.1111/jcpp.12960.

15

Convergence Mental Health Across the Life Span

Advances in Precision Geriatric Psychiatry

Malcolm Forbes, Thomas Rego, Helen Lavretsky, and Charles F. Reynolds III

Introduction

Geriatric mental disorders have become an important public health problem. Globally, there were 703 million elderly adults (individuals older than 65) in 2019. It is predicted there will be 1.5 billion elderly adults in 2050 (United Nations, 2019). It is estimated that one-third of elderly adults have experienced a mental disorder during the past year (Andreas et al., 2018). With changing demographics, the burden of mental disorders is expected to increase over time.

Depression is estimated to affect 29% of elderly Europeans (Horackova et al., 2019) and 30.6% of elderly Chinese (Zhong et al., 2019). In Australia and the United States, the overall prevalence of depressive symptoms was 9.8% in healthy, community-dwelling adults over the age of 65 who had enrolled in a primary prevention clinical trial (Mohebbi et al., 2019). In addition to psychological distress and social and occupational impairment, geriatric depression increases the risk of disability (Dong et al., 2019) and all-cause and cardiovascular mortality (Wei, Hou et al., 2019) and is linked to impaired cognition (Wei, Ying et al., 2019). While there exist effective treatments for geriatric depression, there are high rates of recurrence (Deng et al., 2018), and the course of depression tends to become chronic and unremitting in old age (de la Torre-Luque et al., 2019).

There are fewer data available on other mental disorders affecting geriatric populations. From the available data, there is a substantial and increasing incidence of psychotic disorders after 65 years of age. Recent estimates indicate a pooled incidence of affective psychosis of 30.9 per 100,000 person-years at risk and a pooled incidence of schizophrenia of 7.5 per 100,000 person-years at risk (Stafford et al., 2018). Bipolar 1 and 2 disorders are estimated to affect 1% of elderly adults (Sajatovic et al., 2015).

There are significant gaps in service utilization, with a large European study estimating that only one in five elderly adults with depression were accessing mental health services (Horackova et al., 2019).

Precision psychiatry is defined as an approach for treatment and prevention that incorporates each person's variability in genes, environment, and lifestyle (Fernandes et al., 2017). Psychiatry has long had a personalized approach to individual diagnosis and treatment, incorporating biological, psychological, social, and spiritual dimensions. Precision psychiatry can be distinguished from standard clinical practice in that it emphasizes the role of measurement and utilizes technology in providing holistic, patient-centered care. This chapter will explore current developments and future possibilities in geriatric precision psychiatry.

Machine Learning in the Prevention and Diagnosis of Mental Disorders in Geriatric Populations

Personal Technology Use

Increasing numbers of elderly adults are utilizing social media and mobile phones. Smartphones in particular are almost ubiquitous. The number of elderly adults using social media is likely to increase as more individuals sign up and as the population of digital natives ages. Pilot study data indicate that mobile phone metadata could be used to predict the presence of mood disorders with 90.31% prediction accuracy (Cao et al., 2017). Analysis of social media posts may also provide cues to early diagnosis. One study of 683 individuals visiting a large urban academic emergency department found that reviewing Facebook data over the past six months could identify depressed patients with a fair degree of accuracy (area under the curve of 0.72; Eichstaedt et al., 2018). Similar research using the photo-sharing application Instagram found that using color analysis, metadata, and algorithmic face detection software could successfully identify markers of depression (Reece and Danforth, 2017). This type of research, via passive data collection and machine learning, may enable healthcare providers to target prevention strategies to high-risk groups; diagnose mental disorders earlier in geriatric populations; and intervene earlier in those with existing mental disorders who may be showing early signs of relapse.

Wearable Technology

Wearable technology refers to smart electronic devices that can be incorporated into clothing or worn on the body. Such technology has the benefit of capturing real-time biometric data on autonomic nervous system activity, voice analytics, sleep quality and quantity (Barrett et al., 2017), physical activity (O'Brien et al., 2017), and social activity (Hodgetts et al., 2017), which can assist in diagnosis. One of the most promising areas of research is in speech analysis. There is increasing evidence that tone of voice, choice of words, and length of phrases can be useful in predicting depression (Cummins et al., 2015) and risk of psychosis (Bedi et al., 2015). This speech can be captured via the use of "virtual humans"—computers with animated characters that interact with people in a natural way. Virtual humans appear to be acceptable to patients to talk to and may in fact increase willingness to disclose sensitive information (Lucas et al., 2014). Such technology, combined with facial expression recognition software (Grabowski et al., 2019; Bartlett et al., 2006), which can analyze the physical manifestations of emotions displayed by individuals, may facilitate earlier diagnosis of mental disorders. As wearable technology (both software and hardware) improves with the aid of machine learning, there is great potential for improved prevention and diagnosis of geriatric mental disorders. It may have particular benefit in bipolar disorder where contemporaneous information on circadian and social rhythm and autonomic disturbance can reveal early signs of relapse (Goodday, 2020). However, at present, the use of artificial intelligence in geriatric psychiatry remains experimental, and there have been no large studies in geriatric populations. Furthermore, there are serious privacy issues around sensitive data collection which must first be traversed before widespread adoption of these technologies.

Clinic-Based Tools

More sophisticated tools exist in the clinic to assist in the diagnosis of mental disorders. There is promising research into diffusion tensor magnetic resonance imaging of the brain to diagnose individuals with major depressive disorder (MDD). It is known that structural brain imaging with standard magnetic resonance imaging or computed tomography has little clinical utility in the diagnosis of mental disorders (Forbes et al., 2019). However, diffusion tensor magnetic resonance imaging provides information on the white matter microstructure of the brain, identifying dysfunction across brain networks thought to be involved in the pathogenesis of depression. In a pilot study of young adults, the tool showed fair accuracy (74%) in distinguishing between depressed individuals and healthy controls (Schnyer et al., 2017). It is expected that advances in machine learning and statistical techniques will further refine prediction algorithms for mental disorders.

Analysis of inflammatory biomarkers including interleukins, tumor necrosis factor-alpha, and brain-derived neurotrophic factor with machine learning techniques can differentiate bipolar and unipolar depression from healthy controls with fair accuracy (Wollenhaupt-Aguiar et al., 2020). Future biomarkers will be able to be incorporated into machine learning relevant for geriatric psychiatry.

Analysis of neuroimaging data, along with genetic and clinical information obtained in the clinic, can assist with predicting clinical symptom trajectories in major neurocognitive disorder due to Alzheimer's disease (AD). By using age, apolipoprotein E status, sex, neuroimaging data, and cognitive scores, researchers can stratify individuals into groups to predict degree of decline with a fair degree of accuracy (Bhagwat et al., 2018).

Rich data sources from electronic medical records also present unique opportunities to improve clinical care. It is widely known that many of our current approaches in clinical practice need urgent improvement. Regarding risk assessment, a meta-analysis of 365 studies over the past 50 years found that prediction of suicidal behaviors is only slightly better than chance (Franklin et al., 2017). However, using machine learning algorithms, there is potential to improve accuracy. In one study, researchers were able to accurately (area under the curve = 0.84) predict future suicide attempts using demographic and clinical data from electronic medical records (Walsh et al., 2017). Given the high rate of completed suicide, particularly in elderly adult men, there is an urgent need for enhanced predictive tools to prevent suicide.

There are additional benefits of analyzing electronic medical records. Machine learning methods including deep neural networks, random decision forests, and penalized logistic regressions have been shown to be useful in predicting readmission (Futoma et al., 2015). They may also be able to help determine the likelihood of medical comorbidities that can extend hospital stay. As an example, one study was able to estimate with a fair degree of accuracy hospital-acquired delirium risk using electronic medical record data within 24 hours of hospital admission (Wong et al., 2018).

Treatment of Mental Disorders in Geriatric Populations

In addition to enhancing early detection of mental disorders, precision geriatric psychiatry heralds new approaches to treatment. This is most evident in treatments for MDD. One challenge of treating MDD is that it is a heterogeneous construct. Analysis of STAR*D data found that, of the 3703 depressed outpatients at the beginning of the study, there were 1,030 unique symptom profiles (Fried and Nesse, 2015). This phenotypic variation reflects genetic variation. Depression is caused by an interplay between the monoaminergic, gamma aminobutyric acid, and glutamate systems; hypothalamic–pituitary–adrenal axis; neurotrophic and neuroimmune factors; inflammation; circadian rhythm; extracellular matrix remodeling pathways; and dysfunctional brain networks. However, current clinical practice guidelines recommend that we treat depression largely the same way with a stepwise approach of psychotherapy, pharmacology, and brain stimulation if required. The Research Domain Criteria framework seeks to improve the current state of play and develop objective measures of symptom-linked pathophysiology that can lead to refinement of classification. By using functional magnetic resonance (MRI) in a large multisite sample of patients with depression, researchers were able to divide individuals into four neurophysiological subtypes by examining connectivity between 258 brain regions and using machine learning techniques. Each depression biotype was able to be differentiated from controls with 80% to 90% sensitivity and specificity. They then used these subtypes to predict responsiveness to dorsomedial prefrontal cortex transcranial magnetic stimulation, finding two biotypes responded well (61%–73% response rates) and two did not (25%–30% response rates; Drysdale et al., 2016). Such approaches present significant opportunities to better treat geriatric depression.

Using machine learning by mining existing clinical trial data may soon enable prospective identification of patients who are likely to respond to a specific antidepressant in clinical practice. Using a machine learning multivariate method with a training dataset from STAR*D, researchers have been able to better identify individuals who would remit after citalopram treatment examining 25 variables (Chekroud et al., 2016).

Smartphone Apps and Chatbots

Chatbots are systems that can converse and interact with human users via spoken or written language or visual cues. While the evidence evaluating their use in geriatric mental disorders is sparse, there is potential for chatbots to be used to assist in delivery of digital cognitive behavioral therapy (Abd-Alrazaq et al., 2019). Another avenue to deliver existing psychotherapeutic modalities is via smartphone applications. Given the stigma around mental disorders, personalized and private access via a smartphone in the home environment is one avenue that could lead to more elderly adults receiving treatment. This is already commonplace in youth mental health services. With depressive symptoms, there is evidence that smartphone interventions had a moderate positive effect when compared to inactive controls, with a Hedges' g of 0.56 (Firth et al., 2017). At present these sorts of interventions are best targeted at elderly adults who are technologically literate and with mild depressive symptoms. They may be of particular benefit for those who feel particularly stigmatized and would not seek treatment in a conventional setting and those who are based in rural areas with limited access to specialist services. There needs to be ongoing research in this area to evaluate these tools (Torous et al., 2019).

Pharmacogenetics

Pharmacogenetics (PGx) has emerged as a promising approach to treatment mental illness, particularly MDD, and reduce polypharmacy in elderly adults. There have been a number of studies that have demonstrated the potential efficacy and improved clinical outcomes associated with applying PGx in the treatment of depression (Bousman et al., 2019). To date, most studies of PGx have focused on MDD in adults. However, there is now a focus on PGx applications to enhance treatment of late-life depression (LLD). This corresponds with growing understanding that LLD has a distinct pathophysiology and requires unique considerations (Alexopoulos, 2019). For example, it has been noted that serotonin receptors reduce with age, a physiological occurrence that may potentially impact the pharmacological response to treatments. Moreover, there is more variability in antidepressant concentrations in elderly adults, which has implications for accurately gauging the correlation of a patient's genetically-predicted metabolizer status versus actual antidepressant metabolism (Pollock, 2005). In addition, white matter hyperintensities noted in brain MRI (indicators of vascular dysfunction) are more prominent in LLD whereas in MDD they are rare (Abbott et al., 2018). These cerebral white matter hyperintensities have been proposed to impair neuronal connections, possibly contributing toward the pathogenesis of LLD (Eyre et al., 2016). These differences highlight the importance of understanding the biological and pathophysiological basis of LLD to advance treatment modalities and therapeutic strategies for patients (Lavretsky, 2016).

Pharmacokinetic properties in late life also undergo significant change. Absorption is reduced due to reduced first pass metabolism from structural and functional hepatic changes that are a consequence of aging (Reeve et al., 2017). Progressive atrophy of the gastric mucosa can also lead to decreased absorption in older adults. Moreover, due to the changing gastrointestinal architecture, it has also been suggested that the microbiome is different in older adults, which may subsequently affect medication absorption (Claesson et al., 2011). The blood–brain barrier permeability also increases with age while drug efflux transporters such as P-glycoprotein are decreased (Farrall and Wardlaw, 2009). These changes can result in a more neural exposure to drug treatments.

Changes in metabolism and elimination also occur. Enzymatic activity of important metabolic enzymes such as CYP450 isozymes are decreased leading to reduced Phase I metabolism (Abbott et al., 2018). Most antidepressants are eliminated via the kidneys. Aging is correlated with reduced kidney function and reduced clearance of antidepressant drugs (Gentile et al., 2016). Altogether, the unique pathophysiology and alterations in pharmacokinetics that occur in late life require clinical tools that can take these changes into account.

Advances in Late-Life Depression Pharmacogenetics

Most research has focused on the elucidating the relationship between specific genetic loci related to LLD (e.g., 5-HTTPLR, MDR1, BDNF) and the impact they have on pharmacodynamics and pharmacokinetics of drug treatments such as selective serotonin reuptake inhibitors (SSRIs) and serotonin noradrenaline reuptake inhibitors (SNRIs).

The serotonin transporter gene (SLC6A4) contains a promoter region, 5-HTTLPR, which has been extensively studied for its impact on SSRI efficacy and adverse effects (Abbott et al., 2018). Notably, the promoter region can contain either long (L) or short (S) allele, which corresponds to long or short repeat segments, respectively. Depressed elderly patients carrying the S allele report a higher incidence of gastrointestinal discomfort, fatigue, agitation, sweating, and dizziness (Murphy et al., 2004). A recent randomized controlled trial (RCT) conducted in depressed elderly adults found that certain allele combinations for the serotonin transporter or receptor were associated with increased rates of reported adverse events from the SSRI escitalopram (Garfield et al., 2014). SNRIs are also used commonly in LLD. Specific polymorphisms in the serotonin and norepinephrine transporter genes are associated with higher rates of remission in elderly depressed patients taking the SNRI venlafaxine (Marshe et al., 2017).

Pharmacogenetic Clinical Decision Support Tools for Late-Life Depression Treatment

Pharmacogenetic decision support tools (DSTs) are clinical tools that assessing patient genotype and medications and provide clinical interpretations to assist physicians in optimizing drug prescription. These tools provide information about the anticipated patient phenotype as well as recommendations for drug dosage and cautions about potential drug–drug interactions. Since the introduction of the first DST from Roche in 2004, there has been significant progress in the development of DSTs and to date there are currently over 30 DSTs related to depression management. In an observational study of elderly adults, pharmacogenetic DSTs resulted in a significant decrease in hospitalizations and emergency department visits (Brixner et al., 2016). In another study, DST use in depressed elderly adults was shown to positively impact on the rehospitalization rate (Elliott et al., 2017). This study evaluated the DST called YouScript on its ability to help manage polypharmacy and whether the application of YouScript reduced rehospitalizations. It found that the group of patients whose physician utilized YouScript had reduced hospital visits over a 60 day period (Elliott et al., 2017). Future studies are needed to fully evaluate the clinical potential and utility of DSTs for LLD patients. It is important to note that DSTs are limited to only genetic input—to date, there is no DST that can yet account for comorbidities or psychosocial factors which may influence treatment response.

Other Geriatric Precision Psychiatric Initiatives to Manage Dementias

Virtual Reality

Virtual reality (VR) is its nascent stages in the clinic but shows promise in geriatric mental disorders, in particular in addressing phobias, anxiety, and major neurocognitive disorders (dementias). It can be used to simulate a variety of interactive scenarios and can induce stimulation or relaxation depending on the individual's needs. Small studies suggest that it is accepted positively by individuals with mild to moderately severe dementia and their caregivers (Rose et al., 2019). In a recent meta-analysis of 11 studies on individuals with mild cognitive impairment or dementia, VR interventions were found to have small to medium positive effects on physical fitness, cognition, and emotion (Kim et al., 2019). Further research is required on patient outcomes given the limited number of studies available and uncertainty regarding definitive conclusions (Sayma et al., 2020). Another possibility is for VR to be used in educating doctors, care staff, and families about the experience of dementia to promote empathy and facilitate improved care. There are no high-level studies with controlled design or group comparisons available yet regarding this intervention (Hirt and Beer, 2019).

Robotics

Robots are now commonly used in many countries to assist in screening, assessment, and diagnosis of geriatric mental disorders; support independent living and autonomy; and enhance care and comfort. In Japan, where over 20% of the population is over the age of 65, home based biometric monitoring and robotics are increasingly being utilized. In aged-care facilities, robotic exoskeletons can assist care workers to lift people and humanoid robots can assist with communication by using a microphone and camera to mirror the person's actions and decipher simple language (Leroi et al., 2018). In a cluster RCT, the use of a robotic pet modeled on a harp seal was found to improve pleasure and reduce agitation (Moyle et al., 2017). A meta-analysis of RCTs of pet robot interventions found that the use of pet robots have positive effects on the behavioral and psychological symptoms of dementia (Leng et al., 2019). As with the use of all technology, there are ethical challenges associated with the use of robots in vulnerable elderly populations. Excessive reliance on robots may result in elderly individuals having less meaningful interaction with actual people and may have wider ramifications on society including blinding us to the vulnerable and dependent aspect of our human condition (O'Brolchain, 2019).

Brain Stimulation for Cognitive Enhancement

Transcranial magnetic stimulation (TMS) has been shown in a large number of studies to modulate cortical networks to enhance cognitive performance in healthy human subjects (Luber and Lisanby, 2014). Transcranial direct current stimulation (tDCS) has less evidence (McIntire et al., 2014). These tools are now being explored in elderly adults with cognitive impairment. There are conflicting findings to date. In one randomized sham-controlled pilot study of tDCS, 20 patients with a mean age of 76.1 years (9 patients with minor neurocognitive disorders and 11 with major neurocognitive disorders) were studied and assessed using Mini-Mental State Examination. While tDCS was found to be safe and tolerable, there was no statistically significant cognitive effects. Another small double-blind RCT of rTMS combined with cognitive training in 27 patients with AD (18 and 8 in the treatment and sham groups, respectively, with one dropout) found that the Alzheimer's Disease Assessment Scale—Cognitive Subscale (ADAS-Cog) scores were improved significantly in the treatment group compared to the sham group. The effects were greatest in the domains of memory and language (Lee et al., 2016). There may be some benefit of rTMS in mild cognitive impairment. One small double-blind RCT of rTMS over the dorsolateral prefrontal cortex found improvements on the Rivermead Behavioural Memory Test, which was sustained for one month. However, the absolute effect of the treatment was small (Drumond Marra et al., 2015). All of the studies discussed, as well as another study, that found selective improvement in episodic memory but not in other cognitive domains (Koch et al., 2018) are small. There is a need for further larger, well-designed trials as this technology improves.

Anti-Aging and Disease-Modifying Therapies

Aging is a significant risk factor for many diseases and indeed many neurodegenerative disorders are considered an inevitable consequence of the aging process. There have been recent hypotheses raised that diseases of aging share common pathways and may represent an acceleration of the aging process (Franceschi et al., 2018). A subdivision of the different hallmarks of aging that may be targeted by interventions has been suggested (López-Otín et al., 2013). Considering that neurodegenerative disorders are an inevitable part of the aging process, targeting the aging process itself—or, indeed, particular hallmarks of aging—may delay the onset of neurodegenerative disorders among multiple diseases of aging. This theory is the basis for large medication trials targeting multiple outcomes as nonspecific markers of delayed aging (e.g., the Targeting Aging with Metformin [TAME] Trial). There have also been studies into the neuroprotective effect of anti-inflammatory molecules; as well as interventions targeting other "hallmarks of aging" including protein homeostasis and altered nutrient sensing pathways.

There is some evidence, particularly in animal models, around the repurposing of existing medications to target specific hallmarks of ageing (Heard et al., 2018). One of the most studied molecules is resveratrol (de la Lastra and Villegas, 2005), a natural phenol found in the skin of grapes among other plants. Although widely studied in animal models, there is not sufficient evidence of efficacy in humans (Vang et al., 2011). There have also been trials of novel "senolytic" molecules in animal models (Zhu et al., 2016), which show promise in delaying the onset of age-related symptoms. This is an area of promise for future research targeting multiple diseases of aging such as cardiovascular disease, osteoarthritis, and cataracts, as well as neurodegenerative diseases. Although this area of research targets broad outcomes in the wide domain of "age-related diseases," there is great potential in future research interventions. An example is the role of telomere shortening in aging (Blackburn et al., 2015), and experimental use of telemerase (telomere lengthening) gene therapy in mice resulted in a 24% increase in median lifespan (Bernardes de Jesus et al., 2012).

Brain Imaging

Late-life depression is a known risk factor for cognitive decline, and a common feature of AD and other dementias. AD is the most common cause of dementia and remains incurable. Its prevalence is rising. Currently dementia remains a clinical diagnosis based on standardized criteria. Unfortunately, a common precursor of mild cognitive impairment is often diagnosed late or not diagnosed at all. This highlights the need for improved diagnosis of memory disorders. Imaging remains an important component of diagnosis for AD but traditionally has been limited to excluding "organic" causes of dementia such as brain tumors and strokes (Knopman et al., 2001). However, newer tools exist to extract additional information from brain MRI scans with quantitative analysis. These volumes can be of entire lobes of the brain, such as the frontal lobes or of specific structures known to be abnormal in AD such as the hippocampus. Some tools such as Neuroreader are validated in the computation of hippocampal volumes (Ahdidan et al., 2015) compared to gold standard, expert anatomical tracings. This allows for rapidly quantitative information that clinicians can use in tailoring their diagnostic and therapeutic approaches.

Tools such as Neurostat are in use in clinical practice and research, allowing standardized comparison of functional neuroimaging such as positron-emission tomography. Similar software packages, using automated segmentation in structural neuroimaging, allow comparison of brain volume with standardized datasets (e.g., MorphoBOX from Siemens, NeuroQuant by CorTechs). Automated tools are established in the treatment of multiple sclerosis (Jain et al., 2015) and can flag changes in white matter hyperintensities over time. This kind of automated interpretation of MRI may have a role in the early atrophic changes and longitudinal atrophy characteristic of neurodegenerative conditions.

Initial assessments of persons with cognitive disorders can now include a combination of mental status examination, computerized neuropsychology tests, genomic directed psychopharmacology, quantitative electroencephalography with event-related potential testing (Raicher et al., 2008; Cecchi et al., 2015), and quantitative MRI volumetrics. The imaging component is a key part of initial assessment—not only for identifying hippocampal volume loss that is a key imaging feature of AD (Laasko et al., 2000) but, more important, for identifying other potential causes of memory loss. The importance of this technology is pertinent given the difficulty of identifying either cross sectional or longitudinal atrophy (Ross et al., 2015).

Clinical Implications and Future Directions

A recent debate about whether artificial intelligence could eventually replace psychiatrists highlighted the importance of human interaction in psychiatry (Brown et al., 2019). Precision psychiatry has great potential to improve patient care. However, psychiatry is both a science and an art, and data obtained by technology should be used as an adjunct to enhance doctor–patient connection and therapeutic alliance rather

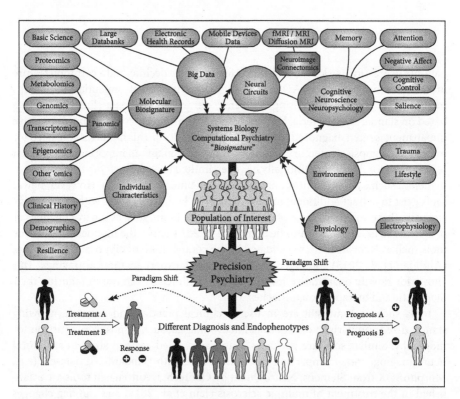

Figure 15.1 A mind map of precision psychiatry with several diverse approaches and techniques converging to produce biosignatures that can be applied to populations to enhance diagnosis and treatment at an individual level.

Fernandes et al. (2017).

than leading to impersonal care from a psychiatrist behind a computer screen. The goal of precision psychiatry is twofold. First, it seeks to improve patient care and outcomes by a deeper and finer grained understanding of the patient and care delivery system characteristics that influence the validity and reliability of diagnosis. Second, it seeks to optimize patient outcomes by targeting multiple mediators of the strength and durability of treatment response—from neurotransmitter systems and specific brain circuits to boosting self-efficacy, social supports, and treatment adherence. It seeks to enhance to science of psychiatry via use of data, without detracting from the art of psychiatry. Much of precision psychiatry pertains to experimental technologies. There is a need to ensure future research incorporates proof-of-concept studies, integration of engineering principles to help research keep pace with technology, and studies around implementation issues (Fortuna et al., 2019). It is essential for the promise of precision geriatric psychiatry to be realized that we implement platforms and systems that enact team-based, multidisciplinary, and measurement-based care. These platforms provide necessary infrastructure for the use of PGx, biomarker and imaging DSTs and collaborate care between psychiatrists, patients and their families, and allied health staff.

Conclusion

When making future predictions, it is helpful to examine past predictions. An article published in the *New England Journal of Medicine* in 1970 predicted that by the year 2000 computers would have an entirely new role in medicine, acting as a powerful extension of the physician's intellect and fundamentally altering the role of the physician (Schwartz, 1970). This has not occurred, at least in the field of psychiatry.

While precision geriatric psychiatry offers significant promise in diagnosis and treatment of geriatric mental disorders, skills in the art of psychiatry remain paramount. Patient outcomes are inextricably linked to therapeutic alliance and advances in diagnosis and treatment should never interfere with the sacrosanct connection between psychiatrist and patient.

The goals of personalized psychiatry are to predict the individual's susceptibility to mental illness, achieve an accurate diagnosis, and provide an efficient and favorable response to treatment. There is value in developing a model for this specifically with geriatric mental disorders. More work is required to refine these approaches.

References

Abbott, R., Chang, D. D., Eyre, H. A., Bousman, C. A., Merrill, D. A. & Lavretsky, H. 2018. Pharmacogenetic decision support tools: A new paradigm for late-life depression? *Am J Geriatr Psychiatry*, 26, 125–133.

Abd-Alrazaq, A. A., Alajlani, M., Alalwan, A. A., Bewick, B. M., Gardner, P. & Househ, M. 2019. An overview of the features of chatbots in mental health: A scoping review. *Int J Med Inform*, 132, 103978.

Ahdidan, J., Raji, C. A., Deyoe, E. A., Mathis, J., Noe, K. O., Rimestad, J., Kjeldsen, T. K., Mosegaard, J., Becker, J. T. & Lopez, O. 2015. Quantitative neuroimaging software for clinical assessment of hippocampal volumes on MR imaging. *J Alzheimers Dis*, 49, 723–32.

Alexopoulos, G. S. 2019. Mechanisms and treatment of late-life depression. *Transl Psychiatry*, 9, 188.

Andreas, S., Schulz, H., Volkert, J., Dehoust, M., Sehner, S., Suling, A., Ausín, B., Canuto, A., Crawford, M., Da Ronch, C., Grassi, L., Hershkovitz, Y., Muñoz, M., Quirk, A., Rotenstein, O., Santos-Olmo, A. B., Shalev, A., Strehle, J., Weber, K., Wegscheider, K., Wittchen, H.-U. & Härter, M. 2018. Prevalence of mental disorders in elderly people: The European MentDis_ICF65+ study. *British Journal of Psychiatry*, 210, 125–131.

Barrett, P. M., Steinhubl, S. R., Muse, E. D. & Topol, E. J. 2017. Digitising the mind. *Lancet*, 389, 1877.

Bartlett, M. S., Littlewort, G. C., Frank, M. G., Lainscsek, C., Fasel, I. R. & Movellan, J. R. 2006. Automatic recognition of facial actions in spontaneous expressions. *J Multimedia*, 1, 22–35 https://doi.org/10.4304/jmm.1.6.22-35.

Bedi, G., Carrillo, F., Cecchi, G. A., Slezak, D. F., Sigman, M., Mota, N. B., Ribeiro, S., Javitt, D. C., Copelli, M. & Corcoran, C. M. 2015. Automated analysis of free speech predicts psychosis onset in high-risk youths. *npj Schizophrenia*, 1, 15030.

Bernardes de Jesus, B., Vera, E., Schneeberger, K., Tejera, A. M., Ayuso, E., Bosch, F. & Blasco, M. A. 2012. Telomerase gene therapy in adult and old mice delays aging and increases longevity without increasing cancer. *EMBO Mol Med*, 4, 691–704 https://doi.org/10.1002/emmm.201200245.

Bhagwat, N., Viviano, J. D., Voineskos, A. N. & Chakravarty, M. M. 2018. Modeling and prediction of clinical symptom trajectories in Alzheimer's disease using longitudinal data. *PLoS Comput Biol*, 14, e1006376.

Blackburn, E. H., Epel, E. S. & Lin, J. 2015. Human telomere biology: A contributory and interactive factor in aging, disease risks, and protection. *Science*, 350, 1193–1198 https://doi.org/10.1126/science.aab3389.

Bousman, C. A., Arandjelovic, K., Mancuso, S. G., Eyre, H. A. & Dunlop, B. W. 2019. Pharmacogenetic tests and depressive symptom remission: A meta-analysis of randomized controlled trials, *Pharmacogenomics*, 20, 37–47 https://doi.org/10.2217/pgs-2018-0142.

Brixner, D., Biltaji, E., Bress, A., Unni, S., YE, X., Mamiya, T., Ashcraft, K. & Biskupiak, J. 2016. The effect of pharmacogenetic profiling with a clinical decision support tool on healthcare resource utilization and estimated costs in the elderly exposed to polypharmacy. *J Med Econ*, 19, 213–228 https://doi.org/10.3111/13696998.2015.1110160.

Brown, C., Story, G. W., Mourao-Miranda, J. & Baker, J. T. 2019. Will artificial intelligence eventually replace psychiatrists? *Br J Psychiatry*. [Epub Ahead of Print] https://doi.org/10.1192/bjp.2019.245

Cao, B., Zheng, L., Zhang, C., Yu, P., Piscitello, A., Zulueta, J., Ajilore, O., Ryan, K., Leow, A. D. & Matwin, S. 2017. Deepmood: Modeling mobile phone typing dynamics for mood detection. In *Proceedings of the 23rd ACM SIGKDD International Conference on Knowledge Discovery and Data Mining—KDD '17* (pp. 747–755). New York, NY: ACM.

Cecchi, M., Moore, D. K., Sadowsky, C. H., Solomon, P. R., Doraiswamy, P. M., Smith, C. D., Jicha, G. A., Budson, A. E., Arnold, S. E. & Fadem, K. C. 2015. A clinical trial to validate event-related potential markers of Alzheimer's disease in outpatient settings. *Alzheimers Dement (Amst)*, 1, 387–94.

Chekroud, A. M., Zotti, R. J., Shehzad, Z., Gueorguieva, R., Johnson, M. K., Trivedi, M. H., Cannon, T. D., Krystal, J. H. & Corlett, P. R. 2016. Cross-trial prediction of treatment outcome in depression: A machine learning approach. *Lancet Psychiat*, 3, 243–250 https://doi.org/10.1016/s2215-0366(15)00471-x.

Claesson, M. J., Cusack, S., O'Sullivan, O., Greene-Diniz, R., de Weerd, H., Flannery, E., Marchesi, J. R., Falush, D., Dinan, T., Fitzgerald, G., Stanton, C., van Sinderen, D., O'Connor, M., Harnedy, N., O'Connor, K., Henry, C., O'Mahony, D., Fitzgerald, A. P., Shanahan, F., Twomey, C., Hill, C., Ross, R. P. & O'Toole, P. W. 2011. Composition, variability, and temporal stability of the intestinal microbiota of the elderly. *Proc Natl Acad Sci U S A*, 108(Suppl 1), 4586–4591.

Cummins, N., Scherer, S., Krajewski, J., Schnieder, S., Epps, J. & Quatieri, T. F. 2015. A review of depression and suicide risk assessment using speech analysis. *Speech Comm*, 71, 10–49 https://doi.org/10.1016/j.specom.2015.03.004.

de la Lastra, C. A. & Villegas, I. 2005. Resveratrol as an anti-inflammatory and anti-aging agent: Mechanisms and clinical implications. *Mol Nutr Food Res*, 49, 405–30.

de la Torre-Luque, A., de la Fuente, J., Sanchez-Niubo, A., Caballero, F. F., Prina, M., Muniz-Terrera, G., Haro, J. M. & Ayuso-Mateos, J. L. 2019. Stability of clinically relevant depression symptoms in old-age across 11 cohorts: A multi-state study. *Acta Psychiatr Scand*, 140, 541–551 https://doi.org/10.1111/acps.13107.

Deng, Y., Mcquoid, D. R., Potter, G. G., Steffens, D. C., Albert, K., Riddle, M., BEYER, J. L. & Taylor, W. D. 2018. Predictors of recurrence in remitted late-life depression. *Depress Anxiety*, 35, 658–667 https://doi.org/10.1002/da.22772.

Dong, L., Freedman, V. A. & Mendes de Leon, C. F. 2019. The association of comorbid depression and anxiety symptoms with disability onset in older adults. *Psychosom Med*, 82, 158–164.

Drumond Marra, H. L., Myczkowski, M. L., Maia Memória, C., Arnaut, D., Leite Ribeiro, P., Sardinha Mansur, C. G., Lancelote Alberto, R., Boura Bellini, B., Alves Fernandes da Silva, A., Tortella, G., Ciampi de Andrade, D., Teixeira, M. J., Forlenza, O. V. & Marcolin, M. A. 2015. Transcranial magnetic stimulation to address mild cognitive impairment in the elderly: A randomized controlled study. *Behav Neurol*, 2015, 287843 https://doi.org/10.1155/2015/287843.

Drysdale, A. T., Grosenick, L., Downar, J., Dunlop, K., Mansouri, F., Meng, Y., Fetcho, R. N., Zebley, B., Oathes, D. J., Etkin, A., Schatzberg, A. F., Sudheimer, K., Keller, J., Mayberg, H. S., Gunning, F. M., Alexopoulos, G. S., Fox, M. D., Pascual-Leone, A., Voss, H. U., Casey, B. J., Dubin, M. J. & Liston, C. 2016. Resting-state connectivity biomarkers define neurophysiological subtypes of depression. *Nat Med*, 23, 28.

Eichstaedt, J. C., Smith, R. J., Merchant, R. M., Ungar, L. H., Crutchley, P., Preoţiuc-Pietro, D., Asch, D. A. & Schwartz, H. A. 2018. Facebook language predicts depression in medical records. *P Nat Acad Sci*, 115, 11203.

Elliott, L. S., Henderson, J. C., Neradilek, M. B., Moyer, N. A., Ashcraft, K. C. & Thirumaran, R. K. 2017. Clinical impact of pharmacogenetic profiling with a clinical decision support tool in polypharmacy home health patients: A prospective pilot randomized controlled trial. *PLOS ONE*, 12, e0170905.

Eyre, H. A., Yang, H., Leaver, A. M., Van Dyk, K., Siddarth, P., Cyr, N. S., Narr, K., Ercoli, L., Baune, B. T. & Lavretsky, H. 2016. Altered resting-state functional connectivity in late-life depression: A cross-sectional study. *J Affect Disord*, 189, 126–133.

Farrall, A. J. & Wardlaw, J. M. 2009. Blood-brain barrier: Ageing and microvascular disease--systematic review and meta-analysis. *Neurobiol Aging*, 30, 337–52.

Fernandes, B. S., Williams, L. M., Steiner, J., Leboyer, M., Carvalho, A. F. & Berk, M. 2017. The new field of "precision psychiatry." *BMC Med*, 15, 80 https://doi.org/10.1186/s12916-017-0849-x.

Firth, J., Torous, J., Nicholas, J., Carney, R., Pratap, A., Rosenbaum, S. & Sarris, J. 2017. The efficacy of smartphone-based mental health interventions for depressive symptoms: A meta-analysis of randomized controlled trials. *World Psychiatr*, 16, 287–298 https://doi.org/10.1002/wps.20472.

Forbes, M., Stefler, D., Velakoulis, D., Stuckey, S., Trudel, J. F., Eyre, H., Boyd, M. & Kisely, S. 2019. The clinical utility of structural neuroimaging in first-episode psychosis: A systematic review. *Aust N Z J Psychiatry*, 53, 1093–1104.

Fortuna, K. L., Torous, J., Depp, C. A., Jimenez, D. E., Arean, P. A., Walker, R., Ajilore, O., Goldstein, C. M., Cosco, T. D., Brooks, J. M., Vahia, I. V. & Bartels, S. J. 2019. A future research agenda for digital geriatric mental healthcare. *Am J Geriatr Psychiatry*, 27, 1277–1285.

Franceschi, C., Garagnani, P., Morsiani, C., Conte, M., Santoro, A., Grignolio, A., Monti, D., Capri, M. & Salvioli, S. 2018. The continuum of aging and age-related diseases: Common mechanisms but different rates. *Front Med*, 5, 61.

Franklin, J. C., Ribeiro, J. D., Fox, K. R., Bentley, K. H., Kleiman, E. M., Huang, X., Musacchio, K. M., Jaroszewski, A. C., Chang, B. P. & Nock, M. K. 2017. Risk factors for suicidal thoughts and behaviors: A meta-analysis of 50 years of research. *Psychol Bull*, 143, 187–232.

Fried, E. I. & Nesse, R. M. 2015. Depression is not a consistent syndrome: An investigation of unique symptom patterns in the STAR*D study. *J Affect Disord*, 172, 96–102.

Futoma, J., Morris, J. & Lucas, J. 2015. A comparison of models for predicting early hospital readmissions. *Journal of Biomedical Informatics*, 56, 229–238.

Garfield, L. D., Dixon, D., Nowotny, P., Lotrich, F. E., Pollock, B. G., Kristjansson, S. D., Dore, P. M. & Lenze, E. J. 2014. Common selective serotonin reuptake inhibitor side effects in older adults associated with genetic polymorphisms in the serotonin transporter and receptors: Data from a randomized controlled trial. *Am J Geriatr Psychiatry*, 22, 971–979.

Gentile, G., Cipolla, F., Capi, M., Simmaco, M., Lionetta, L. & Borro, M. 2016. Precise medical decision making in geriatric anti-depressant therapy. *Expert Rev Precision Med Drug Dev*, 1, 387–396.

Goodday, S. M. 2020. The unique utility of digital technology for bipolar disorder. *Bipolar Disord*, 22, 197.

Grabowski, K., Rynkiewicz, A., Lassalle, A., Baron-Cohen, S., Schuller, B., Cummins, N., Baird, A., Podgorska-Bednarz, J., Pieniazek, A. & Lucka, I. 2019. Emotional expression in psychiatric conditions: New technology for clinicians. *Psychiatry Clin Neurosci*, 73, 50–62.

Heard, D. S., Tuttle, C. S. L., Lautenschlager, N. T. & Maier, A. B. 2018. Repurposing proteostasis-modifying drugs to prevent or treat age-related dementia: A systematic review. *Front Physiol*, 9, 1520.

Hirt, J. & Beer, T. 2019. Use and impact of virtual reality simulation in dementia care education: A scoping review. *Nurse Educ Today*, 84, 104207.

Hodgetts, S., Gallagher, P., Stow, D., Ferrier, I. N. & O'Brien, J. T. 2017. The impact and measurement of social dysfunction in late-life depression: An evaluation of current methods with a focus on wearable technology. *Int J Geriatr Psychiatry*, 32, 247–255.

Horackova, K., Kopecek, M., Machů, V., Kagstrom, A., Aarsland, D., Motlova, L. B. & Cermakova, P. 2019. Prevalence of late-life depression and gap in mental health service use across European regions. *Euro Psychiatr*, 57, 19–25.

Jain, S., Sima, D. M., Ribbens, A., Cambron, M., Maertens, A., Van Hecke, W., de Mey, J., Barkhof, F., Steenwijk, M. D., Daams, M., Maes, F., Van Huffel, S., Vrenken, H. & Smeets, D. 2015. Automatic segmentation and volumetry of multiple sclerosis brain lesions from MR images. *NeuroImage-Clin*, 8, 367–375.

Kim, O., Pang, Y. & Kim, J. H. 2019. The effectiveness of virtual reality for people with mild cognitive impairment or dementia: A meta-analysis. *BMC Psychiatry*, 19, 219.

Knopman, D. S., Dekosky, S. T., Cummings, J. L., Chui, H., Corey-Bloom, J., Relkin, N., Small, G. W., Miller, B. & Stevens, J. C. 2001. Practice parameter: Diagnosis of dementia (an evidence-based review): Report of the Quality Standards Subcommittee of the American Academy of Neurology. *Neurology*, 56, 1143–1153.

Koch, G., Bonni, S., Pellicciari, M. C., Casula, E. P., Mancini, M., Esposito, R., Ponzo, V., Picazio, S., di Lorenzo, F., Serra, L., Motta, C., Maiella, M., Marra, C., Cercignani, M., Martorana, A., Caltagirone, C. & Bozzali, M. 2018. Transcranial magnetic stimulation of the precuneus enhances memory and neural activity in prodromal Alzheimer's disease. *Neuroimage*, 169, 302–311.

Laasko, M. P., Lehtovirta, M., Partanen, K., Riekkinen, P. J. & Soininen, H. 2000. Hippocampus in Alzheimer's disease: A 3-year follow-up MRI study. *Biol Psychiatry*, 47, 557–561.

Lavretsky, H. 2016. Intervention research in late-life depression: Challenges and opportunities. *Am J Geriatr Psychiatry*, 24, 6–10.

Lee, J., Choi, B. H., Oh, E., Sohn, E. H. & Lee, A. Y. 2016. Treatment of Alzheimer's disease with repetitive transcranial magnetic stimulation combined with cognitive training: A prospective, randomized, double-blind, placebo-controlled study. *J Clin Neurol (Seoul)*, 12, 57–64.

Leng, M., Liu, P., Zhang, P., Hu, M., Zhou, H., Li, G., Yin, H. & Chen, L. 2019. Pet robot intervention for people with dementia: A systematic review and meta-analysis of randomized controlled trials. *Psychiatr Res*, 271, 516–525.

Leroi, I., Watanabe, K., Hird, N. & Sugihara, T. 2018. "Psychogeritechnology" in Japan: Exemplars from a super-aged society. *Int J Geriatr Psychiatry*, 33, 1533–1540.

López-Otín, C., Blasco, M. A., Partridge, L., Serrano, M. & Kroemer, G. 2013. The hallmarks of aging. *Cell*, 153, 1194–1217.

Luber, B. & Lisanby, S. H. 2014. Enhancement of human cognitive performance using transcranial magnetic stimulation (TMS). *Neuroimage*, 85 Pt 3, 961–70.

Lucas, G. M., Gratch, J., King, A. & Morency, L.-P. 2014. It's only a computer: Virtual humans increase willingness to disclose. *Comput Hum Behav*, 37, 94–100.

Marshe, V. S., Maciukiewicz, M., Rej, S., Tiwari, A. K., Sibille, E., Blumberger, D. M., Karp, J. F., Lenze, E. J., Reynolds, C. F., 3rd, Kennedy, J. L., Mulsant, B. H. & Muller, D. J. 2017. Norepinephrine transporter gene variants and remission from depression with venlafaxine treatment in older adults. *Am J Psychiatry*, 174, 468–475.

McIntire, L. K., McKinley, R. A., Goodyear, C. & Nelson, J. 2014. A comparison of the effects of transcranial direct current stimulation and caffeine on vigilance and cognitive performance during extended wakefulness. *Brain Stimul*, 7, 499–507.

Mohebbi, M., Agustini, B., Woods, R. L., McNeil, J. J., Nelson, M. R., Shah, R. C., Nguyen, V., Storey, E., Murray, A. M., Reid, C. M., Kirpach, B., Wolfe, R., Lockery, J. E. & Berk, M. 2019. Prevalence of depressive symptoms and its associated factors among healthy community-dwelling older adults living in Australia and the United States. *Int J Geriatr Psychiatry*, 34, 1208–1216.

Moyle, W., Jones, C. J., Murfield, J. E., Thalib, L., Beattie, E. R. A., Shum, D. K. H., O'dwyer, S. T., Mervin, M. C. & Draper, B. M. 2017. Use of a robotic seal as a therapeutic tool to improve dementia symptoms: A cluster-randomized controlled trial. *J Am Med Dir Assoc*, 18, 766–773.

Murphy, G. M., Jr., Hollander, S. B., Rodrigues, H. E., Kremer, C. & Schatzberg, A. F. 2004. Effects of the serotonin transporter gene promoter polymorphism on mirtazapine and paroxetine efficacy and adverse events in geriatric major depression. *Arch Gen Psychiatry*, 61, 1163–9.

O'Brien, J. T., Gallagher, P., Stow, D., Hammerla, N., Ploetz, T., Firbank, M., Ladha, C., Ladha, K., Jackson, D., McNaney, R., Ferrier, I. N. & Olivier, P. 2017. A study of wrist-worn activity measurement as a potential real-world biomarker for late-life depression. *Psychol Med*, 47, 93–102.

O'Brolchain, F. 2019. Robots and people with dementia: Unintended consequences and moral hazard. *Nurs Ethics*, 26, 962–972.

Pollock, B. G. 2005. The pharmacokinetic imperative in late-life depression. *J Clin Psychopharmacol*, 25, S19–S23.

Raicher, I., Yasumasa Takahashi, D., Medeiros Kanda, P. A., Nitrini, R. & Anghinah, R. 2008. qEEG spectral peak in Alzheimer's disease: A possible tool for treatment follow-up. *Dement Neuropsychol*, 2, 9–12.

Reece, A. G. & Danforth, C. M. 2017. Instagram photos reveal predictive markers of depression. *EPJ Data Sci*, 6, 15.

Reeve, E., Trenaman, S. C., Rockwood, K. & Hilmer, S. N. 2017. Pharmacokinetic and pharmacodynamic alterations in older people with dementia. *Expert Opin Drug Metab Toxicol*, 13, 651–668.

Rose, V., Stewart, I., Jenkins, K. G., Tabbaa, L., Ang, C. S. & Matsangidou, M. 2019. Bringing the outside in: The feasibility of virtual reality with people with dementia in an inpatient psychiatric care setting. *Dementia*. https://doi.org/10.1177/1471301219868036.

Ross, D. E., Ochs, A. L., Desmit, M. E., Seabaugh, J. M. & Havranek, M. D.; Alzheimer's Disease Neuroimaging Initiative. 2015. Man versus machine part 2: Comparison of radiologists' interpretations and NeuroQuant measures of brain asymmetry and progressive atrophy in patients with traumatic brain injury. *J Neuropsychiatry Clin Neurosci*, 27, 147–52.

Sajatovic, M., Strejilevich, S. A., Gildengers, A. G., Dols, A., al Jurdi, R. K., Forester, B. P., Kessing, L. V., Beyer, J., Manes, F., Rej, S., Rosa, A. R., Schouws, S. N., Tsai, S. Y., Young, R. C. & Shulman, K. I. 2015. A report on older-age bipolar disorder from the International Society for Bipolar Disorders Task Force. *Bipolar Disord*, 17, 689–704.

Sayma, M., Tuijt, R., Cooper, C. & Walters, K. 2020. Are we there yet? Immersive virtual reality to improve cognitive function in dementia and mild cognitive impairment. *Gerontologist*, 60(7), e502–e512. https://www.doi.org/10.1093/geront/gnz132

Schnyer, D. M., Clasen, P. C., Gonzalez, C. & Beevers, C. G. 2017. Evaluating the diagnostic utility of applying a machine learning algorithm to diffusion tensor MRI measures in individuals with major depressive disorder. *Psychiatr Res-Neuroimag*, 264, 1–9.

Schwartz, W. B. 1970. Medicine and the computer. The promise and problems of change. *N Engl J Med*, 283, 1257–1264.

Stafford, J., Howard, R. & Kirkbride, J. B. 2018. The incidence of very late-onset psychotic disorders: a systematic review and meta-analysis, 1960-2016. *Psychol Med*, 48, 1775–1786.

Torous, J., Cerrato, P. & Halamka, J. 2019. Targeting depressive symptoms with technology. *Mhealth*, 5, 19.

United Nations, Department of Economic and Social Affairs. 2019. *World Population Ageing 2019*. https://www.un.org/en/development/desa/population/publications/pdf/ageing/WorldPopulationAgeing2019-Highlights.pdf [Accessed November 13, 2019].

Vang, O., Ahmad, N., Baile, C. A., Baur, J. A., Brown, K., Csiszar, A., Das, D. K., Delmas, D., Gottfried, C., Lin, H.-Y., Ma, Q.-Y., Mukhopadhyay, P., Nalini, N., Pezzuto, J. M., Richard, T., Shukla, Y., Surh, Y.-J., Szekeres, T., Szkudelski, T., Walle, T. & Wu, J. M. 2011. What is new for an old molecule? Systematic review and recommendations on the use of resveratrol. *PLOS ONE*, 6, e19881–e19881.

Walsh, C. G., Ribeiro, J. D. & Franklin, J. C. 2017. Predicting risk of suicide attempts over time through machine learning. *Clin Psychol Sci*, 5, 457–469.

Wei, J., Hou, R., Zhang, X., Xu, H., Xie, L., Chandrasekar, E. K., Ying, M. & Goodman, M. 2019. The association of late-life depression with all-cause and cardiovascular mortality among community-dwelling older adults: Systematic review and meta-analysis. *Br J Psychiatry*, 215, 449–455.

Wei, J., Ying, M., Xie, L., Chandrasekar, E. K., Lu, H., Wang, T. & Li, C. 2019. Late-life depression and cognitive function among older adults in the U.S.: The National Health and Nutrition Examination Survey, 2011–2014. *J Psychiatr Res*, 111, 30–35.

Wollenhaupt-Aguiar, B., Librenza-Garcia, D., Bristot, G., Przybylski, L., Stertz, L., Kubiachi Burque, R., Cereser, K. M., Spanemberg, L., Caldieraro, M. A., Frey, B. N., Fleck, M. P.,

Kauer-Sant'anna, M., Cavalcante Passos, I. & Kapczinski, F. 2020. Differential biomarker signatures in unipolar and bipolar depression: A machine learning approach. *Aust N Z J Psychiatry*, 54, 393–401.

Wong, A., Young, A. T., Liang, A. S., Gonzales, R., Douglas, V. C. & Hadley, D. 2018. Development and validation of an electronic health record–based machine learning model to estimate delirium risk in newly hospitalized patients without known cognitive impairment. *JAMA Netw Open*, 1, e181018–e181018.

Zhong, B. L., Xu, Y. M., Xie, W. X., Liu, X. J. & Huang, Z. W. 2019. Depressive symptoms in elderly Chinese primary care patients: Prevalence and sociodemographic and clinical correlates. *J Geriatr Psychiatry Neurol*, 32, 312–318.

Zhu, Y., Tchkonia, T., Fuhrmann-Stroissnigg, H., Dai, H. M., Ling, Y. Y., Stout, M. B., Pirtskhalava, T., Giorgadze, N., Johnson, K. O., Giles, C. B., Wren, J. D., Niedernhofer, L. J., Robbins, P. D. & Kirkland, J. L. 2016. Identification of a novel senolytic agent, navitoclax, targeting the Bcl-2 family of anti-apoptotic factors. *Aging Cell*, 15, 428–435.

16

Convergence Neuroscience of Meditative Mind–Body Therapies for Mental Health

Kelsey T. Laird, Felipe A. Jain, and Helen Lavretsky

Mental health disorders account for roughly one third of adult disability worldwide, resulting in enormous personal and socioeconomic costs (Anderson, Jane-Llopis, & Hosman, 2011). Approaches that are minimally invasive, cost-effective, culturally acceptable, and scalable are essential to the successful management of global mental health needs. Many patients engage in meditative therapies as an alternative or in addition to other treatments. Roughly 19% of the U.S. adult population reports currently practicing some form of meditation (Macinko & Upchurch, 2019), and rates among those with a mental health disorder are even higher (Morone, Moore, & Greco, 2017). Results of a national survey indicate that anxiety, stress, and depression are the most common health conditions for which U.S. adults report using meditation (Cramer, Ward, et al., 2016).

The term *meditation* describes any psychosomatic practice that involves training and regulating attention toward interoceptive foci (e.g., sensations of breath or body), exteroceptive foci (e.g., a candle flame or external sound), or intentionally created mental images (e.g., visualization of light or movement; Davidson & Goleman, 1977; F. A. Jain, Walsh, Eisendrath, Christensen, & Cahn, 2015; Walsh & Shapiro, 2006). Meditation can be practiced while stationary or as part of a movement-based practice, as in the case of yoga, tai chi, and qigong.

A growing body of research supports the use of meditative therapies as effective, holistic approaches to the treatment of a variety of mental health conditions (F. A. Jain et al., 2015). Meditative therapies confer a lower risk of side effects compared to more invasive approaches, have been shown to reduce side effects associated with pharmacological treatment (Eyre, Baune, & Lavretsky, 2015; Sprod et al., 2015), and have potential to build life-long skills with benefits far beyond initial training. In the first part of the chapter, we review meditative interventions with evidence of efficacy for the treatment of common mental health disorders. Specifically, we review meta-analyses and randomized controlled trials (RCTs) evaluating the efficacy of meditative therapies for the treatment of mood disorders, anxiety and stress-related disorders, and substance use disorder (SUD), as well as for improving adjustment among heterogenous clinical samples. Following the World Health Organization's (1948) definition of health as "a state of complete physical, mental, and social well-being and not merely the absense of disease or infirmity," we also evaluate the efficacy of these interventions for improving well-being in nonclinical samples. For consistency, positive treatment effects are delineated by positive standardized mean differences (SMDs) regardless of the outcome measure (e.g., well-being vs. depression). In the second part of the chapter, we review candidate neurobiological mechanisms that may account for the potential of meditative therapies to enhnce resilience to a range of mental health disorders.

A Summary of Research Evaluating Clinical Efficacy

Mood Disorders

Mindfulness-Based Therapies

Meditation is a component of many ancient religious traditions, and secular forms of meditation have been more recently adopted in Western culture as a method of reducing depression, pain, and stress. The most widely adopted form of meditation in clinical research and practice focuses on the development of mindfulness, defined as "paying attention on purpose, in the present moment, and nonjudgmentally" (Kabat-Zinn, 2003, p. 145). Of note, mindfulness can take the form of either formal meditation or informal practice in daily life. Mindfulness-based treatment protocols are usually brief (typically eight in-person group sessions) multicomponent interventions incorporating both education and practice. Two of the most commonly available and widely studied forms are mindfulness-based stress reduction (MBSR) and mindfulness-based cognitive therapy (MBCT; Strauss, Cavanagh, Oliver, & Pettman, 2014). MBSR, originally developed by Jon Kabat-Zin in the 1970s, is an intensive multicomponent program comprised of didactic and experiential exercises. Practices typically include mindfulness of breath, eating (the "raisin exercise"), bodily sensations (the "body scan"), and gentle movement (Hatha yoga), as well as the practice of compassion toward self and others ("loving-kindness meditation"; Kabat-Zinn & Hanh, 2009). With its emphasis on stress reduction and enhancement of well-being, MBSR has been successfully applied to a variety of clinical and nonclinical populations (Strauss et al., 2014). MBCT was developed in the 1990s and combines components of MBSR with elements of cognitive therapy for depression.

A meta-analysis of 12 RCTs of mindfulness-based interventions for individuals with a current depressive or anxiety disorder found that mindfulness-based interventions significantly decreased primary symptom severity (i.e., severity of the target clinical problem identified in each study; SMD = 0.59) compared to a mixed control group including both active (e.g., cognitive behavior therapy, psychoeducation; number of trials [k] = 5) and inactive (e.g., treatment as usual; k = 7) control conditions (Strauss et al., 2014). Sensitivity analyses revealed that effects were statistically significant for depression outcomes (but not anxiety outcomes), inactive (but not for active) control conditions, and MBCT (but not MBSR).

Another more recent meta-analysis on individual patient data from nine RCTs examined the efficacy of MBCT compared with usual care and other active treatments (including antidepressants) in treating adults with recurrent depression (Kuyken et al., 2016). Results indicated that patients who received MBCT had a reduced risk of relapse (hazard ratio = 0.69) within a 60-week follow-up period compared with those who did not. Individuals with more severe depression pretreatment experienced greater benefits with MBCT compared to controls. Another meta-analysis investigated the efficacy of mindfulness-based therapies on clinical versus subclinical depression (Khoury et al., 2013). Both pre–post studies (k = 6) and waitlist-controlled studies (k = 8) indicated a significant effect of mindfulness-based therapies targeting depressive symptoms (SMD = 0.66 and 0.53, repectively). As assessed by the 20-item Center for Epidemiological Studies Depression Scale (CES-D), subclinical depression (k=5, mean CESD-D score = 11.03) was further reduced at post-treatment (M = 6.76) and follow-up (M = 8.44). Clinical depression (k =9) at pretreatment (M = 18.31) became subclinical at both posttreatment (M = 13.48) and follow-up (M = 15.49).

Meditative Movement
A 2013 meta-analysis 12 of RCTs of adults with major depressive disorder (MDD) or depressive symptoms found significant effects of yoga for reducing depression compared to usual care (SMD = 0.69), relaxation (SMD = 0.62), and aerobic exercise (SMD = 0.59; Cramer, Lauche, Langhorst, & Dobos, 2013). However, a more recent meta-analysis examining the efficacy of meditative movement interventions in general (including tai chi, qigong, and yoga) on participants meeting criteria for MDD (Zou et al., 2018) identified 15 eligible studies and found that although meditative movement significantly decreased depression severity compared to passive controls (i.e., waitlist, SMD = 0.56), there was no significant benefit compared to active controls (e.g., electroconvulsive therapy, health and wellness education, walking).

In sum, research suggests that meditative movement (e.g., yoga) and multicomponent mindfulness-based interventions such as MBCT are at least as effective, on average, as other forms of psychological interventions for depression. Additional research is needed to identify individual characteristics that predict which interventions will be most effective for individuals with MDD.

Anxiety- and Stress-Related Disorders

Mindfulness-Based Therapies
Khoury et al. (2013) investigated the efficacy of various standardized multi-component mindfulness-based therapies (e.g., MBSR, MBCT) on clinical and subclinical anxiety. Waitlist-controlled studies indicated a significant effect of mindfulness-based therapies targeting anxiety symptoms (k = 4; g = 0.96). As assessed by the State-Trait Anxiety Inventory, subclinical anxiety (k=13, mean State-Trait Anxiety Inventory score = 35.91) was significantly reduced at posttreatment (M = 31.25) and follow-up (M = 29.35). A moderate clinical baseline level of anxiety (k = 22, M = 42.94) was reduced to a subclinical level posttreatment (M = 39.73) and to a mild level at follow-up (M = 40.33). A high clinical baseline level of anxiety (k = 8, M = 52.87) was reduced to moderate levels at both posttreatment (M = 47.20) and follow-up (M = 46.54). The magnitude of these effect may be regarded as ranging from fairly small (mean = 6% improvement) for individuals with subclinical anxiety to more clinically significant for individuals with moderate or high levels of anxiety (18% and 11%, respectively).

Mixed Meditative Therapies
A meta-analysis of 10 RCTs examined the efficacy of various meditation interventions (including MBSR, mantram meditation, and yoga) for adults with posttraumatic stress disorder (Hilton et al., 2017). Compared to mixed control groups (e.g., treatment as usual, waitlist, attention control, or other active treatments), meditative interventions

significantly reduced posttraumatic stress disorder symptoms (SMD = 0.41). Of the included meditative interventions, yoga had the largest between-group effect (yoga SMD = 0.54, k = 2), although this effect was not significantly different in magnitude compared to MBSR (SMD = 0.48, k = 2) or mantram repetition (SMD = 0.27, k = 2). Another meta-analyses investigating this question found a similar pooled effect size (overall SMD=0.39; Gallegos, Crean, Pigeon, & Heffner, 2017). Again, although slightly larger effects were demonstated for yoga (SMD = 0.71) compared to mindfulness interventions (SMD = 0.33) and other forms of meditation (0.37), differences in effect size by modality were not statistically significant.

Substance Use Disorder

Mindfulness-Based Relapse Prevention

Mindfulness-based relapse prevention (MBRP) is a multicomponent intervention developed specifically for SUD that integrates traditional psychotherapeutic relapse prevention strategies with mindfulness-based meditation education and practice, including yoga. A systematic review and meta-analysis of 9 RCTs found that MBRP significantly reduced withdrawal/craving symptoms (SMD = 0.13) and negative consequences of substance use (SMD = 0.23) compared to mixed control conditions (e.g., relapse prevention, health education, cognitive-behavior therapy [CBT], and treatment as usual). No statistically significant differences were detected for any other outcomes (e.g., relapse, frequency of use; Grant et al., 2017). These results suggest that MBRP is similarly effective to other SUD treatments such as traditional psychotherapeutic relapse prevention and CBT.

Meditative Movement

A recent meta-analysis compared the efficacy of meditative movement interventions to standard aerobic exercise for SUD. Physical exercise interventions that incorporated meditative components (e.g., yoga, tai chi quan, and qigong) were effective for increasing abstinence rate (odds ratio = 3.0; k = 3), reducing anxiety (SMD = 0.33; k = 4), and reducing depression (SMD = 0.50; k = 6) compared to mixed control conditions (D. Wang, Wanget al., 2014). Although effects on abstinence were somewhat larger for meditative movement interventions compared to standard aerobic exercise (odds ratio = 1.7), this difference was not statistically significant.

Mixed Clinical and Healthy Samples

Mental health and physical health are bidirectionally related, with poor mental health increasing risk for poor physical health, and vice versa. As such, it makes sense that a number of investigators have tested the efficacy of meditative therapies for improving adjustment in chronic illness. The following section reviews findings of these studies with regards to effects on mental health. However, meditative therapies have also been found to significantly improve physical health. For example, meditative therapies have been shown to improve physical symptoms in conditions such as epilepsy (Arias, Steinberg, Banga, & Trestman, 2006), premenstrual syndrome (Arias et al., 2006), menopause (Innes, Selfe, & Vishnu, 2010), irritable bowel syndrome (Crowe et al., 2016), fibromyalgia (Crowe et al., 2016), tinnitus (Crowe et al., 2016), asthma (Crowe et al., 2016), psoriasis (Gamret, Price, Fertig, Lev-Tov, & Nichols, 2018), hypertension (Hughes et al., 2013), and autoimmune illness (Arias et al., 2006). In the second part of the chapter, we review physiological mechanisms that may mediate the effects of meditative therapies on both mental and physical health.

Mindfulness-Based Interventions

Meta-analysis of 16 waitlist-controlled trials investigating the effects of mindfulness-based therapies in mixed clinical samples found a significant medium-sized effect on combined mental and physical health outcomes (SMD = 0.62; Khoury et al., 2013). Specifically, significant effects were observed for waitlist-controlled studies targeting both psychological disorders (k = 18; SMD = 0.70), and physical health conditions (k = 28; SMD = 0.40). Mindfulness-based therapies were significantly more effective than comparison psychoeducational interventions (k = 9; SMD = 0.61), supportive therapies (k=7; SMD = 0.37), relaxation-based interventions (k=8; SMD = 0.19), and imagery/suppression techniques (k = 2; SMD = 0.26).

Medical illness. A meta-analysis of the effect of MBSR on mental health in adults with chronic medical illness (k = 8) found small, statistically significant effects for depression (SMD = 0.26), anxiety (SMD = 0.47), and distress (SMD = 0.24) compared to (primarily nonactive) control conditions (Bohlmeijer, Prenger, Taal, & Cuijpers, 2010). Similar effect sizes were observed in a meta-analysis of MBSR for adults with fibromyalgia (k = 6; Lauche, Cramer, Dobos, Langhorst, & Schmidt, 2013). Although effects were not robust against bias, short-term improvements were observed with MBSR compared to active control conditions with regard to quality of life (SMD=0.32) and pain (SMD=0.44).

Healthy individuals. A meta-analysis of 7 RCTs investigating the efficacy of MBSR in healthy adults (Chiesa & Serretti, 2009) found that MBSR significantly reduced stress (pre–post SMD = 1.39) compared to inactive control conditions (pre–post SMD = −0.05, t = 18.18, $P < 0.001$). One study examined the efficacy of MBSR compared to standard relaxation and found the two interventions to be similarly effective for reducing stress (Jain et al., 2007). Another trial found that MBSR was significantly more effective than a self-help control group for improving depressive symptoms, anxiety, coping self-efficacy, and mindfulness in family caregivers (all $Ps < 0.05$; Hou et al., 2014). Results of several other studies with healthy populations suggest that MBSR may be effective for decreasing rumination, increasing empathy, self-control, self-compassion, and spirituality, as well as enhancing the quality of personal relationships (Chiesa & Serretti, 2009).

Mixed Meditative Therapies

Another meta-analysis investigated the effect of meditation interventions among adults with a medical illness, mental health diagnosis, or who were experiencing chronic stress (e.g., dementia caregivers; Goyal et al., 2014). Only studies with active control conditions were included. Interventions included any structured meditation program with at least four hours of training and instructions for additional home practice. Meditation programs focused on mindfulness had a significant, medium-sized effect on anxiety (SMD = 0.38 at 8 weeks; k = 8), depression (SMD = 0.30; k = 10), and pain (SMD = 0.33; k = 4) compared to nonspecific active control conditions. By contrast, mantra meditation did not improve any of the outcomes examined, although few mantra meditation trials met the inclusion criteria.

Kindness-Based Meditation

Another meta-analysis investigated the effect of kindness-based meditation (e.g., loving-kindness meditation and compassion meditation) in individuals with health problems as well as in the general population (k = 22; Galante et al., 2014). Kindness-based meditation interventions significantly reduced depressive symptoms compared to passive control groups (SMD = 0.61), but not compared to progressive muscle relaxation or other forms of meditation.

Meditative Movement

Chen et al. (2012) investigated the efficacy of meditative therapies (including meditative movement) for reducing anxiety symptoms in mixed samples (mostly individuals with physical health conditions). Compared to mixed control conditions, meditation therapies significantly reduced anxiety (SMD = 0.53). Subgroup analyses suggested that moving meditation was associated with slightly larger effects (yoga SMD=0.63 and qigong or tai chi SMD = 0.68 vs. mindfulness meditation SMD=0.51 and guided imagery SMD = 0.39); however, differences in effect size by therapy type were not statistically significant. A meta-analysis of RCTs evaluating the efficacy of yoga for improving outcomes in clinical (60% of studies) and subclinical samples (40% of studies; total k = 306) found no significant differences by type of yoga (i.e., hatha yoga, Iyengar yoga, pranayama, and the integrated approach to yoga therapy; Cramer, Lauche, Langhorst, & Dobos, 2016).

   Cancer. Two recent meta-analyses have investigated the efficacy of yoga for improving well-being in cancer patients and survivors. Buffart et al. (2012) identified 13 studies that compared yoga to a nonexercise or waitlist control conditon for individuals with cancer or cancer survivors. After excluding outliers that may have biased the results toward finding a more positive effect of yoga, analyses indicated that yoga resulted in statistically significant medium-sized reductions in distress (SMD = 0.75), anxiety (SMD = 0.77), depression (SMD = 0.69), and fatigue (SMD = 0.51), as well as a statistically significant, small increases in general quality of life (SMD = 0.37), emotional function (SMD = 0.49), social function (SMD = 0.33), and functional well-being (SMD = 0.31). Another analysis focused on individuals with breast cancer specifically and identified 12 eligible RCTs (Cramer, Lange, Klose, Paul, & Dobos, 2012). Compared to mixed (active and nonactive) control conditions, yoga significantly improved symptoms of anxiety (SMD = 1.51), depression (SMD = 1.59), perceived stress (SMD = 1.14), and psychological distress (SMD = 0.86) posttreatment.

   Chronic pain. Another systematic review assessed the efficacy of yoga for chronic pain (Posadzki, Ernst, Terry, & Lee, 2011). Of the 10 RCTs identified, nine studies found a significantly greater reduction in pain with yoga compared to mixed controls (e.g., usual care, therapeutic exercises, touch and manipulation, no intervention). Another meta-analysis of seven trials investigating the efficacy of qigong for improving outcomes in fibromyalgia found significant post-treatment improvements in pain (SMD=0.69), quality of life (QOL; SMD = 0.84), and sleep (SMD = 0.67) compared to usual care or waitlist control groups but not compared to active treatments (i.e., sham qigong, a support group with education, training in awareness of bodily perceptions, or aerobic exercise with stretching; Lauche, Cramer, Häuser, Dobos, & Langhorst, 2013). There is growing evidence of the efficacy of yoga and tai chi on back and knee pain in individuals with arthritis (Field, 2016; Lauche, Hunter, Adams, & Cramer, 2019; Park, Krause-Parello, & Barnes, 2020). Studies of yoga for low-back pain and neck pain have found promising results, and yoga is among the options recommended by the American College of Physicians for first-line treatment of chronic low-back pain (National Center for Complementary and Integrative Health, 2019).

Healthy individuals. A meta-analysis evaluating the effect of yoga on positive mental health among healthy adults found that compared to no intervention, yoga had a significant, moderate-sized effect on well-being (SMD = 0.69; Hendriks, de Jong, & Cramer, 2017). No significant effect was found compared to other forms of physical activity. Another meta-analysis investigated the acute and long-term effects of qigong on stress and anxiety in healthy adults (C.-W. Wang et al., 2014). Compared to attention control sessions, qigong led to significant reductions in state anxiety immediately following practice. Compared to waitlist-control conditions, qigong interventions (ranging in duration from 4–12 weeks) led to significant reductions in anxiety (SMD = 0.75) and stress (SMD = 0.88) at one and three-month follow-up.

Comparative Efficacy of Meditative Therapies Versus Physical Exercise
A recent review of RCTs examined the efficacy of nonactive forms of meditation compared to physical activity in mixed samples (Edwards & Loprinzi, 2018). Of the main outcomes assessed across five eligible studies, meditation was significantly more effective at reducing anxiety, chronic neck pain, and pain-related bothersomeness. Exercise was more effective at improving physical health-related QOL, cholesterol, and blood glucose. Meditation and exercise were similarly effective for improving well-being and perceived stress.

Special Populations

A body of literature also supports the use of mindfulness with certain special populations, including prisoners and adults with mild intellectual disabilities (Singh et al., 2008). A recent systematic review identified 13 studies that investigated the efficacy of mindfulness-based interventions in prisoners (Auty, Cope, & Liebling, 2017). The majority of studies focused on sitting meditation (including mindfulness meditation and vipassana), although a minority of studies included physical postures (yoga). Compared to various control conditions (i.e., waitlist, no treatment, treatment as usual, or alternative treatment programs), mindfulness interventions were found to significantly increase psychological well-being (SMD = 0.46) and behavioral functioning (SMD = 0.30) in prisoners, with less intense programs of longer duration showing larger effects on behavioral functioning.

Technology-Assisted Meditative Therapies

Digital behavioral health interventions have potential to overcome the most common barriers to face-to-face delivery and are frequently cited as cost-effective methods of extending mental healthcare (Mohr, Burns, Schueller, Clarke, & Klinkman, 2013). RCTs show that technology-based tools can produce effects similar to those of in-person psychological treatments (Andersson, Cuijpers, Carlbring, Riper, & Hedman, 2014; Cuijpers et al., 2009; Kuester, Niemeyer, & Knaevelsrud, 2016; Richards & Richardson, 2012; Wagner, Horn, & Maercker, 2014). Video- or app-based interventions that can be self-administered may be particularly scalable by overcoming barriers such as cost, stigma, and access to healthcare providers (Gitlin & Hodgson, 2015). The acceptability of online administration of meditation interventions is evidenced by the 170 million meditation videos available through Google's search engine, with the most popular mindfulness videos on YouTube boasting over 8 million views (The Honest Guys, 2015).

One meta-analysis sought to determine whether mindfulness and acceptance-based interventions can be taught via self-help, which the authors defined as interventions that were either entirely self-administered (via written or pre-recorded materials) or facilitated by a clinician or coach (Cavanagh, Strauss, Forder, & Jones, 2014). As a whole, the 15 identified RCTs demonstrated statistically significant improvements with self-help mindfulness or acceptance interventions compared to control conditions with regard to the target of practice (either mindfulness or acceptance), depression, and anxiety (SMDs = 0.49, 0.37, and 0.33, respectively).

As interest in both meditation and mobile apps ("apps") for health promotion have grown exponentially, an abundance of mental health apps have become available to consumers. A systematic review identified over 200 apps related to mindfulness for Google Android smartphones alone (Plaza, Demarzo, Herrera-Mercadal, & García-Campayo, 2013), although very few of the publicly available apps have been empirically tested (Neary & Schueller, 2018). A 2017 meta-analysis of RCTs testing the efficacy of mental health apps for depression identified six apps that included a mindfulness component (Firth et al., 2017). These apps had a significant medium-sized effect on reducing depressive symptoms (Hedges' g = 0.49)—an effect size similar to those of apps rooted in CBT (g = 0.53).

Determining which apps are most likely to be helpful is a challenge to consumers and providers alike. Consumer ratings assess liking but do not necessarily reflect clinical usefulness or utility. Furthermore, the validity of such ratings is questionable, as app developers can leave ratings for their own apps or pay others to do so (BinDhim, Hawkey, & Trevena, 2015). Resources developed specifically to identify and assess mental health apps using standardized criteria will be incredibly useful for helping consumers choose apps that are most supported by empirical evidence for improving the outcome of interest. Currently, the most active and comprehensive such platform in the United States is PsyberGuide.org, a nonprofit that aims to provide unbiased reviews of mental health app credibility, user experience, and transparency (i.e., degree to which information regarding an app's data storage and collection policy is readily available to users; Neary & Schueller, 2018). Of the apps including a mindfulness component (64 of the 198 products listed on PsyberGuide), currently the app with the highest credibility score (4.64/5.00) is Headspace, which has shown to enhance well-being and compassion in RCTs (Howells, Ivtzan, & Eiroa-Orosa, 2016; Lim, Condon, & DeSteno, 2015).

Technology-Assisted Yoga
A plethora of online yoga videos are readily available; Google's video search engine returns over 400 million hits for the search term "yoga," with the most popular videos boasting 25 million views (Adriene, 2013). However, little research has been conducted to confirm the efficacy of video-based yoga interventions. To our knowledge, only one RCT to date has investigated the effect of a video-based yoga intervention on psychological well-being in adults (Schuver & Lewis, 2016). In that study, 40 women with depression were randomized to 12 weeks of home-based yoga plus telephone-administered mindfulness education versus home-based walking plus telephone-administered health education. Depressive symptoms improved significantly in both groups, and yoga significantly reduced rumination compared to the attention-matched control. Clearly, additional research is needed to better understand the effects of video-based yoga on mental health as well as which individuals are most likely to benefit from these interventions.

Virtual Reality
Recently, developers have begun to test virtual reality (VR) interventions designed to facilitate mindfulness practice (Navarro-Haro et al., 2017). In a pilot study, Navarro-Haro and colleagues investigated the effects of a 10-minute VR experience in which participants listened a guided mindfulness practice while floating down an animated computer-generated river in VR. A convenience (nonclinical) sample of 44 individuals completed mood rating before and after this experience and reported average increases in state mindfulness and relaxation and decreases in sadness, anger, and anxiety. Further research is needed to compare the effects of such interventions to active control conditions, assess feasibility and efficacy in clinical samples, and measure the duration of these effects.

Proposed Neurobiological Mechanisms

As a whole, meditative therapies appear effective for improving psychological well-being in a wide range of populations. However, the psychological mechanisms by which meditative therapies affect clinical outcomes are not entirely understood. Broadly, meditation practice is hypothesized to increase well-being via improvement in self-regulation (Chiesa, Serretti, & Jakobsen, 2013; Dhungel, Malhotra, Sarkar,

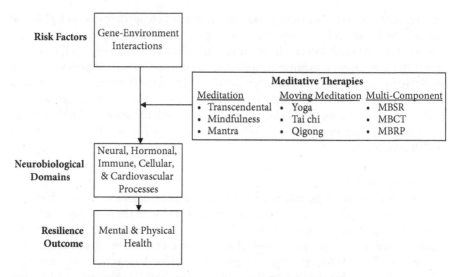

Figure 16.1. Hypothesized mechanisms by which meditative therapies increase resilience.

MBSR = mindfulness-based stress reduction; MBCT = mindfulness-based cognitive therapy; MBRP = mindfulness-based relapse prevention.

& Prajapati, 2008; Gard, Noggle, Park, Vago, & Wilson, 2014; Jovanov, 2005; Sinha, Deepak, & Gusain, 2013; Turankar et al., 2013). However, significant differences in mechanisms may exist depending on the type or component of meditative therapy. For example, biopsychosocial pathways affecting mental health may be very different for mindfulness meditation, chanting meditation, pranayama, or various forms of meditative movement (yoga, tai chi, qigong). A recent systematic review of mindfulness interventions concluded that decreases in cognitive reactivity, emotional reactivity, rumination, and worry may mediate the effect of mindfulness practice on mental health (Gu, Strauss, Bond, & Cavanagh, 2015). Although lack of establishment of temporal precedence precludes firm conclusions, existing research on biological mechanisms offer some support for these findings. A model of the hypothesized mechanisms by which meditative therapies may increase resilience to mental illness is presented in Figure 16.1.

Neural Mechanisms

Neuroimaging studies suggest that mindfulness practice alters both brain structure and function. However, findings are diverse across studies, and methodological limitations are numerous (e.g., small sample sizes, dearth of longitudinal studies, and variability in meditative techniques and other protocol characteristics; Tang, Hölzel, & Posner, 2015). A recent meta-analysis of magnetic resonance imaging (MRI) studies used an activation likelihood estimation approach to identify brain regions that are consistently altered during meditation practice (Boccia, Piccardi, & Guariglia, 2015). Identified regions included those involved in processing self-relevant information (e.g., precuneus); self-regulation, focused problem-solving, and adaptive behavior (anterior cingulate cortex); interoception (insula); reorienting attention (angular gyrus); and experiential self-processing (premotor cortex and superior frontal gyrus). In addition, significant structural differences were observed between expert meditators and novices, with expert meditators showing greater grey matter volume in the right anterior cingulate. One possible interpretation of these data is that these neural differences are the result of long-term meditation practice and account for the superior self-regulatory abilities observed in long-term meditators (Boccia et al., 2015).

The Stress Response and the HPA Axis

Stress can be defined as the perception that demands of the environment exceed one's resources for adapting to the situation (Cohen, Janicki-Deverts, & Miller, 2007). Chronic, uncontrollable stress is a known risk factor for depression and other mental illness (Charney, 2004; Conway, Raposa, Hammen, & Brennan, 2018; Hammen, 2005; Lee & Sawa, 2014; McEwen, 2002), and one prominent hypothesis is that chronic stress increases this risk via sustained activation and ultimate dysregulation of the hypothalamic–pituitary–adrenal axis (HPA) axis (Chopra, Kumar, & Kuhad, 2011). Uncontrollable stress amplifies cortisol secretion, and sustained elevated levels of cortisol eventually suppress output of corticotropin-releasing hormone and adrenocorticotropin hormone (G. E. Miller, Chen, & Zhou, 2007). This ultimate blunting of HPA axis responsivity is proposed to underlie the withdrawal and disengagement behaviors that often accompany chronic uncontrollable stress (Gold & Chrousos, 2002; Heim, Ehlert, & Hellhammer, 2000; Mason et al., 2001). Sustained activation of the HPA axis also results in deficient monoamine transmission, disruption of neurotrophic processes, oxidative stress, widespread inflammatory processes, and neurodegeneration (Chopra et al., 2011; Pfau & Russo, 2015). Once in motion, this stress-related biological cascade can be exacerbated by environmental factors (e.g., social isolation) or maladaptive coping behaviors (sedentary lifestyle, substance abuse; McEwen, 2002).

Although important limitations remain and there is low consistency of findings (O'Leary, O'Neill, & Dockray, 2016), several studies suggest that restoration of HPA axis dysregulation may be one mechanism by which yoga and other meditative therapies improve mental health (Lavretsky et al., 2013; Prakhinkit, Suppapitiporn, Tanaka, & Suksom, 2014; Shahidi et al., 2011; Tsang et al., 2013). Studies of both younger healthy adults (Pascoe & Bauer, 2015; Pascoe, Thompson, & Ski, 2017) as well as sedentary community-dwelling older adults (Gothe, Keswani, & McAuley, 2016) suggest that yoga may lead to both acute reductions in HPA axis activity as well as longer-term changes with repeated practice. Results of several studies (Field, 2011) suggest that yoga reduces cortisol secretion (Kamei et al., 2000; West, Otte, Geher, Johnson, & Mohr, 2004), although not all studies demonstrate this effect and an increase in the cortisol awakening response has also been reported (Cahn, Goodman, Peterson, Maturi, & Mills, 2017). Some forms of meditation practice appear to reduce cortisol secretion (Klimes-Dougan et al., 2019; Vandana, Vaidyanathan, Saraswathy, Sundaram, & Kumar, 2011), although there is some inconsistency of findings here as well. Larger sample sizes and use of standardized methodology will help to clarify these findings.

Immune and Inflammatory Markers

Inflammation is another pathway by which stress is thought to increase risk for depression and other mental health disorders (Couzin-Frankel, 2010; Slavich & Irwin, 2014). Increased levels of inflammation have been observed in both adults with depression (Martinez-Cengotitabengoa et al., 2016; A. H. Miller, Maletic, & Raison, 2009) and in individuals undergoing chronic stress (Danese, Pariante, Caspi, Taylor, & Poulton, 2007; Kiecolt-Glaser et al., 2005; McDade, Hawkley, & Cacioppo, 2006; G. E. Miller et al., 2008). Furthermore, acute psychosocial stress (e.g., public speaking, mental arithmetic) stimulates inflammatory signaling molecules (Bierhaus et al., 2003), and these responses are exaggerated in patients with depression (A. H. Miller et al., 2009). Results of a systematic review of RCTs investigating the effect of mindfulness meditation on the immune system suggest that mindfulness may affect specific markers of inflammation, cell-mediated immunity, and biological aging (Black & Slavich, 2016). Additional research is needed to better understand these effects.

Cellular Protection and Repair Markers

Lavretsky et al. (2013) investigated the mechanisms by which the chanting meditation Kirtan Kriya reduced symptoms of depression in stressed informal caregivers of individuals with dementia. Compared to listening to relaxing music, Kirtan Kriya led to significant improvements in depressive symptoms, QOL, and telomerase activity in peripheral blood mononuclear cells (a stress-activated signal of aging). Furthermore, change in telomerase activity was correlated with depression improvement in the Kirtan Kriya group but not in the control group. These results indicate inflammatory and antiviral transcription pathways as one mechanism by which meditation may buffer against the negative effects of chronic stress on mood (Black et al., 2013). Other studies have shown that mindfulness interventions may protect against cellular aging (Epel, Daubenmier, Moskowitz, Folkman, & Blackburn, 2009). A meta-analysis of four RCTs estimated a moderate-sized effect of mindfulness meditation on increased telomerase activity in peripheral blood mononuclear cells ($d = 0.46$; Schutte & Malouff, 2014).

Brain-derived neurotrophic factor (BDNF) is an important modulator of neural development and plasticity as well as neuronal survival. One pre–post study found increases in BDNF during the course of a three-month yoga and meditation retreat (Cahn et al., 2017). Another study of meditation versus usual care for glaucoma patients observed increases in BDNF in the meditation arm (Gagrani et al., 2018).

Cardiovascular Markers

Prospective studies indicate that individuals with depression are at nearly twice the risk of developing cardiovascular disease, and that cardiovascular disease predicts subsequent depression (Hare, Toukhsati, Johansson, & Jaarsma, 2013; Valkanova & Ebmeier, 2013). Autonomic nervous system dysregulation is one biological mechanism that may explain the link between cardiovascular risk and depression (Carney & Freedland, 2017).

Heart Rate Variability

Heart rate variability (HRV) is a measure of beat-to-beat time or frequency variability of the heart and in part represents the ability of the autonomic nervous system to adapt to a changing psychological, social, and physical environment (Appelhans & Luecken, 2006). Higher HRV is thought to reflect greater self-regulatory capacity (i.e., regulation of behavioral, cognitive, and emotional processes). In neuroimaging studies of both younger and older adults, higher HRV is associated with higher resting-state functional connectivity between the medial prefrontal cortex and amygdala (Jennings, Sheu, Kuan, Manuck, & Gianaros, 2016; Sakaki et al., 2016), a biomarker of emotion regulation (Etkin, Büchel, & Gross, 2015), and with resilience to the development of mental health disorders (Brown et al., 2018; Carnevali, Koenig, Sgoifo, & Ottaviani, 2018; Koenig, Kemp, Beauchaine, Thayer, & Kaess, 2016). Research with pregnant women suggests that yoga has potential to increase the high-frequency band of the HRV spectrum during meditation (an indicator of parasympathetic activity) compared to standard prenatal exercises (Satyapriya, Nagendra, Nagarathna, & Padmalatha, 2009). Another study conducted with healthy older adults assessed parasympathetic activity via baroreflex sensitivity (the alpha index at high frequency) and found that parasympathetic activity increased after yoga, but not after other aerobic exercise (Bowman et al., 1997). However, greater high-frequency HRV is not always associated with positive outcomes, and the factors that moderate this relation is unclear. For example, one study of yoga for adults with depression found reductions in high-frequency HRV in those who remitted versus those who did not remit (Shapiro et al., 2007).

Blood Pressure

Chronic stress (e.g., in the form of work strain, low socioeconomic status, relationship stress, or discrimination) has been associated with hypertension, and several studies have investigated the effect of meditation on blood pressure. One randomized study of mantra meditation for elderly women with hypertension found that chanting significantly reduced blood pressure (in addition to depression, anxiety, and stress; Amin et al., 2016). A recent meta-analysis examined the effect of meditation interventions on blood pressure in mixed populations (11 of 19 studies were of nonhypertensive individuals) compared to mixed controlled groups (primarily health education). Nontranscendental meditation interventions (primarily mindful breathing or MBSR) led to significant reductions in both systolic and diastolic blood pressure (Shi et al., 2017).

Respiration

Although a component of many meditative interventions, the biological mechanisms by which controlled breathing affects self-regulation and mental health remain underexplored. Existing evidence suggests that the short-term practice of yogic breathing (*pranayama*) produces a positive impact on cardiovascular and respiratory systems (Pradhan, 2013; Srinivasan, 1991; Stancák, Kuna, Dostalek, & Vishnudevananda, 1991; Telles, Yadav, Gupta, & Balkrishna, 2013). Slow-paced breathing leads to reduced heart rate and blood pressure (Shavanani & Udupa, 2003), while fast-breathing leads to less robust but consistent increase in heart rate (Bhavanani, Ramanathan, & Kt, 2012; Rajesh, Ilavarasu, & Srinivasan, 2014; Sharma et al., 2014; Vialatte, Bakardjian, Prasad, & Cichocki, 2009). Changes in HRV also support the notion that the practice of pranayama improves respiratory function and cardiac sympatho-vagal balance (Jella & Shannahoff-Khalsa, 1993; Nagendra, 2007). It has been hypothesized that the effects of pranayama are mediated by the vagal nerve system, through interconnections between peripheral sensory organs, the solitary nucleus, thalamus, amygdala and limbic areas and the prefrontal cortex (Marshall, Basilakos, Williams, & Love-Myers, 2014; Telles, Yadav, Kumar, et al., 2013). Research suggests that the increase of parasympathetic activity associated with increased expiration time reduces the release of stress hormones (Marshall et al., 2014; Marshall, Laures-Gore, DuBay, Williams, & Bryant, 2015), reduces amygdala activation via enhanced gamma-aminobutyric acid, inhibition from the prefrontal cortex and insula, and reduces psychological and somatic symptoms associated with stress (Pal, Agarwal, Karthik, Pal, & Nanda, 2014; Shannahoff-Khalsa & Kennedy, 1993). Research on the effects of *pranayama* on the neural networks involved in respiratory control, breath awareness, and emotion regulation is still in its infancy, and this is an area that warrants further study. Our group is working to develop rodent and human models of respiratory control of emotion regulation in anxiety and panic that will become the first translational model of breath-based mind–body interventions that will explore underlying mechanisms by which controlled breathing in pranayama is likely to affect emotions and resilience to stress.

Directions for Future Research

Current models of mental health service delivery fail to adequately address the enormous burden of mental health disorders worldwide (Lake & Turner, 2017). Existing evidence suggests that meditative therapies are a promising approach to improving mental health in a variety of populations, that they can be self-administered, and that they can be used either as stand-alone or adjunct treatments. However, many methodological limitations remain. These include inadequate reporting regarding intervention components, small sample sizes, and lack of standardization across studies (e.g., with regard to assessment measures, inclusion criteria, control conditions, and physiological assessment protocols). In addition, the meditative therapies being investigated have varied greatly in the the type of practice, method of training, and duration of instruction. Determining which meditative therapies are most effective for which disorders, outcomes, and individuals will require greater collaboration between researchers to achieve greater protocol standardization and sample sizes. In addition, inclusion of adverse event monitoring will be important to establish safety of meditative interventions, particularly in the case of self-administered interventions and in vulnerable populations. Finally, carefully designed dismantling studies will be helpful for determining "active ingredients" of meditative interventions and ultimately informing the development of more effective interventions.

Much work also remains in elucidating the neurobiological mechanisms of meditative therapies. Examining mediation and moderation hypotheses requires even larger samples compared to efficacy testing, and yet the expense of neuroimaging and other forms of physiological assessment typically means that such studies comprise even smaller samples compared to clinical trials. In addition, assessment of constructs at multiple time points is necessary to establish a mechanistic timeline. One method of testing possible biological mechanisms is to situate such a study within the context of a larger clinical study. Transdisciplinary collaboration will be extremely helpful in making progress in this area.

Importantly, the biological mechanisms of meditative therapy may vary greatly depending on the type or component of practice. For example, manipulation of breathing is a component of many meditative therapies, and the biological mechanisms by which such practices improve health have received little attention to date. This may be partially due to challenges in visualizing the human brainstem and examining effects of respiratory effort in the MRI due to the influence of changes in breathing on the BOLD signal detection (Brooks, Faull, Pattinson, & Jenkinson, 2013; Faull, Jenkinson, Clare, & Pattinson, 2015; Pattinson et al., 2009). However, neuroimaging can be used to examine two neural pathways (one involving visceral afferents projecting to the insula and another involving skin afferents projecting to somatosensory cortex) by which interoceptive awareness of breath might modulate emotion regulation.

Conclusion

In sum, existing evidence suggests that meditative mind–body therapies have potential to improve mental health in a variety of populations. Effects appear largest among individuals with psychological disorders, although benefits have also been observed in healthy adults as well as those with physical health conditions. Further research is needed to determine which types of interventions are most effective for which disorders and outcomes, identify the active ingredients of interventions, and determine the biological processes that mediate observed effects. Work in each of these areas will inform the development of more potent and individualized interventions to fulfill the mandate of precision medicine. In addition, studies investigating the cost-effectiveness of implementing mind–body therapies for primary or secondary prevention of chronic physical and mental disorders will be important for informing public health policies and may facilitate the integration of such therapies into mainstream Western medicine healthcare.

References

Adriene, Y. W. (2013). Yoga For complete beginners: 20 minute home yoga workout! Retrieved from https://www.youtube.com/watch?v=v7AYKMP6rOE

Amin, A., Kumar, S. S., Rajagopalan, A., Rajan, S., Mishra, S., Reddy, U. K., & Mukkadan, J. K. (2016). Beneficial effects of OM chanting on depression, anxiety, stress and cognition in elderly women with hypertension. *Indian Journal of Clinical Anatomy and Physiology, 3*(3), 253–255 https://doi.org/10.5958/2394-2126.2016.00056.6.

Anderson, P., Jane-Llopis, E., & Hosman, C. (2011). Reducing the silent burden of impaired mental health. *Health Promotion International, 26*(Suppl 1), i4–i9 https://doi.org/10.1093/heapro/dar051.

Andersson, G., Cuijpers, P., Carlbring, P., Riper, H., & Hedman, E. (2014). Guided Internet-based vs. face-to-face cognitive behavior therapy for psychiatric and somatic disorders: A systematic review and meta-analysis. *World Psychiatry, 13*(3), 288–295 https://doi.org/10.1002/wps.20151.

Appelhans, B. M., & Luecken, L. J. (2006). Heart rate variability as an index of regulated emotional responding. *Review of General Psychology, 10*(3), 229 https://doi.org/10.1037/1089-2680.10.3.229.

Arias, A. J., Steinberg, K., Banga, A., & Trestman, R. L. (2006). Systematic review of the efficacy of meditation techniques as treatments for medical illness. *Journal of Alternative & Complementary Medicine, 12*(8), 817–832 https://doi.org/10.1089/acm.2006.12.817.

Auty, K. M., Cope, A., & Liebling, A. (2017). A systematic review and meta-analysis of yoga and mindfulness meditation in prison: Effects on psychological well-being and behavioural functioning. *International Journal of Offender Therapy and Comparative Criminology, 61*(6), 689–710 https://doi.org/10.1177/0306624x15602514.

Bhavanani, A. B., Ramanathan, M., & Kt, H. (2012). Immediate effect of mukha bhastrika (a bellows type pranayama) on reaction time in mentally challenged adolescents. *Indian Journal of Physiology and Pharmacology, 56*(2), 174–180 https://doi.org/10.1177/0306624x15602514.

Bierhaus, A., Wolf, J., Andrassy, M., Rohleder, N., Humpert, P. M., Petrov, D., . . . Rudofsky, G. (2003). A mechanism converting psychosocial stress into mononuclear cell activation. *Proceedings of the National Academy of Sciences, 100*(4), 1920–1925 https://doi.org/10.1073/pnas.0438019100.

BinDhim, N. F., Hawkey, A., & Trevena, L. (2015). A systematic review of quality assessment methods for smartphone health apps. *Telemedicine and e-Health, 21*(2), 97–104 https://doi.org/10.1089/tmj.2014.0088.

Black, D. S., Cole, S. W., Irwin, M. R., Breen, E., St Cyr, N. M., Nazarian, N., . . . Lavretsky, H. (2013). Yogic meditation reverses NF-kappaB and IRF-related transcriptome dynamics in leukocytes of family dementia caregivers in a randomized controlled trial. *Psychoneuroendocrinology, 38*(3), 348–355. https://www.doi.org/10.1016/j.psyneuen.2012.06.011

Black, D. S., & Slavich, G. M. (2016). Mindfulness meditation and the immune system: a systematic review of randomized controlled trials. *Annals of the New York Academy of Science, 1373*(1), 13.

Boccia, M., Piccardi, L., & Guariglia, P. (2015). The meditative mind: a comprehensive meta-analysis of MRI studies. *BioMed Research International, 2015,* 419808. https://doi.org/10.1155/2015/419808.

Bohlmeijer, E., Prenger, R., Taal, E., & Cuijpers, P. (2010). The effects of mindfulness-based stress reduction therapy on mental health of adults with a chronic medical disease: a meta-analysis. *Journal of Psychosomatic Research, 68*(6), 539–544 https://doi.org/10.1016/j.jpsychores.2009.10.005.

Bowman, A. J., Clayton, R. H., Murray, A., Reed, J. W., Subhan, M. M. F., & Ford, G. A. (1997). Effects of aerobic exercise training and yoga on the baroreflex in healthy elderly persons. *European Journal of Clinical Investigation, 27*(5), 443–449 https://doi.org/10.1046/j.1365-2362.1997.1340681.x.

Brooks, J. C. W., Faull, O. K., Pattinson, K. T. S., & Jenkinson, M. (2013). Physiological noise in brainstem FMRI. *Frontiers in Human Neuroscience, 7*, 623 https://doi.org/10.1046/j.1365-2362.1997.1340681.x.

Brown, L., Karmakar, C., Gray, R., Jindal, R., Lim, T., & Bryant, C. (2018). Heart rate variability alterations in late life depression: A meta-analysis. *Journal of Affective Disorders, 235*, 456–466. https://doi.org/10.1016/j.jad.2018.04.071

Buffart, L. M., Van Uffelen, J. G. Z., Riphagen, I. I., Brug, J., van Mechelen, W., Brown, W. J., & Chinapaw, M. J. M. (2012). Physical and psychosocial benefits of yoga in cancer patients and survivors, a systematic review and meta-analysis of randomized controlled trials. *BMC Cancer, 12*(1), 559 https://doi.org/10.1186/1471-2407-12-559.

Cahn, B. R., Goodman, M. S., Peterson, C. T., Maturi, R., & Mills, P. J. (2017). Yoga, meditation and mind-body health: increased BDNF, cortisol awakening response, and altered inflammatory marker expression after a 3-month yoga and meditation retreat. *Frontiers in Human Neuroscience, 11*, 315.

Carnevali, L., Koenig, J., Sgoifo, A., & Ottaviani, C. (2018). Autonomic and Brain Morphological Predictors of Stress Resilience. *Frontiers in Neuroscience, 12*, 228 https://doi.org/10.3389/fnins.2018.

Carney, R. M., & Freedland, K. E. (2017). Depression and coronary heart disease. *Nature Reviews Cardiology, 14*(3), 145 https://doi.org/10.1038/nrcardio.2016.181.

Cavanagh, K., Strauss, C., Forder, L., & Jones, F. (2014). Can mindfulness and acceptance be learnt by self-help? A systematic review and meta-analysis of mindfulness and acceptance-based self-help interventions. *Clinical Psychology Review, 34*(2), 118–129.

Charney, D. S. (2004). Psychobiological mechanisms of resilience and vulnerability: implications for successful adaptation to extreme stress. *American Journal of Psychiatry, 161*(2), 195–216 https://doi.org/10.1176/appi.ajp.161.2.195.

Chen, K. W., Berger, C. C., Manheimer, E., Forde, D., Magidson, J., Dachman, L., & Lejuez, C. W. (2012). Meditative therapies for reducing anxiety: A systematic review and meta-analysis of randomized controlled trials. *Depress Anxiety, 29*(7), 545–562 https://doi.org/10.1002/da.21964.

Chiesa, A., & Serretti, A. (2009). Mindfulness-based stress reduction for stress management in healthy people: A review and meta-analysis. *Journal of Alternative and Complementary Medicine, 15*(5), 593–600 https://doi.org/10.1089/acm.2008.0495.

Chiesa, A., Serretti, A., & Jakobsen, J. C. (2013). Mindfulness: Top–down or bottom–up emotion regulation strategy? *Clinical Psychology Revie, 33*(1), 82–96 https://doi.org/10.1089/acm.2008.0495.

Chopra, K., Kumar, B., & Kuhad, A. (2011). Pathobiological targets of depression. *Expert Opinion on Therapeutic Targets, 15*(4), 379–400 https://doi.org/10.1517/14728222.2011.553603.

Cohen, S., Janicki-Deverts, D., & Miller, G. E. (2007). Psychological stress and disease. *JAMA, 298*(14), 1685–1687 https://doi.org/10.1001/jama.298.14.1685.

Conway, C. C., Raposa, E. B., Hammen, C., & Brennan, P. A. (2018). Transdiagnostic pathways from early social stress to psychopathology: A 20-year prospective study. *Journal of Child Psychology and Psychiatry, 59*(8), 855–862 https://doi.org/10.1111/jcpp.12862.

Couzin-Frankel, J. (2010). Inflammation bares a dark side. *Science, 220*(6011), 1621. https://doi.org/10.1126/science.330.6011.1621.

Cramer, H., Lange, S., Klose, P., Paul, A., & Dobos, G. (2012). Yoga for breast cancer patients and survivors: a systematic review and meta-analysis. *BMC Cancer, 12*(1), 412 https://doi.org/10.1186/1471-2407-12-412.

Cramer, H., Lauche, R., Langhorst, J., & Dobos, G. (2013). Yoga for depression: A systematic review and meta-analysis. *Depress Anxiety, 30*(11), 1068–1083 https://doi.org/10.1002/da.22166.

Cramer, H., Lauche, R., Langhorst, J., & Dobos, G. (2016). Is one yoga style better than another? A systematic review of associations of yoga style and conclusions in randomized yoga trials. *Complementary Therapies in Medicine, 25*, 178–187 https://doi.org/10.1002/da.22166.

Cramer, H., Ward, L., Steel, A., Lauche, R., Dobos, G., & Zhang, Y. (2016). Prevalence, patterns, and predictors of yoga use: results of a US nationally representative survey. *American Journal of Preventive Medicine, 50*(2), 230–235 https://doi.org/10.1016/j.amepre.2015.07.037.

Crowe, M., Jordan, J., Burrell, B., Jones, V., Gillon, D., & Harris, S. (2016). Mindfulness-based stress reduction for long-term physical conditions: A systematic review. *Australian & New Zealand Journal of Psychiatry, 50*(1), 21–32 https://doi.org/10.1177/0004867415607984.

Cuijpers, P., Marks, I. M., van Straten, A., Cavanagh, K., Gega, L., & Andersson, G. (2009). Computer-aided psychotherapy for anxiety disorders: a meta-analytic review. *Cognitive Behaviour Therapy, 38*(2), 66–82 https://doi.org/10.1080/16506070802694776.

Danese, A., Pariante, C. M., Caspi, A., Taylor, A., & Poulton, R. (2007). Childhood maltreatment predicts adult inflammation in a life-course study. *Proceedings of the National Academy of Sciences, 104*(4), 1319–1324 https://doi.org/10.1073/pnas.0610362104.

Davidson, R. J., & Goleman, D. J. (1977). The role of attention in meditation and hypnosis: A psychobiological perspective on transformations of consciousness. *International Journal of Clinical and Experimental Hypnosis, 25*(4), 291–308 https://doi.org/10.1080/00207147708415986.

Dhungel, K. U., Malhotra, V., Sarkar, D., & Prajapati, R. (2008). Effect of alternate nostril breathing exercise on cardiorespiratory functions. *Nepal Medical College Journal, 10*(1), 25–27 https://doi.org/10.1080/00207147708415986.

Edwards, M. K., & Loprinzi, P. D. (2018). Comparative effects of meditation and exercise on physical and psychosocial health outcomes: a review of randomized controlled trials. *Postgraduate Medicine, 130*(2), 222–228 https://doi.org/10.1080/00325481.2018.1409049.

Epel, E., Daubenmier, J., Moskowitz, J. T., Folkman, S., & Blackburn, E. (2009). Can meditation slow rate of cellular aging? *Cognitive stress, mindfulness, and telomeres. Annals of New York Academy of Science, 1172*(1), 34–53 https://doi.org/10.1111/j.1749-6632.2009.04414.x.

Etkin, A., Büchel, C., & Gross, J. J. (2015). The neural bases of emotion regulation. *Nature Reviews Neuroscience, 16*(11), 693–700 https://doi.org/10.1038/nrn4044.

Eyre, H. A., Baune, B., & Lavretsky, H. (2015). Clinical advances in geriatric psychiatry: a focus on prevention of mood and cognitive disorders. *Psychiatric Clinics of North America, 38*(3), 495–514 https://doi.org/10.1016/j.psc.2015.05.002.

Faull, O. K., Jenkinson, M., Clare, S., & Pattinson, K. T. S. (2015). Functional subdivision of the human periaqueductal grey in respiratory control using 7 tesla fMRI. *NeuroImage, 113*, 356–364 https://doi.org/10.1016/j.neuroimage.2015.02.026.

Field, T. (2011). Yoga clinical research review. *Complementary Therapies in Clinical Practice, 17*(1), 1–8 https://doi.org/10.1016/j.neuroimage.2015.02.026.

Field, T. (2016). Knee osteoarthritis pain in the elderly can be reduced by massage therapy, yoga and tai chi: a review. *Complementary Therapies in Clinical Practice, 22*, 87–92.

Firth, J., Torous, J., Nicholas, J., Carney, R., Pratap, A., Rosenbaum, S., & Sarris, J. (2017). The efficacy of smartphone-based mental health interventions for depressive symptoms: A meta-analysis of randomized controlled trials. *World Psychiatry, 16*(3), 287–298 https://doi.org/10.1002/wps.20472.

Gagrani, M., Faiq, M. A., Sidhu, T., Dada, R., Yadav, R. K., Sihota, R., . . . Dada, T. (2018). Meditation enhances brain oxygenation, upregulates BDNF and improves quality of life in patients with primary open angle glaucoma: A randomized controlled trial. *Restorative Neurology and Neuroscience, 36*(6), 741–753 https://doi.org/10.3233/rnn-180857.

Galante, J., Galante, I., Bekkers, M.-J., & Gallacher, J. (2014). Effect of kindness-based meditation on health and well-being: A systematic review and meta-analysis. *Journal of Consulting and Clinical Psychology, 82*(6), 1101 https://doi.org/10.1037/a0037249.

Gallegos, A. M., Crean, H. F., Pigeon, W. R., & Heffner, K. L. (2017). Meditation and yoga for posttraumatic stress disorder: A meta-analytic review of randomized controlled trials. *Clinical Psychology Review, 58,* 115–124.

Gamret, A. C., Price, A., Fertig, R. M., Lev-Tov, H., & Nichols, A. J. (2018). Complementary and alternative medicine therapies for psoriasis: A systematic review. *JAMA Dermatology, 154*(11), 1330–1337 https://doi.org/10.1001/jamadermatol.2018.2972.

Gard, T., Noggle, J. J., Park, C. L., Vago, D. R., & Wilson, A. (2014). Potential self-regulatory mechanisms of yoga for psychological health. *Frontiers in Human Neuroscience, 8,* 770 https://doi.org/10.3389/fnhum.2014.00770.

Gitlin, L. N., & Hodgson, N. (2015). Caregivers as therapeutic agents in dementia care: the context of caregiving and the evidence base for interventions. In J. E. Gaugler & R. L. Kane (Eds.), *Family caregiving in the new normal* (pp. 305–353). London: Elsevier.

Gold, P. W., & Chrousos, G. P. (2002). Organization of the stress system and its dysregulation in melancholic and atypical depression: High vs low CRH/NE states. *Molecular Psychiatry, 7*(3), 254 https://doi.org/10.1038/sj.mp.4001032.

Gothe, N. P., Keswani, R. K., & McAuley, E. (2016). Yoga practice improves executive function by attenuating stress levels. *Biological Psychology, 121*(Pt A), 109–116. https://doi.org/10.1016/j.biopsycho.2016.10.010.

Goyal, M., Singh, S., Sibinga, E. M. S., Gould, N. F., Rowland-Seymour, A., Sharma, R., . . . Shihab, H. M. (2014). Meditation programs for psychological stress and well-being: a systematic review and meta-analysis. *JAMA Internal Medicine, 174*(3), 357–368.

Grant, S., Colaiaco, B., Motala, A., Shanman, R., Booth, M., Sorbero, M., & Hempel, S. (2017). Mindfulness-based relapse prevention for substance use disorders: A systematic review and meta-analysis. *Journal of Addiction Medicine, 11*(5), 386 https://doi.org/10.1097/adm.0000000000000338.

Gu, J., Strauss, C., Bond, R., & Cavanagh, K. (2015). How do mindfulness-based cognitive therapy and mindfulness-based stress reduction improve mental health and wellbeing? A systematic review and meta-analysis of mediation studies. *Clinical Psychology Review, 37,* 1–12.

Hammen, C. (2005). Stress and depression. *Annual Review of Clinical Psychology, 1,* 293–319.

Hare, D. L., Toukhsati, S. R., Johansson, P., & Jaarsma, T. (2013). Depression and cardiovascular disease: a clinical review. *European Heart Journal, 35*(21), 1365–1372.

Heim, C., Ehlert, U., & Hellhammer, D. H. (2000). The potential role of hypocortisolism in the pathophysiology of stress-related bodily disorders. *Psychoneuroendocrinology, 25*(1), 1–35 https://doi.org/10.1016/s0306-4530(99)00035-9.

Hendriks, T., de Jong, J., & Cramer, H. (2017). The effects of yoga on positive mental health among healthy adults: A systematic review and meta-analysis. *Journal of Alternative and Complementary Medicine, 23*(7), 505–517 https://doi.org/10.1089/acm.2016.0334.

Hilton, L., Maher, A. R., Colaiaco, B., Apaydin, E., Sorbero, M. E., Booth, M., . . . Hempel, S. (2017). Meditation for posttraumatic stress: Systematic review and meta-analysis. *Psychological Trauma, 9*(4), 453 https://doi.org/10.1037/tra0000180.

The Honest Guys. (2015). Mindfulness meditation: Guided 10 minutes. Retrieved from https://www.youtube.com/watch?v=6p_yaNFSYao

Hou, R. J., Wong, S. Y.-S., Yip, B. H.-K., Hung, A. T. F., Lo, H. H.-M., Chan, P. H. S., . . . Mak, W. W. S. (2014). The effects of mindfulness-based stress reduction program on the mental health of family caregivers: A randomized controlled trial. *Psychotherapy and Psychosomatics, 83*(1), 45–53.

Howells, A., Ivtzan, I., & Eiroa-Orosa, F. J. (2016). Putting the "app" in happiness: a randomised controlled trial of a smartphone-based mindfulness intervention to enhance wellbeing. *Journal of Happiness Studies, 17*(1), 163–185 https://doi.org/10.1007/s10902-014-9589-1.

Hughes, J. W., Fresco, D. M., Myerscough, R., van Dulmen, M., Carlson, L. E., & Josephson, R. (2013). Randomized controlled trial of mindfulness-based stress reduction for prehypertension. *Psychosomatic Medicine, 75*(8) https://doi.org/10.1097/psy.0b013e3182a3e4e5.

Innes, K. E., Selfe, T. K., & Vishnu, A. (2010). Mind-body therapies for menopausal symptoms: A systematic review. *Maturitas, 66*(2), 135–149 https://doi.org/10.1016/j.maturitas.2010.01.016.

Jain, F. A., Walsh, R. N., Eisendrath, S. J., Christensen, S., & Cahn, B. R. (2015). Critical analysis of the efficacy of meditation therapies for acute and subacute phase treatment of depressive disorders: A systematic review. *Psychosomatics, 56*(2), 140–152 https://doi.org/10.1016/j.psym.2014.10.007.

Jain, S., Shapiro, S. L., Swanick, S., Roesch, S. C., Mills, P. J., Bell, I., & Schwartz, G. E. R. (2007). A randomized controlled trial of mindfulness meditation versus relaxation training: Effects on distress, positive states of mind, rumination, and distraction. *Annals of Behavioral Medicine, 33*(1), 11–21 https://doi.org/10.1207/s15324796abm3301_2.

Jella, S. A., & Shannahoff-Khalsa, D. S. (1993). The effects of unilateral forced nostril breathing on cognitive performance. *International Journal of Neuroscience, 73*(1–2), 61–68 https://doi.org/10.3109/00207459308987211.

Jennings, J. R., Sheu, L. K., Kuan, D. C. H., Manuck, S. B., & Gianaros, P. J. (2016). Resting state connectivity of the medial prefrontal cortex covaries with individual differences in high-frequency heart rate variability. *Psychophysiology, 53*(4), 444–454 https://doi.org/10.1111/psyp.12586.

Jovanov, E. (2005). On spectral analysis of heart rate variability during very slow yogic breathing. *Conference Proceedings: IEEE Engineering in Medicine and Biology Society, 2005,* 2467–2470.

Kabat-Zinn, J. (2003). Mindfulness-based interventions in context: past, present, and future. *Clinical Psychology: Science and Practice, 10*(2), 144–156 https://doi.org/10.1093/clipsy.bpg016.

Kabat-Zinn, J., & Hanh, T. N. (2009). *Full catastrophe living: Using the wisdom of your body and mind to face stress, pain, and illness.* New York, NY: Delta Trade.

Kamei, T., Toriumi, Y., Kimura, H., Kumano, H., Ohno, S., & Kimura, K. (2000). Decrease in serum cortisol during yoga exercise is correlated with alpha wave activation. *Perceptual and Motor Skills, 90*(3), 1027–1032 https://doi.org/10.2466/pms.2000.90.3.1027.

Khoury, B., Lecomte, T., Fortin, G., Masse, M., Therien, P., Bouchard, V., . . . Hofmann, S. G. (2013). Mindfulness-based therapy: A comprehensive meta-analysis. *Clinical Psychology Review, 33*(6), 763–771 https://doi.org/10.2466/pms.2000.90.3.1027.

Kiecolt-Glaser, J. K., Loving, T. J., Stowell, J. R., Malarkey, W. B., Lemeshow, S., Dickinson, S. L., & Glaser, R. (2005). Hostile marital interactions, proinflammatory cytokine production, and wound healing. *Archives of General Psychiatry, 62*(12), 1377–1384 https://doi.org/10.1001/archpsyc.62.12.1377.

Klimes-Dougan, B., Chong, L. S., Samikoglu, A., Thai, M., Amatya, P., Cullen, K. R., & Lim, K. O. (2019). Transcendental meditation and hypothalamic–pituitary–adrenal axis functioning: A pilot, randomized controlled trial with young adults. *Stress.* https://doi.org/10.1001/archpsyc.62.12.1377.

Koenig, J., Kemp, A. H., Beauchaine, T. P., Thayer, J. F., & Kaess, M. (2016). Depression and resting state heart rate variability in children and adolescents: A systematic review and meta-analysis. *Clinical Psychology Review, 46*, 136–150.

Kuester, A., Niemeyer, H., & Knaevelsrud, C. (2016). Internet-based interventions for post-traumatic stress: A meta-analysis of randomized controlled trials. *Clinical Psychology Review, 43*, 1–16.

Kuyken, W., Warren, F. C., Taylor, R. S., Whalley, B., Crane, C., Bondolfi, G., . . . Schweizer, S. (2016). Efficacy of mindfulness-based cognitive therapy in prevention of depressive relapse: An individual patient data meta-analysis from randomized trials. *JAMA Psychiatry, 73*(6), 565–574.

Lake, J., & Turner, M. S. (2017). Urgent need for improved mental health care and a more collaborative model of care. *Permanente Journal, 21*, 17-024.

Lauche, R., Cramer, H., Dobos, G., Langhorst, J., & Schmidt, S. (2013). A systematic review and meta-analysis of mindfulness-based stress reduction for the fibromyalgia syndrome. *Journal of Psychosomatic Research, 75*(6), 500–510 https://doi.org/10.1016/j.jpsychores.2013.10.010.

Lauche, R., Cramer, H., Häuser, W., Dobos, G., & Langhorst, J. (2013). A systematic review and meta-analysis of qigong for the fibromyalgia syndrome. *Evidence-Based Complementary and Alternative Medicine, 2013*, 635182 https://doi.org/10.1155/2013/635182.

Lauche, R., Hunter, D. J., Adams, J., & Cramer, H. (2019). Yoga for osteoarthritis: A systematic review and meta-analysis. *Current Rheumatology Reports, 21*(9), 47 https://doi.org/10.1007/s11926-019-0846-5.

Lavretsky, H., Epel, E. S., Siddarth, P., Nazarian, N., Cyr, N. S., Khalsa, D. S., . . . Irwin, M. R. (2013). A pilot study of yogic meditation for family dementia caregivers with depressive symptoms: Effects on mental health, cognition, and telomerase activity. *International Journal of Geriatric Psychiatry, 28*(1), 57–65 https://doi.org/10.1002/gps.3790.

Lee, R. S., & Sawa, A. (2014). Environmental stressors and epigenetic control of the hypothalamic–pituitary–adrenal axis. *Neuroendocrinology, 100*(4), 278–287. https://doi.org/10.1159/000369585.

Lim, D., Condon, P., & DeSteno, D. (2015). Mindfulness and compassion: an examination of mechanism and scalability. *PloS One, 10*(2), e0118221 https://doi.org/10.1371/journal.pone.0118221.

Macinko, J., & Upchurch, D. M. (2019). Factors associated with the use of meditation, US adults 2017. *Journal of Alternative and Complementary Medicine, 25*(9), 920–927 https://doi.org/10.1089/acm.2019.0206.

Marshall, R. S., Basilakos, A., Williams, T., & Love-Myers, K. (2014). Exploring the benefits of unilateral nostril breathing practice post-stroke: Attention, language, spatial abilities, depression, and anxiety. *Journal of Alternative and Complementary Medicine, 20*(3), 185–194 https://doi.org/10.1089/acm.2013.0019.

Marshall, R. S., Laures-Gore, J., DuBay, M., Williams, T., & Bryant, D. (2015). Unilateral forced nostril breathing and aphasia—exploring unilateral forced nostril breathing as an adjunct to aphasia treatment: A case series. *Journal of Alternative and Complementary Medicine, 21*(2), 91–99 https://doi.org/10.1089/acm.2013.0285.

Martinez-Cengotitabengoa, M., Carrascon, L., O'Brien, J. T., Diaz-Gutierrez, M. J., Bermudez-Ampudia, C., Sanada, K., . . . Gonzalez-Pinto, A. (2016). Peripheral inflammatory parameters in late-life depression: A systematic review. *International Journal of Molecular Science, 17*(12) https://doi.org/10.3390/ijms17122022.

Mason, J. W., Wang, S., Yehuda, R., Riney, S., Charney, D. S., & Southwick, S. M. (2001). Psychogenic lowering of urinary cortisol levels linked to increased emotional numbing and a shame-depressive syndrome in combat-related posttraumatic stress disorder. *Psychosomatic Medicine, 63*(3), 387–401 https://doi.org/10.1097/00006842-200105000-00008.

McDade, T. W., Hawkley, L. C., & Cacioppo, J. T. (2006). Psychosocial and behavioral predictors of inflammation in middle-aged and older adults: The Chicago health, aging, and
social relations study. *Psychosomatic Medicine, 68*(3), 376–381 https://doi.org/10.1097/
01.psy.0000221371.43607.64.

McEwen, B. S. (2002). Sex, stress and the hippocampus: Allostasis, allostatic load and
the aging process. *Neurobiology of Aging, 23*(5), 921–939 https://doi.org/10.1016/
S0197-4580(02)00027-1.

Miller, A. H., Maletic, V., & Raison, C. L. (2009). Inflammation and its discontents: The role of
cytokines in the pathophysiology of major depression. *Biological Psychiatry, 65*(9), 732–741
https://doi.org/10.1016/j.biopsych.2008.11.029.

Miller, G. E., Chen, E., Sze, J., Marin, T., Arevalo, J. M. G., Doll, R., . . . Cole, S. W. (2008).
A functional genomic fingerprint of chronic stress in humans: Blunted glucocorticoid and
increased NF-κB signaling. *Biological Psychiatry, 64*(4), 266–272. https://doi.org/10.1016/
j.biopsych.2008.03.017.

Miller, G. E., Chen, E., & Zhou, E. S. (2007). If it goes up, must it come down? Chronic stress and
the hypothalamic-pituitary-adrenocortical axis in humans. *Psychological Bulletin, 133*(1), 25
https://doi.org/10.1037/0033-2909.133.1.25.

Mohr, D. C., Burns, M. N., Schueller, S. M., Clarke, G., & Klinkman, M. (2013). Behavioral
intervention technologies: evidence review and recommendations for future research in
mental health. *General Hospital Psychiatry, 35*(4), 332–338.

Morone, N. E., Moore, C. G., & Greco, C. M. (2017). Characteristics of adults who used mindfulness meditation: United States, 2012. *Journal of Alternative and Complementary Medicine,
23*(7), 545–550 https://doi.org/10.1089/acm.2016.0099.

Nagendra, H. R. (2007). *Pranayama—The art and science.* Bangalore: Swami Vivekananda Yoga
Prakashana.

National Center for Complementary and Integrative Health. (2019). Yoga: What you need to
know. Retrieved from https://nccih.nih.gov/health/yoga/introduction.htm#hed4

Navarro-Haro, M. V., López-del-Hoyo, Y., Campos, D., Linehan, M. M., Hoffman, H. G.,
García-Palacios, A., . . . García-Campayo, J. (2017). Meditation experts try virtual reality
mindfulness: A pilot study evaluation of the feasibility and acceptability of virtual reality
to facilitate mindfulness practice in people attending a mindfulness conference. *PloS One,
12*(11), e0187777 https://doi.org/10.1371/journal.pone.0187777.

Neary, M., & Schueller, S. M. (2018). State of the field of mental health apps. *Cognitive and
Behavioral Practice, 25*(4), 531–537 https://doi.org/10.1016/j.cbpra.2018.01.002.

O'Leary, K., O'Neill, S., & Dockray, S. (2016). A systematic review of the effects of mindfulness
interventions on cortisol. *Journal of Health Psychology, 21*(9), 2108–2121 https://doi.org/
10.1177/1359105315569095.

Pal, G. K., Agarwal, A., Karthik, S., Pal, P., & Nanda, N. (2014). Slow yogic breathing through
right and left nostril influences sympathovagal balance, heart rate variability, and cardiovascular risks in young adults. *North American Journal of Medical Sciences, 6*(3), 145 https://doi.
org/10.4103/1947-2714.128477.

Park, J., Krause-Parello, C. A., & Barnes, C. M. (2020). A narrative review of movement-based
mind-body interventions: Effects of yoga, tai chi, and qigong for back pain patients. *Holistic
Nursing Practice, 34*(1), 3–23 https://doi.org/10.1097/hnp.0000000000000360.

Pascoe, M. C., & Bauer, I. E. (2015). A systematic review of randomised control trials on the
effects of yoga on stress measures and mood. *Journal of Psychiatric Research, 68*, 270–282.
doi:10.1016/j.jpsychires.2015.07.013

Pascoe, M. C., Thompson, D. R., & Ski, C. F. (2017). Yoga, mindfulness-based stress reduction
and stress-related physiological measures: A meta-analysis. *Psychoneuroendocrinology, 86*,
152–168 https://doi.org/10.1016/j.psyneuen.2017.08.008.

Pattinson, K. T. S., Mitsis, G. D., Harvey, A. K., Jbabdi, S., Dirckx, S., Mayhew, S. D., . . . Wise, R. G. (2009). Determination of the human brainstem respiratory control network and its cortical connections in vivo using functional and structural imaging. *NeuroImage, 44*(2), 295–305 https://doi.org/10.1016/j.neuroimage.2008.09.007.

Pfau, M. L., & Russo, S. J. (2015). Peripheral and central mechanisms of stress resilience. *Neurobiology of Stress, 1*, 66–79 https://doi.org/10.1016/j.ynstr.2014.09.004.

Plaza, I., Demarzo, M. M. P., Herrera-Mercadal, P., & García-Campayo, J. (2013). Mindfulness-based mobile applications: Literature review and analysis of current features. *JMIR mHealth and uHealth, 1*(2), e24 https://doi.org/10.2196/mhealth.2733.

Posadzki, P., Ernst, E., Terry, R., & Lee, M. S. (2011). Is yoga effective for pain? A systematic review of randomized clinical trials. *Complementary Therapies in Medicine, 19*(5), 281–287.

Pradhan, B. (2013). Effect of kapalabhati on performance of six-letter cancellation and digit letter substitution task in adults. *International Journal of Yoga, 6*(2), 128 https://doi.org/10.4103/0973-6131.113415.

Prakhinkit, S., Suppapitiporn, S., Tanaka, H., & Suksom, D. (2014). Effects of Buddhism walking meditation on depression, functional fitness, and endothelium-dependent vasodilation in depressed elderly. *Journal of Alternative and Complementary Medicine, 20*(5), 411–416 https://doi.org/10.1089/acm.2013.0205.

Rajesh, S. K., Ilavarasu, J. V., & Srinivasan, T. M. (2014). Effect of Bhramari Pranayama on response inhibition: Evidence from the stop signal task. *International Journal of Yoga, 7*(2), 138 https://doi.org/10.4103/0973-6131.133896.

Richards, D., & Richardson, T. (2012). Computer-based psychological treatments for depression: a systematic review and meta-analysis. *Clinical Psychology Review, 32*(4), 329–342.

Sakaki, M., Yoo, H. J., Nga, L., Lee, T.-H., Thayer, J. F., & Mather, M. (2016). Heart rate variability is associated with amygdala functional connectivity with MPFC across younger and older adults. *NeuroImage, 139*, 44–52 https://doi.org/10.1016/j.neuroimage.2016.05.076.

Satyapriya, M., Nagendra, H. R., Nagarathna, R., & Padmalatha, V. (2009). Effect of integrated yoga on stress and heart rate variability in pregnant women. *International Journal of Gynecology & Obstetrics, 104*(3), 218–222 https://doi.org/10.1016/j.ijgo.2008.11.013.

Schutte, N. S., & Malouff, J. M. (2014). A meta-analytic review of the effects of mindfulness meditation on telomerase activity. *Psychoneuroendocrinology, 42*, 45–48 https://doi.org/10.1016/j.psyneuen.2013.12.017.

Schuver, K. J., & Lewis, B. A. (2016). Mindfulness-based yoga intervention for women with depression. *Complementary Therapies in Medicine, 26*, 85–91 https://doi.org/10.1016/j.psyneuen.2013.12.017.

Shahidi, M., Mojtahed, A., Modabbernia, A., Mojtahed, M., Shafiabady, A., Delavar, A., & Honari, H. (2011). Laughter yoga versus group exercise program in elderly depressed women: A randomized controlled trial. *International Journal of Geriatric Psychiatry, 26*(3), 322–327 https://doi.org/10.1002/gps.2545.

Shannahoff-Khalsa, D. S., & Kennedy, B. (1993). The effects of unilateral forced nostril breathing on the heart. *International Journal of Neuroscience, 73*(1–2), 47–60 https://doi.org/10.3109/00207459308987210.

Shapiro, D., Cook, I. A., Davydov, D. M., Ottaviani, C., Leuchter, A. F., & Abrams, M. (2007). Yoga as a complementary treatment of depression: Effects of traits and moods on treatment outcome. *Evidence-Based Complementary and Alternative Medicine, 4*(4), 493–502 https://doi.org/10.1093/ecam/nel114.

Sharma, V. K., Rajajeyakumar, M., Velkumary, S., Subramanian, S. K., Bhavanani, A. B., Madanmohan, A. S., & Thangavel, D. (2014). Effect of fast and slow pranayama practice on cognitive functions in healthy volunteers. *Journal of Clinical and Diagnostic Research, 8*(1), 10 https://doi.org/10.1093/ecam/nel114.

Shavanani, A. B., & Udupa, K. (2003). Acute effect of Mukh bhastrika (a yogic bellows type breathing) on reaction time. *Indian Journal of Physiology and Pharmacology, 47*, 297–300.

Shi, L., Zhang, D., Wang, L., Zhuang, J., Cook, R., & Chen, L. (2017). Meditation and blood pressure: A meta-analysis of randomized clinical trials. *Journal of hypertension, 35*(4), 696–706 https://doi.org/10.1097/hjh.0000000000001217.

Singh, N. N., Lancioni, G. E., Winton, A. S. W., Singh, A. N., Adkins, A. D., & Singh, J. (2008). Clinical and benefit–cost outcomes of teaching a mindfulness-based procedure to adult offenders with intellectual disabilities. *Behavior Modification, 32*(5), 622–637 https://doi.org/10.1177/0145445508315854.

Sinha, A. N., Deepak, D., & Gusain, V. S. (2013). Assessment of the effects of pranayama/alternate nostril breathing on the parasympathetic nervous system in young adults. *Journal of Clinical and Diagnostic Research, 7*(5), 821 https://doi.org/10.7860/JCDR/2013/4750.2948.

Slavich, G. M., & Irwin, M. R. (2014). From stress to inflammation and major depressive disorder: A social signal transduction theory of depression. *Psychological Bulletin, 140*(3), 774–815 https://doi.org/10.1037/a0035302.

Sprod, L. K., Fernandez, I. D., Janelsins, M. C., Peppone, L. J., Atkins, J. N., Giguere, J., . . . Mustian, K. M. (2015). Effects of yoga on cancer-related fatigue and global side-effect burden in older cancer survivors. *Journal of Geriatric Oncology, 6*(1), 8–14 https://doi.org/10.1016/j.jgo.2014.09.184.

Srinivasan, T. M. (1991). Pranayama and brain correlates. *Ancient Science of Life, 11*(1–2), 2 https://doi.org/10.1016/j.jgo.2014.09.184.

Stancák, J. A., Kuna, M., Dostalek, C., & Vishnudevananda, S. (1991). Kapalabhati--yogic cleansing exercise. II. EEG topography analysis. *Homeostasis in Health and Disease, 33*(4), 182–189.

Strauss, C., Cavanagh, K., Oliver, A., & Pettman, D. (2014). Mindfulness-based interventions for people diagnosed with a current episode of an anxiety or depressive disorder: A meta-analysis of randomised controlled trials. *PloS One, 9*(4), e96110 https://doi.org/10.1371/journal.pone.0096110.

Tang, Y.-Y., Hölzel, B. K., & Posner, M. I. (2015). The neuroscience of mindfulness meditation. *Nature Reviews Neuroscience, 16*(4), 213 https://doi.org/10.1038/nrn3916.

Telles, S., Yadav, A., Gupta, R. K., & Balkrishna, A. (2013). Reaction time following yoga bellows-type breathing and breath awareness. *Perceptual and Motor Skills, 117*(1), 89–98 https://doi.org/10.2466/22.25.pms.117x10z4.

Telles, S., Yadav, A., Kumar, N., Sharma, S., Visweswaraiah, N. K., & Balkrishna, A. (2013). Blood pressure and Purdue pegboard scores in individuals with hypertension after alternate nostril breathing, breath awareness, and no intervention. *Medical Science Monitor, 19*, 61 https://doi.org/10.12659/msm.883743.

Tsang, H. W., Tsang, W. W., Jones, A. Y., Fung, K. M., Chan, A. H., Chan, E. P., & Au, D. W. (2013). Psycho-physical and neurophysiological effects of qigong on depressed elders with chronic illness. *Aging and Mental Health, 17*(3), 336–348. https://doi.org/10.1080/13607863.2012.732035.

Turankar, A. V., Jain, S., Patel, S. B., Sinha, S. R., Joshi, A. D., Vallish, B. N., . . . Turankar, S. A. (2013). Effects of slow breathing exercise on cardiovascular functions, pulmonary functions & galvanic skin resistance in healthy human volunteers: A pilot study. *Indian Journal of Medical Research, 137*(5), 916.

Valkanova, V., & Ebmeier, K. P. (2013). Vascular risk factors and depression in later life: A systematic review and meta-analysis. *Biological Psychiatry, 73*(5), 406–413 https://doi.org/10.1016/j.biopsych.2012.10.028.

Vandana, B., Vaidyanathan, K., Saraswathy, L. A., Sundaram, K. R., & Kumar, H. (2011). Impact of integrated amrita meditation technique on adrenaline and cortisol levels in healthy volunteers. *Evidence-Based Complementary and Alternative Medicine, 2011,* 379645 https://doi.org/10.1155/2011/379645.

Vialatte, F. B., Bakardjian, H., Prasad, R., & Cichocki, A. (2009). EEG paroxysmal gamma waves during Bhramari Pranayama: A yoga breathing technique. *Consciousness and cognition, 18*(4), 977–988 https://doi.org/10.1016/j.concog.2008.01.004.

Wagner, B., Horn, A. B., & Maercker, A. (2014). Internet-based versus face-to-face cognitive-behavioral intervention for depression: A randomized controlled non-inferiority trial. *Journal of Affective Disorders, 152,* 113–121 https://doi.org/10.1016/j.jad.2013.06.032.

Walsh, R., & Shapiro, S. L. (2006). The meeting of meditative disciplines and Western psychology: A mutually enriching dialogue. *American Psychologist, 61*(3), 227 https://doi.org/10.1037/0003-066x.61.3.227.

Wang, C.-W., Chan, C. H. Y., Ho, R. T. H., Chan, J. S. M., Ng, S.-M., & Chan, C. L. W. (2014). Managing stress and anxiety through qigong exercise in healthy adults: A systematic review and meta-analysis of randomized controlled trials. *BMC Complementary and Alternative Medicine, 14*(1), 8.

Wang, D., Wang, Y., Wang, Y., Li, R., & Zhou, C. (2014). Impact of physical exercise on substance use disorders: A meta-analysis. *PloS One, 9*(10), e110728 https://doi.org/10.1371/journal.pone.0110728.

West, J., Otte, C., Geher, K., Johnson, J., & Mohr, D. C. (2004). Effects of Hatha yoga and African dance on perceived stress, affect, and salivary cortisol. *Annals of Behavioral Medicine, 28*(2), 114–118 https://doi.org/10.1207/s15324796abm2802_6.

World Health Organization. (1948). *Preamble to the Constitution of the WHO as Adopted by the International Health Conference, New York, 1946.* Geneva: WHO.

Zou, L., Yeung, A., Li, C., Wei, G.-X., Chen, K., Kinser, P., . . . Ren, Z. (2018). Effects of meditative movements on major depressive disorder: A systematic review and meta-analysis of randomized controlled trials. *Journal of Clinical Medicine, 7*(8), 195 https://doi.org/10.3390/jcm7080195.

17

The Use of Bioinformatics and Big Data for the In Silico Study of Psychiatric Disorders

Wei Zhang, Gabriel R. Fries, and Joao L. de Quevedo

Introduction

Psychiatry is a medical field that aims to understand and treat mental disorders, which includes anxiety disorders, mood disorders, psychotic disorders, personality disorders, and posttraumatic stress disorders, among others. In general terms, psychiatric disorders have been typically associated not only with functions of the human brain, but also with social and experiential factors,[1] which makes them highly complex diseases that interact with and depend on many concurrent variables. Accordingly, most of these disorders are thought to result from the interaction between a genetic risk and environmental exposures, which makes them highly heterogeneous in nature with both clinical and public health implications.[2]

Although much progress has been made in the past several years, the underlying bases of mental disorders are largely unknown, which has hindered the development and implementation of highly successful treatments. From a biological perspective, these disorders are thought to lack quantifiable and objective phenotypes, and often groups identified by biological studies do not directly match those categorized by the clinical diagnostic criteria (such as the widely used *Diagnostic and Statistical Manual of Mental Disorders, 5th Edition* [DSM-5]).[3] In contrast, in medical fields such as oncology, tumors can be detected and classified by imaging and pathological tests, removed by surgery, and further examined so that oncologists can track the health conditions of their patients. In psychiatry, the diagnosis is typically built upon self-reported symptoms, which are often subjective in nature, and neuroimaging has, so far, not been decisive and largely useful to aid in diagnosis and prognosis decisions.[4] In this scenario, it is a consensus in the field that we need a deeper unbiased focus on biology-based measurements spanning from genes and proteins to cells, to neuron synapse and, finally, to behaviors, to ultimately better understand what is behind these disorders.[5]

In the past few decades, the development of cutting-edge biological technologies, especially those based on high throughput data, has enabled the rapid collection of unprecedented amounts of data. Biologists and bioengineers have amassed countless terabytes of high-resolution videos of microscopic cells as they wiggle and grow and interact, sequenced millions of genomes, as well as generated large data sets containing genomic, transcriptomic (RNA-sequencing), proteomic, chromatin immunoprecipitation sequencing (ChIP-seq), and epigenomic data.[6] Such big data differs from traditional data sets in their volume, velocity, and variety, and they often refer to extremely large and complex data sets. In addition to their complexity and potential influence on human decision-making processes, these data can be obtained by providing usable and accurate data in a short amount of time.

Due to the particularity of studying highly complex and heterogeneous disorders, such as psychiatric disorders, large numbers of patients and healthy controls are typically needed for case-control and longitudinal studies of their biological bases. In this sense, the sharing and discovering as well as reuse of the data, such as by forming consortia and making data available for the general public through online databases, is extremely important for the advancement of the field. In this chapter, we will focus on a discussion of existing databases containing big data in psychiatry. Based on the nature of the data, we have divided the existing data sets into four distinct categories, which will be discussed in more details in the next sessions and are presented in Table 17.1: genomic data, proteomics data, imaging data, and integrated data.

Big Data Datasets in Psychiatry

Genomic Data

The transcriptome is the full set of RNA transcripts expressed in a cell or by an organism or a specific tissue type. The transcriptome is not as stable as the genome and varies depending on many factors, including but not limited to type of the cell or tissue, development stage, and the environment. The aim of studying the transcriptome in a given sample is to catalogue and quantify all transcripts, including messenger RNAs, noncoding RNAs, microRNAs, and other small RNAs.

The most widely used technologies for the study of transcriptomes are RNA-sequencing (RNA-seq) and microarray. As a successor of microarray, RNA-seq has the ability to detect novel transcripts, a wider dynamic range, and higher specificity and sensitivity. RNA-seq can study the gene expression profile between multiple samples/conditions, as well as investigate alternative splicing events and gene fusions taking place in a particular biological system. Because the brain is comprised of many different kinds of cell, the traditional sequencing of bulk tissue gets sequencing reads from a mixture of different cells, which is an approach considered problematic for many reasons.[18] As an alternative, "single-cell" sequencing technologies have been developed to help scientists further understand the mechanisms of the brain and the biological basis of psychiatry disorders with better cell specificity and less cellular heterogeneity (which is thought to dilute group differences and increase heterogeneity). As technologies for single-cell sequencing improve and slowly become more affordable, more and more single-cell sequencing data are becoming available. So far, however, the vast majority of available data is focused on bulk tissue transcriptomic assessments by microarrays or RNA-seq.

There are two general (not specific to psychiatry disorders) RNA-seq/microarray data repositories: GEO[19] (Gene Expression Omnibus) and ArrayExpress.[20] They are hosted by the US National Institutes of Health's National Center for Biotechnology

Table 17.1. Public Databases

Resource	URL	Description
Genomic data		
NIMH	nimh.nih.gov/index.shtml	Largest research organization in the world specializing in mental illness, focuses on mental health and psychiatric disorders[7].
SMRI	stanleyresearch.org/	Nonprofit organization supporting research focusing on understanding and treating serious mental illness. There are RNA-seq data from specific brain regions available.
Common Mind Consortium	commonmind.org	Partnership that aims to generate and analyze large-scale genomic data, such as RNA-seq, ATAC-seq, genotypes and clinical data from human subjects with neuropsychiatric disease.
PsychENCODE	synapse.org//#! Synapse: syn4921369/wiki/ 235539	Founded by the NIMH in 2015 to study the role of rare genetic variants involved in several psychiatric disorders. The goal is to sequence the noncoding genomic elements in brains of human, mouse, chimpanzee and macaque, and investigating their role by the combination of ChIP-seq, ATAC-seq and genotype data.
GWAS Catalog	https://www.ebi.ac.uk/gwas/	Online, freely available database created by the NHGRI in 2008 that compiles the results of genome-wide association studies (GWAS).
dbGap	ncbi.nlm.nih.gov/gap	Developed by NCBI to archive the individual-level phenotype, exposure, genotype, and sequence data, and results from studies that have investigated the interaction of genotype and phenotype. There are many large scale GWAS data available.
Braincloud	braincloud.jhmi.edu/	Free application developed by the Lieber Institute and NIMH designed for exploring the temporal dynamics and genetic control of transcription in the human brain across the lifespan. There are genome-wide gene expression data and methylation data.
PGC	med.unc.edu/pgc	International consortium of scientists dedicated to conducting meta- and mega-analyses of genomic-wide genetic data, with a focus on psychiatric disorders. It provides summary statistics of GWAS studies.
ChIP-Atlas	chip-atlas.org	Integrative and comprehensive database for visualizing and making use of public ChIP-seq data.
ChIPBase v2.0	rna.sysu.edu.cn/chipbase/	Open database for studying transcription factor binding sites and motifs, and decoding the transcriptional regulatory networks of lncRNAs, microRNAs, other ncRNAs and protein-coding genes from ChIP-seq data. Their database currently contains ~10,200 curated peak datasets derived from ChIP-seq methods in 10 species.

(continued)

Table 17.1. Continued

Resource	URL	Description
Synapse	synapse.org/	Technology platform developed by Sage Bionetworks. It provides a set of web services and tools that make it easier for researchers to aggregate, organize, analyze, and share scientific data, code, and insights.
GEO	ncbi.nlm.nih.gov/geo/	The Gene Expression Omnibus (GEO) is a database that archives and distributes gene expression data including microarray, next-generation sequencing and other high-throughput functional genomics data submitted by the research community.
AE	ebi.ac.uk/arrayexpress/	ArrayExpress (AE) is founded to archive functional genomics data from microarray and sequencing to support reproducible research.
PD_NGSAtlas	bioinfo.hrbmu.edu.cn/pd_ngsatlas/	Focuses on the efficient storage of epigenomic and transcriptomic data based on next-generation sequencing and on the quantitative analyses of epigenetic and transcriptional alterations involved in psychiatric disorders.[8]
The Brain Atlas	proteinatlas.org/humanproteome/brain	Explored the protein expression in the mammalian brain by visualization and integration of data from three mammalian species (human, pig and mouse). Transcriptomics data combined with affinity-based protein in situ localization. The data focuses on human genes and one-to-one orthologues in pig and mouse.[9]
Cistrome Data Browser	cistrome.org/db/	The Cistrome Data Browser (DB) is a resource of human and mouse cis-regulatory information derived from ChIP-seq, DNase-seq and ATAC-seq chromatin profiling assays, which map the genome-wide locations of transcription factor binding sites, histone post-translational modifications and regions of chromatin accessible to endonuclease activity.[10]
DataMed	datamed.org/	Open source biomedical data discovery system. It contains two major components: DatA Tag Suite, a data ingestion pipeline, which can collect and transform original metadata information into a unified model, and a search engine that finds relevant data according to user-entered queries.[11]
Image data		
OpenNeuro (previously OpenfMRI)	openneuro.org/ (https://openfmri.org/)	Neuroimaging data sharing platform that provides curated datasets. It is a repository of human brain imaging data collected using MRI and EEG techniques. It provides a resource for researchers to share their MRI data, make the data openly available to the research community.

Table 17.1. Continued

Resource	URL	Description
Internet Brain Volume Database (IBVD)	ibvd.virtualbrain.org/	Web-based database of brain neuroanatomic volumetric data. It also provides the electronic access to both group volumetric results as well as volume observations in individual cases from the published literature.[12]
GEMMA	chibi.ubc.ca/Gemma/	Website and database that provides a set of tools for the meta-analysis and re-use of genomics data. It currently focuses on the analysis of gene expression profiles.[13]
Neuroscience Information Framework (NIF)	neuinfo.org/	Initiative of the NIH Blueprint Consortium, NIF has been cataloguing and investigating the neuroscience resource landscape since 2006. NIF includes >4500 curated resources and access to>100 databases.[14]
Proteomics data		
Metabolomics Workbench (MW)	metabolomicswork bench.org/	Funded by NIH to address key barriers and difficulties in the discovery of biomedical research as well as its translation into improved human health. A repository for metabolomics data and metadata, MW provides analysis tools and access to metabolite standards, protocols, tutorials and training, as well as promotes data sharing and collaboration.
PRIDE	ebi.ac.uk/pride/archive/	Founded by European Bioinformatics Institute to provide a centralized and standard public data repository for proteomics data. It is the world's largest data repository of mass spectrometry-based proteomics data, and is one of the founding members of the global ProteomeXchange (PX) consortium.
Metabolights	ebi.ac.uk/metabolights/	An open-access database repository for cross-platform and cross-species metabolomics research at the European Bioinformatics Institute. It provides Metabolomics Standard Initiative compliant metadata and raw experimental data associated with metabolomics experiments.
Human Connectome Project (HCP)	humanconnectome.org/	The goal of the Human Connectome Project is to build a "network map" (connectome) that will shed light on the anatomical and functional connectivity within the healthy human brain, as well as to produce a body of data that will facilitate research into neurological disorders such as dyslexia, autism, Alzheimer's disease, and schizophrenia.[15]
Integrated data		
OmicsDI	omicsdi.org	Open source platform that can be used to access, discover and disseminate omics datasets. It provides a unique infrastructure to integrate datasets coming from multiple omics studies, including proteomics, genomics, metabolomics, and transcriptomics data sets.

(*continued*)

Table 17.1. Continued

Resource	URL	Description
SNCID	sncid. stanleyresearch.org/	An integrative database that includes 1749 neuropathological markers measured in 12 different brain regions in 60 human subjects (15 each schizophrenia, bipolar disorder, depression, and unaffected controls). It also includes three independent Genome-wide expression microarray datasets. It integrates statistical analysis tools such as correlation analysis, variance analysis, as well as functional annotation tools.[16]
GTEx Portal	gtexportal.org/ home/	Comprehensive public resource to study tissue-specific gene expression and regulation. Samples were collected from 54 nondiseased tissue sites across nearly 1000 individuals, primarily for molecular assays including WGS, WES, and RNA-Seq. Remaining samples are available from the GTEx Biobank. The GTEx Portal provides open access to data including gene expression, QTLs, and histology images.
Braineac	braineac.org	Exon-specific eQTL data set comprised of 134 brains from individuals free of neurodegenerative disorders, covering ten human brain regions.
Enhancing Neuro Imaging Genetics Through Meta Analysis (ENIGMA)	enigma.ini.usc.edu/ ongoing/enigma-schizophrenia-workinggroup/	Collaborative network of researchers in imaging genomics, neurology and psychiatry, to understand brain structure and function, based on MRI, fMRI, DTI, genetic data from many patients.
PharmGKB	pharmgkb.org	Pharmacogenomics knowledge resource that encompasses clinical information including clinical guidelines and drug labels, potentially clinically actionable gene-drug associations and genotype-phenotype relationships. PharmGKB collects, curates and disseminates knowledge about the impact of human genetic variation on drug responses.[17]

Abbreviations: dbGaP, database of genotypes and phenotypes; DTI, diffusion tensor imaging; EEG, electroencephalogram; eQTL, expression quantitative trait *loci*; GTEx, genotype-tissue expression; MRI, magnetic resonance imaging; NCBI, National Center for Biotechnology Information; NHGRI, National Human Genome Research Institute; NIMH, National Institute of Mental Health; PGC, Psychiatric Genomics Consortium; PRIDE, PRoteomics IDEntifications; SMRI, Stanley Medical Research Institute; SNCID, Stanley Neuropathology Consortium Integrative Database.

Informatics (NCBI) and the European Bioinformatics Institute within the European Molecular Biology Laboratory, respectively. In both cases, microarray data, next-generation sequencing, and other high-throughput data are submitted by the authors of scientific papers and the research community, and the data become freely available and open to the public without any applications or request.

There are also such data repositories that are specific to psychiatry disorders and neuroscience. These are established by federal agencies such as the National Institute of Mental Health and nonprofit organizations such as the Stanley Medical Research Institute. These data repositories include PsychENCODE,[21] CommonMind,[22] and the Psychiatric Genomics Consortium[23] (PGC). Some of them are more than just a data storage and act as a proper platform, such as the Synapse, which is a technology platform developed by Sage Bionetworks that provides a set of web services and tools that make it easier for researchers to aggregate, organize, analyze, and share scientific data, code, and insights.

In addition to traditional RNA sequencing, chromatin immunoprecipitation (ChIP)-sequencing (ChIP-seq) has been developed as a high throughput method for investigating DNA–protein interactions. It combines chromatin immunoprecipitation assays with next-generation sequencing, allowing for the identification of genome-wide DNA binding sites for transcription factors and other DNA-binding proteins. Transcription of genes are regulated by the binding of transcription factors (TF) at promoters and distal regulatory elements, as well as the accessibility of these elements, which is controlled by histone modifications. ChIP-seq can detect both TFs and histone modifications, having the potential to predict gene expression, and can be integrated with RNA-seq data to decipher the basic regulatory control of gene expression.[24]

There are two publicly available data sets containing ChIP-seq data: ChIPBase and ChIP-Atlas.[25,26] ChIPBase currently contains ~10,200 curated peak data sets derived from ChIP-seq methods in 10 species, and provides a co-expression tool to investigate the co-expression patterns between DNA-binding proteins and genes, as well as a ChIP-function tool to predict the functions of genes. ChIP-Atlas is able to show alignment and peak-call results for all public ChIP-seq and DNase-seq data and visualize them. It contains the NCBI Sequence Read Archive, which encompasses data derived from GEO, ArrayExpress, ENCODE,[27] Roadmap Epigenomics,[28] and the scientific literature.

Genome-wide association studies (GWA study or GWAS), also known as whole genome association studies (WGA study or WGAS) are observational studies of a genome-wide set of genetic variants in different individuals to check whether any DNA variant may associated with a specific trait.[29] Over 100 GWAS focused on neuropsychiatric disorders have been reported, mostly on schizophrenia, Alzheimer's disease, and bipolar disorder. Since a typical GWAS evaluates hundreds of thousands of single nucleotide polymorphism (SNP) markers (normally millions of markers after imputation), it normally requires an extremely large sample size to achieve reliable results. Because the need of large sample sizes for GWAS discovery and replication are beyond the reach of single groups, multiple consortia have emerged to foster scientific discovery. The major player is the PGC,[30] which has more than 300 investigators and more than 75,000 subjects with GWAS data under analysis. The achievement of PGC is quite significant: it has published many GWAS papers on several psychiatry disorders such as schizophrenia[31] (36,989 cases and 113,075 controls), autism spectrum disorder[32] (7387 cases and 8567 controls), and bipolar disorder[33] (20,352 cases and 31,358 controls), among others.

The major GWAS data repositories include the Genotypes and Phenotypes (dbGaP) database from NCBI,[34] the European Genome-Phenome Archive[35] from

European Bioinformatics Institute, and the Centre for Genomic Regulation, as well as the GWAS Catalog[36] created by the National Human Genome Research Institute. They contain archived data and full *P*-value summary statistics for eligible studies from GWAS. Likewise, the PGC has made the full *P*-value summary statistics results from all published PGC studies downloadable as well.

Proteomic Data Sets

Proteomic technologies have been increasingly used, especially in the search for diagnostic and prognostic protein biomarkers in neuropsychiatric disorders. Proteomics produce high-throughput data revealing proteins expression levels, posttranslational modifications, and protein–protein interaction networks. Proteomics provide the modifications and interactions data at the protein level, which might be more closely related to pathophysiological processes underlying the psychiatric disorders, in contrast to other methods such as molecular genetics, since proteins are the players that fulfill most of the biological functions.[37]

The major technique in proteomic is protein mass spectrometry.[38] Its applications include the quantitation of proteins and their posttranslational modifications, as well as the identification of protein–protein interactions. Proteomic studies usually use blood serum/plasm protein as input, and there are many papers published.[39]

The two major metabolomics data repositories are European Bioinformatics Institute's Metabolights[40] and NCBI's Metabolomics Workbench.[41] Besides these two repositories is the PRIDE (Proteomics Identifications).[42] This leading proteomics data repository is a centralized, standards compliant, public data repository for proteomics data, including protein and peptide identifications, posttranslational modifications, and supporting spectral evidence.

Imaging Data Sets

There are a few general brain imaging repositories available for the scientific community, such as the OpenNeuro (formerly OpenfMRI)[43] and the Neuroimaging Informatics Tools and Resources Clearinghouse Image Repository (NITRC IR).[44] However, very limited publicly available image data sets are available specifically for psychiatric disorders.

IMAGEN[45] is a European research project examining how biological, psychological, and environmental factors during adolescence may influence brain development and mental health. Using brain imaging and genetics, the project will help develop prevention strategies and improved therapies for mental health disorders in the future. The project has been initially funded by the European Commission and has subsequently received funding from various agencies including the European Research Council, Medical Research Council, National Institute for Health Research (UK),

Swedish Research Council (Vetenskapsrådet), German Federal Ministry of Research & Education (BMBF), National Institute for Health Research (US) and the National Institute on Drug Abuse. The IMAGEN project spans eight sites across four EU countries: the United Kingdom, Germany, France, and Ireland.

Integrated Data Sets

Brain tissues are extremely complex, and the integration of data coming multiple parallel approaches and omics is thought to significantly inform biologically relevant mechanisms in a systematic way. For example, GWAS of human complex diseases have identified a large number of disease-associated genetic loci, distinguished by an altered frequency of specific SNPs among individuals with a particular disease compared to controls. However, most of these risk loci do not provide direct information on the biological basis of a disease or on their underlying mechanisms. Recent genome-wide expression quantitative trait loci (eQTLs) association studies have provided information on genetic factors, especially SNPs, associated with gene expression variation.[46] The most common used eQTL data set is GTEx.[47] The GTEx project was proposed in 2008 with the goal of establishing a database and associated tissue biobank to catalogue genetic variation and its influence on gene expression in all major human tissues across 1,000 individuals. This nearly decade-long effort now brings the largest multitissue research study using postmortem donors.

Another common integrative approach in this field is the combination of genomic data with imaging data. The Enhancing NeuroImaging Genetics through Meta-Analysis (ENIGMA) consortium is a collaborative network of researchers in imaging genomics, neurology, and psychiatry to understand brain structure and function based on magnetic resonance imaging, functional magnetic resonance imaging, diffusion tensor, and genetic data from many patients. The very first project of ENIGMA was a GWAS identifying common variants associated with hippocampal volume. Continuing work is exploring genetic variant that associated with subcortical volumes (ENIGMA2) and white matter microstructure (ENIGMA-DTI).[48] It provides tools and protocols to analyze genome-wide and neuroimaging data from research teams worldwide.

Studies Using Nontraditional Big Data

Big data is transforming psychiatric studies. Table 17.2 enumerates several examples of recent projects and shows how big data may have potential impacts in the field. These studies investigate very large populations, and some of them are cohort studies with very long range. They also include the analysis of some data that are not traditionally used in biomedical research, such as private insurance claims database,[49] and electronic health record.[50-54]

Table 17.2. Examples of Studies Using Novel Big Data

Description	Data Used	Number of Subjects (n)
Explore prevalence of substance use disorders among psychiatric patients in large university system[54]	Electronic health records data	40,999 psychiatric patients aged 18–64 years who sought treatment between 2000 and 2010
Used a private insurance claims database to examine the use of psychotropic medications by patients without a psychiatric diagnosis[49]	Private insurance claims database	5,132,789 individuals who received psychotropic prescription medication
The authors used linkable Danish nationwide population-based registers to investigate the relationship between head injury and subsequent psychiatric disorders[55]	Linkable Danish nationwide population-based registers	113,906 people who were born between 1977 and 2000 had suffered head injuries
Integrate depression screening, prescription fulfillment and electronic medical records to improve care in primary care[52]	Electronic medical records	61,464 patients in primary care in 14 clinical organizations
Natural language processing was applied to classify notes from patients with major depressive disorder[53]	Electronic medical records	127,504 patients with a billing diagnosis of major depressive disorder
Use natural language processing to train a diagnostic algorithm then use it to investigate electronic health records electronic medical records to assist with phenotyping in bipolar disorder[56]	Electronic medical records	52,235 patients who have one or more diagnosis of bipolar or mania within 20 years

Concluding Remarks

In this chapter, we review the data resources and platforms available with big data for the study of psychiatry disorders. Noteworthy, the data availability and convenience of access for psychiatry-associated data is still limited nowadays compared to other medical fields, such as oncology. To generate larger data sets requires wider collaborations among experimental researchers, data scientists, clinicians, engineers, patients, and others, not only to generate and analyze data, but also to properly integrate and interpret them in a meaningful way.

Big data is extremely different from small data in size and verity, and it therefore requires different and advanced tools for its analysis. There is an emerging field called "computational psychiatry,"[57] which applies machine learning to these big data and tries to find patterns and associations in mental illness. Although it is still very young, it sets the ambitious goals to model mental processes computationally and to draw connections between symptoms and causes, regardless of diagnoses, with the ultimate goal of developing tools for use by psychiatrists. Overall, despite the many technical challenges, the sizes and access of big data in psychiatry are rapidly increasing, and this will likely contribute to a better understanding of existing and new questions in psychiatry.

References

1. Goldberg D, Bridges K, Cook D, Evans B, Grayson D. The influence of social factors on common mental disorders: Destabilisation and restitution. *Brit J Psychiatry,* 1990;156(6):704–713.
2. Uher R. Gene-environment interactions in severe mental illness. *Front Psychiatry.* 2014;5:48 https://doi.org/10.3389/fpsyt.2014.00048.
3. Krystal JH, State MW. Psychiatric disorders: diagnosis to therapy. *Cell.* 2014;157(1):201–214 https://doi.org/10.1016/j.cell.2014.02.042.
4. Rego T, Velakoulis D. Brain imaging in psychiatric disorders: target or screen? *BJPsych Open.* 2019;5(1):e4–e4 https://doi.org/10.1192/bjo.2018.79.
5. Jollans L, Whelan R. Neuromarkers for mental disorders: harnessing population neuroscience. *Front Psychiatry.* 2018;9:242 https://doi.org/10.3389/fpsyt.2018.00242.
6. Wang Z, Gerstein M, Snyder M. RNA-Seq: a revolutionary tool for transcriptomics. *Nat Rev Genet.* 2009;10(1):57–63 https://doi.org/10.1038/nrg2484.
7. Barch DM, Gotlib IH, Bilder RM, et al. Common measures for national institute of mental health funded research. *Biol Psychiatry.* 2016;79(12):e91–e96 https://doi.org/10.1016/j.biopsych.2015.07.006.
8. Zhao Z, Li Y, Chen H, et al. PD_NGSAtlas: a reference database combining next-generation sequencing epigenomic and transcriptomic data for psychiatric disorders. *BMC Med Genomics.* 2014;7:71 https://doi.org/10.1186/s12920-014-0071-z.
9. Sunkin SM, Ng L, Lau C, et al. Allen Brain Atlas: an integrated spatio-temporal portal for exploring the central nervous system. *Nucleic Acids Res.* 2013;41(Database issue):D996–D1008 https://doi.org/10.1093/nar/gks1042.
10. Zheng R, Wan C, Mei S, et al. Cistrome Data Browser: expanded datasets and new tools for gene regulatory analysis. *Nucleic Acids Res.* 2019;47(D1):D729–D735 https://doi.org/10.1093/nar/gky1094.
11. Ohno-Machado L, Sansone S-A, Alter G, et al. Finding useful data across multiple biomedical data repositories using DataMed. *Nat Genet.* 2017;49(6):816–819 https://doi.org/10.1038/ng.3864.
12. Kennedy DN, Hodge SM, Gao Y, Frazier JA, Haselgrove C. The internet brain volume database: a public resource for storage and retrieval of volumetric data. *Neuroinformatics.* 2012;10(2):129–140 https://doi.org/10.1007/s12021-011-9130-1.
13. Zoubarev A, Hamer KM, Keshav KD, et al. Gemma: a resource for the reuse, sharing and meta-analysis of expression profiling data. *Bioinformatics.* 2012;28(17):2272–2273 https://doi.org/10.1093/bioinformatics/bts430.
14. Gardner D, Akil H, Ascoli GA, et al. The neuroscience information framework: a data and knowledge environment for neuroscience. *Neuroinformatics.* 2008;6(3):149–160 https://doi.org/10.1007/s12021-008-9024-z.
15. Marcus DS, Harms MP, Snyder AZ, et al. Human Connectome Project informatics: quality control, database services, and data visualization. *Neuroimage.* 2013;80:202–219 https://doi.org/10.1016/j.neuroimage.2013.05.077.
16. Kim S, Webster MJ. The stanley neuropathology consortium integrative database: a novel, web-based tool for exploring neuropathological markers in psychiatric disorders and the biological processes associated with abnormalities of those markers. *Neuropsychopharmacology.* 2010;35(2):473–482 https://doi.org/10.1038/npp.2009.151.
17. Gong L, Owen RP, Gor W, Altman RB, Klein TE. PharmGKB: an integrated resource of pharmacogenomic data and knowledge. *Curr Protoc Bioinformatics.* 2008;23(1):14.7.17 https://doi.org/10.1002/0471250953.bi1407s23.

18. Hwang B, Lee JH, Bang D. Single-cell RNA sequencing technologies and bioinformatics pipelines. *Exp Mol Med.* 2018;96:50 https://doi.org/10.1038/s12276-018-0071-8.
19. Barrett T, Wilhite SE, Ledoux P, et al. NCBI GEO: archive for functional genomics data sets--update. *Nucleic Acids Res.* 2013;41(Database issue):D991–D995 https://doi.org/10.1002/0471250953.bi1407s23.
20. Parkinson H, Kapushesky M, Shojatalab M, et al. ArrayExpress: a public database of microarray experiments and gene expression profiles. *Nucleic Acids Res.* 2007;35(Database issue):D747–D750 https://doi.org/10.1093/nar/gkl995.
21. Akbarian S, Liu C, Knowles JA, et al. The PsychENCODE project. *Nucleic Acid Res.* 2007;35(Suppl 1):D747–D750 https://doi.org/10.1093/nar/gkl995.
22. Hoffman GE, Bendl J, Voloudakis G, et al. CommonMind Consortium provides transcriptomic and epigenomic data for schizophrenia and bipolar disorder. *Scientific Data.* 2019;6(1):180 https://doi.org/10.1038/s41597-019-0183-6.
23. Sullivan PF. The psychiatric GWAS consortium: big science comes to psychiatry. *Neuron.* 2010;68(2):182–186 https://doi.org/10.1016/j.neuron.2010.10.003.
24. Park PJ. ChIP–seq: advantages and challenges of a maturing technology. *Nat Rev Genet.* 2009;10(10):669–680 https://doi.org/10.1038/nrg2641.
25. Oki SA-O, Ohta TA-O, Shioi G, et al. ChIP-Atlas: a data-mining suite powered by full integration of public ChIP-seq data. *EMBO Rep.* 2018;19:e46255 https://doi.org/10.15252/embr.201846255.
26. Zhou K-R, Liu S, Sun W-J, et al. ChIPBase v2.0: decoding transcriptional regulatory networks of non-coding RNAs and protein-coding genes from ChIP-seq data. *Nucleic Acids Res.* 2017;45(D1):D43–D50 https://doi.org/10.1093/nar/gkw965.
27. Dunham I, Kundaje A, Aldred SF, et al. An integrated encyclopedia of DNA elements in the human genome. *Nature.* 2012;489(7414):57–74 https://doi.org/10.1093/nar/gkw965.
28. Bernstein BE, Stamatoyannopoulos JA, Costello JF, et al. The NIH Roadmap Epigenomics Mapping Consortium. *Nat Biotechnol.* 2010;28(10):1045–1048 https://doi.org/10.1038/nbt1010-1045.
29. Hancock DB, Markunas CA, Bierut LJ, Johnson EO. Human genetics of addiction: new insights and future directions. *Curr Psychiatry Rep.* 2018;20(2):8 https://doi.org/10.1007/s11920-018-0873-3.
30. Psychiatric GWAS Consortium Steering Committee. A framework for interpreting genome-wide association studies of psychiatric disorders. *Mol Psychiatry.* 2009;14(1):10-7.
31. Ripke S, Neale BM, Corvin A, et al. Biological insights from 108 schizophrenia-associated genetic loci. *Nature.* 2014;511(7510):421–427.
32. Anney RJL, Ripke S, Anttila V, et al. Meta-analysis of GWAS of over 16,000 individuals with autism spectrum disorder highlights a novel locus at 10q24.32 and a significant overlap with schizophrenia. *Molecular Autism.* 2017;8(1):21.
33. Stahl EA, Breen G, Forstner AJ, et al. Genome-wide association study identifies 30 loci associated with bipolar disorder. *Nat Genet.* 2019;51(5):793–803.
34. Mailman MD, Feolo M Jin Y, et al. The NCBI dbGaP database of genotypes and phenotypes. *Nat Genet.* 2007; 39(10):1181–1186.
35. Lappalainen I, Almeida-King J, Kumanduri V, et al. The European Genome-Phenome Archive of human data consented for biomedical research. *Nat Genet.* 2015;47(7):692–695 https://doi.org/10.1038/ng.3312.
36. Buniello A, MacArthur JAL, Cerezo M, et al. The NHGRI-EBI GWAS Catalog of published genome-wide association studies, targeted arrays and summary statistics 2019. *Nucleic Acids Res.* 2019;47(D1):D1005–D1012 https://doi.org/10.1093/nar/gky1120.

37. Sokolowska I, Ngounou Wetie AG, Wormwood K, Thome J, Darie CC, Woods AG. The potential of biomarkers in psychiatry: focus on proteomics. *J Neural Transm.* 2015;122, 9–18 https://doi.org/10.1007/s00702-013-1134-6.

38. Han X, Aslanian A, Yates JR, 3rd. Mass spectrometry for proteomics. *Curr Opin Chem Biol.* 2008;12(5):483–490 https://doi.org/10.1016/j.cbpa.2008.07.024.

39. Bot M, Chan MK, Jansen R, et al. Serum proteomic profiling of major depressive disorder. *Transl Psychiatry.* 2015;5:e599 https://doi.org/10.1038/tp.2015.88.

40. Haug K, Salek RM, Conesa P, et al. MetaboLights: an open-access general-purpose repository for metabolomics studies and associated meta-data. *Nucleic Acids Res.* 2013;41(Database issue):D781–D786 https://doi.org/10.1093/nar/gks1004.

41. Sud M, Fahy E, Cotter D, et al. Metabolomics Workbench: an international repository for metabolomics data and metadata, metabolite standards, protocols, tutorials and training, and analysis tools. *Nucleic Acids Res.* 2016;44(D1):D463–D470 https://doi.org/10.1093/nar/gkv1042.

42. Vizcaíno JA, Côté RG, Csordas A, et al. The PRoteomics IDEntifications (PRIDE) database and associated tools: status in 2013. *Nucleic Acids Res.* 2013;41(Database issue):D1063–D1069 https://doi.org/10.1093/nar/gkv1042.

43. Poldrack RA, Gorgolewski KJ. OpenfMRI: open sharing of task fMRI data. *Neuroimage.* 2017;144(Pt B):259–261 https://doi.org/10.1016/j.neuroimage.2015.05.073.

44. Kennedy DN, Haselgrove C, Riehl J, Preuss N, Buccigrossi R. The NITRC image repository. *Neuroimage.* 2016;124(Pt B):1069–1073 https://doi.org/10.1016/j.neuroimage.2015.05.074.

45. Cury C, Glaunès JA, Toro R, et al. Statistical shape analysis of large datasets based on diffeomorphic iterative centroids. *Front Neurosci.* 2018;12:803 https://doi.org/10.1016/j.neuroimage.2015.05.074.

46. Gorlov I, Xiao X, Mayes M, Gorlova O, Amos C. SNP eQTL status and eQTL density in the adjacent region of the SNP are associated with its statistical significance in GWA studies. *BMC Genet.* 2019;20(1):85 https://doi.org/10.1186/s12863-019-0786-0.

47. Gorlov I, Xiao X, Mayes M, et al. The Genotype-Tissue Expression (GTEx) project. *BMC Genet.* 2019;20:85 https://doi.org/10.1186/s12863-019-0786-0.

48. Thompson PM, Stein JL, Medland SE, et al. The ENIGMA Consortium: large-scale collaborative analyses of neuroimaging and genetic data. *Brain Imaging Behav.* 2014;8(2):153–182.

49. Wiechers IR, Leslie DL, Rosenheck RA. Prescribing of psychotropic medications to patients without a psychiatric diagnosis. *Psychiatric Serv.* 2013;64(12):1243–1248 https://doi.org/10.1176/appi.ps.201200557.

50. Castro VM, Minnier J Murphy SN, et al. Validation of electronic health record phenotyping of bipolar disorder cases and controls. *Am J Psychiatry*, 2015;172(4):363–372.

51. Ghassemi M, Marshall J, Singh N, Stone DJ, Celi LA. Leveraging a critical care database: selective serotonin reuptake inhibitor use prior to ICU admission is associated with increased hospital mortality. *Chest.* 2014;145(4):745–752.

52. Valuck RJ, Anderson HO, Libby AM, et al. Enhancing electronic health record measurement of depression severity and suicide ideation: a Distributed Ambulatory Research in Therapeutics Network (DARTNet) study. *J Am Board Fam Med.* 2012;25(5):582–593 https://doi.org/10.3122/jabfm.2012.05.110053.

53. Perlis RH, Iosifescu DV Castro VM, et al. Using electronic medical records to enable large-scale studies in psychiatry: treatment resistant depression as a model. *Psychol Med.* 2012;42(1):41–50 https://doi.org/10.1017/s0033291711000997.

54. Wu LT, Gersing KR, Swartz MS, Burchett B, Li T-K, Blazer DG. Using electronic health records data to assess comorbidities of substance use and psychiatric diagnoses and

treatment settings among adults. *J Psychol Res.* 2013;47(4):555–563 https://doi.org/10.1016/j.jpsychires.2012.12.009.

55. Orlovska S, Pedersen MS, Benros ME, Mortensen PB, Agerbo E, Nordentoft M. Head injury as risk factor for psychiatric disorders: a nationwide register-based follow-up study of 113,906 persons with head injury. *Am J Psychiatry.* 2014;171(4):463–469 https://doi.org/10.1176/appi.ajp.2013.13020190.

56. Castro VM, Minnier J, Murphy SN, et al. Validation of electronic health record phenotyping of bipolar disorder cases and controls. *Am J Psychiatry.* 2015;172(4):363–372 https://doi.org/10.3122/jabfm.2012.05.110053.

57. Wang X-J, Krystal JH. Computational psychiatry. *Neuron.* 2014;84(3):638–654 https://doi.org/10.1016/j.neuron.2014.10.018.

18

Converging Technologies Between the Space Mars Mission and Earth Global Mental Health

Donald D. Chang, Ryan Abbott, and Harris A. Eyre

Introduction

The first Mars mission is expected to take place this century and with it comes a whole new wave of mental health challenges. One study models a round trip travel time of days approximately 930 days, which is nearly 500 days more than the current record for continuous duration in Space, underscoring the potential mental health burden that might arise [1]. In another study that simulated a 520-day Mars mission, the authors highlighted the significant psychosocial challenges that arise from such small work areas and quarters. In this study, a six-member crew simulated the 520 day Space travel with one crew member (20%) developing depressive symptoms and three (50%) displaying confusion [2,3]. These findings are underscored by the psychiatry problems observed to occur from existing Space missions, which include symptoms of anxiety and depression [4,5].

Understandably, these mental stressors can be traced to the challenges of Space travel including extreme isolation, confinement, constant danger, circadian disruption, boredom, and monotony. Further, Mars mission Space crew face unprecedented autonomy given the significant delay in communication. This has important implications for their healthcare as medical support will be delayed or possibly ineffective by the time consults are received [4]. Currently, the technologies available are not sufficient to address these challenges nor provide the support required for such a demanding and prolonged travel in Space. Thus, there is a direct unmet need for innovation.

In parallel to this Space effort is the need to resolve existing mental health challenges on Earth. Besides the debilitating effects of mental health disorders on individuals, there is also a significant global burden from incapacity and reduced productivity secondary to mental illness [6]. It is anticipated that the burden of mental health disorders will cost \$16 trillion by 2030 [7]. Unfortunately, modern therapy remains limited in terms of treatment options. Most pharmacological strategies rely on trial-and-error approaches and preventative strategies are scarce due to a limited evidence base. Further complicating care is stigma and discrimination often associated with mental health disorders, inadequate healthcare financing, and a limited workforce of licensed psychiatry providers. National organizations such as the US National Council for Behavioral Health Medication Director Institute and the Lancet Commission for Global Mental Health have said that the current trajectory is unsustainable.

The realization that mental health challenges in Space and Earth share innovation needs lead us to speculate: *Can there be convergence between Earth and Space applications of technological innovations in mental health?* We argue there are, and in this chapter we highlight the bidirectional value of mental health technology transfer between Earth and Space.

The Biological Impact of Spaceflight on Mental Health

To appreciate the value of technological innovation toward mental health in Space, and the subsequent relations to mental health on Earth, it is important to first understand the physiological changes that occur in Space. We highlight a few notable studies here as the subject has been extensively reviewed in other publications [8,9].

A recent study evaluated anatomical changes in the brains of astronauts who underwent long-duration Space residency on the International Space Station [10]. Using magnetic resonance imaging, the study compared before and after images from the Space flight and found that postflight, there was narrowing of the central sulcus narrowing and cerebrospinal fluid (CSF) spaces at the vertex. This is an interesting observation given that it goes against the aging progression of enlarging CSF spaces. The consequence of such anatomical changes are that postflight astronauts are at risk of "visual impairment and intracranial pressure" syndrome, recently renamed as Spaceflight Associated Neuro-ocular Syndrome, which presents as a decrease in near-field visual acuity [11]. Elucidating the physiological basis of this syndrome remains an active area of research. Another recent study also found changes in brain white matter for subjects undergoing a 520 day confinement that simulated a Mars mission [12]. Noticeably, a reduction in fractional anisotropy was observed in the corpus callosum region and temporo-parietal-junction zone in the right hemisphere, suggesting changes in axonal structural integrity.

Recently, a landmark study was done on a pair of 50-year-old male monozygotic twins in which one spent 340 days about the International Space Station while his identical twin remained on Earth [13]. The study applied an exhaustive approach and collected telomeric, transcriptomic, epigenetic, proteomic, and metabolic data. The results unequivocally demonstrated that there were definite physiological changes that occur differently in Space relative to Earth, proving what many have long suspected while also spurring a new wave of research to translate these scientific findings into applications that be used to improve Space travel.

Converging Innovative Technologies Between
Space and Earth Mental Health

In the following sections, we explore and cite examples of how technological advances in mental health in either Space or Earth can be reciprocally insightful. In doing so, we hope to illustrate how these two seemingly disparate environments do in fact share overlapping interests when it comes to advancing mental health therapies and outcomes. We begin by exploring how Earth technologies can inform Space.

Innovative Earth Technologies Translatable to in Mental Health on Long-Duration Space Missions

As can be expected, extrapolating Earth-based technologies toward Space technologies has been the traditional approach given the ease at which studies can be done on Earth. However, designing research projects and clinical trials specific toward mental health is challenging given the constraints of testing and difficulty in reciprocating all the nuances of a long-duration spaceflight. Nonetheless, there are noteworthy examples tackling the issue head-on such as MyCompass, a web-based cognitive behavioral therapy (CBT) platform that is being test for its application in Spaceflight. MyCompass is a running a trial that recruits individuals similar to astronauts (i.e., high performing, healthy, intelligent) and then assigns them to groups based on how delayed therapist contact is, mimicking the time lapse that between Earth and astronauts while on long-duration Space flights with some delays up to 44 minutes, similar to what would be expected for a Mars mission. This clinical trial will be the first time this technology will be tested among "astronaut-like" adults. The research will assess how effective such programs are with and without video or text-based messaging, when real-time and face-to-face psychological assistance is unavailable, mimicking constraints of long-term Spaceflight. This clinical trial is significant for the first time that "astronaut-like" adults are being used as test subjects for a mental health application.

In addition to clinical trials, there are a number of Earth technologies that are well-positioned as potential Space technologies. A brief overview, relation to Space missions, and transferrable insights are described in Table 18.1.

Innovative Space Technologies Translatable to Mental Health on Earth

There is a rich history of technologies developed for Space use being applied to Earthly matters. The value of Space technologies for global health is underscored by its recognition in global organizations such as the United Nation's Sustainable Development Goals [14]. For example, Space exploration relies heavily on satellite technology, and there are efforts to leverage this technology to study and forecast the trajectories of communicable and noncommunicable disease.

Specific to mental health, we organize translatable technologies from Space into two broad categories: (i) technologies derived from engineering advances (e.g., satellite communications, sensing devices) and (ii) technologies derived from medical advances (e.g., nutritional recommendations, chronotherapies, cognitive training).

Table 18.1 Earth Mental Health Technologies Translatable to Long-Duration Space Missions

Technology Type	Overview	Significance in Space Mental Health
Chronotherapies	Chronotherapy is a behavioral technique that incorporates interventions based on the body's natural cycles. The association of chronotherapy with circadian rhythms and light therapy has been known to researchers since a seminal paper in 1981 demonstrated the ability to treat delayed sleep phase insomnia with altered light schedules.	It has long been recognized that astronauts often struggle to obtain adequate sleep while in orbit. Since the International Space Station circles earth every 90 minutes, astronauts can experience up to 16 sunrises and sunsets per 24-hour window, resulting in an average sleep of 6 hours. Successful long-duration Space travel will necessitate improved astronaut sleep quality and quantity. NASA has developed novel light-emitting diodes (LEDs) that emit three types of light with each one tailored for a different purpose; one for daily work, one to promote alertness, and another to assist in sleep. The effects of these new LED lights on astronaut sleep will be recorded and published in the forthcoming Lighting Effects study. Underscoring the importance of sleep, a recent study also suggests that the use of melatonin in Space might help prevent bone loss in Space, in addition to its therapeutic effects on correcting circadian rhythm. And lastly, actigraphy may be an important tool to reliably document sleep as previous studies have shown that actigraphy via wrist worn accelerometers can help corroborate subjective sleep diaries.
Sensors and monitoring devices	Salience monitoring using electronic communication for emotional cues has been shown to be a feasible and reliable way of monitoring mental health markers. This allows for real time monitoring of changes in mental state that are detected automatically in real time, which can be communicated to base or to the astronaut. As such, sensors and monitoring devices hold promise for augmenting standard clinical diagnosis, and have particular relevance in the context of the extreme isolation settings of deep Space travel.	As Space missions become farther in distance, the paradigm of relatively direct and immediate communication with on-ground medical staff will be hindered by increasingly prolonged delays in message transmission with the Space crew growing increasingly isolated. Current estimates have predicted a 3–22 minute delay between Mars site and Earth control center. This poses an increased risk of delayed treatment and management suggestions for depression, anxiety and behavioral changes. To this end, the monitoring devices and vital sensors may be utilized to pick up nonverbal and physiological changes, respectively. In addition to informing medical teams on Earth, the information can also be transferred laterally to other astronauts to watch out for each other.

Table 18.1 Continued

Technology Type	Overview	Significance in Space Mental Health
Nutritional mental health	Nutritional Mental Health offers promise as a nonpharmacological treatment approach. There is a large body of evidence suggesting that the quality of individuals' diets is related to their risk for common mental disorders, such as depression. Moreover, new intervention studies implementing dietary changes suggest promise for the prevention and treatment of depression.	Nutrition has numerous roles during Spaceflight including providing metabolic needs to optimizing physiological functions to counteract negative effects of Spaceflight can include radiation, immune deficits, oxidative stress, and bone and muscle loss. As missions increase in duration, any dietary/nutritional deficiencies will be amplified. Adequate nourishment is also vital toward an astronaut's mental function during long Space travel and has been extensively reviewed. Beyond the direct nutritional benefits, the meal itself has been cited as one of the primary conduits for strengthening team relationships.
Physical activity and health	Physical activity has long been recognized to be correlated to mental health with even 20–40 minutes of exercise showing improvement over depressive symptoms.	The importance of physical activity on long-duration Space missions is primarily 2-fold: (i) muscle and aerobic fitness and (ii) mental health benefits. With regards to mental health, exercising has been identified as an important factor in helping astronauts adjust to Space. The benefits of exercise toward anxiety are also valuable given the high stress environment and mental strain placed on the astronauts, all while in isolation.
Voicebot conversational agents	Voicebot agents are defined as software applications that respond to users with natural language, often with the goal of helping a user complete a task such as Apple's Siri, Amazon's Alexa, Samsung's S Voice, and Microsoft's Cortana. Importantly, conversational agents are being used to deliver mental health information in some instances such as the Woebot, 7Cups, and Koko and have been demonstrated to be efficacious and reducing depressive symptoms. However, a criticism of their use is their inability to display empathy and acceptability.	In long Space missions, voicebots are a promising tool to provide instructional guidance and feedback to astronauts that utilizes audio channels. This may be a refreshing change from the immense amount of screen time and readings that an astronaut must interpret and thus, provide some visual relief. All this together may be important in reducing the mental health stressors in Space. Moreover, voicebots may potential be integrated with sensing devices and help provide suggestions to astronauts on how to manage their mental health. And lastly, in Space, the sheer length of time and duration a voicebot may have with a single crew member offers a unique environment in which to adapt and truly learn a crew member's nonverbal cues—an opportunity not necessarily present at Earth where continuity of a single voice bot is relatively rare. That said, research done specific on Earth can continue to provide the necessary improvements to refine the voicebots.

(continued)

Table 18.1 Continued

Technology Type	Overview	Significance in Space Mental Health
Automated psychiatric screenings tools	While traditional psychiatric screening tools (e.g., Montreal cognitive assessment, mental state exam), require a clinician to be physically present, there are options being researched that employ a more automated approach. For example, an analytic approach using voice prosody was studied to assess major depressive disorder (MDD) severity and found to be able to detect symptom changes. There have also been studies evaluating whether subtle nonverbal cues of psychiatric illness can be captured using audiovisual devices and running diagnostic algorithms on them.	The challenge in Space is regular assessments with the convenience of in-person physicals. To this end, automated tools using actigraphy, salience detection of verbal communication, biometrics and audiovisual inputs are a promising approaches. If developed successfully, these tools may provide the robust clinical diagnostic help needed to capture early signs of deteriorating mental health and warn crew members of mental health risks.
Biological diagnostic tools	Researchers have long known that there are underlying biological changes that occur in the pathophysiology of psychiatric disorders yet reliant biomarkers still remain elusive. There is ongoing research in this area including one study found that found the serum of MDD patients had an elevated count of a nine specific biomarkers, which was correlated with a diagnostic accuracy of 94%.	In the context of long Space travel, diagnostic biomarkers for psychiatric conditions would be a valuable tool as it allows for the ability to track trends and have the ability to monitor and compare prior measurements in a quantitative manner. The importance of an objective measurement is further emphasized in the absence of clinical in-person assessments. One important point to consider though are the physiological changes that occur in Space versus that on Earth. Recently, the year-long Space study between twins (one on Earth, one in Space) was conducted. Important biological and biochemical changes were observed when comparing the biological between the twins including changes in telomere length, body weight, serum metabolites, and immune response networks. Thus, it is important to keep in mind that any biological diagnostic tool developed on Earth, may need a different set of guidelines in Space.

Table 18.1 Continued

Technology Type	Overview	Significance in Space Mental Health
Pharmaco-genetic guidance	Psychiatric pharmacogenetics tools assess genetic factors that influence individual variability in combinations of genes involved in pharmacokinetic (i.e., the effect that the body has on a drug) and pharmacodynamic (i.e., the effect that a drug has on the body) reactions. To date, seven commercial tests have published studies examining clinical usefulness, including the ABCB1 test, CNSDose, GeneSight, Genecept, NeuroIDgenetix, Neuropharmagen, and Pathway Genomics. Five commercial pharmacogenetic tools have been evaluated in randomized controlled trials in participants with MDD, all of which were industry-sponsored and there is preliminary evidence that pharmacogenetic-guided therapy improves response and remission rates in MDD.	There is significant potential for pharmacogenetic decision support tools to be utilized in prolonged Spaceflight. The goal of these tools is to optimize recovery time for astronauts and minimize side effects associated with these medications. The formulary on Space Shuttle flights included anti-anxiety medications, such as diazepam; antipsychotic medications, such as haloperidol; pain medications, such as codeine and morphine; medications for sleep, such as flurazepam and temazepam; stimulants, such as dextroamphetamine; and promethazine for Space motion sickness—all of which are known to have significant adverse effects. Traditionally, medications are ground-tested to determine if the pilot or astronaut will experience adverse effects that could result in the inability to pilot the craft. With pharmacogenetic decision support, the formulary may be even further refined to include medications that are likely to have the greatest clinical impact with the least amount of adverse effects.

Tables 18.2 and 18.3 outline these categories of technology respectively and provide an overview as well the significance they hold to mental health on Earth.

The Mars Mental Health Model: Bidirectional Technology Transfer at the Intersection of the Mars Mission and Global Mental Health

To tie in all the potential opportunities of cross-pollination for technologies between Earth mental health and long-duration Space travel mental health, we propose a bidirectional model for technology transfer (Figure 18.1).

Table 18.2 Fundamental Space Engineering and Physics Advances Translatable to Earth Mental Health

Technology Type	Overview	Significance to Earth Mental Health
Noninvasive and remote sensing devices	Remote sensing refers to data collection at distance, usually from a satellite or an aircraft, as opposed to on-site sensing. The electromagnetic radiation may be the reflection of an external source of energy (usually the sun) or of a source of energy carried by the satellite or aircraft itself. Examples of parameters that can be derived from Space via remote sensing include land temperature, humidity, air pollutants, and population density.	The ability to track our environmental health using satellite imagery and remote Space sensing devices can have important implications to global mental health given the ties of environmental green exposure to psychiatric disorders. Indeed, one recent study investigated the association between residential green exposure and prevalence of major depressive disorders and found a protective effect of greenness on depression. Lavretsky also describes the need to be aware of our environment as it relates to mental health: "The acceleration of profoundly stressful global natural disasters and growing urbanization with the negative impacts on mental and physical health force clinicians, researchers, and general public alike to become more aware of our deep connection to and dependence on our planet" (p. 2). Thus, remote sensing from Space on environmental cues can provide important data toward the effort to reduce global mental burden.
Global navigation satellite systems (GNSS)	GNSS describes satellite navigation systems that provide geospatial positioning with global coverage. GNSSs are most commonly used on Earth to determine one's position.	Geospatial activity may be a useful metric for the detection and tracking of mental health disorders. A recent study examined whether the information captured with multi-modal smartphone sensors could serve as behavioral markers for one's mental health. A total of 47 young adults were provided with smartphones embedded with a range of sensors and software that enabled continuous tracking of their geospatial activity (using GPS and WiFi), kinesthetic activity (using multi-axial accelerometers), sleep duration (modeled using device use data, accelerometer inferences, ambient sound features, and ambient light levels), and time spent proximal to human speech (i.e., speech duration using microphone and speech detection algorithms). The study found most of the metrics tracked including sleep duration, activity, and time spent with human speech proximity were all strongly associated with clinical manifestations of stress symptoms. Thus, the study suggests that geospatial tracking through smartphones may potentially be used to monitor behavioral indicators of mental health.

Table 18.2 Continued

Technology Type	Overview	Significance to Earth Mental Health
Satellite communications	Satellite communication is the technology detailing the transfer of information via orbiting satellites in orbit around earth.	Utilizing Space satellite communications is important in telemedicine for mental health as this is an important tool for patients where psychotherapy and psychiatrist contact is necessary for care, but an in-person meeting may not be possible, which can be particularly relevant in rural settings.

In this model, the aim is to provide a framework for which to identify relevant technologies toward mental health in one area that might benefit another, which, in our case, refers to Earth and Space. By fostering an open exchange of ideas and technology, we hope that mental health outcomes will improve in both sectors—Earth and Space. To further describe this model, we provide specific recommendations, discussed next. Recommendations for Developing the Bidirectional Technology Transfer Model of Mental Health Between Earth and Space

Establish Initiatives to Facilitate Earth Mental Health Technologies Into the Space Market
Conventional research has a notorious reputation of moving slow and being a tedious process whereas industrial innovation is recognized to move faster. However, to encourage cross-pollination of Earth health technologies toward Space applications, Earth health technologies need to accelerate their processes to match the industrial pace of Space development. Fortunately, there are a number of initiatives heading this direction.

Founded in 1997, the National Space Biomedical Research Institute (NSBRI) is a research organization that collaborates with NASA as well as over 70 agencies and universities. Their aim is to develop novel approaches to address Space health-related problems including mental health and psychosocial challenges that are unique to long-duration Space missions [15]. Notable developments arising from the NSBRI that were accelerated into the Space applications include ultrasound therapy for back pain [16] and devices to monitor CSF pressure as a marker for brain health [17].

Another example is the Translational Research Institute for Space Health (TRISH) based at Baylor College of Medicine. They are notable for the TRISH Launch Pad program, which targets companies entering the Space medicine industry and provides a 10-week intensive training program to give them the skills needed to sustain their companies in the field [18]. By doing so, TRISH Launch Pad positions companies in an ideal position to accelerate their technologies from Earth to Space applications.

Table 18.3 Space Medicine Advances Translatable to Earth Mental Health

Technology Type	Overview	Significance to Earth Mental Health
Virtual conflict resolution and depression devices	Given the social and psychological problems encountered on long Space missions, researchers are working on novel solutions by using a Virtual Space Station interface. This type of therapy involves a computer helping the user achieve conflict resolution and develop steps to achieve them. The Virtual Space Station is also equipped with a tool specialized for role-playing interpersonal to help simulate scenarios.	Insights from astronauts utilizing virtual conflict devices can be translated to help create new technology specific to these fields on Earth in addition to those who lack in-person capabilities for psychiatric treatment.
Nutritional advances	A recent review on nutritional and metabolism priorities for human exploration of Space suggested there could be major benefits of Space research on Earth. The suggestion is that being able to manage energy balance for an astronaut requires completing the development of an accurate system for nutritional status monitoring in Space. This may be of tremendous interest to multiple groups on the ground, ranging from the military to the physicians working with obese patients and hospital doctors dealing with patients with nutritional issues.	The importance of cross-talk between Earth and Space nutrition research has been recognized with the formation of a dedicated nutrition group within THESEUS—an international consortium of experts who aim to gain insight by Space and Earth research in tandem. Studies in Space would further require very accurate and reliable approaches to assess nutrition in a minimal resource setting and the technologies used to achieve such precise measurements could certainly find use on Earth.
Case Example: "The 33" Chilean Miners	In 2010, the NASA Engineering and Safety Center came to the aid of 33 miners trapped for more than two months under the stone walls of a Chilean copper mind. NASA's initial support for "The 33" included recommendations on medical care, nutrition, and psychological support which was advice was based on expertise developed from working with the International Space Station.	Guidance offered by NASA's Engineering and Safety Center to "The 33" Chilean Miners and Chilean officials: 1. Recommending methods for replacing Vitamin D since the miners, much like astronauts confined to a Space station, were without direct sunlight. 2. Encouraging moderate exercise to increase the miners' muscle contractility and help prepare their bodies for the stress of the rescue mission.

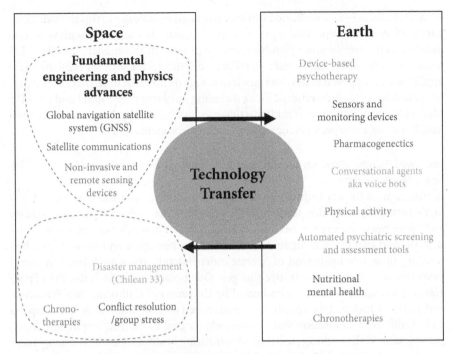

Figure 18.1 A bidirectional model for technology transfer between Space technology for Mars mission (L box) and Earth technology (R box) to improve mental health outcomes. The middle "Technology Transfer" icon represents the various avenues and approaches for facilitating this transfer (see the section The Mars Mental Health Model).

Adapted from Chang, et al. *Promoting Tech Transfer Between Space and Global Mental Health*. Aerosp Med Hum Perform, 2020 Sep 1. *91*(9): p. 737–745. doi:10.3357/AMHP.5589.2020

Establish Initiatives to Facilitate Space Technologies Into the Earth Mental Health Market

One of the difficulties of each Space mission is the huge amounts of primary data to sift through which is a barrier that must be overcome before extrapolating that data to other applications. Given that NASA is the primary effort for Space exploration in the United States, it perhaps comes as no surprise that they are also spearheading the effort to extrapolate their data toward Earth mental health applications. Notably, NASA Spinoff is a catalogue of Space technologies that are being applied toward Earth. Similarly, the NSBRI has also developed technologies from Space to the Earth applications including an ultrasound treatment to resolve nephrolithiasis.

Bidirectional Training Programs

Currently, there is no formal training program with the specific objective of developing a bidirectional mindset and skill set for technology transfer between Space and Earth mental health focuses. Such a formal training program would benefit the field as there would now be a dedicated workforce trained specifically in this multidisciplinary field. Another important aspect that this program should aim to achieve is train individuals to identify other possible technologies that fit this model. The latter skill would be useful as it is much easier to tailor an existing technology for Earth or Space applications as opposed to developing a technology de novo. Of note, there are conferences that have this bidirectional focus including one hosted by TRISH and the MIT Media Lab Space Exploration Initiative that specifically aimed to "optimize behavioral health and cognitive performance in confined environments" [19].

Improve Dialogue Between Mental Health Technology Innovators and
Space Medicine Experts
A critical piece for any technology transfer model is open communication and dialogue between key opinion leaders and field experts. As such, mental health leaders and Space medicine experts necessarily need to foster a healthy, communicative relationship to effectively facilitate the transfer of technologies and ideas. While historically, these two fields tend to operate independently, there are forums in recent years that are attempting to bridge this gap. One notable example is the 2019 Space Health Innovation Conference co-hosted by University of California, San Francisco, and TRISH, which had the specific aim to convene a diverse audience of Space experts and Health Tech Innovation stakeholders with a goal to inform, inspire and invite participation in the exciting challenge of optimizing health and medical management in Space environments. Developing future forums and similar collaborative environments will help promote the dialogue to enable this bidirectional technology transfer.

Track Outcomes
Lastly, the success of any initiative is only as good as the metrics and objectives defined beforehand. Too many cross-disciplinary efforts begin with good intentions only to fall short because their objectives and aims are not clearly defined. As such, it is important that what is considered success for this bidirectional technology transfer model is defined clearly and beforehand. However, this model faces a unique challenge inherent to working with Space medicine, namely, the infrequent Space missions relative to the pace of studies on Earth. For instance, a study on the efficacy of a technology proposed to improve mental health stressors could be completed in a span of months on earth. However, a Space mission to measure the same outcomes would be the order of years. Thus, milestones and check points must be put in place to ensure that even though the pace is different, both Earth and Space efforts are in tune with each other.

Conclusion

Mental health continues to emerge as one of the most highly discussed challenges both on Earth and in long-duration Space travel. Converging the technologies that benefit mental health in both environments can potentially allow for a synergistic and bidirectional relationship with the ultimate result of improved mental health outcomes in both environments.

Conflict of Interest

HE owns shares in CNSdose Pty Ltd. RA has consulted for CNSdose Pty Ltd. No other authors note conflict of interest.

References

1. Aleksandrovskiy, Y. and M. Novikov, Psychological prophylaxis and treatments for Space crews, in *Space Biology and Medicine III: Humans in Spaceflight. Book 2.*, A. Nicogossian et al., Editors. Reston, VA: American Institute of Aeronautics and Astronautics, 1996: p. 433–444. https://doi.org/10.1016/j.neuron.2014.10.018
2. Baisden, D. L., et al., *Human health and performance for long-duration Spaceflight.* Aviat Space Environ Med, 2008. *79*(6): p. 629–635.
3. Ball, J. R. and C. H. Evans, *Safe passage: Astronaut care for exploration missions.* Washington, DC: National Academies Press, 2001.
4. Kanas, N., et al., *Psychology and culture during long-duration Space missions.* Acta Astronautica, 2009. *64*(7–8): p. 659–677 https://doi.org/10.1016/j.actaastro.2008.12.005.
5. Kanas, N. and D. Manzey, *Space psychology and psychiatry.* El Segundo, Calif. Microcosm Press, 2008.
6. Vigo, D., G. Thornicroft, and R. Atun, *Estimating the true global burden of mental illness.* Lancet Psychiatry, 2016. *3*(2): p. 171–178 https://doi.org/10.1016/s2215-0366(15)00505-2.
7. Patel, V., et al., *The Lancet Commission on global mental health and sustainable development.* Lancet, 2018. *392*(10157): p. 1553–1598 https://doi.org/10.1016/s0140-6736(18)32270-0.
8. Vico, L. and A. Hargens, *Skeletal changes during and after Spaceflight.* Nat Rev Rheumatol, 2018. *14*(4): p. 229–245 https://doi.org/10.1038/nrrheum.2018.37.
9. Shen, M. and W. H. Frishman, *Effects of Spaceflight on cardiovascular physiology and health.* Cardiol Rev, 2019. *27*(3): p. 122–126 https://doi.org/10.1097/crd.0000000000000236.
10. Roberts, D. R., et al., *Effects of Spaceflight on Astronaut Brain Structure as indicated on MRI.* N Engl J Med, 2017. *377*(18): p. 1746–1753 https://doi.org/10.1056/nejmoa1705129.
11. Zhang, L. F. and A. R. Hargens, *Spaceflight-induced intracranial hypertension and visual impairment: pathophysiology and countermeasures.* Physiol Rev, 2018. *98*(1): p. 59–87 https://doi.org/10.1152/physrev.00017.2016.
12. Brem, C., et al., *Changes of brain DTI in healthy human subjects after 520 days isolation and confinement on a simulated mission to Mars.* Life Sci Space Res (Amst), 2020. *24*: p. 83–90 https://doi.org/10.1016/j.lssr.2019.09.004.
13. Garrett-Bakelman, F. E., et al., *The NASA Twins Study: a multidimensional analysis of a year-long human Spaceflight.* Science, 2019. *364*(6436) https://doi.org/10.1016/j.lssr.2019.09.004.
14. Dietrich, D., et al., *Applications of Space technologies to global health: scoping review.* J Med Internet Res, 2018. *20*(6): p. e230 https://doi.org/10.2196/jmir.9458.
15. NASA. National Space Biomedical Research Institute. [Home page]. June 20, 2019. Available from: https://www.nasa.gov/exploration/humanresearch/HRP_NASA/research_at_nasa_NSBRI.html

16. BioSpace.com. *National Space Biomedical Research Institute (NSBRI) Release: Clinical Study to Treat Lower Back Pain on Earth May Help Astronauts in Space.* August 13, 2014. Available from: https://www.bioSpace.com/article/releases/national-Space-biomedical-research-institute-nsbri-release-clinical-study-to-treat-lower-back-pain-on-earth-may-help-astronauts-in-Space-/.

17. BioSpace.com. *National Space Biomedical Research Institute (NSBRI) Funds Cerebrotech to Accelerate Development of Brain Monitoring Device.* March 13, 2013. Available from: https://www.biospace.com/article/releases/national-space-biomedical-research-institute-nsbri-funds-b-cerebrotech-b-to-accelerate-development-of-brain-monitoring-device-/.

18. Translational Research Institute for Space Health. *TRISH Launch Pad.* [Home page]. Available from: https://colab.secure-platform.com/a/page/TRISH-home. Accessed August 27, 2019.

19. Translational Research Institute for Space Health. *Spaces in Space: optimizing behavioral health & cognitive performance in confined environments.* February 6–7, 2019. Available from: https://www.media.mit.edu/events/space-workshop/.

19
Innovation Diplomacy in the Clinical Neurosciences

Kylie Ternes, Walter Dawson, and Harris A. Eyre

Health diplomacy is based on negotiations that influence the policy environment for global health by leveraging the disciplines of global health, international affairs, management, law, and economics.[1-3] Health diplomacy uses conventional approaches to optimize global health by working to strengthen healthcare systems and leveraging public and not-for-profit sectors. It is an important means of exercising large-scale reform due to its ability to have cultural and economic impact on multiple nations. Health diplomacy has made numerous important contributions to solving global healthcare crises in the past, including the President's Emergency Plan for AIDS Relief, projects addressing Ebola and Zika viruses, the concerning rise of antimicrobial resistance, and the Sustainable Development Goals aiming to impact chronic disease deaths.[4,5]

Clinical neuroscience is a branch of neuroscience that focuses on the scientific study of fundamental pathophysiological mechanisms that underlie diseases and disorders of the brain and central nervous system. It seeks to develop new ways of understanding, diagnosing, and treating such disorders. For the purposes of this book, we will focus on brain health disorders (i.e., dementias and geriatric neurocognitive disorders) as the primary clinical neuroscience disorders.

The population of people with neurologic and psychiatric illness (i.e., depression, dementia and geriatric cognitive disorders) is increasing rapidly around the world. Current estimates of the global societal and economic cost of these disorders is approximately US$ 1 trillion per year.[6,7] Not only is the rate of dementia growing, but the related disease's associated economic burden are as well.[7,8] Advanced age remains one of the most important primary risk factors for developing dementia. In the coming decades, experts believe the rising numbers of aging populations will occur most rapidly in low- and middle-income countries (LMICs), and therefore these countries will disproportionately shoulder the burden of dementia.[9-11] Incidence of dementia is driven largely by the same social determinants of health that drive other major health problems that are rooted in socioeconomic inequities such as low educational attainment, poor diet, less access to healthcare, inadequate treatment of hypertension, and other medical diseases.[9,12,13] An alarmingly small number of countries have developed a plan to combat this rise in dementia, and dementia still is often assumed to be a normal part of aging leading to its underrecognition and underdiagnosis.[9,12,14]

Epidemiological modeling has projected that a population-level approach to dementia risk reduction could prevent up to 30% of dementia cases around the world in the next 20 years.[15] Additionally, individual-level factors such as healthcare access and personal beliefs about neurological and psychiatric health can have a significant impact on health and wellbeing. On a larger scale population-based level, social determinants such as air pollution and mass migration due to fleeing conflicts can affect disease course by either hastening disease onset[16] or preventing access to care,[17] respectively. Current global factors that may be exacerbating brain health disorders include climate change, air pollution, large-scale war and conflicts and associated refugee migration, food insecurity, and lost productivity due to communicable and noncommunicable health conditions (for reviews, see Livingston et al[12]; Ledoux, Pilot, Diaz and, Krafft[17]; Jung, Lin, and Hwang[18]; Carey et al[19]; Chen et al[20]; Killin, Starr, Shiue, and Russ[21]; and Wei et al.[22] Given the breadth of factors that affect neurological health, large-scale diplomatic activity is necessary to improve such societal conditions. These activities will help to coordinate and enhance projects in research, advocacy, clinical care, and public health across the globe spanning both high-income and low-income countries.

We propose these traditional health diplomacy approaches to clinical neuroscience should be referred to as "clinical neuroscience diplomacy." We suggest a version of clinical neuroscience diplomacy that aims to influence the global policy environment for clinical neuroscience disorders by leveraging the disciplines of global health, international affairs, management, law, and economics.

While the current field of clinical neuroscience diplomacy is valuable as it is, it is not likely to make a large enough impact on global clinical brain health outcomes. In its current state, clinical neuroscience diplomacy specifically does not adequately consider the growing importance of technological innovation and entrepreneurship, as these may augment the impact of more conventional clinical neuroscience diplomacy mechanisms. With increasing technological ubiquity, decreasing costs of production, and speed of innovation, the impact of technology on society is arguably more visible now than ever. This is evidenced by the European Union establishing the Digital Health Society,[23] an open multi-stakeholder conglomerate of member states, regional governments, healthcare providers, industry, research organizations, and advocacy groups with the goal of exchanging knowledge, experiences and best practices and to accelerate research, innovation, and novel solutions. It is clear that with the rapidity of recent and future technological innovation, it will be paramount to recognize how these changes and movements can be adapted for the future of clinical neuroscience diplomacy.

A novel model of clinical neuroscience innovation diplomacy (CNID) is proposed in this chapter. This model of CNID is adapted from a recently proposed model of brain health innovation diplomacy.[24] CNID aims to improve global clinical neuroscience outcomes by leveraging technological innovation, entrepreneurship, and innovation diplomacy. CNID will broaden the scope of health diplomacy by bringing together the disciplines of clinical neuroscience, brain health, health diplomacy, and science diplomacy with the emerging disciplines of precision medicine, digital health, convergence science, innovation diplomacy (aka iDiplomacy), technology diplomacy (aka techplomacy) and consumer participation.[9,25–34] Each of these disciplines provides critical input to the field of CNID, but none alone are sufficient.

The Role of Technology and Innovation in Global Health, Clinical Neurosciences, and Aging

If a model of CNID aims to emphasize the promise and mitigate the dangers of technological advancements in the realm of clinical neuroscience, it is important to first review the role technology and innovation in this context.

Innovation Ecosystems Influencing Global Health

There are a number of examples of new health technologies that have been adapted to address the needs of neglected global disease and health conditions.[35,36] These specific innovations and innovation ecosystems that arise as a result of this repurposed technology are important frameworks to build upon when creating a novel model of health diplomacy. One example is the use of low-cost tablet computers like Aakash, which was developed by Datawind and the Government of India and sold to Indian university students for US$35 with the intention of reaching rural communities via e-learning.[35] Another useful platform created specifically for brain health innovation is the newly established Global Health Technologies Coalition (GHTC).[37] GHTC is an advocacy organization funded by the Bill and Melinda Gates Foundation, focusing on global health research and development for new tools and technologies. It is a coalition of more than 25 nonprofit organizations, academic institutions, and aligned businesses advancing policies to accelerate the creation of new vaccines, drugs, diagnostics, and other tools. The GHTC educates policymakers and stakeholders and convenes members to facilitate innovation and advocacy for policy solutions and investment to spur innovation.

Innovation in Aging and Clinical Neuroscience

A 2019 report from the Task Force on Research and Development for Technology to Support Aging Adults, White House National Science and Technology Council[38] convened U.S. federal government experts to identify emerging technologies to meet the needs of older adults. The report identified "a range of emerging technologies that have significant potential to assist older adults with successfully aging in place, each categorized by their role in supporting a set of primary capabilities."[38p2] These emerging technology areas included nutrition, hygiene, medication management, cognition, financial security, hearing, and telehealth. The report then provided recommendations as a guide for research and development. One possible method of reducing the issue of polypharmacy is pharmacogenetic-based clinical decision support tools. Polypharmacy is a risk factor for hospitalizations and unnecessary emergency department visits, and thus reducing the overall number of medications that individuals, specifically the elderly, take on a regular basis could therefore reduce these types of hospital admissions.[39,40]

Clinical Neuroscience Health Innovation in Action: Trends and Key Examples

There are several areas of value for clinical neuroscience technologies.[41] A recent review published by members of the U.S. Alzheimer's Association Technology Professional Interest Area included three broad categories of useful technologies[42]:

1. *Dementia risk reduction technologies*: Technology that can be used to address lifestyle-based dementia risk reduction factors.[43] For example, a recent meta-analysis of web-based multidomain lifestyle programs for brain health demonstrated these programs can positively influence brain health outcomes.[44]
2. *Remote monitoring and care for individuals with dementia*: Technologies such as apps, wearables, and smart home systems could allow clinicians to remotely monitor patients and support maintenance of cognitive, social, and physical functioning.
3. *Technology for dementia caregivers*: An example is the Supporting Family Caregivers with Technology for Dementia Home Care (FamTechCare) intervention.[45] This intervention provides individualized dementia care strategies to in-home caregivers based on video recordings that the caregiver creates of complex and challenging care situations.[45] A team of dementia care experts review videos submitted by caregivers and provide interventions to improve care for the experimental group.

A recent dementia technology report from Britain included additional health economic analysis and revealed dementia technology would be cost-effective from both a health and social care perspective in two core scenarios: postponing nursing home admission by at least three months and reducing unpaid care hours by about 8% or improved carer quality of life by 0.06 to 0.08 quality-adjusted life years per year.[46]

Investment into the clinical neuroscience health innovation industry is increasing,[47] yet some technology may be advancing without clear theoretical frameworks, ethical and privacy considerations, or proof of concept. This is not to say that technology should not be part of the solution, but rather development and scaling should proceed with caution.

Effects of Computer and Internet Use on Brain Health

Internet access has been designated a human right by the United Nations.[48] Access to broadband internet has significant potential impacts on the brain health of aging adults. However, increasing rates of cybercrime and digital exploitation has come with the rising rates of older adults using the internet.[49]

Internet utilization and access amongst older adults is greatly affected by education, income level, geography, and other social determinants.[50] Older populations with high disease burdens living in rural areas are particularly at-risk of lacking reliable internet access. The U.S. Federal Communications Commission tracks broadband access and prevalence of chronic health conditions such as diabetes and obesity.[51] Geo-mapping these overlapping characteristics demonstrates a stark inequality. A lack of internet access—particularly broadband internet—undermines the platform needed to run and access new technological innovations, which in turn limits the opportunity to receive care, support, and education that these innovations offer. Ensuring internet access is widely accessible to all persons as they age is a key step in promoting health innovation and health equity.

Internet use has a number of recognized brain health benefits, including reducing depression, increased health literacy, and increased social engagement, particularly in advanced age.[52,53] Previously, older adults who regularly used computers were often white and had higher levels of education and income. However, those demographics are changing. A recent study examining the effects of computer use in older adults in and out of the home (e.g., libraries, friend's homes) found that those who access computers from social resources were more likely to report higher self-efficacy and better self-reported health.[53] Compared to occasional or never-users, regular computer users also reported higher self-efficacy, indicating that computer and internet access are associated with more positive views of self by older adults.[54]

Internet assessment of brain health and disease is also growing. The Brain Health Registry uses online strategies to assess cognitive function and refer potential participants to clinical trials.[55] The Alzheimer Prevention Trial web study uses similar approaches to online assessment with the goal of referring cognitively normal persons to clinical trials for the prevention of Alzheimer's disease. The Cleveland Clinic's Healthy Brains website (healthbrains.org) provides its Brain Heath Index based on six pillars of brain health to guide users to more brain-healthy lifestyles.[56]

Social Media and the Aging Brain

Some studies suggest social media platforms may have a positive effect by promoting interpersonal connectedness[57] while many others show that loneliness and social isolation can negatively impact overall health in older adults.[58] Social media platforms such as Facebook and Twitter are known to enhance social connectedness, and a recent Pew Research report showed that about one-third of all adults over age 65 reported using them.[59] Given the established relationship between the frequency of supportive social interactions and the delayed onset of cognitive decline, there are hypotheses that social media may be protective against some forms of dementia,[60] although reverse causation may be occurring. A 2018 waitlist control trial demonstrated that teaching older adults to use social media improved their executive functioning significantly as measured by their inhibitory control and improved their overall cognition as measured by the Mini-Mental State Examination compared to controls. These data suggest that social media may have impacts on brain health beyond those of social and emotional connection.[61]

Alternatively, social media may also have adverse effects on older adults. Lonely adults have a more difficult time maintaining vigilance and self-regulating and demonstrate a heightened awareness of social threats, as well as paying greater attention to negative social stimuli.[54,62] This broad constellation of behaviors likely predisposes older, lonely adults to gravitate toward information on social media that mirrors their own world view, a trend amplified further by the algorithms of social media platforms that are constructed to keep users on the platforms for as long as possible. These ideas could explain recent reports showing that individuals over age 65 are seven times more likely to share and disseminate fake news domains on social media than their younger counterparts.[63] These results are particularly concerning given the increased numbers of aging adults on social media and the fact that political and policy decisions are now often shaped by information publicly available on these platforms. Furthermore, other findings suggest that "memory and other cognitive domains deteriorate in some elders in a way that particularly undermines resistance to 'illusions of truth' and other effects related to belief persistence and the availability heuristic, especially in relation to source cues."[64,65] The severity of these issues would hypothetically increase with the prevalence of misinformation and the complexity of the information. This wealth of data demonstrates the overwhelming interest in social media as an influential technological tool of our society and its potential positive and negative effects. More research and monitoring are needed to strike an optimal balance, however the difficulty of balancing protected free speech and protection from negative effects of social media is an ongoing debate.

Finally, the role of social media in optimizing sociability is a nuanced one. A 2018 review[66] suggests social media can influence sociability in three core ways depending on whether it allows for a deeper understanding of peoples thoughts and feelings. The suggestion is that social media "a) benefits sociability when it compliments already deep offline engagement with others, b) impairs sociability when it supplants deeper offline engagement for superficial online engagement and c) enhanced sociability when deep offline engagement is otherwise difficult to attain."[66p473] Clearly further exploration of this issue is needed.

Ethical Considerations of Technological Innovation

New and potentially valuable technologies targeted toward improving the lives of either patients or caregivers include memory and communication aids, global positioning satellites (GPS) tracking devices, "smart home" technologies, and even companion robots.[67-69] Although these technologies were developed with positive intentions, it is important to recognize the fact that the ethical implications of such technologies are only just beginning to be studied. Many assistive technologies were developed as a response to the traditionally restrictive means of dementia care (i.e., physical restraints, medication); however, these technologies may implement new and unprecedented levels of surveillance, privacy limitation, and movement restriction.[70] Very little consideration has been given to how these technologies should be regulated to be in compliance with human rights obligations or how they should be incorporated into advance care planning while an individual may still retain their decision-making capacity.[70] Even the use of care or companion robots have ethical considerations, as some have argued these robots may eventually devalue care and reduce person-to-person contact with older adults, which would restrict rather than enhance social interaction.[71] Furthermore, there are philosophical, ethical, and policy considerations that have gone previously unexplored when developing assistive technologies for those with dementia[72] such as, How can we balance the need for safety and monitoring against the potential feelings of objectification and lack of control? Is there an element of deception and infantilization created in addition to the loss of privacy and personal liberties when technology is responsible for caring and monitoring a human? Are there circumstances under which a person living with dementia should be able to control their own devices?

With middle-aged and older adults being among the fastest growing demographics creating social media profiles, ethical issues will undoubtedly arise in concurrence with the pending dementia epidemic.[73] Although older adults may be registering for profiles while they still have capacity to accept the terms and conditions of a social media account, what happens if they develop a neurocognitive disorder and can no longer understand the implications of their digital footprint?[73] How can we support digital autonomy while also protecting privacy? Clearly, there is a need to develop and integrate emerging ethicolegal frameworks into new technologies and innovation diplomacy to protect and promote neurological health in the most vulnerable populations.

Introducing the Clinical Neuroscience Innovation Diplomacy Model

CNID aims to improve global neurological health outcomes by leveraging innovation in technological, entrepreneurship, and diplomacy spheres while simultaneously recognizing the significant role that technology, entrepreneurship and digitization will play in the future of brain health on micro and macro scales. The goal of CNID includes highlighting the positive role of novel solutions and mitigating the potential and actual risks of digital platforms. The CNID model also acknowledges the economic, cultural, and political influences that clinical neuroscience technological innovation and entrepreneurship has, and will continue to have, in the 21st century.

As recognition of the economic and productivity impact of neurocognitive disorders increases, greater economic influence will come from direct investment into brain and mental health-related technologies. Cultural influences may similarly develop as CNID advocates for improved healthcare equity, destigmatization, access to care, and socioeconomic inclusion for people with neurological disorders. In the same vein, it is possible that further awareness and education around brain health may reduce human rights violations (e.g., force restraints, physical and sexual violence, and torture) that can be found in in community or institutional settings in LMICs or high-income countries. It is imperative that the private sector increase engagement, which would therefore allow for greater trade and investment linkages for global clinical neuroscience innovation and avenues for cross-cultural understanding. Ultimately, with this model, it is likely that these linkages will foster further innovation and investment and allow brain healthcare to be scaled up.

Clinical Neuroscience Diplomacy and Traditional Disciplines

Clinical neuroscience health diplomacy draws strengths from health diplomacy, science diplomacy, and global brain health. Each are summarized next with descriptions of frameworks for developing future practitioners in these fields.

Health Diplomacy
The field of health diplomacy fuses the disciplines of public health, international affairs, economics, management and law, with a particular focus on negotiations that impact the global public health policy.[26] Health diplomacy has been formally categorized in three broad levels: core, multi-stakeholder, and informal.[74,75] Each level has varying tools, roles, actors, and levels of accreditation. Core health diplomacy practitioners are officially accredited "health attachés" who connect public health organizations in one government to public health and related organizations in another (e.g., departments of innovation, industry, science, aging, trade and investment, and social services). Health attachés require formal credentialing, which typically involves obtaining agreements between representative state foreign affairs ministries. Multi-stakeholder health diplomacy practitioners include multilateral representatives and government employees. Informal health diplomacy includes host country officials as well as a wide array of other stakeholders including nongovernmental organizations, universities, private enterprises, and, ultimately, the general public.

Science Diplomacy
Science diplomacy is a field that uses science as an instrument and method of communication to achieve foreign policy objectives that aims to promote peace, ethical research, and sustainable development.[25] In 2008, the American Association for the Advancement of Science established the Center for Science Diplomacy, which became a major source for further capacity building for science diplomacy.[76] The Center excels as a leader in positioning science diplomacy as a key element of science and international affairs in the 21st century. The Center has strengthened connections between the scientific and diplomatic communities and developed the framework to support and train the future of science diplomacy. Perhaps its most significant contribution has been its ability to illustrate how science can strengthen relationships between countries amidst global geopolitical conflict.

Global Neurologic Health
The goals of global neurologic or brain health is ultimately to protect the world's aging populations from risks and threats to brain health such as dementia and stroke.[9,27] To do so, the field aims to strengthen collaborations in developing preventions and therapies, share knowledge, and advocate for all of the major neurodegenerative disorders of late life.

In 2019, the American Association of Retired Persons established the Global Council on Brain Health. The Council was created to be an independent collaborative resource to provide up-to-date information on how individuals can maintain and improve their neurologic health as they age.[27]

Clinical Neuroscience Innovation Diplomacy and Emerging Disciplines

With the growth of technological innovation and entrepreneurship in clinical neuroscience, it is imperative to incorporate emerging disciplines into standard working models. An overview of these emerging disciplines is presented next.

Digital Health

Digital health describes a field that leverages digital technologies as tools for optimizing screening, diagnostic, treatment, and prevention of health disorders.[77] Digital health solutions can be used alone or in conjunction with pharmaceuticals, biologics, or other products. Digital health is well positioned to facilitate patient and healthcare provider empowerment by connecting each with useful data and can be used in public health/epidemiological projects. Digital biomarkers, or "digitomics" can be used in parallel with other biological, environmental and lifestyle factors to illuminate novel insights into disease course and treatment.

Precision Medicine

In recent years, the fields of clinical neurosciences have been transformed by embracing precision medicine and systems biology. Utilizing such models has helped to create novel therapeutic solutions for proteinopathies, neurodegenerative disease (such as Alzheimer's disease), protein misfolding disorders, and other dementias.[28] Precision medicine is based on the idea of targeted treatments to meet the specific needs of individuals based on technologies using multi-omics inputs from genomics, epigenomics, connectomics, lipidomics, proteomics, metabolomics, digitomics, and phenomics. These new treatments may include novel drug compounds, pharmacogenomic strategies or other diagnostic methods, such as new neuroimaging biomarkers.[28] This discipline is currently most relevant in high-income countries as opposed to LMICs but aims to be useful worldwide as LMICs social, economic, and healthcare systems improve.

Convergence Medicine

Convergence science in medicine involves leveraging transdisciplinary science to achieve improved outcomes for patients and healthcare systems. This concept necessitates a robust integration of scientists, clinicians, bioinformaticists, global health experts, engineers, technology entrepreneurs, medical educators, caregivers, and patients.[30,31]

Innovation Diplomacy

Innovation diplomacy describes the practice of using diplomacy to further innovation for a country, as well as the ability to leverage innovation to improve foreign relations among countries in bi-, multi-, or transnational setting.[32] Innovation diplomacy includes supporting partnerships with industry, academic, and nongovernmental organizations. Innovation diplomacy is built on the idea that supporting open innovation and collaboration will lead to more effective global value chains, intellectual property rights, ethical regulation, and use of technology, as well as developing, deploying, and scaling innovative solutions to global problems.[78]

Technology Diplomacy

Technology diplomacy acknowledges "the key role that technology and digitalization will play now and in the future for individuals and societies alike.d"[33] The "TechPlomacy Initiative", launched by the Danish government in 2017, suggests "technology will contribute to solving some of the most acute global challenges and bring about a positive transformation with enormous potential for people around the world."[33] In establishing this initiative, the Danish government established a "tech ambassador" office between Silicon Valley, Copenhagen, and Beijing with a mandate to rethink traditional diplomatic representation.[33] The tech ambassador is tasked with developing strategic partnerships with entrepreneurs and executives, tech ecosystems and hubs, biotechnology organizations, governments, international organizations, civil society, cities, regions, and universities. Relevant initiatives include security, cyber, biotechnology, development, export, and investment promotion. Opportunities and challenges arising with this technology agenda are then also addressed in relevant and complementary bi-, multi-, and transnational fora.

Complex Technological Issues Justifying Clinical Neuroscience Innovation Diplomacy

There are a range of complex technology-related issues that justify the need for and value of CNID. For example, a recent paper highlighted some of the key issues slowing the use of computing technology in aging populations.[79] Core issues noted were lack of appreciation for technology as a useful source of therapeutic benefits in aging, lack of evidence-based technologies and lack of sustaining investment in the field. The discipline of CNID will be uniquely positioned to understand and integrate these issues. Training practitioners in CNID will supply specific and essential knowledge to help optimize the effects of these various platforms on clinical neuroscience health.

Recommendations

To increase the value and sustainable practice of CNID, training and education should be developed and scaled up. The following recommendations to support the emergence and growth of this field are as follows:

Involve Consumers in Innovation Design, Research, Ethics, and Advocacy
Individuals, especially those at risk of developing neurodegenerative disorders, should be involved in research, advocacy, policy, clinical care, ethical discussions, and novel solution development. This idea is advocated for by Alzheimer Europe, an organization that has issued a specific position on patient and public involvement in the context of dementia research.[80] Novel solution development should prioritize

end-user needs as patients and caregivers can make valuable contributions to product design and testing. Current research practices can make validating new technologies prior to implementation difficult, however consumers are in a useful position to help expand research practices through research prioritization and resource advocacy. It is also important to involve the consumer and the patient when exploring models for joint clinical decision-making. Patients also have an invaluable perspective on ethical issues unique to innovative brain health technologies as both research subjects and the ultimate beneficiaries of new technologies.[38,81] The definition of who constitutes "patients" is continuing to evolve as the course of dementia is increasingly shown to begin decades prior to onset of cognitive decline, implying that interventions must similarly begin earlier in life and involve advocacy by healthy at-risk individuals.[82]

Create Clinical Neuroscience Innovation Diplomacy Training Opportunities
Educational and training opportunities are critical to developing the field of CNID. These opportunities must be tailored to be relevant to the various stakeholders in the model, including clinicians, policy makers, scientists, innovators, technology executives, philanthropists and diplomats. Examples of education and training opportunities could include incorporating innovation into school curricula, offering postgraduate fellowship opportunities in clinical neuroscience innovation for trainees in various disciplines, and creating certificate programs for current clinicians or researchers that are interested in pursuing leadership positions in the field. To optimally support a varied breadth of ideas and innovations, clinical neuroscience technological innovation and entrepreneurship engagements should occur across departments in universities. This should include departments of neurology, psychiatry, regulatory science, geriatrics, psychology, politics, sociology, public policy, public health schools, law schools, business schools, international studies programs, and design schools. It is critical to develop educational and training opportunities to create a sustainable and dynamic network of clinical neuroscience innovation diplomats.

Advance Global Policy Change via Clinical Neuroscience Innovation Diplomacy
To reach its full potential, CNID must engage with national and global policymakers. Building on the expertise of existing programs and partnerships, there is a clear opportunity to become the trusted resource for knowledge and expertise on all matters related to clinical neuroscience innovation to whom policymakers can turn to during decision-making processes. One possible approach to help facilitate this idea would be via a global forum where a consensus of policy ideas is agreed on, such as a white paper. Policymakers as well as intragovernmental organizations (such as the World Health Organization) should be invited to participate in this forum to maximize its efficacy. The translation of these consensus recommendations to policymakers is essential to implementation and success, and an active engagement of the CNID community is critical to this step. Actions of the community should include advocacy to address the issues identified within the consensus agreements and consensus building and stakeholder engagement so that a coalition of relevant stakeholders will support recommendations made. This requires a visible role within the policymaking process as experts, innovators, and advocates.

Develop Measurable Outcomes to Track

In developing the CNID model, it is critical to also have measurable outcomes to best to track the value and production of the model. It is important to consider the number of individuals and investigators trained in innovation diplomacy, but also where these investigators and their companies are located. It would be feasible and useful to track these numbers and also the countries where these innovative companies are head-quartered to ensure maximal global interest and diversity. Similarly, ecosystem scan-ning of accelerators and incubators should be performed to ensure support for clinical neuroscience companies. It will also be valuable to track the numbers of multina-tional projects initiated and completed in addition to the clinical tools developed and scaled into the market. Readership and utilization of guidelines for clinical neurosci-ence innovation and entrepreneurship can and should also be tracked as a measure of training future practitioners and leaders in the field. Finally, measuring contributions for funding foreign governments and/or foreign owned nonprofits and for-profit cor-porations dedicated to innovative clinical neuroscience diplomacy projects should also be encouraged.

Conclusions

CNID is a novel model that, if implemented effectively, has the potential to bring about valuable positive changes via its role in economic and cultural influence. The field will continue to extend its influence as further technologic advances in data an-alytics, "-omic" analyses and more ubiquitous and affordable use of smart devices are coupled with increasing globalization and decreasing neurological disease stigma in the modern world. It is therefore imperative that we develop new frameworks to har-ness the power of economic and technologic innovation in clinical neuroscience and train future practitioners to benefit the widest array of individuals across the globe and produce a sustainable model.

References

1. Kennedy PJ, Manju H, Staglin G. Unlocking global action on mental health. *Diplomatic Courier*, 2017; https://www.diplomaticourier.com/issue/unlocking-global-action-mental-health.
2. Turekian VC, Moore A, Rasenick MM. Mental health diplomacy: building a global re-sponse. *Science & Diplomacy*, June 23, 2014; https://www.sciencediplomacy.org/editorial/2014/mental-health-diplomacy-building-global-response.
3. World Health Organization. *WHO iSupport: A Programme for Carers of People with Dementia*. Geneva: World Health Organization; 2019.
4. Colglazier EW. Science diplomacy and future worlds. *Science & Diplomacy*, September 13, 2018; http://sciencediplomacy.org/editorial/2018/science-diplomacy-and-future-worlds.
5. Gomez-Olive FX, Thorogood M. Sustainable Development Goal 3 is unlikely to be achieved without renewed effort. *Lancet Glob Health*. 2018;6(8):e824–e825 https://doi.org/10.1016/s2214-109x(18)30297-3.

6. Alzheimer's Disease International. World Alzheimer Report 2018: the state of the art of dementia research: new frontiers. September 2018; https://www.alz.co.uk/research/WorldAlzheimerReport2018.pdf.

7. Cantarero-Prieto D, Leon PL, Blazquez-Fernandez C, Juan PS, Cobo CS. The economic cost of dementia: a systematic review. *Dementia (London)*. 2019:1471301219837776.

8. Alzheimer's Disease International. World Alzheimer Report 2015: the global impact of dementia: an analysis of prevalence, incidence, cost and trends. August 2015; https://www.alz.co.uk/research/WorldAlzheimerReport2015.pdf.

9. Global Brain Health Institute. [Home page]. www.gbhi.org. Accessed May 7, 2019.

10. United Nations. World Population Ageing 2015 (ST/ESA/SER.A/390). 2015; https://www.un.org/en/development/desa/population/publications/pdf/ageing/WPA2015_Report.pdf.

11. Alzheimer's Disease International. *Policy brief for heads of government: the global impact of dementia 2013–2050.* December 2013; https://www.alz.co.uk/research/GlobalImpactDementia2013.pdf.

12. Livingston G, Sommerlad A, Orgeta V, et al. Dementia prevention, intervention, and care. *Lancet.* 2017;390(10113):2673–2734 https://doi.org/10.1016/s0140-6736(17)31363-6.

13. Sukumaran P. Addressing the social determinants of brain health. *Salud! America*, April 29, 2019; https://salud-america.org/addressing-the-social-determinants-of-brain-health/.

14. Valcour VG, Masaki KH, Curb JD, Blanchette PL. The detection of dementia in the primary care setting. *Arch Intern Med.* 2000;160(19):2964–2968 https://doi.org/10.1001/archinte.160.19.2964.

15. Norton S, Matthews FE, Barnes DE, Yaffe K, Brayne C. Potential for primary prevention of Alzheimer's disease: an analysis of population-based data. *Lancet Neurol.* 2014;13(8):788–794 https://doi.org/10.1016/s1474-4422(14)70136-x.

16. Peters R, EE N, Peters J, Booth A, Mudway I, Anstey KJ. Air pollution and dementia: a systematic review. *J Alzheimers Dis.* 2019;70(Suppl 1):S145–S163 https://doi.org/10.3233/jad-180631.

17. Ledoux C, Pilot E, Diaz E, Krafft T. Migrants' access to healthcare services within the European Union: a content analysis of policy documents in Ireland, Portugal and Spain. *Global Health.* 2018;14(1):57 https://doi.org/10.1186/s12992-018-0373-6.

18. Jung CR, Lin YT, Hwang BF. Ozone, particulate matter, and newly diagnosed Alzheimer's disease: a population-based cohort study in Taiwan. *J Alzheimers Dis.* 2015;44(2):573–584 https://doi.org/10.3233/jad-140855.

19. Carey IM, Anderson HR, Atkinson RW, et al. Are noise and air pollution related to the incidence of dementia? A cohort study in London, England. *BMJ Open.* 2018;8(9):e022404 https://doi.org/10.1136/bmjopen-2018-022404.

20. Chen H, Kwong JC, Copes R, et al. Living near major roads and the incidence of dementia, Parkinson's disease, and multiple sclerosis: a population-based cohort study. *Lancet.* 2017;389(10070):718–726 https://doi.org/10.1016/s0140-6736(16)32399-6.

21. Killin LO, Starr JM, Shiue IJ, Russ TC. Environmental risk factors for dementia: a systematic review. *BMC Geriatr.* 2016;16(1):175 https://doi.org/10.1186/s12877-016-0342-y.

22. Wei Y, Wang Y, Lin C-K, et al. Associations between seasonal temperature and dementia-associated hospitalizations in New England. *Environ Intl.* 2019;126:228–233 https://doi.org/10.1016/j.envint.2018.12.054.

23. Digital Health Society. *The Digital Health Society 2018 action plan.* December 2018; https://ehff.eu/wp-content/uploads/2018/09/2d.-DHS_2018-Action-plan_v2.pdf.

24. Ternes K, Iyengar V, Lavretsky H, et al. Brain health Innovation diplomacy: a model binding diverse disciplines to manage the promise and perils of technological innovation. *Int Psychogeriatr.* 2020. [Epub Ahead of Print]. https://doi.org/10.1017/S1041610219002266

25. UNESCO. Science, technology and innovation policy. http://www.unesco.org/new/en/natural-sciences/science-technology/science-policy-and-society/science-diplomacy/. Accessed November 14, 2018.

26. Drage N, Fidler DP. Foreign policy, trade and health: at the cutting edge of global health diplomacy. *Bull World Health Org*. 2007;85(3):161–244.

27. AARP, Global Council on Brain Health. About the council. https://www.aarp.org/health/brain-health/global-council-on-brain-health/about-us/. Accessed November 8, 2019.

28. Hampel H, Toschi N, Babiloni C, et al. Revolution of Alzheimer precision neurology: passageway of systems biology and neurophysiology. *J Alzheimers Dis*. 2018;64(Suppl 1):S47–S105.

29. Coravos A, Goldsack JC, Karlin DR, et al. Digital medicine: a primer on measurement. *Digital Biomarkers*. 2019;3:31–71 https://doi.org/10.1159/000500413.

30. Eyre HA, Lavretsky H, Forbes M, et al. Convergence science arrives: how does it relate to psychiatry? *Acad Psychiatry*. 2017;41(1):91–99 https://doi.org/10.1007/s40596-016-0496-0.

31. Eyre HA, al. e. Strengthening the role of convergence science in medicine. *Converg Sci Phys Oncol*. 2015;1(2) https://doi.org/10.1088/2057-1739/1/2/026001.

32. Miremadi T. A model for science and technology diplomacy: how to align the rationales of foreign policy and science. *SSRN*. 2016 https://doi.org/10.1007/s40596-016-0496-0.

33. Udenrigsministeriet. About TechPlomacy. http://techamb.um.dk/en/techplomacy/ Accessed January 39, 2019.

34. Michalak EE, Jones S, Lobban F, et al. Harnessing the potential of community-based participatory research approaches in bipolar disorder. *Int J Bipolar Dis*. 2016;4(1):4.

35. Staruch RM, Beverly A, Sarfo-Annin JK, Rowbotham S. Calling for the next WHO Global Health Initiative: the use of disruptive innovation to meet the health care needs of displaced populations. *J Glob Health*. 2018;8(1):010303 https://doi.org/10.7189/jogh.08.010303.

36. Juma C. Exponential innovation and human rights: implications for science and technology diplomacy (HKS Working Paper No. RWP18-011). February 2018; https://www.hks.harvard.edu/publications/exponential-innovation-and-human-rights-implications-science-and-technology-diplomacy.

37. Global Health Technologies Coalition. [Home page]. https://www.ghtcoalition.org/. Accessed June 4, 2019.

38. Task Force on Research and Development for Technology to Support Aging Adults, Committee on Technology, National Science and Technology Council. Emerging technologies to support an aging population. March 2019; https://www.whitehouse.gov/wp-content/uploads/2019/03/Emerging-Tech-to-Support-Aging-2019.pdf.

39. Abbott R, Chang DD, Eyre HA, Bousman CA, Merrill DA, Lavretsky H. Pharmacogenetic decision support tools: a new paradigm for late-life depression? *Am J Geriatr Psychiatry*. 2018;26(2):125–133 https://doi.org/10.1016/j.jagp.2017.05.012.

40. Chang DD, Eyreeuro HA, Abbott R, et al. Pharmacogenetic guidelines and decision support tools for depression treatment: application to late-life. *Pharmacogenomics*. 2018;19(16):1269–1284 https://doi.org/10.2217/pgs-2018-0099.

41. Lund C, Brooke-Sumner C, Baingana F, et al. Social determinants of mental disorders and the Sustainable Development Goals: a systematic review of reviews. *Lancet Psychiatry*. 2018;5(4):357–369 https://doi.org/10.1016/s2215-0366(18)30060-9.

42. Astell AJ. Technology and dementia: the future is now. *Dement Geriatr Cogn Disord*. 2019;47(3):129–130 https://doi.org/10.1159/000497799.

43. Hartin PJ, Nugent CD, McClean SI, et al. The empowering role of mobile apps in behavior change interventions: the Gray Matters randomized controlled trial. *JMIR Mhealth Uhealth*. 2016;4(3):e93 https://doi.org/10.2196/mhealth.4878.

44. Wesselman LM, Hooghiemstra AM, Schoonmade LJ, de Wit MC, van der Flier WM, Sikkes SA. Web-based multidomain lifestyle programs for brain health: comprehensive overview and meta-analysis. *JMIR Ment Health*. 2019;6(4):e12104 https://doi.org/10.2196/12104.

45. Williams K, Blyler D, Vidoni ED, et al. A randomized trial using telehealth technology to link caregivers with dementia care experts for in-home caregiving support: FamTechCare protocol. *Res Nurs Health*. 2018;41(3):219–227 https://doi.org/10.1002/nur.21869.

46. Knapp M, Barlow J, Comas-Herrera A, et al. The case for investment in technology to manage the global costs of dementia (PIRU Publication 2016-18). November 2015; https://piru.lshtm.ac.uk/assets/files/Dementia_IT_PIRU_publ_18.pdf.

47. SharpBrains. *The digital brain health market 2012–2020: Web-based, mobile and biometrics-based technology to assess, monitor and enhance cognition and brain functioning*. San Francisco, CA: Author, 2013. http://www.sharpbrains.com

48. United Nations General Assembly. Human Rights Council, 32nd Session. June 27, 2016; https://www.article19.org/data/files/Internet_Statement_Adopted.pdf.

49. Iyengar V, Ghosh D, Smith T, Krueger F. Age-related changes in interpersonal trust behavior: can neuroscience inform public policy? *National Academy of Medicine*, July 1, 2019; https://nam.edu/age-related-changes-in-interpersonal-trust-behavior-can-neuroscience-inform-public-policy/.

50. Pew Research Center. Older adults and technology use. April 4, 2014; https://www.pewinternet.org/2014/04/03/older-adults-and-technology-use/.

51. Federal Communications Commission. Mapping broadband health in America. *Connect2HealthFCC*. https://www.fcc.gov/health/maps. Accessed August 19, 2019.

52. Choi NG, Dinitto DM. Internet use among older adults: association with health needs, psychological capital, and social capital. *J Med Internet Res*. 2013;15(5):e97 https://doi.org/10.2196/jmir.2333.

53. Shim H, Crimmins E, Ailshire J. Internet use and social capital: findings from the National Health and Aging Trends study. *Innov Aging*. 2018;2(Suppl 1):560–561 https://doi.org/10.1093/geroni/igy023.2074.

54. Cacioppo JT, Hawkley LC. Perceived social isolation and cognition. *Trends Cogn Sci*. 2009;13(10):447–454 https://doi.org/10.1016/j.tics.2009.06.005.

55. Weiner MW, Nosheny R, Camacho M, et al. The Brain Health Registry: an internet-based platform for recruitment, assessment, and longitudinal monitoring of participants for neuroscience studies. *Alzheimers Dement*. 2018;14(8):1063–1076 https://doi.org/10.1016/j.jalz.2018.02.021.

56. Zhong K, Cummings J. Healthybrains.org: from registry to randomization. *J Prev Alzheimers Dis*. 2016;3(3):123–126.

57. Boll F, Brune P. Online support for the elderly: why service and social network platforms should be integrated. *Procedia Comput Sci*. 2016;98:395–400 https://doi.org/10.1016/j.procs.2016.09.060.

58. Landeiro F, Barrows P, Nuttall Musson E, Gray AM, Leal J. Reducing social isolation and loneliness in older people: a systematic review protocol. *BMJ Open*. 2017;7(5):e013778 https://doi.org/10.1136/bmjopen-2016-013778.

59. Anderson M, Perrin A. Tech adoption climbs among older adults. Pew Research Center, May 17, 2017; https://www.pewresearch.org/internet/2017/05/17/tech-adoption-climbs-among-older-adults/.

60. Seeman TE, Lusignolo TM, Albert M, Berkman L. Social relationships, social support, and patterns of cognitive aging in healthy, high-functioning older adults: MacArthur studies of successful aging. *Health Psychol*. 2001;20(4):243–255 https://doi.org/10.1037/0278-6133.20.4.243.

61. Quinn K. Cognitive effects of social media use: a case of older adults. *Social Media and Society*. 2018;4(3) https://doi.org/10.1177/2056305118787203.

62. Hawkley LC, Cacioppo JT. Loneliness matters: a theoretical and empirical review of consequences and mechanisms. *Ann Behav Med*. 2010;40(2):218–227 https://doi.org/10.1007/s12160-010-9210-8.

63. Guess A, Nagler J, Tucker J. Less than you think: prevalence and predictors of fake news dissemination on Facebook. *Sci Adv*. 2019;5(1):eaau4586 https://doi.org/10.1126/sciadv.aau4586.

64. Swire B, Ecker UKH, Lewandowsky S. The role of familiarity in correcting inaccurate information. *J Exp Psychol Learn Mem Cogn*. 2017;43(12):1948–1961 https://doi.org/10.1037/xlm0000422.

65. Glisky EL, Rubin SR, Davidson PS. Source memory in older adults: an encoding or retrieval problem? *J Exp Psychol Learn Mem Cogn*. 2001;27(5):1131–1146 https://doi.org/10.1037//0278-7393.27.5.1131.

66. Waytz A, Gray K. Does online technology make us more or less sociable? A preliminary review and call for research. *Perspect Psychol Sci*. 2018;13(4):473–491 https://doi.org/10.1177/1745691617746509.

67. Landau R, Werner S. Ethical aspects of using GPS for tracking people with dementia: recommendations for practice. *Int Psychogeriatr*. 2012;24(3):358–366 https://doi.org/10.1017/s1041610211001888.

68. Shibata T, Wada K. Robot therapy: a new approach for mental healthcare of the elderly—a mini-review. *Gerontology*. 2011;57(4):378–386 https://doi.org/10.1159/000319015.

69. Majumder S, Aghayi E, Noferesti M, et al. Smart homes for elderly healthcare: recent advances and research challenges. *Sensors (Basel)*. 2017;17(11) https://doi.org/10.3390/s17112496.

70. Bennett B, McDonald F, Beattie E, et al. Assistive technologies for people with dementia: ethical considerations. *Bull World Health Organ*. 2017;95(11):749–755 https://doi.org/10.2471/blt.16.187484.

71. Elder A. False friends and false coinage: a tool for navigating the ethics of sociable robots. *SIGCAS Comput Soc*. 2015;45(3):248–254.

72. Sharkey A, Sharkey N. Granny and the robots: ethical issues in robot care for the elderly. *Ethics Inf Technol*. 2012;14(1):27–40 https://doi.org/10.1007/s10676-010-9234-6.

73. Batchelor R, Bobrowicz A, Mackenzie R, Milne A. Challenges of ethical and legal responsibilities when technologies' uses and users change: social networking sites, decision-making capacity and dementia. *Ethics Inf Technol*. 2012;14:99–108 https://doi.org/10.1007/s10676-012-9286-x.

74. Katz R, Kornblet S, Arnold G, Lief E, Fischer JE. Defining health diplomacy: changing demands in the era of globalization. *Milbank Q*. 2011;89(3):503–523 https://doi.org/10.1111/j.1468-0009.2011.00637.x.

75. Brown MDM, Tim K, Shapiro CN, Kolker J, Novotny TE. Bridging public health and foreign affairs: the tradecraft of global health diplomacy and the role of health attachés. *Science & Diplomacy*, September 8, 2014. https://www.sciencediplomacy.org/article/2014/bridging-public-health-and-foreign-affairs.

76. American Association for the Advancement of Science. Programs: Center for Science Diplomacy. https://www.aaas.org/programs/center-science-diplomacy/about. Accessed October 28, 2018.

77. The Digital Medicine Society. [Home page]. www.dimesociety.org. Accessed July 9, 2019.

78. Leijten J. Exploring the future of innovation diplomacy. *Eur J Futures Res*. 2017;5:20 https://doi.org/10.1007/s40309-017-0122-8.

79. Kaye J. Making pervasive computing technology pervasive for health and wellness in aging. *Public Policy Aging Rep.* 2017;27(2):53–61 https://doi.org/10.1093/ppar/prx005.

80. Gove D, Diaz-Ponce A, Georges J, et al. Alzheimer Europe's position on involving people with dementia in research through PPI (patient and public involvement). *Aging Ment Health.* 2018;22(6):723–729.

81. Arandjelovic K, Eyre HA, Lenze E, Singh AB, Berk M, Bousman C. The role of depression pharmacogenetic decision support tools in shared decision making. *J Neural Transm (Vienna).* 2019;126(1):87–94.

82. Brookmeyer R, Abdalla N, Kawas CH, Corrada MM. Forecasting the prevalence of preclinical and clinical Alzheimer's disease in the United States. *Alzheimers Dement.* 2018;14(2):121–129 https://doi.org/10.1016/j.jalz.2017.10.009.

SECTION IV
CONVERGENT MENTAL HEALTH TECHNOLOGIES

20

Toward Multi-Omic–Informed Psychotropic Prescribing

Abdullah Al Maruf and Chad Bousman

Introduction

Mental health disorders are a major public health concern worldwide. These disorders collectively account for approximately one-third of disability globally and cause enormous personal and societal burden.[1,2] The Lancet Commission on Global Mental Health and Sustainable Development reported that mental health disorders are on the rise in every country in the world and will cost the global economy approximately $16 trillion between 2010 and 2030.[3] Given these sobering figures, increased focus has been given to early identification and treatment of mental health disorders. Both pharmacotherapies and non-pharmacotherapies (e.g., cognitive behavioral therapy) are used to treat mental health disorders. Unfortunately, matching an individual to both a tolerable and efficacious therapy has proven challenging, with consensus that a "one-size-fits-all" approach to treating mental health disorders is not sufficient. As such, concerted efforts to identify tools for personalizing therapy have emerged.

The personalization of pharmacotherapies in mental health has received considerable attention over the past decade. This attention has been fueled by technological advances in genomics, specifically pharmacogenomics, and, more recently, epigenomics, transcriptomics, proteomics, and metabolomics that have facilitated the identification of clinically useful biological markers to guide medication selection and dosing. The convergence of these omic technologies is arguably the future of personalized psychotropic prescribing. However, the prospect of multi-omic informed psychotropic prescribing is still largely unexplored and unrealized. In this chapter, we provide an overview of the current genomic, epigenomic, transcriptomic, proteomic, and metabolomic knowledgebase as it relates to psychotropic drug response in an effort to identify promising linkages between and facilitate convergence across these approaches.

Genomic Markers of Psychotropic Drug Response

An extensive literature has been published covering the association between common genetic markers and psychotropic drug response. The most studied drugs are those classified as antidepressants and antipsychotics.[4–9] Altar et al.[10] in their systematic review examining genes encoding for cytochrome P450 (CYP) drug metabolizing enzymes (CYP2D6, CYP2C19, CYP2C9, CYP1A2, CYP3A4), serotonin receptors (HTR2C, HTR2A), and the serotonin transporter (SLC6A4) identified that the strongest gene associations for 26 commonly prescribed antipsychotic and antidepressant medications involved the CYP2D6 and CYP2C19 genes. In addition, a recent narrative review[11] of 92 original articles and six systematic reviews and meta-analyses identified a strong association between CYP2D6 metabolizer status and antipsychotic drug response. CYP2D6 and CYP2C19 enzymes are involved in the metabolism of most psychotropic drugs, and polymorphisms in the genes encoding for these enzymes can lead to altered metabolism of these drugs. Altered metabolism can result in low or high drug blood levels that can lead to decreased efficacy or increased adverse drug reactions, respectively. Common variation in the genes encoding these enzymes are often used to predict an individual's drug metabolizing phenotype (e.g., poor, intermediate, normal, rapid, or ultrarapid metabolizer).[12]

The US Food and Drug Administration (FDA) recommends using the pharmacogenomics information provided in the Food and Drug Administration–approved drug labeling to guide treatment. Currently, 24 psychotropic medications have pharmacogenomic information on their labeling based on polymorphisms in CYP450 enzymes, mostly polymorphisms in *CYP2D6* and *CYP2C19*.[13] The Pharmacogenomics Knowledgebase (PharmGKB)[14] has catalogued more than 400 gene–drug interactions relevant to psychiatry based on the current scientific literature, drug labels, and pharmacogenetic-based implementation guidelines, for example, the evidence-based guidelines published by the Clinical Pharmacogenetics Implementation Consortium, the Royal Dutch Association for the Advancement of Pharmacy—Pharmacogenetics Working Group, the Canadian Pharmacogenomics Network for Drug Safety, and other professional societies. In psychiatry, pharmacogenetics (PGx)-based guidelines currently exist for 13 antidepressants (i.e., amitriptyline, citalopram, clomipramine, desipramine, doxepin, escitalopram, fluvoxamine, imipramine, nortriptyline, paroxetine, sertraline, trimipramine, venlafaxine), 4 antipsychotics (i.e., aripiprazole, haloperidol, pimozide, zuclopenthixol), 3 anticonvulsants (i.e., carbamazepine, oxcarbazepine, phenytoin), and the attention-deficit/hyperactivity disorder medication, atomoxetine.[15-19] The antidepressant, antipsychotic, and atomoxetine guidelines are linked to CYP2D6 and/or CYP2C19, while CYP2C9, HLA-A and HLA-B (human leukocyte antigens) and POLG (DNA polymerase gamma) are relevant to anticonvulsants and mood stabilizers.[20]

Armed with these PGx-based guidelines, a number of medical centers are routinely implementing pharmacogenetics.[21] Commercial offerings of pharmacogenetic testing are also on the rise and may facilitate the wider use of PGx-based guidelines in psychiatry.[22] In fact, a recent horizon scan identified 76 laboratories in the United States that offer PGx services.[23] Furthermore, the perception of PGx testing is favorable among clinicians, patients and the public.[24-27] Walden et al.[28] recently reported that genetic testing for *CYP2D6* and *CYP2C19* improved the outcome for antidepressant and antipsychotic medication and the majority of clinicians who used the test to guide treatment provided positive feedback. A systematic review and meta-analysis of randomized controlled trials reported that major depressive disorder (MDD) patients receiving PGx-guided dynamical systems therapy were 1.71 (95% confidence interval: 1.17–2.48; $P = 0.005$) times more likely to achieve symptom remission compared to patients who received treatment as usual.[29] Despite these encouraging findings, clinical adoption of PGx testing has been slow due to a number of outstanding hurdles (e.g., standardization, feasibility, cost, and healthcare provider readiness). For example, the gene and allele contents among commercial PGx tests vary significantly,[22,30,31] which may lead to considerable differences in medication recommendations.[32] In an effort to inform providers and advocate for better standardization across PGx tests, we recently proposed a minimum gene and allele set for PGx testing in psychiatry that includes 16 variant alleles within five genes (*CYP2C9*, *CYP2C19*, *CYP2D6*, *HLA-A*, *HLA-B*).[20] As the commercial PGx tests are mostly unstandardized and unregulated, we also recently published test selection guidance for providers based on eight critical points—analytical validity, accessibility, test ordering methods, delivery of test results, turnaround time, cost, clinical trial evidence, and gene/allele content.[33]

In summary, pharmacogenomics is progressing rapidly and holds a strong promise to be incorporated as a standard clinical tool for psychotropic medication selection and dosing. There are several actionable genes relevant to psychiatry (e.g., *CYP2C19*, *CYP2D6*, *CYP2C9*, *HLA-A*, *HLA-B*), and evidence-based drug and dose selection guidelines from professional societies are facilitating the clinical implementation of PGx tools.

Epigenomic Markers of Psychotropic Drug Response

Epigenetics involves the study of changes in gene expression by factors other than changes to the underlying DNA sequence which can be significantly influenced by environmental exposures. Epigenetic mechanisms, such as DNA methylation (the addition of methyl groups from *S*-adenylyl methionine to the fifth carbon position of the cytosine residue in DNA by a family of DNA methyltransferase enzymes), histone modifications (enzymatic attachment to or removal of chemical groups from lysine and arginine residues on histones' *N*-terminal tails), chromatin remodeling (rearrangement of chromatin from a condensed state to a transcriptionally accessible state), and noncoding RNA (e.g., microRNAs [miRNAs]) dysregulation can contribute to alterations in gene expression and these mechanisms have been reviewed extensively.[34,35]

Epigenetic changes can occur throughout a person's lifetime by multiple environmental factors, including exposure to pharmacotherapy.[36] Pharmacoepigenomics is an emerging field of research that deals with the effects of epigenetic alterations on drug efficacy and safety, and also how drugs may have an effect on the epigenetic machinery. Epigenetic effects on genes encoding drug-metabolizing enzymes (e.g., CYP1A2, CYP 2C19, CYP2D6), UDP glucuronosyltransferase 1, glutathione S-transferase 1, drug transporters (e.g., p-glycoprotein), solute carrier transporters (SLC19A1, SLC22A8), and nuclear receptors (e.g., estrogen receptor 1) have been documented and extensively reviewed.[37,38] However, the identification of clear mechanisms of these epigenetic marks on drug response and subsequent development of pharmacotherapy optimization is still in its infancy.

The potential role of epigenetics has been explored in relation to drug response for almost all classes of psychotropic medications, including antidepressants, antipsychotics, and mood stabilizers. A systematic review[39] identified 31 studies (in animal and cellular models as well as in humans) where DNA methylation has been implicated as a potential marker for treatment response to antipsychotics, mood stabilizers (anticonvulsants and lithium carbonate), and antidepressants in the treatment of bipolar, schizophrenia, and MDD. This is particularly important because response to these psychotropic drugs is variable, both in terms of efficacy and tolerability. Tang et al.[40] reported that DNA methylation at the thirteenth CpG site (a site where cytosine and guanine appearing consecutively on the same strand of DNA) on the 5-HTR1A (serotonin 1A receptor) correlated with negative symptom treatment response after 10 weeks of treatment with antipsychotic drugs in 82 patients with first-episode schizophrenia. In a whole-genome DNA methylation study that looked at differences in methylation profiles in male schizophrenia patients before and after achieving complete remission, six genes were found to be hypermethylated (*APIS3, C16orf59, KCNK15, LOC146336, MGC16384,* and *XRN2*) and were identified as good markers of treatment-induced effects.[39,41] The functions of *C16orf59, LOC146336, and MGC1638* are not known, whereas *AP1S3* is reported to be involved in protein sorting and intracellular transport and *KCNK15* encodes a potassium channel.[41] In another study, Ju et al.[42] conducted a genome-wide DNA methylation using the Canadian Biomarker Integration Network in Depression (CAN-BIND) patient cohort. They investigated genome-wide DNA methylation patterns in peripheral blood between responders and non-responders to an eight-week escitalopram treatment for MDD patients. Their findings suggest that differential methylation at CpG sites upstream of the *CHN2* (encodes beta-chimaerin, a protein that is important for cell proliferation) and *JAK2* (encodes anus kinase 2, a protein that promotes the growth of cells) transcriptional start site regions are potential peripheral predictors of antidepressant treatment response as the sites were significantly associated with messenger RNA expression changes and subsequently validated.

In a recent narrative review, Hack et al.[43] identified the most studied epigenetic factors in relation to antidepressant response, including DNA methylation, histone modifications, and the control of gene expression by noncoding RNAs. The review identified that the majority of studies of antidepressant pharmacoepigenetics has examined selective serotonin reuptake inhibitor (SSRIs) in relation to epigenetic marks, although some studies looked at other antidepressants, such as serotonin-norepinephrine reuptake inhibitors, tricyclic antidepressants, monoamine oxidase inhibitors, and mirtazapine (a tetracyclic piperazino-azepine antidepressant). Genes that were studied in humans included the brain-derived neurotrophic factor (*BDNF*), serotonin transporters (*SLC6A4*), norepinephrine transporter (*SLC6A2*), serotonin receptors (*HTR1A, HTR1B*), interleukin 11 (*IL-11*), monoamine oxidase A (*MAO-A*), liprin-alpha-4 (*PPFIA4*), and heparan sulfate-glucosamine 3-sulfotransferase 1 (*HS3ST1*). DNA methylation and histone modifications are implicated as the most important epigenetic markers which can predict antidepressant response from the reviewed articles. However, the overall pharmacoepigenetics literature of antidepressant response in humans and animal models have inconsistent findings with limited power, heterogeneity of patient characteristics and loci studied as well as lack of replication.[43]

Several reviews[44–47] have discussed the role of miRNAs as potential biomarkers in antidepressant treatment response. miRNAs are a small noncoding RNA molecule containing about 17 to 22 nucleotides, which are involved in RNA silencing and posttranscriptional regulation of gene expression.[48] Two main reasons are behind the enthusiasm of using miRNAs as biomarkers in antidepressant treatment response. First, there are relatively a limited number of miRNAs in humans (approximately 4,000); therefore, miRNA-focused studies will have better statistical power. Second, miRNAs are known to be released into circulation, which would make it possible to be measured from blood.[45,47,49] Although no miRNA has yet been identified as a validated biomarker to predict or monitor antidepressant response, Belzeaux et al.[45] in their systematic review identified several miRNAs having a translational impact in MDD disease diagnosis and antidepressant treatment response. From the identified miRNAs, the authors selected miR-1202, miR-124, miR-135a, miR-145, and miR-20b as the best candidates to be developed as potential biomarkers. The same group also demonstrated differential expression of miR-146a-5p, miR-146b-5p, miR-425-3p and miR-24-3p to antidepressant treatment response in a landmark study, which were replicated in two independent clinical trials of MDD (the Genome Based Therapeutic Drugs for Depression study[50] and the CAN-BIN) study[51] as well as an animal model of depression and in postmortem human brains.[44,52]

Current evidence suggests that epigenetics plays a role in regulating cytochrome P450 enzyme expression, major transporter function, and in interactions with nuclear receptors.[38] However, unlike genetic tools, developing epigenetic decision support tools for psychotropic drug response is a tough task due to the tissue-specific nature and the environmental influences on epigenetic changes. As such, the path to developing clinically useful epigenetic decision support tools will require the development and use of reproducible epigenetic assays and careful selection of tissues to be assayed.[43]

Transcriptomic Markers of Psychotropic Drug Response

Transcriptomics, or gene expression profiling, is the study of how genes are regulated and expressed in a given biological state. Transcriptomic approaches have historically used microarrays or target quantitative polymerase chain reaction assays but have more recently begun to transition to RNA sequencing.[53] A recent narrative review[46] on the transcriptomics of antidepressant response identified three primary types of studies, (a) messenger RNA-based candidate biomarker studies, (b) messenger RNA-based whole transcriptome analyses, and (c) network analysis of gene expression.

In the first type of studies, which are hypothesis-driven, researchers used the current knowledge regarding the pathophysiology of MDD and antidepressant response mechanisms to target well-known protein-coding genes. The genes that were reported to have significant findings relevant to antidepressant response are *SLC6A4* (encoding the serotonin transporter), *IL1β* (interleukin 1β), *TNF* (tumor necrosis factor), and

FKBP5 (FK 506 binding protein 5), which is also implicated in the epigenetic regulation of BDNF (reviewed in Belzeaux et al.[46]).

The second type of studies are hypothesis-free, genome-wide full transcriptome analysis to identify new loci and biological pathways. For example, Mamdani et al.[54] investigated peripheral gene expression patterns associated with response to antidepressants in MDD patients and identified interferon regulatory factor 7 (*IRF7*) was upregulated among citalopram responders. In another study, Guilloux et al.[55] used machine learning approaches to identify a set of 13 genes that predicted remission with an accuracy of 79.4%, which was replicated in another independent cohort of depressive patients with a corrected accuracy of 76%. In the case of antipsychotic drug response, Crespo-Facorro et al.[56] analyzed the blood transcriptome of 22 schizophrenic patients before and after treatment with atypical antipsychotics and identified 17 genes that had significantly altered expression upon drug treatment. In a subsequent study by the same group identified four genes with the highest predictive value (best response vs worst response) before treatment with antipsychotics. The four identified genes were *SLC9A3* (encodes a Na/H exchanger, which uses an inward sodium ion gradient to expel acids from the cell), *HMOX1* (encodes heme oxygenase 1, which mediates the first step of heme catabolism), *SLC22A16* (encodes a transporter protein, which transports carnitine), and *LOC284581* (uncharacterized).[57]

The third type of studies used gene coexpression network analyses (i.e., sets of genes displaying correlated expression).[46] Using this approach, Belzeaux et al.[58] did a global gene coexpression analysis and found the importance of gene modules related to immune response, acute inflammatory response and C-X-C motif chemokine ligand 8 receptor activity using three independent cohorts of depressive patients. Using the data from the Genome-Based Therapeutic Drugs for Depression (GENDEP) study, Hogson et al.[59] concluded that changes in gene expression are related to antidepressant treatment and are a result of a number of smaller changes acting across a network of co-expressed genes, rather than single genes showing large changes in gene expression levels.

To date, no marker from the current collection of transcriptomic studies has the robustness required for clinical use. However, the dynamic nature of RNA and the arrival of more precise transcript measurement techniques (e.g., RNA sequencing and digital PCR), suggests the contribution of this technology will be important for personalized psychotropic prescribing.

Proteomic Markers of Psychotropic Drug Response

The tools and methods, either alone or in combinations, that have been used for proteomic analyses for discovery of markers for treatment response are two-dimensional gel electrophoresis with mass spectrometry (MS), shotgun proteomics using liquid chromatography–tandem mass spectrometry, antibody-based assays like western blots or enzyme-linked immunosorbent assays, and the newest technology, multiplex immunoassay (advanced multiplex Luminex-based technologies allow measurement of multiple analytes in individual small-volume samples). The techniques/

tools, including commercially available ones and their limitations, are described elsewhere.[60,61]

Proteomic profiling has been limited to the investigation of changes in the levels of specific proteins, mostly focusing on pathways such as cell communication and signaling, inflammation and cellular growth, and maintenance in response to psychotropic drugs in both preclinical models and clinical samples (extensively reviewed by Cassoli et al.[62] and Guest el al.[63]). Compared to preclinical models, where numerous proteomic biomarkers or combinations of biomarkers have been identified, studies in clinical samples are limited. Most of the studies have looked at changes in protein levels due to antipsychotic treatment in schizophrenia patients. It has been reported that schizophrenia patients with a higher serum prolactin level have a better outcome after five years of antipsychotic treatment.[64] Using multiplex immunoassay profiling, Schwarz et al.[65] reported that the serum levels of seven proteins (interleukin-16, fatty acid binding protein, ferritin, C-reactive protein (CRP), myoglobin, prolactin, and complement factor H) could predict the improvement in positive symptoms, and two proteins (matrix metalloproteinase 2 and insulin) could be used for prediction of improved negative symptoms in 77 first-onset schizophrenia patients upon treatment with antipsychotics who were followed up over 25 months. Their study using the same antipsychotic-treated patient cohort also reported that increased levels of transforming growth factor beta and reduced levels of insulin and leptin were indicative of relapse.

In the case of antidepressant drug response, the most studied protein and probably the most promising is CRP. CRP is a well-characterized protein found in blood plasma, which is a good marker of global inflammation. Using the Genome-Based Therapeutic Drugs for Depression study cohort, Uher et al.[50] reported that patients with lower levels of CRP (<1 mg/L) would respond better to escitalopram (a serotonin reuptake inhibitor) than nortriptyline (a norepinephrine reuptake inhibitor). On the other hand, higher CRP levels were associated with a greater reduction in depression severity with nortriptyline treatment. Using the Combining Medications to Enhance Depression Outcomes (CO-MED) trial participants, Jha et al.[66] reported that depressed patients with low CRP level (<1 mg/L) respond better to SSRI monotherapy, whereas those with higher levels respond better to a combination of bupropion and SSRI. These results indicate the potential use of plasma CRP level as a peripheral biomarker in assisting the selection of an antidepressant.[50] Furthermore, Gadad et al.[67] identified two potential inflammatory markers, eotaxin/CCL11 and interferon gamma) Increased levels of eotaxin were reported to be associated with remission, whereas decreased interferon gamma was associated with non-remission after 12 weeks of treatment with antidepressants. Other proteins studied in relations to antidepressant drug response are tumor necrosis factor alpha; interleukins 6, 10, and 1 beta; and BDNF (reviewed in Gadad et al.[61]).

Until now, no validated proteomic marker is available to predict psychotropic drug response. However, further studies investigating these proteins may lead to validated biomarkers (and subsequent development of molecular tests) that can assist in selecting an ideal psychotropic drug as well as patients who would be an ideal candidate for a specific psychotropic drug. This also raises the possibility of using adjunct therapies targeting inflammatory, metabolic, or other molecular pathways based on individual patients.[63]

Metabolomic Markers of Psychotropic Drug Response

Pharmacometabolomics is the study of interindividual differences in the metabolic state and is an important tool to study both the mechanism of action of drugs and response to drug treatment.[68] The use of metabolomic profiling to discover drug response phenotypes has been pioneered by the Pharmacometabolomics Research Network (http://pharmacometabolomics.duhs.duke.edu) in partnership with the Pharmacogenomics Research Network (http://pgrn.org). The tools used for metabolic profiling (e.g., MS, high-performance liquid chromatography, gas chromatography, targeted electrochemistry-based MS platforms, nuclear magnetic resonance spectroscopy, and multiplex-based metabolites screening) and their limitations are reviewed in Gadad et al.[61]

Although promising, metabolomic studies in psychiatry are sparse. However, the Pharmacometabolomics Research Network published a series of studies identifying genetic and metabolic variants of response to multiple drugs, including antidepressants (e.g., citalopram/escitalopram, sertraline, and ketamine/esketamine) in clinical samples. "Pharmacometabolomics-informed pharmacogenomics" is a concept coined by the network that enables the identification of novel genetic variants associated with drug-response phenotypes based on metabolic profiles (reviewed in Neavin et al.[68] and Kaddurah-Daouk et al.[69]). The group recently published a metabolomic profiling study using 290 unipolar MDD patients from the Mayo Clinic and National Institutes of Health's Pharmacogenomics Research Network-Antidepressant Pharmacogenomics Medication Study (PGRN-AMPS). An electrochemistry-based targeted metabolomics platform was used to identify and quantify 31 neurotransmitter-related metabolites primarily from the tryptophan, tyrosine, and tocopherol pathways, including serotonin. Plasma samples were collected at baseline, after four and eight weeks of citalopram/escitalopram treatment and metabolic pathways related to tryptophan, tyrosine, and purine metabolism were found to be activated after the drug exposure compared to baseline. The study also reported that depressed patients who responded well to citalopram/escitalopram differ in their baseline levels as well as in the trajectories of several metabolites, including several gut–microbiota related metabolites (compared to those who did not respond to citalopram/escitalopram). These findings raise the possibility that exposure to these drugs can alter gut–microbial ecology. A deeper discussion of pharmacomicrobiomics, (i.e., how exposure to drugs alters a person's microbiome or how a person's microbiome alters a drug's response) can be found elsewhere in this book.

Convergence of Omic Markers for Psychotropic
Drug Response

The ultimate goal of personalized psychotropic prescribing is to identify the right drug for the right patient at the right dose. However, no single omic technology is sufficient to meet this goal and as such efforts to facilitate convergence of available technologies will be required. We envision that these efforts will utilize rapidly emerging artificial intelligence approaches (e.g., machine learning) capable of sifting through large sets of omic data to identify personalized prescribing signatures (Figure 20.1). For this to be realized however, large amounts of omic data from diverse populations will be required to train machine learning algorithms. Furthermore, the three core object-ives of convergence neuroscience (i.e., focus on a common challenge, encourage con-vergence through structural change, and expand educational and training programs that teach convergence) presented by Turnbull and Freeman in Chapter 5 of this book must be embraced by the psychiatric omics community. Finally, addressing the four major barriers to achieving convergence (i.e., insufficient scientific evidence, insuf-ficient data sharing, lack of field-wide coordination, and difficulties with access to technologies) discussed by Randall and Altimus in Chapter 35 of this book are also integral to the success of personalized psychotropic prescribing. Fortunately, the clin-ical implementation of pharmacogenomic technologies has or is currently addressing these objectives and barriers.[70] Thus, there are opportunities to learn from these ex-periences and devise solutions that will facilitate the convergence of technologies and move multi-omic informed psychotropic prescribing from a notion to a clinical reality.

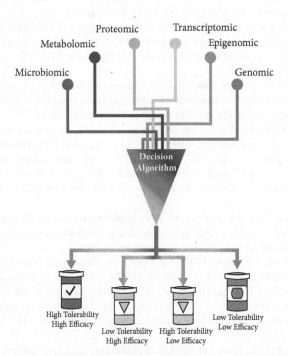

Figure 20.1 Conceptualization of multi-omic informed medication selection.

References

1. Collins PY, Patel V, Joestl SS, et al. Grand challenges in global mental health. *Nature.* 2011;475(7354):27–30. doi:10.1038/475027a

2. Menke A. Precision pharmacotherapy: psychiatry's future direction in preventing, diagnosing, and treating mental disorders. *Pharmgenomics Pers Med.* 2018; 11:211–222. doi:10.2147/PGPM.S146110

3. Patel V, Saxena S, Lund C, et al. The Lancet Commission on global mental health and sustainable development. *Lancet (London, England).* 2018;392(10157):1553–1598. doi:10.1016/S0140-6736(18)31612-X

4. Tansey KE, Guipponi M, Hu X, et al. Contribution of common genetic variants to antidepressant response. *Biol Psychiatry.* 2013;73(7):679–682. doi:10.1016/j.biopsych.2012.10.030

5. Ising M, Lucae S, Binder EB, et al. A Genomewide Association study points to multiple loci that predict antidepressant drug treatment outcome in depression. *Arch Gen Psychiatry.* 2009;66(9):966. doi:10.1001/archgenpsychiatry.2009.95

6. Arranz MJ, Rivera M, Munro JC. Pharmacogenetics of response to antipsychotics in patients with schizophrenia. *CNS Drugs.* 2011;25(11):933–969. doi:10.2165/11595380-000000000-00000

7. Fabbri C, Porcelli S, Serretti A. From pharmacogenetics to pharmacogenomics: the way toward the personalization of antidepressant treatment. *Can J Psychiatry.* 2014;59(2):62. doi:10.1177/070674371405900202

8. Brandl EJ, Müller DJ, Richter MA. Pharmacogenetics of obsessive–compulsive disorders. *Pharmacogenomics.* 2012;13(1):71–81. doi:10.2217/pgs.11.133

9. Fabbri C, Hosak L, Mössner R, et al. Consensus paper of the WFSBP Task Force on Genetics: genetics, epigenetics and gene expression markers of major depressive disorder and antidepressant response. *World J Biol Psychiatry.* 2017;18(1):5–28. doi:10.1080/15622975.2016.1208843

10. Altar CA, Hornberger J, Shewade A, Cruz V, Garrison J, Mrazek D. Clinical validity of cytochrome P450 metabolism and serotonin gene variants in psychiatric pharmacotherapy. *Int Rev Psychiatry.* 2013;25(5):509–533. doi:10.3109/09540261.2013.825579

11. Yoshida K, Müller DJ. Pharmacogenetics of antipsychotic drug treatment: update and clinical implications. *Mol Neuropsychiatry.* 2019;5:1–26. doi:10.1159/000492332

12. Caudle KE, Dunnenberger HM, Freimuth RR, et al. Standardizing terms for clinical pharmacogenetic test results: consensus terms from the Clinical Pharmacogenetics Implementation Consortium (CPIC). *Genet Med.* 2017;19(2):215–223. doi:10.1038/gim.2016.87

13. US Food and Drug Administration. Table of pharmacogenomic biomarkers in drug labeling. https://www.fda.gov/drugs/science-and-research-drugs/table-pharmacogenomic-biomarkers-drug-labeling. Accessed November 10, 2019

14. Thorn CF, Klein TE, Altman RB. PharmGKB: the Pharmacogenomics Knowledge Base. *Methods Mol Biol.* 2013;1015:311–320. doi:10.1007/978-1-62703-435-7_20

15. Hicks J, Bishop J, Sangkuhl K, et al. Clinical Pharmacogenetics Implementation Consortium (CPIC) guideline for CYP2D6 and CYP2C19 genotypes and dosing of selective serotonin reuptake inhibitors. *Clin Pharmacol Ther.* 2015;98(2):127–134. doi:10.1002/cpt.147

16. Hicks J, Sangkuhl K, Swen J, et al. Clinical pharmacogenetics implementation consortium guideline (CPIC) for CYP2D6 and CYP2C19 genotypes and dosing of tricyclic antidepressants: 2016 update. *Clin Pharmacol Ther.* 2017;102(1):37–44. doi:10.1002/cpt.597

17. Swen JJ, Nijenhuis M, de Boer A, et al. Pharmacogenetics: from bench to byte—an update of guidelines. *Clin Pharmacol Ther.* 2011;89(5):662–673. doi:10.1038/clpt.2011.34

18. Phillips EJ, Sukasem C, Whirl-Carrillo M, et al. Clinical Pharmacogenetics Implementation Consortium guideline for HLA genotype and use of carbamazepine and oxcarbazepine: 2017 update. *Clin Pharmacol Ther.* 2018;103(4):574–581. doi:10.1002/cpt.1004

19. Caudle KE, Rettie AE, Whirl-Carrillo M, et al. Clinical Pharmacogenetics Implementation Consortium guidelines for CYP2C9 and HLA-B genotypes and phenytoin dosing. *Clin Pharmacol Ther.* 2014;96(5):542–548. doi:10.1038/clpt.2014.159

20. Bousman C, Maruf A Al, Müller DJ. Towards the integration of pharmacogenetics in psychiatry. *Curr Opin Psychiatry.* 2018;32(1):1. doi:10.1097/YCO.0000000000000465

21. Dunnenberger HM, Crews KR, Hoffman JM, et al. preemptive clinical pharmacogenetics implementation: current programs in five US medical centers. *Annu Rev Pharmacol Toxicol.* 2015;55(1):89–106. doi:10.1146/annurev-pharmtox-010814-124835

22. Fan M, Bousman C. Commercial pharmacogenetic tests in psychiatry: do they facilitate the implementation of pharmacogenetic dosing guidelines? *Pharmacopsychiatry.* 2020;53(4):174–178. doi:10.1055/a-0863-4692

23. Haga SB, Kantor A. Horizon scan of clinical laboratories offering pharmacogenetic testing. *Health Aff.* 2018;37(5):717–723. doi:10.1377/hlthaff.2017.1564

24. Stanek EJ, Sanders CL, Taber KAJ, et al. Adoption of pharmacogenomic testing by US physicians: results of a nationwide survey. *Clin Pharmacol Ther.* 2012;91(3):450–458. doi:10.1038/clpt.2011.306

25. Walden LM, Brandl EJ, Changasi A, et al. Physicians' opinions following pharmacogenetic testing for psychotropic medication. *Psychiatry Res.* 2015;229(3):913–918. doi:10.1016/j.psychres.2015.07.032

26. Haga SB, O'Daniel JM, Tindall GM, Lipkus IR, Agans R. Survey of US public attitudes toward pharmacogenetic testing. *Pharmacogenomics J.* 2012;12(3):197–204. doi:10.1038/tpj.2011.1

27. McKillip R, Borden B, Galecki P, et al. Patient perceptions of care as influenced by a large institutional pharmacogenomic implementation program. *Clin Pharmacol Ther.* 2017;102(1):106–114. doi:10.1002/cpt.586

28. Walden LM, Brandl EJ, Tiwari AK, et al. Genetic testing for CYP2D6 and CYP2C19 suggests improved outcome for antidepressant and antipsychotic medication. *Psychiatry Res.* 2019;279:111–115. doi:10.1016/j.psychres.2018.02.055

29. Bousman CA, Arandjelovic K, Mancuso SG, Eyre HA, Dunlop BW. Pharmacogenetic tests and depressive symptom remission: a meta-analysis of randomized controlled trials. *Pharmacogenomics.* 2019;20(1):37–47. doi:10.2217/pgs-2018-0142

30. Bousman CA, Hopwood M. Commercial pharmacogenetic-based decision-support tools in psychiatry. *Lancet Psychiatry.* 2016;3(6):585–590. doi:10.1016/S2215-0366(16)00017-1

31. Bousman CA, Jaksa P, Pantelis C. Systematic evaluation of commercial pharmacogenetic testing in psychiatry. *Pharmacogenet Genomics.* 2017;27(11):387–393. doi:10.1097/FPC.0000000000000303

32. Bousman CA, Dunlop BW. Genotype, phenotype, and medication recommendation agreement among commercial pharmacogenetic-based decision support tools. *Pharmacogenomics J.* 2018;18(5):613–622. doi:10.1038/s41397-018-0027-3

33. Bousman CA, Zierhut H, Müller DJ. Navigating the labyrinth of pharmacogenetic testing: a guide to test selection. *Clin Pharmacol Ther.* 2019;106(2):309–312. doi:10.1002/cpt.1432

34. Zhang G, Pradhan S. Mammalian epigenetic mechanisms. *IUBMB Life.* 2014;66(4):240–256. doi:10.1002/iub.1264

35. Allis CD, Jenuwein T. The molecular hallmarks of epigenetic control. *Nat Rev Genet.* 2016;17(8):487–500. doi:10.1038/nrg.2016.59

36. Kanherkar RR, Bhatia-Dey N, Csoka AB. Epigenetics across the human lifespan. *Front cell Dev Biol.* 2014;2:49. doi:10.3389/fcell.2014.00049

37. Cacabelos R, Torrellas C. Pharmacoepigenomics. In: Tollefsbol, T. O., ed. *Medical Epigenetics*. Amsterdam: Elsevier; 2016:585–617. doi:10.1016/B978-0-12-803239-8.00032-6

38. Kim I-W, Han N, Burckart GJ, Oh JM. Epigenetic changes in gene expression for drug-metabolizing enzymes and transporters. *Pharmacother J Hum Pharmacol Drug Ther.* 2014;34(2):140–150. doi:10.1002/phar.1362

39. Goud Alladi C, Etain B, Bellivier F, Marie-Claire C. DNA methylation as a biomarker of treatment response variability in serious mental illnesses: a systematic review focused on bipolar disorder, schizophrenia, and major depressive disorder. *Int J Mol Sci.* 2018;19(10):3026. doi:10.3390/ijms19103026

40. Tang H, Dalton CF, Srisawat U, Zhang ZJ, Reynolds GP. Methylation at a transcription factor-binding site on the 5-HT1A receptor gene correlates with negative symptom treatment response in first episode schizophrenia. *Int J Neuropsychopharmacol.* 2014;17(04):645–649. doi:10.1017/S1461145713001442

41. Rukova B, Staneva R, Hadjidekova S, Stamenov G, Milanova V, Toncheva D. Whole genome methylation analyses of schizophrenia patients before and after treatment. *Biotechnol Equip.* 2014;28(3):518–524. doi:10.1080/13102818.2014.933501

42. Ju C, Fiori LM, Belzeaux R, et al. Integrated genome-wide methylation and expression analyses reveal functional predictors of response to antidepressants. *Transl Psychiatry.* 2019;9(1):254. doi:10.1038/s41398-019-0589-0

43. Hack LM, Fries GR, Eyre HA, et al. Moving pharmacoepigenetics tools for depression toward clinical use. *J Affect Disord.* 2019;249:336–346. doi:10.1016/j.jad.2019.02.009

44. Lopez JP, Kos A, Turecki G. Major depression and its treatment. *Curr Opin Psychiatry.* 2018;31(1):7–16. doi:10.1097/YCO.0000000000000379

45. Belzeaux R, Lin R, Turecki G. Potential use of microRNA for monitoring therapeutic response to antidepressants. *CNS Drugs.* 2017;31(4):253–262. doi:10.1007/s40263-017-0418-z

46. Belzeaux R, Lin R, Ju C, et al. Transcriptomic and epigenomic biomarkers of antidepressant response. *J Affect Disord.* 2018;233:36–44. doi:10.1016/j.jad.2017.08.087

47. Fiori LM, Lin R, Ju C, Belzeaux R, Turecki G. Using epigenetic tools to investigate antidepressant response. *Progr Mol Biol Translat Sci.* 2018;158:255–272. doi:10.1016/bs.pmbts.2018.04.004

48. Wahid F, Shehzad A, Khan T, Kim YY. MicroRNAs: synthesis, mechanism, function, and recent clinical trials. *Biochim Biophys Acta-Mol Cell Res.* 2010;1803(11):1231–1243. doi:10.1016/J.BBAMCR.2010.06.013

49. Valadi H, Ekström K, Bossios A, Sjöstrand M, Lee JJ, Lötvall JO. Exosome-mediated transfer of mRNAs and microRNAs is a novel mechanism of genetic exchange between cells. *Nat Cell Biol.* 2007;9(6):654–659. doi:10.1038/ncb1596

50. Uher R, Maier W, Hauser J, et al. Differential efficacy of escitalopram and nortriptyline on dimensional measures of depression. *Br J Psychiatry.* 2009;194(3):252–259. doi:10.1192/bjp.bp.108.057554

51. Lam RW, Milev R, Rotzinger S, et al. Discovering biomarkers for antidepressant response: protocol from the Canadian biomarker integration network in depression (CAN-BIND) and clinical characteristics of the first patient cohort. *BMC Psychiatry.* 2016;16(1):105. doi:10.1186/s12888-016-0785-x

52. Lopez JP, Fiori LM, Cruceanu C, et al. MicroRNAs 146a/b-5 and 425–3p and 24–3p are markers of antidepressant response and regulate MAPK/Wnt-system genes. *Nat Commun.* 2017;8(1):15497. doi:10.1038/ncomms15497

53. Pedrotty DM, Morley MP, Cappola TP. Transcriptomic biomarkers of cardiovascular disease. *Prog Cardiovasc Dis*. 2012;55(1):64–69. doi:10.1016/j.pcad.2012.06.003

54. Mamdani F, Berlim MT, Beaulieu M-M, Labbe A, Merette C, Turecki G. Gene expression biomarkers of response to citalopram treatment in major depressive disorder. *Transl Psychiatry*. 2011;1(6):e13-e13. doi:10.1038/tp.2011.12

55. Guilloux J-P,. Bassi S, Ding Y, et al. Testing the predictive value of peripheral gene expression for nonremission following citalopram treatment for major depression. *Neuropsychopharmacology*. 2015;40(3):701–710. doi:10.1038/npp.2014.226

56. Crespo-Facorro B, Prieto C, Sainz J. Schizophrenia gene expression profile reverted to normal levels by antipsychotics. *Int J Neuropsychopharmacol*. 2015;18(4). doi:10.1093/ijnp/pyu066

57. Sainz J, Prieto C, Ruso-Julve F, Crespo-Facorro B. Blood gene expression profile predicts response to antipsychotics. *Front Mol Neurosci*. 2018;11:73. doi:10.3389/fnmol.2018.00073

58. Belzeaux R, Lin C-W, Ding Y, et al. Predisposition to treatment response in major depressive episode: a peripheral blood gene coexpression network analysis. *J Psychiatr Res*. 2016;81:119–126. doi:10.1016/J.JPSYCHIRES.2016.07.009

59. Hodgson K, Tansey KE, Powell TR, et al. Transcriptomics and the mechanisms of antidepressant efficacy. *Eur Neuropsychopharmacol*. 2016;26(1):105–112. doi:10.1016/J.EURONEURO.2015.10.009

60. Belzeaux R, Lefebvre M-N, Lazzari A, et al. How to: measuring blood cytokines in biological psychiatry using commercially available multiplex immunoassays. *Psychoneuroendocrinology*. 2017;75:72–82. doi:10.1016/j.psyneuen.2016.10.010

61. Gadad BS, Jha MK, Czysz A, et al. Peripheral biomarkers of major depression and antidepressant treatment response: Current knowledge and future outlooks. *J Affect Disord*. 2018;233:3–14. doi:10.1016/j.jad.2017.07.001

62. Cassoli JS, Guest PC, Santana AG, Martins-de-Souza D. Employing proteomics to unravel the molecular effects of antipsychotics and their role in schizophrenia. *Proteomics-Clin Appl*. 2016;10(4):442–455. doi:10.1002/prca.201500109

63. Guest PC, Martins-de-Souza D, Schwarz E, et al. Proteomic profiling in schizophrenia: enabling stratification for more effective treatment. *Genome Med*. 2013;5(3):25. doi:10.1186/gm429

64. Shrivastava A, Johnston M, Bureau Y, Shah N. Baseline serum prolactin in drug-naive, first-episode schizophrenia and outcome at five years: is it a predictive factor? *Innov Clin Neurosci*. 2012;9(4):17–21. doi:10.1186/gm429

65. Schwarz E, Guest PC, Steiner J, Bogerts B, Bahn S. Identification of blood-based molecular signatures for prediction of response and relapse in schizophrenia patients. *Transl Psychiatry*. 2012;2(2):e82–e82. doi:10.1038/tp.2012.3

66. Jha MK, Minhajuddin A, Gadad BS, et al. Can C-reactive protein inform antidepressant medication selection in depressed outpatients? Findings from the CO-MED trial. *Psychoneuroendocrinology*. 2017;78:105–113. doi:10.1016/J.PSYNEUEN.2017.01.023

67. Gadad BS, Jha MK, Grannemann BD, Mayes TL, Trivedi MH. Proteomics profiling reveals inflammatory biomarkers of antidepressant treatment response: Findings from the CO-MED trial. *J Psychiatr Res*. 2017;94:1–6. doi:10.1016/J.JPSYCHIRES.2017.05.012

68. Neavin D, Kaddurah-Daouk R, Weinshilboum R. Pharmacometabolomics informs pharmacogenomics. *Metabolomics*. 2016;12(7):121. doi:10.1007/s11306-016-1066-x

69. Kaddurah-Daouk R, Weinshilboum R; Pharmacometabolomics Research Network. Metabolomic signatures for drug response phenotypes: pharmacometabolomics enables precision medicine. *Clin Pharmacol Ther*. 2015;98(1):71–75. doi:10.1002/cpt.134

70. Klein ME, Parvez MM, Shin JG. Clinical implementation of pharmacogenomics for personalized precision medicine: barriers and solutions. *J Pharm Sci*. 2017;106(9):2368–2379. doi:10.1016/j.xphs.2017.04.051

21

Biobehavioral Sensing for Objective Evaluation of OCD Patients

Gary Liu, Patrick J. Hunt, Amruta Pai, Sophie C. Schneider,
Ashutosh Sabharwal, Nidal J. Moukaddam, Wayne K. Goodman,
and Eric A. Storch

Introduction

Obsessive-compulsive disorder (OCD) is a chronic and highly debilitating psychiatric condition in which distressing and unwanted thoughts, images, or impulses (obsessions) trigger patients to perform compensatory thoughts or actions (rituals) or avoidance [1]. Time-consuming obsessive-compulsive symptoms and associated distress impairs patients' lives significantly, causing disruption in social functioning, health, and attainment in educational and occupational domains [2–5]. Importantly, patients with OCD demonstrate substantial quality of life (QOL) impairment across all life domains [6], and with a lifetime prevalence of 2.3% in U.S. adults [5], OCD negatively affects a significant number of individuals.

Unfortunately, the efficacy of current treatment options is inadequate. Randomized controlled studies demonstrate that 14% to 31% of OCD patients do not respond to the first-line OCD treatment, a type of psychotherapy termed exposure and response prevention [7,8]. Similarly, only about 50% to 60% of patients respond to pharmacotherapy. Most responders to both approaches do not achieve remission [9,10], and relapse is common among responders [9,10]. Treatment nonresponders also experience significantly decreased QOL across multiple life domains following treatment when compared to their own pretreatment QOL [6].

Clearly, there is significant scope to improve outcomes for those with OCD receiving first-line treatments. Decisions regarding exposure strategy, degree of response prevention, supplementation with pharmacotherapy, and the timing of therapy can all be tailored to fit each patient [11,12]. However, a central challenge for clinicians in selecting or refining treatment options to each individual is the lack of tools that can be used to quickly and objectively gauge the effectiveness of therapies. This is primarily due to the heavy reliance on subjective measures—clinical interviews and self-report questionnaires—to examine patients' symptoms. Reliance on subjective measures could thus result in incorrect treatment decisions, either terminating intervention too early or too late, thereby negatively influencing treatment outcomes. Similarly, inaccurate assessments of severity may translate into incorrect treatment decisions such as initiating or discontinuing interventions inappropriately (i.e., switching medications or not maximizing exposure tasks) [13,14].

The gold standard for assessing the severity of illness in OCD patients is the clinician-administered Yale–Brown Obsessive Compulsive Scale (YBOCS) [15]. A decrease in the YBOCS score correlates well with decreases in OCD symptoms, making this an effective tool for monitoring treatment efficacy [16]. However, subjective measures like the YBOCS and other questionnaires, may also be imprecise, difficult to compare across individuals, and vulnerable to inaccurate reporting [17]. Clinical judgement can also be prone to errors [18]. Clinicians typically make decisions by learning a certain prototypical patient for a diagnosis, which each patient is then compared to. This prototype can be influenced by recent exposures to other patients and therefore, may not be objectively formed. Thus, if a new patients' characteristics do not match this prototype, this mismatch can lead to misdiagnosis [18]. This is particularly problematic in OCD given the significant heterogeneity of symptoms [19,20], and the intense stigma associated with common symptoms (e.g. intrusive thoughts of harm, sexual obsessions) [21,22]. Unbiased objective measurements could therefore help clinicians if they encounter patients who are outside their own prototypical patients.

Furthermore, recent work demonstrates that in-session subjective measurements have limited predictive value regarding treatment outcome. For example, one commonly used mode of assessment called Subject Units of Distress Scale (SUDS) involves asking the patient to describe their evoked fear level during exposures or other therapeutic tasks on a numeric rating scale (e.g. 0–10 or 0–100). This scale can be used in concert with YBOCS, as YBOCS measures global symptoms over the prior week while SUDS measures the patient's status at the moment of measurement. However, studies demonstrate that SUDS and other in-session subjective measures of distress are not reliable predictors of treatment efficacy. That is, they do not correlate closely with changes in global OCD severity [7]. Consequently, there is great need to develop objective measures of OCD severity and treatment-related distress that can be employed inexpensively and in frontline settings to enhance assessment, treatment delivery, and patient outcomes.

Biobehavioral sensing uses engineering tools to objectively measure patients' biological, behavioral, and psychosocial makeup, thereby better characterizing patients with mental health disorders [23]. By using these data, we may be able to uncover more robust and reliable markers to assess obsessive-compulsive symptoms. Additionally, tracking how these objective markers change throughout treatment may allow us to discover markers that predict treatment efficacy. The following sections outline some emerging areas in which biobehavioral sensing may be of use in obtaining objective markers to better characterize OCD patients. We acknowledge that using biobehavioral sensing to further mental health is a relatively new idea and that many of the ideas presented in this chapter are proposals that require rigorous assessment prior to use. However, we believe that, once validated, these techniques will enhance the surveys and clinical observations that currently drive the field of psychiatry. Many of the proposed ideas have a strong foundation in human physiology and behavior. Thus, the determination of predictive biomarkers using the technologies outlined next may be able to one day further early detection, diagnosis, and to monitor treatment efficacy.

Physiology Measurements

A robust literature supports the mind and body connection. For example, during times of excitation or stress, one can sometimes feel their heart racing or their face filling with blood. This change in body physiology during times of stress is due to a well-studied component of the central nervous system called the autonomic nervous system [24]. The autonomic nervous system can be divided into the parasympathetic and the sympathetic systems. During calm periods of daily life, the parasympathetic system is more active. For example, while eating, the parasympathetic system stimulates the gastrointestinal tract to promote food digestion. However, once a fear-evoking stimulus presents itself, the sympathetic system takes over, leading to decreased gastrointestinal activity, increased cardiac output, and dilated bronchi. Thus, an active sympathetic system allows one to react quickly. In this way, body physiology is intimately tied to the balance of relaxation and stress within the mind [24–26].

Patients with OCD exhibit aberrant body physiology linked to their disorder [27,28]. Patients with OCD experience decreased heart rate responses when compared to those without OCD during periods of stress [27]. Furthermore, OCD patients experience significantly less autonomic arousal than patients with generalized anxiety disorder or panic disorder [28]. This decrease in responsivity during stress has been partially attributed to physiological inflexibility; the body physiology of patients with OCD cannot change to the same degree as patients without OCD [27].

Measuring relevant physiology and using this to assess the mental status of patients with OCD in a clinical setting have become more feasible in recent years. This is due in part to the advancement of noninvasive technologies for recording body metrics [23]. For example, video recordings of patients can now be used to measure blood flow and heart rate, thus precipitating the discovery of potential biomarkers of OCD. Traditionally, these noninvasive camera-based methods were limited by inadequate lighting conditions, variable skin tones in patients, and motion artifacts [29].

Recently, however, a novel video processing pipeline termed DistancePPG has been developed, which corrects for these limitations by improving the signal to noise ratio via two mechanisms [29]. The first is by accounting for the ambient light intensity and the second is by partitioning each patient's face and processing each partition independently. This approach has substantially improved upon previous generations of video processing that have been used for recording physiological changes. This therefore has the potential to give the scientific and clinical community the ability to use ordinary video recordings to gather physiological data such as the blood flow and heart rate of the patients without requiring physical contact.

The implications of gathering physiological measurements from the patient without direct contact is incredibly powerful. Not only can cardiovascular activity be measured, but many other parameters can be determined as well. For example, the movement of the individual can be tracked as he or she is interacting with the environment. By recording and processing the way in which individuals move as a reaction to various types of stimuli, OCD patients' kinetic data can be monitored remotely. While wearable devices may offer more precision in motion tracking, camera technology is continuing to improve. Due to the overwhelming availability of video-based data, further development in video analysis may lead to greater ability for clinicians to obtain movement data from simple recordings, which can then be processed for various feature extractions. Certain features from these recordings such as speed and directionality of the movements may then correlate to the severity of symptoms experienced by OCD patients. By recording and then processing these movements, the clinician may have more objective data in regard to treatment efficacy.

Wearable devices have also become common, opening new avenues to track physiology [23]. For example, fitness watches like the Apple Watch and the Fitbit can facilitate recording the heart rate of patients, even to the point of detecting atrial fibrillation [26]. Within hospitals, pulse oximeters are readily available and can simply clip onto a patient's fingertip to monitor both heart rate and blood oxygenation. These wearable technologies can be used to track cardiovascular activity during both baseline and stressful activities. For example, the variability of the heart beat itself, which decreases in response to stress, can be measuring using wearable devices (Figure 21.1).

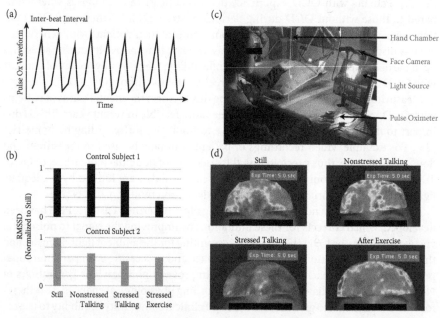

Figure 21.1. (a) Physiological differences between different stress conditions in control subjects. (b) Example pulse oximeter tracings from a healthy control subject. Root mean square of successive interbeat interval differences analysis shows decreased heart rate variability in stressed conditions when compared to nonstressed conditions. (c) Example setup to capture face and hand videos for DistancePPG analysis. (d) Example DistancePPG analysis under different stress conditions

By measuring a patient's baseline heart rate variability and then comparing this to the heart rate variability at various time points of stress, a clinician may be able to objectively quantify the stress that a patient is under. This can then be tracked throughout different therapy sessions to assess treatment efficacy. While these physiological measurements alone may not be able to diagnose mental health disorders, they may be able to augment clinical care and assessments.

Kinetic Measurements

Another physiological difference between those with and without OCD can be observed in the way that these patients move. Patients with OCD utilize a greater repertoire of nonfunctional acts to accomplish the same goal as those without OCD [30]. This can be seen in task engagements, at which point patients with OCD introduce significantly more unnecessary movements. One study found that these unnecessary movements account for over 60% of OCD motor behavior, leading to reduced functionality in patients with OCD [30]. Therefore, identifying movement differences between OCD patients and control subjects in a clinical setting may aid diagnostic efforts and allow for more reliable monitoring of treatment efficacy.

One possible avenue for measuring OCD kinetics is to utilize the Legsys sensor to record the hand motions of patients with and without OCD during a series of directed tasks [31]. With the sensor worn on the wrist, subjects can stand facing an object within arm's reach. The object can either be a control or a fear-inducing object, which can be tailored to the fears of each patient with OCD. While being recorded, the participants can be directed to perform a series of tasks centered around the objects. Hand movements from these recordings can then be analyzed to calculate the time of onset, speed, fluidity, and path of motion of the hand. Comparing these metrics between trials of the control object and the fear-inducing object will allow for the quantification of movement responses. Comparing the responses of patients with and without OCD may uncover disorder-specific movement differences. By comparing these differences to other metrics, such as the YBOCS or SUDS, one may be able to determine if movement differences correlate with symptom severity, thus providing an objective complementary marker of severity.

The implications of utilizing wearable technologies to augment current diagnostic approaches is quite substantial. Besides the previously outlined clinical setting, it may be feasible to track the continuous movement of patients throughout their everyday lives [32]. Due to the increase in nonpurposeful movements of OCD patients, it follows that some parameter of total movement will be different between patients with and without OCD [30]. However, the real power of this technology may be in the longitudinal tracking of patient symptoms. For example, first-line pharmacotherapy of OCD includes selective serotonin reuptake inhibitors (SSRIs) [33]. These pharmacologic interventions typically take a few weeks before noticeable symptomatic improvements, and, more important, 40% to 50% of patients do not experience a satisfactory outcome with SSRI monotherapy [33]. To track symptom progression in an unbiased manner, a clinician may be able to track the kinetic movements of his or her OCD patients both at the start of therapy and as treatment progresses. As long as some feature of purposeless movements corresponds to OCD symptom severity, measuring those features may allow clinicians to assess symptomatology throughout time. This may also be useful in tracking adverse side effects such as behavioral activation [34,35], as actigraphy research has identified distinct patterns of daytime and nighttime activity in those with emerging activation symptoms following SSRI therapy [36].

Behavioral Measurements

The ability to monitor behavior is critical yet challenging in the field of psychiatry. Due to the subjective nature of self-reporting, patients may not be cognizant of their own behaviors. Therefore, what a patient tells their clinician may be very different than their actual behaviors. One reason may be that alterations in memory and concentration are cardinal features in many neuropsychiatric conditions [1]. For example, patients with major depressive disorder have impairments in memory and concentration. Furthermore, in delirious patients, there is altered sensorium, which waxes and wanes. Among individuals with OCD, reporting may be impacted by variable levels of insight [37] or secondary to other co-occurring symptoms such as tics. Thus, any self-reported symptoms must be considered within the overall presenting context. Behavioral tracking may therefore facilitate adequate diagnosis in the field of psychiatry by providing unique information beyond available clinical assessments.

By nature, obsessive-compulsive symptoms are time-consuming. For example, patients with obsessions about cleanliness will spend much time handwashing or cleaning. Clinicians typically rely only on their patients for behavioral reports, and if a patient does not accurately identify or recall the duration of OCD-related behaviors over time, then the efficacy of treatment is difficult to monitor. This is furthermore compounded if a patient's own self-reporting is different than the clinician's clinical observation. Thus, for OCD especially, the ability to accurately monitor behavior outside of a clinical setting may be beneficial in assessing symptom severity.

As smartphone and smartwatch adoption continues to increase, more patients have a tool that can potentially track their OCD-related behaviors. Inherent to these technologies are applications that already seek to track behavior, such as screen time, number of hours slept, and actigraphy. As the computing power of these types of devices improves, it will be hard for clinicians to ignore the advantages that these devices can bring toward tracking patient behavior. For example, one study has already suggested that mood states in bipolar disorder appear to correlate with specific changes in mobile phone usage [38].

The specific parameters of interest to clinicians may be dependent on the type of compulsion inherent to each OCD patient. For example, if the patient feels compelled to check and recheck their home throughout the day, the GPS tracker in their phone or smartwatch can inform their clinician of this type of ritualized behavior. These data can then be tracked to gauge treatment efficacy. This type of individualized measurements can be tailored for each patient to supplement existing approaches.

There may also be more general behaviors that act as biomarkers for symptom progression or remission. One such metric may be sleep. Altered sleep patterns are a hallmark of many psychiatric disorders, including anxiety disorders [1,18] and OCD [39]. While monitoring sleep is not sufficient to diagnose OCD, tracking its patterns may be a way of monitoring the symptom severity of patients with OCD. For example, a recent study showed that OCD patients who sleep later show increases in symptom severity [40], suggesting that sleep may be a marker of OCD symptoms.

Another behavioral symptom of OCD patients is impulsivity [41,42]. In fact, OCD and impulse control disorders overlap on many levels, including comorbidity, neurocircuitry, and family history [41]. Thus, impulsivity may be a behavioral proxy for overall OCD burden on the patient. One such area may be the impulsive use of mobile phones overall or during dangerous situations such as driving. A recent study suggested that the motivations for dangerous mobile phone usage are similar to the motivations that encourage compulsive checking behaviors [43]. Therefore, the monitoring of smartphone usage during driving may give significant insight to clinicians regarding the symptoms experienced by patients with OCD, which may also improve safety.

Affective Measurements

Affective computing is computing that relates to, arises from, or influences emotions [44]. The ability of computers to recognize human emotions can assist in many areas of human health. Recently, advances in affective computing have allowed for the diagnosis of major depressive disorder using both audio and video recordings from affected individuals and healthy controls [45]. Aided by machine learning, computers are able to discover indicators of depression. These indicators can be visual in the form of body movements and facial expressions.

One such methodology is the Facial Action Coding System (FACS), which divides each face into subdomains [46] and the movements of each subdomain are analyzed. The combination of movements can then be attributed to an expression. Building off the idea that facial expressions correlate with internal psychological states, this analysis may reflect the internal state of patients. It is also important to note that the FACS is able to reveal subtypes of facial expressions. For example, smiling when subjects are experiencing pleasant feelings shows activation of muscles around the eyes, whereas smiling to mask disgust, fear, contempt, or sadness does not [47]. This utilization of visual cues can be further extrapolated to include other body parts as well, such as nodding or shrugging. By adding more visual cues and therefore more data points, one group utilized a multimodal approach that included intrafacial muscle analysis as well as movements of the head and shoulders from 30 patients and 30 healthy controls. Using this approach, they were able to detect depression with 76.7% accuracy [48].

The ability for computers to detect depression leads the way for affective computing to aid in the diagnosis of OCD. For example, the facial expressions of OCD patients may be analyzed when presented with various stimuli. One could hypothesize that the expression of patients to a neutral stimulus may be very different than their reaction to a stimulus related to their obsession. A dirty plate versus a clean plate may elicit very different visual cues for someone with obsessions about cleanliness. Thus, with the aid of a video recorder and a computer, a clinician can videotape patients' facial responses as various stimuli are presented. Then by utilizing the FACS as well as body language, a clinician can track evoked distress over time. Therefore, the quantification of facial expressions may be able to supplement existing diagnostic approaches.

Audio indicators are also powerful tools for affective computing toward diagnosing depression [49,50]. Depressed speech, for instance, is different in rate, pause time, and pitch variation [45]. One group found that acoustic measures in speaking rate, pitch variability, and percentage pause time are all correlated with the Hamilton Depression Rating Scale [51]. Accuracy in diagnosis for depression have been shown to be as high as 91% accurate for male speakers and 96% accurate for female speakers [45,52].

The utilization of both audio and visual indicators could dramatically advance the care of OCD patients. Given its accuracy in the diagnosis of depression, there may be features in both facial movements and speech which may be useful in monitoring the efficacy of treatment of OCD. For example, one group found that clinicians' judgements of nonverbal cues such as smiles and frowns, are less predictive of psychological distress than the automatically quantified measurements of these same cues [53]. Utilizing a multimodal approach including facial movements, head movements, and vocal prosody, one group was able to reach 86% accuracy in diagnosing moderate to severe depression [54]. Interestingly, in that same study, facial dynamic expression alone was able to achieve 84% accuracy in diagnosing moderate to severe depression.

Ethics

While the potential applications of the technologies outlined in this chapter are broad, the ethical implications for such technologies will be crucial for society to debate. The ability of machines to understand human mentation comes with it the potential for abuse. With the aid of a simple video-capturing device, anyone's facial expressions can be captured, and their mentation analyzed. For example, if an interviewer captures a interviewee's facial expressions, that interviewer may also have the ability to diagnose the interviewee with a mental health disorder. The moral implications of such powerful tools would be incredibly complicated. At what point can the inferences made by a computer on a person's mentation be categorized as breeching the privacy of personal health information? Also, once a diagnosis is uncovered, to what extent is the interviewer obliged to disclose this information to the affected individual?

Additionally, there would be a need to develop ethically considerate ways of implementing these techniques in the clinic and laboratory. For example, there is dramatic diversity in the appearance of faces throughout the world. Algorithms will need to be adequately trained on faces of all backgrounds, which will require purposeful programming. Many minorities already experience barriers to mental healthcare. At the outset of using this new technology, it is important that we intentionally work to remove these barriers before they arise in this new context. Additionally, many patients may have facial deformities due to trauma, birth defects, etc. These facial structures may be difficult to predict, so these technologies will ideally be able to adapt to unique faces relatively quickly. A patient who cannot use a therapeutic technology due to a facial deformity may even experience increased stress and feelings of isolation.

Finally, it is nearly impossible to separate these data from personally identifiable information, as the data are face-based, and the face is inherent to each person's identity. Thus, as we collect these data, and share these data with other labs for the purposes of analysis and education, we will need to devise creative and thoughtful strategies for protecting the identity and privacy of our patients. The greater the capacity of biobehavioral sensing, the more urgently these matters will need to be addressed.

Conclusion

Many of the current technologies outlined herein are powerful tools to monitor patient movement, physiology, behavior, and affect. However, described are just the initial steps of biobehavioral sensing. The real challenge ahead is to uncover precise markers that can aid in diagnosing OCD and tracking treatment efficacy. The identification of these markers will take time and effort, as clinical trials will be crucial in their development. Once identified, markers must also be scaled in ways that are economically suitable, such as implementing affective computing programs through mobile devices. Perhaps most crucially, these data need to be clinically useful, reliable, and without significant administrative burden.

A multimodal approach may one day result in the most accurate diagnosis and monitoring of OCD patients. In the case of affective computing, a multimodal approach has already been shown to yield the highest accuracy in diagnosis [54]. Thus, a combined strategy utilizing various parameters may one day be necessary for maximal gain. Additionally, the use of modern brain imaging tools and the use of pharmacogenomically informed decision-making may also contribute to this multimodal approach.

Many other fields of medicine have objective, psychometrically sound tools at their disposal for tracking disease states. In cardiology, for example, clinicians have blood pressure, electrocardiography, blood markers, angiograms, and echocardiograms. Unfortunately, psychiatry is currently lacking in comparable tools and is predominantly dependent on either self-reporting by the patient or the clinical judgement and assessment of the clinician. To further the accuracy of diagnosis and monitoring of treatment efficacy, one approach may be to implement more objective measurements. We believe that this will be possible due to the predominance of these tools in many other fields of medicine. With the recent increase in research showing meaningful applications of biobehavioral sensing in mental health, we believe that this technology has great potential to contribute to the field of psychiatry.

References

1. Association, A. P., *Diagnostic and statistical manual of mental disorders (DSM-5®).* 2013: American Psychiatric Pub.
2. Pérez-Vigil, A., et al., *Association of obsessive-compulsive disorder with objective indicators of educational attainment: a nationwide register-based sibling control study.* JAMA Psychiatry, 2018. 75(1): p. 47–55 https://doi.org/10.1001/jamapsychiatry.2017.3523.
3. Isomura, K., et al., *Metabolic and cardiovascular complications in obsessive-compulsive disorder: a total population, sibling comparison study with long-term follow-up.* Biological Psychiatry, 2018. 84(5): p. 324–331 https://doi.org/10.1016/j.biopsych.2017.12.003.
4. Fineberg, N. A., et al., *Early intervention for obsessive compulsive disorder: an expert consensus statement.* European Neuropsychopharmacology, 2019. 29(4): p. 549–565 https://doi.org/10.1016/j.euroneuro.2019.02.002.
5. Ruscio, A. M., et al., *The epidemiology of obsessive-compulsive disorder in the National Comorbidity Survey Replication.* Molecular Psychiatry, 2010. 15(1): p. 53 https://doi.org/10.1038/mp.2008.94.
6. Norberg, M. M., et al., *Quality of life in obsessive-compulsive disorder: an evaluation of impairment and a preliminary analysis of the ameliorating effects of treatment.* Depression and Anxiety, 2008. 25(3): p. 248–259 https://doi.org/10.1002/da.20298.
7. Jacoby, R. J. and J. S. Abramowitz, *Inhibitory learning approaches to exposure therapy: a critical review and translation to obsessive-compulsive disorder.* Clinical Psychology Review, 2016. 49: p. 28–40 https://doi.org/10.1016/j.cpr.2016.07.001.
8. Foa, E. B., et al., *Randomized, placebo-controlled trial of exposure and ritual prevention, clomipramine, and their combination in the treatment of obsessive-compulsive disorder.* American Journal of Psychiatry, 2005. 162(1): p. 151–161.
9. Simpson, H. B., et al., *Standard criteria for relapse are needed in obsessive–compulsive disorder.* Depression and Anxiety, 2005. 21(1): p. 1–8 https://doi.org/10.1002/da.20052.
10. Eisen, J. L., et al., *Five-year course of obsessive-compulsive disorder: predictors of remission and relapse.* The Journal of Clinical Psychiatry, 2013. 74(3): p. 233 https://doi.org/10.4088/jcp.12m07657.
11. Dougherty, D. D., et al., *Neuroscientifically informed formulation and treatment planning for patients with obsessive-compulsive disorder: a review.* JAMA Psychiatry, 2018. 75(10): p. 1081–1087 https://doi.org/10.1001/jamapsychiatry.2018.0930.
12. Wu, M. S. and E. A. Storch, *Personalizing cognitive-behavioral treatment for pediatric obsessive-compulsive disorder.* Expert Review of Precision Medicine and Drug Development, 2016. 1(4): p. 397–405 https://doi.org/10.1080/23808993.2016.1209972.
13. McGuire, J. F., et al., *The nature, assessment, and treatment of obsessive–compulsive disorder.* Postgraduate Medicine, 2012. 124(1): p. 152–165 https://doi.org/10.3810/pgm.2012.01.2528.
14. Storch, E. A., et al., *Defining clinical severity in adults with obsessive–compulsive disorder.* Comprehensive Psychiatry, 2015. 63: p. 30–35 https://doi.org/10.1016/j.comppsych.2015.08.007.
15. Goodman, W. K., et al., *The Yale–Brown obsessive compulsive scale: I. Development, use, and reliability.* Archives of General Psychiatry, 1989. 46(11): p. 1006–1011 https://doi.org/10.1001/archpsyc.1989.01810110048007.
16. Goodman, W. K., et al., *The Yale–Brown obsessive compulsive scale: II. Validity.* Archives of General Psychiatry, 1989. 46(11): p. 1012–1016 https://doi.org/10.1001/archpsyc.1989.01810110054008.
17. Rapp, A. M., et al., *Evidence-based assessment of obsessive–compulsive disorder.* Journal of Central Nervous System Disease, 2016. 8 https://doi.org/10.4137/jcnsd.s38359.

18. Abbott, D., et al., *Biobehavioral assessment of the anxiety disorders: current progress and future directions.* World Journal of Psychiatry, 2017. **7**(3): p. 133 https://doi.org/10.5498/wjp.v7.i3.133.

19. Glazier, K. and L. McGinn, *Non-contamination and non-symmetry OCD obsessions are commonly not recognized by clinical, counseling and school psychology doctoral students.* J Depress Anxiety, 2015. **4**(190) https://doi.org/10.4172/2167-1044.1000190.

20. Glazier, K., M. Swing, and L. K. McGinn, *Half of obsessive-compulsive disorder cases mis-diagnosed: vignette-based survey of primary care physicians.* Journal of Clinical Psychiatry, 2015. **76**(6): p. e761–e767 https://doi.org/10.4088/jcp.14m09110.

21. Bruce, S. L., T. H. Ching, and M. T. Williams, *Pedophilia-themed obsessive–compulsive disorder: assessment, differential diagnosis, and treatment with exposure and response prevention.* Archives of Sexual Behavior, 2018. **47**(2): p. 389–402 https://doi.org/10.1007/s10508-017-1031-4.

22. Sharma, V. and C. Sommerdyk, *Obsessive–compulsive disorder in the postpartum period: diagnosis, differential diagnosis and management.* Women's Health, 2015. **11**(4): p. 543–552 https://doi.org/10.2217/whe.15.20.

23. Sabharwal, A. and A. Veeraraghavan, *Bio-behavioral sensing: an emerging engineering area.* GetMobile: Mobile Computing and Communications, 2017. **21**(3): p. 11–18 https://doi.org/10.1145/3161587.3161591.

24. Costanzo, L. C. L. and W. Wydawnictwo, *BRS Physiology.* Pediatria, 2010. **1**: p. 2.

25. Jacobs, G. D., *The physiology of mind–body interactions: the stress response and the relaxation response.* Journal of Alternative & Complementary Medicine, 2001. **7**(1): p. 83–92 https://doi.org/10.1089/107555301753393841.

26. Dusek, J. A. and H. Benson, *Mind–body medicine: a model of the comparative clinical impact of the acute stress and relaxation responses.* Minnesota Medicine, 2009. **92**(5): p. 47.

27. Hoehn-Saric, R., D. R. McLeod, and P. Hipsley, *Is hyperarousal essential to obsessive-compulsive disorder? Diminished physiologic flexibility, but not hyperarousal, characterizes patients with obsessive-compulsive disorder.* Archives of General Psychiatry, 1995. **52**(8): p. 688–693 https://doi.org/10.1001/archpsyc.1995.03950200078017.

28. Pruneti, C., et al., *Autonomic arousal and differential diagnosis in clinical psychology and psychopathology.* Journal of Psychopathology, 2010. **16**: p. 43–52.

29. Kumar, M., A. Veeraraghavan, and A. Sabharwal, *DistancePPG: robust non-contact vital signs monitoring using a camera.* Biomedical Optics Express, 2015. **6**(5): p. 1565–1588 https://doi.org/10.1364/boe.6.001565.

30. Zor, R., et al., *Obsessive–compulsive disorder: a disorder of pessimal (non-functional) motor behavior.* Acta Psychiatrica Scandinavica, 2009. **120**(4): p. 288–298 https://doi.org/10.1111/j.1600-0447.2009.01370.x.

31. Chen, B.-R., *LEGSys: wireless gait evaluation system using wearable sensors.* In *Proceedings of the 2nd Conference on Wireless Health.* 2011. ACM.

32. Moukaddam, N., et al., *Findings from a trial of the Smartphone and OnLine Usage-based eValuation for Depression (SOLVD) application: what do apps really tell us about patients with depression? concordance between app-generated data and standard psychiatric questionnaires for depression and anxiety.* Journal of Psychiatric Practice, 2019. **25**(5): p. 365–373 https://doi.org/10.1097/pra.0000000000000420.

33. Pallanti, S., et al., *Treatment non-response in OCD: methodological issues and operational definitions.* International Journal of Neuropsychopharmacology, 2002. **5**(2): p. 181–191.

34. Murphy, T. K., et al., *SSRI adverse events: how to monitor and manage.* International Review of Psychiatry, 2008. **20**(2): p. 203–208 https://doi.org/10.1080/09540260801889211.

35. Goodman, W. K., T. K. Murphy, and E. A. Storch, *Risk of adverse behavioral effects with pediatric use of antidepressants.* Psychopharmacology, 2007. **191**(1): p. 87–96 https://doi.org/10.1007/s00213-006-0642-6.

36. Bussing, R., et al., *A pilot study of actigraphy as an objective measure of SSRI activation symptoms: results from a randomized placebo controlled psychopharmacological treatment study.* Psychiatry Research, 2015. **225**(3): p. 440–445 https://doi.org/10.1016/j.psychres.2014.11.070.

37. Selles, R. R., E. A. Storch, and A. B. Lewin, *Variations in symptom prevalence and clinical correlates in younger versus older youth with obsessive–compulsive disorder.* Child Psychiatry & Human Development, 2014. **45**(6): p. 666–674 https://doi.org/10.1007/s10578-014-0435-9.

38. Zulueta, J., et al., *Predicting mood disturbance severity with mobile phone keystroke metadata: a biaffect digital phenotyping study.* Journal of Medical Internet Research, 2018. **20**(7): p. e241 https://doi.org/10.2196/jmir.9775.

39. Paterson, J. L., et al., *Sleep and obsessive-compulsive disorder (OCD).* Sleep Medicine Reviews, 2013. **17**(6): p. 465–474 https://doi.org/10.1016/j.smrv.2012.12.002.

40. Schubert, J. R., E. Stewart, and M. E. Coles, *Later bedtimes predict prospective increases in symptom severity in individuals with obsessive compulsive disorder (OCD): an initial study.* Behavioral Sleep Medicine, 2019: p. 1–13 https://doi.org/10.1080/15402002.2019.1615490.

41. Fontenelle, L. F., et al., *Obsessive-compulsive disorder, impulse control disorders and drug addiction.* Drugs, 2011. **71**(7): p. 827–840 https://doi.org/10.2165/11591790-000000000-00000.

42. Grant, J. E., et al., *Impulse control disorders in adults with obsessive compulsive disorder.* Journal of Psychiatric Research, 2006. **40**(6): p. 494–501 https://doi.org/10.1016/j.jpsychires.2005.11.005.

43. Steelman, Z., et al., *Obsessive compulsive tendencies as predictors of dangerous mobile phone usage.* In: AMCIS Proceedings. 2012: Curran; p. 2687–2700).

44. Picard, R. W., *Affective computing.* 2000: MIT press.

45. Morales, M., S. Scherer, and R. Levitan, *A cross-modal review of indicators for depression detection systems.* In: Proceedings of the Fourth Workshop on Computational Linguistics and Clinical Psychology—From Linguistic Signal to Clinical Reality. 2017: Association for Computational Linguistics https://www.aclweb.org/anthology/W17-3101.pdf

46. Cohn, J. F., Z. Ambadar, and P. Ekman, *Observer-based measurement of facial expression with the Facial Action Coding System.* In: The Handbook of Emotion Elicitation and Assessment, 2007: Oxford; p. 203–221.

47. Ekman, P., W. V. Friesen, and M. O'Sullivan, *Smiles when lying.* Journal of Personality and Social Psychology, 1988. **54**(3): p. 414 https://doi.org/10.1037/0022-3514.54.3.414.

48. Joshi, J., et al., *Multimodal assistive technologies for depression diagnosis and monitoring.* Journal on Multimodal User Interfaces, 2013. **7**(3): p. 217–228 https://doi.org/10.1007/s12193-013-0123-2.

49. Cummins, N., et al., *Analysis of acoustic space variability in speech affected by depression.* Speech Communication, 2015. **75**: p. 27–49 https://doi.org/10.1016/j.specom.2015.09.003.

50. Cummins, N., et al., *A review of depression and suicide risk assessment using speech analysis.* Speech Communication, 2015. **71**: p. 10–49 https://doi.org/10.1016/j.specom.2015.03.004.

51. Cannizzaro, M., et al., *Voice acoustical measurement of the severity of major depression.* Brain and Cognition, 2004. **56**(1): p. 30–35 https://doi.org/10.1016/j.bandc.2004.05.003.

52. Moore, E. II, et al., *Critical analysis of the impact of glottal features in the classification of clinical depression in speech.* IEEE Transactions on Biomedical Engineering, 2007. **55**(1): p. 96–107.

53. Lucas, G. M., et al., *Towards an affective interface for assessment of psychological distress.* In: *2015 International Conference on Affective Computing and Intelligent Interaction (ACII), Xi'an.* 2015. p. 539–545, doi:10.1109/ACII.2015.7344622.

54. Dibeklioğlu, H., Z. Hammal, and J. F. Cohn, *Dynamic multimodal measurement of depression severity using deep autoencoding.* IEEE Journal of Biomedical and Health Informatics, 2017. **22**(2): p. 525–536.

22

An Introduction to Antidepressant Pharmacomicrobiomics and Implications in Depression

Lisa C. Brown, Chelsea L. Cockburn, and Harris A. Eyre

Introduction

Major depressive disorder (MDD) is a leading cause of disability worldwide and is marked by symptoms such as decreased mood, hopelessness, feelings of guilt, and changes in sleep.[1] Currently, only 50% to 60% of patients with MDD will respond to their first antidepressant and even fewer reach remission of symptoms.[2,3] With approximately 21% of individuals experiencing depression in a lifetime, MDD incurs a high burden of illness economically and on quality of life.[4,5] In addition to the burden of a depressive episode, with each medication trial, individuals risk becoming treatment resistant and experiencing increased adverse events.[3,6] There are many factors that can affect response to medication including genetics, epigenetics, environment, diagnosis, comorbidities, and others. It is therefore critical to develop tools that can lead to better treatment selection resulting in remission of depressive symptoms.

Even with new tools such as machine learning, pharmacogenetics, artificial intelligence, pharmacoepigenetics, and others, personalized medication selection is still lacking.[7-11] The full mechanism of most antidepressants is poorly understood and therefore treatment decisions usually rely on clinical features and clinician expertise rather than definitive tests. Another area of medicine that has become popular in the last decade is how a person's microbiome can affect health and investigators have begun to examine ways in that microbiomic markers moderate antidepressant response as part of the field of pharmacomicrobiomics (PMx).

The microbiome consists of the microorganisms such as fungi, bacteria, viruses, and protozoa, which live in and on the human body, including the gastrointestinal tract, skin, mucosal membranes and other body parts. The microbiome has been described as the second genome, "a source of genetic diversity, a modifier of disease, an essential component of immunity, and a functional entity that influences metabolism and modulates drug interactions."[12p151] The microbiome is highly dynamic, and can be altered by diet, exercise, stress, and other factors. PMx is described as the effect of the microbiome on drug action, fate, and toxicity and, in addition to tools like pharmacogenetics, has the potential to personalize medication treatments and outcomes.[13] One must also consider that, in turn, medications can also affect the gut microbiome, making the story of PMx even more convoluted.[13,14] For example, antibiotics disturb the gut microflora leading to antibiotic resistant infections and susceptibility to infections.[15] In addition, the microbiome also has a profound effect on the immune system and inflammation, which has also been implicated in the pathology of mental illness in causation and treatment response.[16,17]

There are a few ways that PMx can be valuable in patients with MDD (Figure 22.1):

1. How the microbiome causes or modulates the disease and how the disease affects the microbiome.
2. How medications affect the microbiome and how the microbiome affects medications.
3. How medications affect the disease.
4. How drug–drug interactions affects the microbiome.
5. How medications affect phenoconversion and therefore the microbiome and disease.
6. How drug-drug interactions affects the disease.
7. How the microbiome affects pharmacogenetics of medications and how the pharmacogenetics of medications affect the microbiome.

PMx may play an important role in antidepressant efficacy, and therefore, a strong understanding of the interplay between the microbiome and antidepressants may lead to tools to help personalize treatments for patients with depression. In this chapter, we discuss the current state of PMx of antidepressant therapy and present a roadmap for the future.

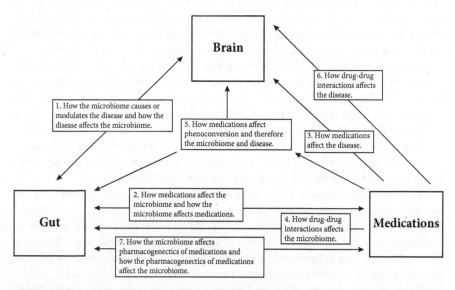

Figure 22.1 Interplay between the microbiome and major depressive disorder. The interactions between the microbiome and major depressive disorder are incredibly complex, including interplays with medications, pharmacogenomics, and other bodily processes.

Microbiomics

Origins and Implications in Depression

The human microbiome is comprised of a complex, interconnected group of bacterial, viral, protozoal, and fungal species that play a major role in the maintenance of health. Dysbiosis of this microbiome can lead to a myriad of symptoms and diseases. In the human gut, only a few phyla have been continuously identified, including *Firmicutes, Bacteroidetes, Proteobacteria, Verrucomicrobia, Actinobacteria*, and *Fusobacteria*.[18] The *Firmicutes/Bacteroidetes* ratio has been implicated in the dysbiosis of the microbiome leading to weight gain, irritable bowel syndrome, and other disorders.[19,20] Lower levels of *Firmicutes* is also hypothesized to cause low level inflammation and depressive symptoms.[21] Indeed, the microbiome of patients with MDD, is different from that of healthy controls.[17] A recent analysis of patients with either untreated MDD, treated MDD, or healthy controls exhibited an increase in *Bacteriodetes, Proteobacteria*, and *Actinobacteria* and a decrease in *Firmicutes* in patients with both untreated and treated MDD.[17] Another study found a lack of diversity in the bacterial flora of patients with severe mental illness and MDD.[22] Specifically, a reduction in *Bifidobacterium* and *Lactobacillus* was found in patients with MDD compared to controls.[23] Most interestingly, even when controlling for covariates that have been shown to predict remission in inpatients, the bacterial diversity predicted remission for these patients. Notable, the study also found that a specific bacterium, *Coprococcus catus*, was depleted in more severely depressed patients as well as patients who did not reach remission, possibly indicating a role in MDD pathology and response for this organism.

Additionally, dysbiosis associated with antibiotic treatment or chronic inflammation can induce depressive symptoms.[24,25] In the case of chronic inflammation, these symptoms can be alleviated by treatment with selective serotonin reuptake inhibitors (SSRIs), implicating the serotonergic system in depression pathophysiology, including a direct connection between infection-induced inflammation and serotonin metabolism.[26,27] The microbiota-inflammasome theory of MDD provides that an increase in inflammatory pathways through the activation of the intrinsic inflammasome response to changes in the microbiota perpetuates depressive symptoms.[28]

The interactions between the gut microbiome and medications can play out in two ways: (i) medications that are more effective with specific gut flora and (ii) the ability for specific flora to breakdown and reduce drug-related toxicity.[29,30] Further, the microbiome can modulate medication pharmacokinetics every step of the way through absorption, distribution, metabolism, and elimination.[31] Risperidone and olanzapine, both of which cause weight gain in patients, have been implicated in changes of the gut microbiome, particularly an increased *Firmicutes* to *Bacterioides* ratio, leading to altered metabolism and subsequent weight gain.[32-34] Additional psychotropics, such as nitrazepam and ketamine have been shown to directly alter the gut microbiome.[35,36]

The microbiome may also have a direct effect on metabolic enzymes such as cytochrome (CYP) P450s and other xenobiotic enzymes.[29,31] Differences in expression of CYP450 enzymes were found between germ-free and normal mice with the same CYP450 genotyping.[30,37] Notably, bacteria also synthesize CYP-like genes and other enzymes, which could even have the capacity to increase drug metabolism separate from the individual's enzymatic system.[38,39] Interestingly, inflammation caused by infection can decrease the expression of CYPs, which may also have an effect on the metabolism of psychotropics.[38] Production of p-cresol by bacterial flora can compete with drugs like acetaminophen for metabolic breakdown by *SULT1A1*, resulting in acetaminophen hepatotoxicity.[40]

Various therapeutic modalities exist to alter the microbiome in depressed patients, including dietary interventions, probiotic interventions, and fecal transplants. A recent analysis of published studies revealed that in addition to various genetic and environmental components, diet plays a major role in gut dysbiosis that occurs in MDD and associated comorbidities.[41] Additionally, probiotics, in particular 1910 lacto-producing bacteria, have been identified as a potential therapeutic target for treating depression and anxiety.[42] Therefore, the hypothesis being that altering the gut microbiome will alleviate depressive symptoms is plausible and requires additional study.[43]

In Vitro

A range of psychotropics have antimicrobial activity against bacteria, fungi, and parasites and have been studied in rodents and humans.[44] Psychotropics have antimicrobial activity via three core mechanisms: (i) direct antimicrobial activity, (ii) direct effect on microorganism pathogenicity, and/or (iii) modulating antibiotic activity.[45] Furthermore, psychotropics have also been shown to decrease antibiotic resistance, which would play an important role in hospital acquired infections and multidrug resistant microbes.[44]

SSRIs are the most common antidepressants used in the healthcare setting. In addition to their psychotropic effects, SSRIs can exhibit antimicrobial properties across the spectrum of Gram-positive and Gram-negative bacteria, fungi, and parasites.[44] In particular, SSRIs are especially effective against Gram-positive organisms, which are notoriously difficult to treat.[45] While the exact mechanisms are poorly understood, SSRIs are thought to potentiate their antimicrobial effect through efflux inhibition leading to synergistic effects with certain antibiotics.[46,47] This synergy is confirmed when examining the decrease in minimum inhibitory concentrations (MIC) that occurs when antimicrobials and antidepressants are combined.

The SSRI, sertraline, was found to be effective against a wide range of pathogens in vivo and in vitro.[48] Sertraline kills *Trypanosoma cruzi* in vitro through metabolic disruption of the parasite and is effective in killing *Leishmania donovani* both in vitro and in mice.[49,50] Sertraline was shown to be effective against *Brucella* spp. but the MIC was much higher than plasma sertraline levels, indicating a limitation to these in vitro studies. Antimicrobial activity are not necessarily translatable to human disease as the in vitro MIC concentrations are much higher than what would be tolerable in human plasma levels.[51] SSRIs are effective against various fungal pathogens as well. Sertraline, fluoxetine, and paroxetine were effective against *Aspergillus* spp. and *Candida albicans* in vitro with sertraline and fluoxetine being the most effective.[52,53]

Additionally, sertraline in combination with amphotericin B, caspofungin, or fluconazole is able to kill and disrupt the biofilm of *Trichosporon asahii*, a common cause of hospital acquired opportunistic infections and biofilm growth on medical devices.[54] Furthermore, citalopram reduced chloroquine resistance in *P. falciparum*, indicating that some psychotropics, in addition to new antimicrobials, treat disease and can reduce the development of antimicrobial resistance.[55]

While most SSRIs have been found to have antimicrobial activity and synergize with antibiotics, one study demonstrated that fluoxetine can induce antibiotic resistance in *Escherichia coli* through induction of mutagenesis in efflux protein machinery.[56] The tricyclic antidepressant (TCA), amitriptyline, also reduced chloroquine resistance in *P. falciparum*.[55] These data only complicate the threat of antimicrobial resistance. Previously, it was thought that the majority of anti-microbial-resistant species arose from selective pressure on beneficial mutations, however, certain psychotropics may actually mutagenize the organism, thus increasing the capability and rate of resistance.

TCAs were among the first generation of antidepressants. While their frequency of use to treat various mood disorders has decreased, research has emerged indicating that they may be efficacious in the treatment of various microbial pathogens. TCAs inhibit growth of the intestinal pathogens, *E. coli*, *Yersinia enterocolitica*, and *Giardia lamblia* due, in part, to their antiplasmid activity.[57,58] Plasmids tend to carry antibiotic-resistant genes; this, again, emphasizes the potential for psychotropics to play a role in the creation of, and battle against antibiotic resistance.[57] Additionally, TCAs exhibit in vitro activity against the parasites, *P. falciparum* and *Leishmania* spp.[59-61] Mianserin was found to effectively kill *Leishmania donovani*, presenting the idea of repurposing the drug to treat visceral leishmaniasis, which is significantly more fatal compared to cutaneous disease.[62] Clomipramine was shown to be effective against *Brucella* spp. as well as *Mycobacterium tuberculosis* at concentrations relevant to those in vivo.[44,51]

Animal Models

Sertraline is not only effective against many microbial species in vitro but it is also effective in animal models.[48] Sertraline kills *L. donovani* both in vitro and in mice.[50] Furthermore, sertraline reduced *Cryptococcus neoformans* fungal burden in the brain, kidney, and spleen of mice at clinical concentrations and was shown to work synergistically with fluconazole.[63-65] The synergistic antimicrobial effect of sertraline and fluconazole to *Cryptococcus* spp has therefore been suggested as a treatment for cryptococcal infection. Interestingly, this combination was antagonistic in strains of *Candida* spp.[65]

Recently, TCAs have been shown to be functional inhibitors of acid sphingomyelinase, which are important machinery of intracellular pathogens.[66] TCAs have been shown to clear infections of the obligate intracellular bacteria, *Anaplasma phagocytophilum*, *Coxiella burnetii*, *Chlamydia pneumoniae*, and *C. trachomatis* both in vitro and in vivo.[67] These results indicate a potential role in treating intracellular pathogen infections as well as recalcitrant infection, which is especially important since many of these pathogens are incredibly difficult to treat.

Additionally, the effect of the microbiome, medications, and the immune system have also been studied. Toll-like receptors interact with commensal and pathogenic bacteria to modulate gut homeostasis resulting in low level inflammation from commensal bacteria and higher inflammation from pathogens.[68,69] Interleukin 6 blockade in mice resulted in reduced depressive symptoms as well as a reduction of *Firmicutes/Bacteroidetes* ratio.[70] These data suggest that reducing interleukin 6 inflammation may improve the microbiome and, subsequently, reduce depressive symptoms.

The effect of the microbiome on inflammation may be especially important during neural development. In one study, neonatal rats with increased inflammation from bacterial lipopolysaccharide challenge resulted in learning difficulties as adults; hence, inflammation caused by bacterial lipopolysaccharide in the microbiome can affect neurodevelopment down the road.[71] This work illustrates the potential effect that the microbiome and environmental challenge as a neonate or in early childhood could affect learning and neurodevelopment into adulthood.

With the recent Food and Drug Administration approval of esketamine nasal spray for the treatment of treatment resistant depression, the interplay within the gut, ketamine, and depressive symptoms is in the spotlight. Personalizing esketamine is especially important as there is a heterogeneous response and side effects that patients may experience with the drug. In mice, ketamine was found to reduce the concentration of *Mollicutes* and *Butyricimonas* in the gut, with (*R*)-ketamine being more potent than (*S*)-ketamine.[35] The reduction of these genera may help perpetuate ketamine's antidepressant effect. Other studies have also found that ketamine alters abnormal gut microbiota and therefore may be a marker for ketamine response.[72,73] Levels of *Lactobacillus* in patients with MDD are usually lower than in healthy controls and recent study found that ketamine increased *Lactobacillus* in mice, potentially affecting inflammation and potentiating antidepressant effects.[74,75]

Another emerging area of PMx is related to the potential for fecal transplants to treat MDD. Mice and rats that received fecal transplantation from patients with MDD exhibited higher depression-like behavior than control animals, indicating a role for the gut microbiome in MDD.[76-78] It is therefore logical to conclude that fecal transplantation could be utilized as a treatment modality for depressed patients by which they receive transplantation from a healthy donor.[79,80]

Human Studies

PMx studies in relation to antidepressant use is a relatively new concept. As such, there are a limited number of completed human studies from which to elucidate the role of antidepressants in the human microbiome. Today, most studies looking at PMx revolve around the use of probiotics. An early study from 2007 showed that individuals who consumed a milk drink containing *Lactobacillus casei* showed significantly improved mood in individuals with low mood at baseline compared to individuals taking placebo.[81]

As one might expect since studies have shown a reduction in *Bifidobacterium* and *Lactobacillus* in patients with MDD compared to controls, that supplementation with *Bifidobacterium* and *Lactobacillus* resulted in decreased depressive symptoms in patients with MDD.[23,82] The Probiotics in Pregnancy study also showed that *Lactobacillus rhamnosus* significantly improved mood in women one-year postpartum.[83,84] One trial, exploring the effect of *Lactobacillus acidophilus*, *L. casei*, and *Bifidobacterium bifidum* compared to placebo showed a significant reduction in depression symptoms.[85] Another study, also found that the probiotics, *Lactobacillus helveticus* and *Bifidobacterium longum* significantly reduced depressive symptoms; however, the prebiotic, galactooligosaccharide, did not.[86] However, not all studies found that probiotics improve outcomes for patients with depression. Romijn et al. found that supplementation with *L. helveticus* and *B. longum* probiotics did not significantly affect mood outcome compared to placebo.[87] A pilot study examining a combination therapy of probiotics and magnesium orotate to treat SSRI-resistant depression indicated that while clinical symptoms improved after treatment, relapse occurred following removal of the probiotics and continuation of SSRIs.[88]

A recent meta-analysis found that probiotics as an attempt to regulate the microbiome are only effective in mild to moderate depression; however, levels of inflammation were not considered in many of the studies.[89] This begs the question that if MDD symptoms are modulated by inflammation changes caused by changes in the microbiome, can targeting modulation in the microbiome treat depressive symptoms by reducing inflammation? One may also wonder if antidepressant modulation of the microbiome is what perpetuates some of the medication effects on depressive symptoms.

Pharmacomicrobiomics: Current Clinical Trials

There are currently quite a few ongoing studies to explore the microbiome of individuals suffering from depression (NCT03062332, NCT04211467); however, there are very few interventional studies being performed (Table 22.1). Neerthless, one exciting study is looking at the effect of fecal transplants on depressive symptoms in patients with moderate to severe depression (NCT03281044). Two other studies are exploring the effect of probiotics on depressive symptoms and mood (NCT03893162, NCT02957591) One of these studies is led by the Canadian Biomarker Integration Network in Depression group, which seeks to identify and integrate biomarkers to personalize depression treatment (NCT03277586).[43] More specific to PMx, one study is evaluating the microbiome effect on treatment response to the antidepressant citalopram (NCT02330068). Ideally, additional studies like this will lead the way to understanding how PMx may predict response to medications and therefore personalize treatments for patients with depression.

Table 22.1. Current PMx Clinical Trials

Study Title	Condition/Disease	Study Design	Sample Size	Intervention/Treatment	Primary Outcome	Reference
Altered Fecal Microbiota Composition in Patients With Major Depressive Disorder and Bipolar Disorder	Bipolar Disorder, Major Depressive Disorder	Observational cohort	240	Genetic: Fecal genome	Composition of the gut microbiota [Time Frame: 3 months]	NCT03062332
A Non-Interventional Pilot Study to Explore the Role of Gut Flora in Depression	Depression	Observational case-only	100	None	Correlation of Microbiome to Disease via Relative Abundance Found in Microbiome Sequencing [Time Frame: Three years]	NCT04211467
Oral Frozen Fecal Microbiota Transplantation (FMT) Capsules for Depression: a Double-blind, Placebo-controlled, Randomized Parallel Group Study	Major Depressive Disorder	Interventional randomized, parallel assignment	40	Drug: Fecal microbiota capsules Drug: Placebo oral c apsule	Depressive symptoms as measured with the Hamilton Rating Scale for Depression [Time Frame: Change from baseline score to follow-up measurements at 1, 2 and 8 months]	NCT03281044
Gut Feeling: Understanding the Mechanisms Underlying the Antidepressant Properties of Probiotics	Major Depressive Disorder	Interventional randomized, parallel assignment	50	Dietary Supplement: Multistrain probiotic Other: Placebo	1. Gut microbiota in major depressive disorder [time frame: baseline] 2. Differences in gut microbiota between MDD and healthy volunteers [Time Frame: baseline] 3. Gut microbiota changes in MDD following probiotic intervention [Time frame: change from baseline to week 8]	NCT03393162

Title	Condition	Design	Enrollment	Intervention	Outcome	NCT Number
The Effect of Probiotic Supplementation on the Efficacy of Antidepressant Treatment in Depression	Severe Depression	Interventional randomized, parallel assignment	60	Dietary Supplement: Vivomixx® Other: Placebo	Hamilton Depression Score [Time Frame: Change from baseline at week four]	NCT02957591
Effects of Probiotics on Symptoms of Depression	Depression, Anxiety	Interventional randomized, parallel assignment	108	Drug: Probio'Stick Drug: Placebo	Montgomery- Asberg Depression Rating Scale Mood [Time Frame: 16 weeks]	NCT03277586
Microbiome of Depression and Treatment Response to Citalopram: A Feasibility Study	Major Depressive Disorder, Bipolar I, Bipolar II	Observational case-only	34	Drug: citalopram	The potential differences in the microbiome between depressed patients and healthy controls [Time Frame: Over 12 weeks]	NCT02330068

Pharmacomicrobiomics: The Future

Various therapeutic modalities exist to alter the microbiome in depressed patients, including dietary interventions, probiotic interventions, and fecal transplants.[90,91] A recent analysis of published studies revealed that in addition to various genetic and environmental components, diet plays a major role in gut dysbiosis that occurs in MDD and associated comorbidities.[41] Additionally, probiotics, in particular lacto-producing bacteria, have been identified as a potential therapeutic target for treating depression and anxiety.[42] While the exact mechanism is unknown, recent evidence suggests that probiotics may increase brain derived neurotrophic factor leading to increased neurogenesis.[92,93] Work has also studied the effect of neurodevelopment during puberty and the effect on brain pathologies in adulthood.[94] It is thought that increased inflammation from stress, diet, antibiotics, etc. can have a profound effect during the vulnerable time of neurodevelopment in puberty leading to cognitive impairment and risk for mental and neurological disorders. Therefore supplementation with probiotics during puberty may also have a protective effect against cognitive impairment and depression.

Multiple studies have demonstrated that mice and rats that received fecal transplantation from patients with MDD exhibited higher depression-like behavior than control animals.[76-78] It is therefore feasible that future work should explore the role of fecal transplantation from not-depressed donor patients as a treatment modality for depressed patients.[79,80]

An emerging area of interest in PMx may also be the study of the interaction between the gut and extracellular vesicles (EVs) produced by microbes.[95] EVs are produced by both Gram-negative and Gram-positive bacteria as well as many fungal species and are thought to act as "vehicles" for the packaging, delivery, and/or release of various proteins, DNA, RNA, and toxins.[96] Interestingly, one study in mice showed that cell-free EVs from *Lactobacillus reuteri* increased gut motility in mice, indicating the biological effects of EVs separate from the presence of bacterial cells.[97] Future work should explore the role of EVs in depression and PMx.

Conclusion

In conclusion, new treatments and treatment strategies are desperately needed to improve outcomes in patients suffering from major depressive disorder. Recent work has shown the relationship among the microbiome, inflammation, disease, and psychopharmacological treatment. There is a huge opportunity to expand research into these interactions in preventing and treating depression.

Acknowledgments

We thank Chad Bousman for his review of the manuscript.

Disclosure/Conflict of Interest

Lisa Brown was an employee of Myriad Neuroscience during synthesis of this chapter and is a current stockholder of Myriad Genetics.

References

1. Mrazek DA, Hornberger JC, Altar CA, Degtiar I. A review of the clinical, economic, and societal burden of treatment-resistant depression: 1996–2013. *Psychiatric Serv.* 2014;65(8):977–987 https://doi.org/10.1176/appi.ps.201300059.
2. Papakostas GI, Fava M. Does the probability of receiving placebo influence clinical trial outcome? A meta-regression of double-blind, randomized clinical trials in MDD. *Eur Neuropsychopharmacol.* 2009;19(1):34–40 https://doi.org/10.1016/j.euroneuro.2008.08.009.
3. Warden D, Rush AJ, Trivedi MH, Fava M, Wisniewski SR. The STAR*D Project results: a comprehensive review of findings. *Curr Psychiatry Rep.* 2007;9(6):449–459 https://doi.org/10.1007/s11920-007-0061-3.
4. Hasin DS, Sarvet AL, Meyers JL, et al. Epidemiology of Adult DSM-5 Major Depressive Disorder and Its Specifiers in the United States. *JAMA Psychiatry.* 2018;75(4):336–346 https://doi.org/10.1001/jamapsychiatry.2017.4602.
5. Tanner JA, Hensel J, Davies PE, Brown LC, Dechairo BM, Mulsant BH. Economic burden of depression and associated resource use in Manitoba, Canada. *Can J Psychiatry.* 2019:706743719895342.
6. Sussman M, O'Sullivan A K, Shah A, Olfson M, Menzin J. Economic burden of treatment-resistant depression on the U.S. health care system. *J Manag Care Specialty Pharm.* 2019;25(7):823–835 https://doi.org/10.18553/jmcp.2019.25.7.823.
7. Hack LM, Fries GR, Eyre HA, et al. Moving pharmacoepigenetics tools for depression toward clinical use. *J Affect Disord.* 2019;249:336–346 https://doi.org/10.1016/j.jad.2019.02.009.
8. Rutledge RB, Chekroud AM, Huys QJ. Machine learning and big data in psychiatry: toward clinical applications. *Current Opin Neurobiol.* 2019;55:152–159 https://doi.org/10.1016/j.conb.2019.02.006.
9. Athreya AP, Iyer R, Wang L, Weinshilboum RM, Bobo WV. Integration of machine learning and pharmacogenomic biomarkers for predicting response to antidepressant treatment: can computational intelligence be used to augment clinical assessments? *Pharmacogenomics.* 2019;20(14):983–988 https://doi.org/10.2217/pgs-2019-0119.
10. Arandjelovic K, Eyre HA, Lenze E, Singh AB, Berk M, Bousman C. The role of depression pharmacogenetic decision support tools in shared decision making. *J Neural Transmiss (Vienna, Austria: 1996).* 2017 https://doi.org/10.1007/s00702-017-1806-8.
11. Bousman CA, Arandjelovic K, Mancuso SG, Eyre HA, Dunlop BW. Pharmacogenetic tests and depressive symptom remission: a meta-analysis of randomized controlled trials. *Pharmacogenomics.* 2019;20(1):37–47 https://doi.org/10.2217/pgs-2018-0142.
12. Grice EA, Segre JA. The human microbiome: our second genome. *Annu Rev Genomics Hum Genet.* 2012;13:151–170 https://doi.org/10.1146/annurev-genom-090711-163814.
13. Saad R, Rizkallah MR, Aziz RK. Gut Pharmacomicrobiomics: the tip of an iceberg of complex interactions between drugs and gut-associated microbes. *Gut Pathog.* 2012;4(1):16 https://doi.org/10.1186/1757-4749-4-16.
14. Doestzada M, Vila AV, Zhernakova A, et al. Pharmacomicrobiomics: a novel route towards personalized medicine? *Protein Cell.* 2018;9(5):432–445 https://doi.org/10.1007/s13238-018-0547-2.

15. Francino MP. Antibiotics and the human gut microbiome: dysbioses and accumulation of resistances. *Front Microbiol.* 2016;6(1543) https://doi.org/10.3389/fmicb.2015.01543.

16. Clapp M, Aurora N, Herrera L, Bhatia M, Wilen E, Wakefield S. Gut microbiota's effect on mental health: the gut–brain axis. *Clinic Pract.* 2017;7(4):987 https://doi.org/10.4081/cp.2017.987.

17. Jiang H, Ling Z, Zhang Y, et al. Altered fecal microbiota composition in patients with major depressive disorder. *Brain Behav Immun.* 2015;48:186–194 https://doi.org/10.1016/j.bbi.2015.03.016.

18. Zoetendal EG, Rajilic-Stojanovic M, de Vos WM. High-throughput diversity and functionality analysis of the gastrointestinal tract microbiota. *Gut.* 2008;57(11):1605–1615 https://doi.org/10.1136/gut.2007.133603.

19. Mariat D, Firmesse O, Levenez F, et al. The Firmicutes/Bacteroidetes ratio of the human microbiota changes with age. *BMC Microbiol.* 2009;9:123 https://doi.org/10.1186/1471-2180-9-123.

20. De Filippo C, Cavalieri D, Di Paola M, et al. Impact of diet in shaping gut microbiota revealed by a comparative study in children from Europe and rural Africa. *P Natl Acad Sci U S A.* 2010;107(33):14691–14696 https://doi.org/10.1073/pnas.1005963107.

21. Huang Y, Shi X, Li Z, et al. Possible association of Firmicutes in the gut microbiota of patients with major depressive disorder. *Neuropsychiatr Dis Treat.* 2018;14:3329–3337.

22. Madan A, Thompson D, Fowler JC, et al. The gut microbiota is associated with psychiatric symptom severity and treatment outcome among individuals with serious mental illness. *Journal of Affective Disorders.* 2020;264:98–106 https://doi.org/10.1016/j.jad.2019.12.020.

23. Aizawa E, Tsuji H, Asahara T, et al. Possible association of Bifidobacterium and Lactobacillus in the gut microbiota of patients with major depressive disorder. *J Affect Disord.* 2016;202:254–257 https://doi.org/10.1016/j.jad.2016.05.038.

24. Lurie I, Yang YX, Haynes K, Mamtani R, Boursi B. Antibiotic exposure and the risk for depression, anxiety, or psychosis: a nested case-control study. *J Clin Psychiatry.* 2015;76(11):1522–1528 https://doi.org/10.4088/jcp.15m09961.

25. Kohler O, Petersen L, Mors O, et al. Infections and exposure to anti-infective agents and the risk of severe mental disorders: a nationwide study. *Acta Psychiatr Scand.* 2017;135(2):97–105 https://doi.org/10.1111/acps.12671.

26. Capuron L, Miller AH. Cytokines and psychopathology: lessons from interferon-alpha. *Biologic Psychiatr.* 2004;56(11):819–824 https://doi.org/10.1016/j.biopsych.2004.02.009.

27. Capuron L, Ravaud A, Miller AH, Dantzer R. Baseline mood and psychosocial characteristics of patients developing depressive symptoms during interleukin-2 and/or interferon-alpha cancer therapy. *Brain, behavior, and immunity.* 2004;18(3):205–213 https://doi.org/10.1016/j.bbi.2003.11.004.

28. Inserra A, Rogers GB, Licinio J, Wong ML. The microbiota-inflammasome hypothesis of major depression. *BioEssays.* 2018;40(9):e1800027 https://doi.org/10.1002/bies.201800027.

29. Enright EF, Gahan CG, Joyce SA, Griffin BT. The impact of the gut microbiota on drug metabolism and clinical outcome. *Yale J Biol Med.* 2016;89(3):375–382.

30. Wilson ID, Nicholson JK. Gut microbiome interactions with drug metabolism, efficacy, and toxicity. *Transl Res.* 2017;179:204–222 https://doi.org/10.1016/j.trsl.2016.08.002.

31. Zhang J, Zhang J, Wang R. Gut microbiota modulates drug pharmacokinetics. *Drug Metabol Rev.* 2018;50(3):357–368 https://doi.org/10.1080/03602532.2018.1497647.

32. Bahra SM, Weidemann BJ, Castro AN, et al. Risperidone-induced weight gain is mediated through shifts in the gut microbiome and suppression of energy expenditure. *EBioMedicine.* 2015;2(11):1725–1734 https://doi.org/10.1016/j.ebiom.2015.10.018.

33. Kao AC-C, Spitzer S, Anthony DC, Lennox B, Burnet PWJ. Prebiotic attenuation of olanzapine-induced weight gain in rats: analysis of central and peripheral

biomarkers and gut microbiota. *Transl Psychiatry.* 2018;8(1):66 https://doi.org/10.1038/s41398-018-0116-8.

34. Skonieczna-Zydecka K, Loniewski I, Misera A, et al. Second-generation antipsychotics and metabolism alterations: a systematic review of the role of the gut microbiome. *Psychopharmacology.* 2019;236(5):1491–1512.

35. Yang C, Qu Y, Fujita Y, et al. Possible role of the gut microbiota-brain axis in the antidepressant effects of (R)-ketamine in a social defeat stress model. *Transl Psychiatry.* 2017;7(12):1294 https://doi.org/10.1038/s41398-017-0031-4.

36. Takeno S, Sakai T. Involvement of the intestinal microflora in nitrazepam-induced teratogenicity in rats and its relationship to nitroreduction. *Teratology.* 1991;44(2):209–214 https://doi.org/10.1002/tera.1420440209.

37. Bjorkholm B, Bok CM, Lundin A, Rafter J, Hibberd ML, Pettersson S. Intestinal microbiota regulate xenobiotic metabolism in the liver. *PLoS One.* 2009;4(9):e6958 https://doi.org/10.1371/journal.pone.0006958.

38. Stavropoulou E, Pircalabioru GG, Bezirtzoglou E. The role of cytochromes P450 in infection. *Front Immunol.* 2018;9:89 https://doi.org/10.3389/fimmu.2018.00089.

39. Das A, Srinivasan M, Ghosh TS, Mande SS. Xenobiotic metabolism and gut microbiomes. *PloS One.* 2016;11(10):e0163099 https://doi.org/10.1371/journal.pone.0163099.

40. Clayton TA, Baker D, Lindon JC, Everett JR, Nicholson JK. Pharmacometabonomic identification of a significant host-microbiome metabolic interaction affecting human drug metabolism. *P Natl Acad Sci U S A.* 2009;106(34):14728–14733 https://doi.org/10.1073/pnas.0904489106.

41. Slyepchenko A, Maes M, Jacka FN, et al. Gut microbiota, bacterial translocation, and interactions with diet: pathophysiological links between major depressive disorder and noncommunicable medical comorbidities. *Psychother Psychosomat.* 2017;86(1):31–46 https://doi.org/10.1159/000448957.

42. Slyepchenko A, Carvalho AF, Cha DS, Kasper S, McIntyre RS. Gut emotions: mechanisms of action of probiotics as novel therapeutic targets for depression and anxiety disorders. *CNS Neurol Dis Drug Target.* 2014;13(10):1770–1786.

43. Wallace CJK, Foster JA, Soares CN, Milev RV. The effects of probiotics on symptoms of depression: protocol for a double-blind randomized placebo-controlled trial. *Neuropsychobiology.* 2020;79(1):108–116.

44. Kalaycı S, Demirci S, Sahin F. Antimicrobial properties of various psychotropic drugs against broad range microorganisms. *Curr Psychopharmacol.* 2014;3(3):195–202.

45. Munoz-Bellido JL, Munoz-Criado S, Garcia-Rodriguez JA. Antimicrobial activity of psychotropic drugs: selective serotonin reuptake inhibitors. *Int J Antimicrob Agents.* 2000;14(3):177–180 https://doi.org/10.1016/s0924-8579(99)00154-5.

46. Bohnert JA, Szymaniak-Vits M, Schuster S, Kern WV. Efflux inhibition by selective serotonin reuptake inhibitors in Escherichia coli. *J Antimicrob Chemother.* 2011;66(9):2057–2060 https://doi.org/10.1093/jac/dkr258.

47. Ayaz M, Subhan F, Ahmed J, et al. Citalopram and venlafaxine differentially augments antimicrobial properties of antibiotics. *Acta Poloniae Pharmaceutica-Drug Res.* 2015;72(6):1269–1278.

48. Samanta A, Debprasad C, Chandrima S, et al. Evaluation of in vivo and in vitro antimicrobial activities of a selective serotonin reuptake inhibitor sertraline hydrochloride. *Anti-Infective Agents.* 2012;10(2):95–104 https://doi.org/10.2174/2211362611208020095.

49. Ferreira DD, Mesquita JT, da Costa Silva TA, et al. Efficacy of sertraline against Trypanosoma cruzi: an in vitro and in silico study. *J Venom Animal Toxin.* 2018;24(1):30 https://doi.org/10.1186/s40409-018-0165-8.

50. Palit P, Ali N. Oral therapy with sertraline, a selective serotonin reuptake inhibitor, shows activity against Leishmania donovani. *J Antimicrob Chemother*. 2008;61(5):1120–1124 https://doi.org/10.1093/jac/dkn046.

51. Munoz-Criado S, Munoz-Bellido JL, Garcia-Rodriguez JA. In vitro activity of nonsteroidal anti-inflammatory agents, phenotiazines, and antidepressants against Brucella species. *Eur J Clin Microbiol Infect Dis*. 1996;15(5):418–420.

52. Lass-Florl C, Dierich MP, Fuchs D, Semenitz E, Jenewein I, Ledochowski M. Antifungal properties of selective serotonin reuptake inhibitors against Aspergillus species in vitro. *J Antimicrob Chemother*. 2001;48(6):775–779 https://doi.org/10.1093/jac/48.6.775.

53. Lass-Florl C, Ledochowski M, Fuchs D, et al. Interaction of sertraline with Candida species selectively attenuates fungal virulence in vitro. *FEMS Immunol Med Microbiol*. 2003;35(1):11–15 https://doi.org/10.1016/s0928-8244(02)00422-4.

54. Cong L, Liao Y, Yang S, Yang R. In vitro antifungal activity of sertraline and synergistic effects in combination with antifungal drugs against planktonic forms and biofilms of clinical *Trichosporon asahii* isolates. *PloS One*. 2016;11(12):e0167903 https://doi.org/10.1371/journal.pone.0167903.

55. Taylor D, Walden JC, Robins AH, Smith PJ. Role of the neurotransmitter reuptake-blocking activity of antidepressants in reversing chloroquine resistance in vitro in *Plasmodium falciparum*. *Antimicrob Agents Chemother*. 2000;44(10):2689–2692 https://doi.org/10.1128/aac.44.10.2689-2692.2000.

56. Jin M, Lu J, Chen Z, et al. Antidepressant fluoxetine induces multiple antibiotics resistance in Escherichia coli via ROS-mediated mutagenesis. *Environ Int*. 2018;120:421–430 https://doi.org/10.1016/j.envint.2018.07.046.

57. Molnar J. Antiplasmid activity of tricyclic compounds. *Methods Find Exp Clin Pharmacol*. 1988;10(7):467–474.

58. Csiszar K, Molnar J. Mechanism of action of tricyclic drugs on Escherichia coli and Yersinia enterocolitica plasmid maintenance and replication. *Anticancer Res*. 1992;12(6B):2267–2272.

59. Bitonti AJ, Sjoerdsma A, McCann PP, et al. Reversal of chloroquine resistance in malaria parasite *Plasmodium falciparum* by desipramine. *Science*. 1988;242(4883):1301–1303 https://doi.org/10.1126/science.3057629.

60. Salama A, Facer CA. Desipramine reversal of chloroquine resistance in wild isolates of *Plasmodium falciparum*. *Lancet*. 1990;335(8682):164–165 https://doi.org/10.1016/0140-6736(90)90034-3.

61. Zilberstein D, Dwyer DM. Antidepressants cause lethal disruption of membrane function in the human protozoan parasite Leishmania. *Science*. 1984;226(4677):977–979 https://doi.org/10.1126/science.6505677.

62. Dinesh N, Kaur PK, Swamy KK, Singh S. Mianserin, an antidepressant kills Leishmania donovani by depleting ergosterol levels. *Experiment Parasitol*. 2014;144:84–90 https://doi.org/10.1016/j.exppara.2014.06.004.

63. Nayak R, Xu J. Effects of sertraline hydrochloride and fluconazole combinations on *Cryptococcus neoformans* and *Cryptococcus gattii*. *Mycology*. 2010;1(2):99–105 https://doi.org/10.1080/21501203.2010.487054.

64. Trevino-Rangel Rde J, Villanueva-Lozano H, Hernandez-Rodriguez P, et al. Activity of sertraline against *Cryptococcus neoformans*: in vitro and in vivo assays. *Med Mycology*. 2016;54(3):280–286.

65. Zhai B, Wu C, Wang L, Sachs MS, Lin X. The antidepressant sertraline provides a promising therapeutic option for neurotropic cryptococcal infections. *Antimicrob Agents Chemother*. 2012;56(7):3758–3766 https://doi.org/10.1128/aac.00212-12.

66. Kornhuber J, Tripal P, Reichel M, et al. Functional inhibitors of acid sphingomyelinase (FIASMAs): a novel pharmacological group of drugs with broad clinical applications. *Cell Physiol Biochem.* 2010;26(1):9–20 https://doi.org/10.1159/000315101.

67. Cockburn CL, Green RS, Damle SR, et al. Functional inhibition of acid sphingomyelinase disrupts infection by intracellular bacterial pathogens. *Life Sci Alliance.* 2019;2(2):e201800292 https://doi.org/10.26508/lsa.201800292.

68. Cebra JJ. Influences of microbiota on intestinal immune system development. *Am J Clin Nutri.* 1999;69(5):1046s–1051s https://doi.org/10.1093/ajcn/69.5.1046s.

69. Neish AS. Microbes in gastrointestinal health and disease. *Gastroenterology.* 2009;136(1):65–80 https://doi.org/10.1053/j.gastro.2008.10.080.

70. Zhang JC, Yao W, Dong C, et al. Blockade of interleukin-6 receptor in the periphery promotes rapid and sustained antidepressant actions: a possible role of gut-microbiota-brain axis. *Translation Psychiatry.* 2017;7(5):e1138 https://doi.org/10.1038/tp.2017.112.

71. Williamson LL, Sholar PW, Mistry RS, Smith SH, Bilbo SD. Microglia and memory: modulation by early-life infection. *J Neurosci.* 2011;31(43):15511–15521 https://doi.org/10.1523/jneurosci.3688-11.2011.

72. Huang N, Hua D, Zhan G, et al. Role of *Actinobacteria* and Coriobacteriia in the antidepressant effects of ketamine in an inflammation model of depression. *Pharmacol Biochem Behav.* 2019;176:93–100 https://doi.org/10.1016/j.pbb.2018.12.001.

73. Qu Y, Yang C, Ren Q, Ma M, Dong C, Hashimoto K. Comparison of (R)-ketamine and lanicemine on depression-like phenotype and abnormal composition of gut microbiota in a social defeat stress model. *Sci Rep.* 2017;7(1):15725 https://doi.org/10.1038/s41598-017-16060-7.

74. Getachew B, Aubee JI, Schottenfeld RS, Csoka AB, Thompson KM, Tizabi Y. Ketamine interactions with gut-microbiota in rats: relevance to its antidepressant and anti-inflammatory properties. *BMC Microbiol* 2018;18(1):222 https://doi.org/10.1186/s12866-018-1373-7.

75. Bravo JA, Forsythe P, Chew MV, et al. Ingestion of Lactobacillus strain regulates emotional behavior and central GABA receptor expression in a mouse via the vagus nerve. *P Natl Acad Scie U S A.* 2011;108(38):16050–16055 https://doi.org/10.1073/pnas.1102999108.

76. Liang S, Wu X, Hu X, Wang T, Jin F. Recognizing depression from the microbiota(–)gut(–) brain axis. *Int J Mol Sci.* 2018;19(6) https://doi.org/10.3390/ijms19061592.

77. Zheng P, Zeng B, Zhou C, et al. Gut microbiome remodeling induces depressive-like behaviors through a pathway mediated by the host's metabolism. *Mol Psychiatry.* 2016;21(6):786–796 https://doi.org/10.1038/mp.2016.44.

78. Kelly JR, Borre Y, C OB, et al. Transferring the blues: depression-associated gut microbiota induces neurobehavioural changes in the rat. *J Psychiatric Res.* 2016;82:109–118 https://doi.org/10.1016/j.jpsychires.2016.07.019.

79. Evrensel A, Ceylan ME. Fecal microbiota transplantation and its usage in neuropsychiatric disorders. *Clin Psychopharmacol Neurosci.* 2016;14(3):231–237 https://doi.org/10.9758/cpn.2016.14.3.231.

80. Bastiaanssen TFS, Cowan CSM, Claesson MJ, Dinan TG, Cryan JF. Making sense of … the microbiome in psychiatry. *Int J Neuropsychopharmacol.* 2019;22(1):37–52 https://doi.org/10.1093/ijnp/pyy067.

81. Benton D, Williams C, Brown A. Impact of consuming a milk drink containing a probiotic on mood and cognition. *Euro J Clin Nutrition.* 2007;61(3):355–361 https://doi.org/10.1038/sj.ejcn.1602546.

82. Messaoudi M, Violle N, Bisson JF, Desor D, Javelot H, Rougeot C. Beneficial psychological effects of a probiotic formulation (*Lactobacillus helveticus* R0052 and *Bifidobacterium longum* R0175) in healthy human volunteers. *Gut Microbes.* 2011;2(4):256–261 https://doi.org/10.4161/gmic.2.4.16108.

83. Barthow C, Wickens K, Stanley T, et al. The Probiotics in Pregnancy Study (PiP Study): rationale and design of a double-blind randomised controlled trial to improve maternal health during pregnancy and prevent infant eczema and allergy. *BMC Pregn Childbirth*. 2016;16(1):133 https://doi.org/10.1186/s12884-016-0923-y.

84. Slykerman RF, Hood F, Wickens K, et al. Effect of *Lactobacillus rhamnosus* HN001 in pregnancy on postpartum symptoms of depression and anxiety: a randomised double-blind placebo-controlled trial. *EBioMedicine*. 2017;24:159–165 https://doi.org/10.1016/j.ebiom.2017.09.013.

85. Akkasheh G, Kashani-Poor Z, Tajabadi-Ebrahimi M, et al. Clinical and metabolic response to probiotic administration in patients with major depressive disorder: a randomized, double-blind, placebo-controlled trial. *Nutrition (Burbank, Calif)*. 2016;32(3):315–320 https://doi.org/10.1016/j.nut.2015.09.003.

86. Kazemi A, Noorbala AA, Azam K, Eskandari MH, Djafarian K. Effect of probiotic and prebiotic vs placebo on psychological outcomes in patients with major depressive disorder: a randomized clinical trial. *Clin Nutrition (Edinburgh, Scotland)*. 2019;38(2):522–528 https://doi.org/10.1016/j.clnu.2018.04.010.

87. Romijn AR, Rucklidge JJ, Kuijer RG, Frampton C. A double-blind, randomized, placebo-controlled trial of *Lactobacillus helveticus* and *Bifidobacterium longum* for the symptoms of depression. *Austr N Z J Psychiatry*. 2017;51(8):810–821 https://doi.org/10.1177/0004867416686694.

88. Bambling M, Edwards SC, Hall S, Vitetta L. A combination of probiotics and magnesium orotate attenuate depression in a small SSRI resistant cohort: an intestinal anti-inflammatory response is suggested. *Inflammopharmacology*. 2017;25(2):271–274 https://doi.org/10.1007/s10787-017-0311-x.

89. Ng QX, Peters C, Ho CYX, Lim DY, Yeo WS. A meta-analysis of the use of probiotics to alleviate depressive symptoms. *J Affect Disord*. 2018;228:13–19 https://doi.org/10.1016/j.jad.2017.11.063.

90. Liu RT, Walsh RFL, Sheehan AE. Prebiotics and probiotics for depression and anxiety: a systematic review and meta-analysis of controlled clinical trials. *Neurosci Biobehav Rev*. 2019;102:13–23 https://doi.org/10.1016/j.neubiorev.2019.03.023.

91. Rea K, Dinan TG, Cryan JF. Gut microbiota: a perspective for psychiatrists. *Neuropsychobiology*. 2020;79(1):50–62.

92. Savignac HM, Corona G, Mills H, et al. Prebiotic feeding elevates central brain derived neurotrophic factor, N-methyl-D-aspartate receptor subunits and D-serine. *Neurochem Int*. 2013;63(8):756–764 https://doi.org/10.1016/j.neuint.2013.10.006.

93. Lee BH, Kim YK. The roles of BDNF in the pathophysiology of major depression and in antidepressant treatment. *Psychiatry Investig*. 2010;7(4):231–235 https://doi.org/10.4306/pi.2010.7.4.231.

94. Yahfoufi N, Matar C, Ismail N. Adolescence and aging: impact of adolescence inflammatory stress and microbiota alterations on brain development, aging and neurodegeneration. *J Gerontol Series A Biol Sci Med Sci*. 2020 https://doi.org/10.1093/gerona/glaa006.

95. Chang X, Wang S, Zhao S, et al. Extracellular vesicles with possible roles in gut intestinal tract homeostasis and IBD. *Mediator Inflamm*. 2020;2020:1945832. https://doi.org/10.1155/2020/1945832.

96. Brown L, Wolf JM, Prados-Rosales R, Casadevall A. Through the wall: extracellular vesicles in gram-positive bacteria, mycobacteria and fungi. *Nat Rev Microbiol*. 2015;13(10):620–630 https://doi.org/10.1038/nrmicro3480.

97. West CL, Stanisz AM, Mao Y-K, Champagne-Jorgensen K, Bienenstock J, Kunze WA. Microvesicles from *Lactobacillus reuteri* (DSM-17938) completely reproduce modulation of gut motility by bacteria in mice. *PloS One*. 2020;15(1):e0225481 https://doi.org/10.1371/journal.pone.0225481.

23

Blockchain for Convergence Science in Mental Health

Wendy Charles

Blockchain is a data management technology that brings together many older forms of record-keeping in a novel way. The concept of blockchain was popularized in a white paper written by an individual (or individuals) using the pseudonym Satoshi Nakamoto.[1] Written during the peak of the 2008 recession, this paper advocated for a trustless peer-to-peer financial transaction system that did not rely on a central intermediary. The white paper's resulting interest led to the creation of the bitcoin network and the first practical use of a blockchain.[2] As blockchain technology has evolved, applications were developed for manufacturing, banking, supply chain, healthcare, and many other industries.[3,4]

Blockchain Introduction

To introduce blockchain concepts to an audience that may not have had much exposure, these concepts are introduced with basic examples, but the reader is cautioned that the actual technology is considerably more sophisticated. Because there is some disagreement about definition of blockchain,[5,6] the term *blockchain* in this chapter refers to all forms of digital ledger technologies. The term *transaction* in a healthcare setting is defined as any new data created, exchanged, or uploaded as part of a healthcare interaction.[7] Other blockchain definitions are provided as applicable concepts are introduced.

Blockchain Features

Ledgers

The core of blockchain technology involves ledgers.[8] A ledger is a record-keeping strategy that first appeared in ancient Babylon to record trades of goods and commodities.[9] Similar to writing an entry with ink on a separate line on a piece of paper, each new transaction on a blockchain is recorded as a new separate line on the ledger. In nearly all uses of blockchain, information cannot be deleted from the ledger, but corrections can be appended as new lines.[10] When the number of transactions reaches a prescribed limit, the ledger is wrapped into a block using the programming determined by the nature of blockchain platform so that no more transactions can be added to the block.[11] This activity is analogous to writing entries of a piece on paper until the page is full, tearing the page off the notepad, and folding it up so that no additional lines can be written to the page.

Cryptography

The second primary feature of blockchain involves cryptography, an old methodology of delivering messages in secret code.[12] Blockchain platforms use cryptography "keys" analogous to a password for electronic addresses and/or electronic signatures,[13] with frequent uses of cryptographic "hash" functions. The National Institute of Standards and Technology describes "hashing" as "a method of applying a cryptographic hash function to data, which calculates a relatively unique output (called a *message digest* or just *digest*) for an input of nearly any size (e.g., a file, text, or image)." [14p7] These one-way hashes are created so that it would be impossible to calculate the hash input using only the resulting hash output.

The cryptographic hashes are the critical component of how blocks are linked together in a chain. As shown in Figure 23.1, the block header contains basic information about each block, including a single hash that summarizes all contents of the block. The header also includes the summary hash for the previous block in the sequence and typically includes a "Merkle Tree," which is a single hash that represents the entire blockchain structure.[14] Because the summary hash of a block is included in the header of subsequent block, it would be extremely difficult to change the contents within a

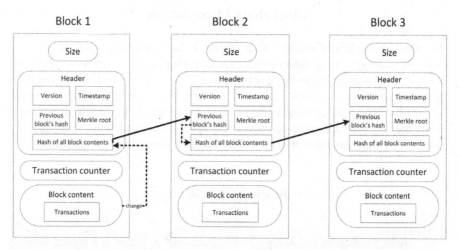

Figure 23.1 Nature and organization of information stored in a typical block. Blocks are linked as a chain when the hash representing all block contents in one block is also saved in next generated block, and so on (shown with solid arrows). The blockchain is tamper-resistant because if there is an attempt to change the contents in one block (shown with the dashed arrow), it would change the hash representing all block contents in that block. Because that hash is also saved in the next block, that block's hash representing all block contents must be changed, and so on for all subsequent blocks in the chain.

block. (While many blockchain publications describe blockchain as being "immutable," the National Institute of Standards and Technology[14] explains that there are situations where a blockchain could be modified and instead asserts that blockchain technology should be described as "tamper evident" and "tamper resistant.")

Distribution

The third primary feature of blockchain involves the nature and distribution of storage. For most medical record storage, computing devices login to a central server. However, with use of any single server, the server is vulnerable to accidental data deletion, data corruption, downtime, computer viruses, and malware and could be taken ransom by a malicious external party.[10] To preserve data integrity with redundancy, the entire blockchain ledger is stored on all of the computing devices, referred to as "nodes," that serve as data hosts for the network.[14] Further, in this peer-to-peer network, all computing devices can communicate directly with one another instead of having to go through a central intermediary.[14]

Public and Private Networks

There are two common types of blockchain networks: public (permissionless) and private (permissioned). With public blockchains, such as the Bitcoin and Ethereum networks, anyone can join the network without receiving permission to do so, and individuals or groups provide their own computers and processing power to support their roles as nodes on the network. Transactions are publicly available and participants' identities are known only by their hash addresses.[1] As of October 2019, there were nearly 10,000 active nodes on the Bitcoin network, demonstrating strength in numbers to resist data tampering.[15]

Private blockchains are maintained by individual organizations. Consensus blockchains are private blockchains shared among trusted organizations.[16] To join a private blockchain, individuals or organizations must receive permission to participate in the blockchain. With consortia, there is shared governance and support for blockchain operations. Roles are assigned to perform approval and/or maintenance functions,[17] and access to private information is typically limited within organizations to their own data. As an example of a private blockchain, Hyperledger was founded by the Linux Foundation as an open source private enterprise blockchain to allow for private and secure transactions commonly used in banking and healthcare.[18]

Consensus

Because blockchain ledgers are verified and (typically) stored by all nodes on the network, it is critical that all nodes can reach agreement about which blocks can be added to the blockchain. This form of agreement is referred to as "consensus."[19] There are currently 66 different types of consensus protocols across blockchain networks that all offer consistency, network support, and fault tolerance.[16] As examples of

---

[1] To view examples of hash addresses and visible transactions, perform an internet search using the terms "Blockchain.com," "hash," and "address." Click on one of the addresses to view the address's hash identification and the nature of information stored with each transaction.

consensus protocols, the Bitcoin network uses Proof of Work where nodes perform intensive computing (using high quantities of electricity) to solve difficult computational puzzles.[14] The other nodes on the network must compute the hash to verify the requirements. Private, permissioned blockchains use a variety of efficient consensus protocols (that do not require intensive computation) where only authorized nodes participate in consensus and have read/write permissions.[16]

Smart Contracts
Contrary to the term applied to this concept, smart contracts are neither "smart" nor "contracts." Smart contracts involve adding programming code to the blockchain that executes when predetermined conditions are met.[20] As an example, smart contracts are envisioned for remote health monitoring to alert healthcare providers of critical health events.[21] Because smart contracts can improve efficiency by eliminating human involvement, they offer the potential for cost savings and increased accuracy.[22]

How Blocks Are Added to the Chain

Taking into account all the previously discussed features of blockchain, the process of adding a block to a chain is illustrated in Figure 23.2. When a new transaction is formed (say, by generating new healthcare data from a patient visit to a psychiatrist's

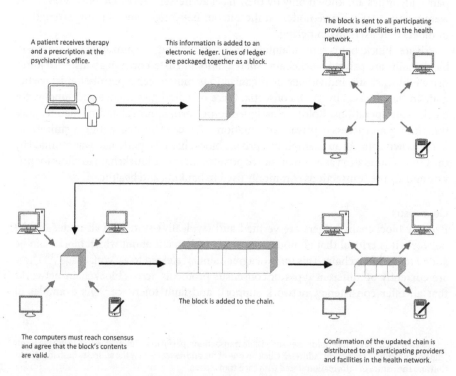

Figure 23.2 Typical steps of block formation in a blockchain.

office), the new information is added to the ledger. When there are enough ledger entries, the ledger is packaged together as a block. The block is transmitted to all participating nodes on the network. The nodes must then reach consensus and agree that the block's contents are valid. The block is added to the chain, and the updated chain is distributed to all participating nodes in the network.[23]

Real-World Uses of Blockchain in Healthcare

Because most uses of blockchain in mental health are in pilot stages of development, this chapter will first describe a few blockchains in production.

Securing Access to Medical Records

Starting in 2016, the Republic of Estonia used blockchain technology to secure the privacy of health records by adding a blockchain layer that tracks access to a patient's health records within the Estonian eHealth system.[24] The electronic health records are stored in a traditional database. Each time the patient's medical record is accessed or altered, the activity is stored with a timestamp on the blockchain.[25] At any point, patients can see which individuals had accessed their health records. The blockchain also adds granular consent mechanisms for future access to health records.[26] Specifically, any patient can explicitly authorize or restrict access to family members and/or care providers, including one's own family physician. Patients also have the opportunity to allow or deny uses of their health data for clinical research.[26]

Consolidations of HHS Contracts

The U.S. Department of Health and Human Services (HHS) implemented a blockchain to improve contract efficiency. This federal department executes nearly 1 million contracts over an 18-month period.[27] With five disparate contracting systems, there were inefficiencies of data collection and business processes. HHS chief information officer, Jose Arrieta, placed a blockchain on top of the contracting systems to pull and clean contract-related data.[27] Adding a microservices model that performs natural language processing and machine learning (forms of artificial intelligence [AI]) to read the conditions of contracts pulled from the blockchain, the model analyzes the terms and determines ranges of prices.[28] The blockchain/AI layer performs analyses in seconds that would have taken an HHS employee several months.[27] Arrieta estimated that the blockchain/AI implementation realized an 800% return on investment.[28]

Consortium of Colorado Health Data Organizations

In a project funded by the Colorado State Innovation Model, a federally funded initiative through the Colorado Governor's Office, three health data organizations in

Colorado placed their clinical quality measures on a blockchain.[29-31] According to Amber Hartley, the chief corporate development officer for BurstIQ (the blockchain platform provider), the blockchain allows each organization to have direct control over its own data, while allowing each to perform analyses on the aggregate data of all three organizations without being able to access the individual data points from the other organizations (personal communication, October 9, 2019). The blockchain-based partnership has allowed for tremendous efficiency in creating consolidated reports with deep contextualization in a manner that protects the confidentiality of each organization's data.[31]

Food Safety

Food-borne contamination frequently creates risk of widespread illness. For instance, the Centers for Disease Control and Prevention's most recent food safety alert (November 26, 2019) cautions that romaine lettuce from a particular growing region has resulted in *E. coli* infections in 67 people in 19 states, resulting in 39 hospitalizations. In an abundance of caution, grocery stores normally clear their grocery shelves of that type of produce. However, to eliminate national recalls and improve food traceability, IBM Food Trust created a blockchain-based food supply tracking system currently used by Walmart, Dole, Wegmans, and Unilever.[32] In a pilot experiment to assess blockchain efficiency for tracking mangos to their originating farm, Walmart compared the traditional track-and-trace method to a blockchain query. Walmart staff needed seven days using conventional methods to locate the particular farm in Mexico versus 2.2 seconds with the blockchain.[33] Starting September 2019, all Walmart suppliers of leafy green produce were required to use this blockchain or be dropped as suppliers.[32] Walmart has found the use of blockchain to be so effective for improving food traceability and safety that the corporation has expanded blockchain-based pilot projects to track meat, packaged vegetables, seafood, and prescription medications.[33,34]

Potential Uses of Blockchain in Mental Health

As blockchain is increasingly used for healthcare, blockchain utilizes transdisciplinary convergence of expertise. Convergence has created environments of innovation and knowledge sharing to develop specific approaches to blockchain applications. For example, blockchain projects for mental health include representatives from psychiatry and psychology, software engineering, health informatics, robotics, artificial intelligence, regulatory agencies, and computer science.[35,36] Collaborations from these diverse fields are creating innovative methods of treating and diagnosing mental health conditions as shared in the upcoming section.

Blockchain technologies are being developed for many aspects of mental healthcare and delivery—not to replace current data management strategies—but as an additional layer of technology intended to reduce some of the technology limitations of current databases. First, blockchain offers integration of multiple sources of information that would not otherwise be compatible or interoperable.[37] Granular consent mechanisms allow for more control of record access and offer intricate privacy controls not available with other databases.[7] Because blockchain reduces—or can eliminate—intermediaries to manage information, this technology reduces unintentional loss or modification inherent with many records databases, instead delivering a high level of transparency and trust.[11]

The following are examples of how convergence blockchain solutions allow for more innovative mental healthcare, but few of these examples are available commercially as of the date of this publication.

Cybertherapy

Cybertherapy, a reference to internet-based therapy, is a popular option for patients with mental illness seeking information and support. In fact, Barak et al.[38] found that the internet is the primary location where people with mental health concerns sought support and consultation. However, the internet does not offer these individuals sufficient privacy or control regarding how their information is managed. A blockchain-based cybertherapy forum, mHealth-BlockC,[7] was proposed to offer single-session mental health consultations, online peer support, and communication in an pseudonymous manner on the Ethereum network. Individuals could provide granular consent of potential access and uses, which offers extensive control.[7]

Artificial Intelligence

Topol[39] predicts that almost every type of care provider—from psychiatrist to paramedic—will be using AI at some point in the future. The term *artificial intelligence* is intended to encompass many computational domains, such as natural language processing, machine learning, and image processing.[40] AI uses data algorithms to identify predictive relationships between datasets and outcomes.[41] There is another chapter in this book devoted to uses of AI in mental health applications, so AI examples unique for mental health will not be repeated in this chapter. However, because AI is often added to uses of blockchain, this section describes the combination of blockchain and AI.

In a pilot study involving wearable biosensors where data were transmitted to the Ethereum network, Lopez et al.[42] found that AI algorithms could detect and classify mental stress from the data profiles of common consumer wearables. The authors suggest that smart contracts on the blockchain could offer automatic mental health referrals to the type of mental health services that best meet the individuals' needs.[42]

The combination of blockchain and a fog computing framework has been proposed for activity recognition to classify normal versus abnormal activities. Using video monitoring piloted by Islam et al.,[43] machine learning was used to provide safety assessments of patients suffering from mental illness. The AI system extracted frames from the video images to identify and classify activities and then translated these images into action vocabularies. The authors found that the blockchain-based pilot was computationally efficient and promoted high accuracy of activity assessment.[43]

Transaction Identity

Blockchain can provide a unique solution to track highly transient individuals with mental illness. Transaction identity involves a collection of interactions that create an individual's history and standing in society.[37] Individuals with mental illness are often high utilizers of medical services and community interventions, yet their mental illness and sometimes transient living arrangements create the high risk of misdiagnosis, fragmented medical records, and duplication of services.[37] Khurshid et al.[37] proposed a blockchain-based transaction identity management solution. The proposed technology platform—accessible with a smart phone—plans to integrate and store healthcare and social services so that an individual could share any information about services with medical providers and/or social workers.

Management of Mental Health Information

In their paper, "Digital Revolution in Depression: a Technologies Update for Clinicians," Lazar et al.[44] introduced blockchain-based methods of securing medical records to fellow psychiatrists. The authors emphasized that blockchain-based records promote patient ownership. Specifically, healthcare records could be shared at the patient's direction to psychiatrists, researchers, or other parties, reducing the likelihood of fragmented healthcare records.[44] Further, Sanyal[45] suggested that a blockchain-based system for mental health records could provide patients with evidence of the progress they've made and strategies for continuing their progress.

A blockchain company, VitalHub,[46] created a new blockchain-based electronic health record, WellLinc, using the Hyperledger network. The company believes it is the first blockchain-based record storage system specifically designed for mental health services. WellLinc allows for exchange of mental health records and services for easy interoperability across the care providers.[47]

Blockchain-based methods are also proposed for collecting patient reported outcome measures related to management of psychiatric conditions. Because blockchain can provide integration and standardization of incoming information, blockchains can collect data from a wide range of mobile mental health apps.[48] As an example, Ichikawa et al.[49] created an app-based assessment of depression symptoms and added the reported outcomes to the Hyperledger network. Further, patient reported outcomes were found to be tamper-resistant and maintained greater integrity by being distributed among many blockchain nodes.[49]

To enhance privacy and security of standardized questionnaires for mental health conditions, Goldwater[48] proposed a blockchain-based collection platform. Because patients often answer the same standard psychological instruments with many care providers—even within a short period of time—a blockchain-based collection system would allow patients and caregivers to determine when, and to whom, they'd like to share questionnaire results.[48]

Future Directions

When considering addition of blockchain for mental health data management or efficiencies, mental health professionals are advised to consider implementation strategies as well and plan for cultural and technological challenges unique to blockchain.

Implementation

While blockchain seems to offer useful features, blockchain should only be pursued if it could address a specific need in a manner not achievable with available technologies. In the report "Blockchain Beyond the Hype: A Practical Framework for Business Leaders," the World Economic Forum[50] offers a framework of business questions and considerations to determine if blockchain would add value to business models and processes. While blockchain could be implemented in a healthcare organization in a manner similar to traditional health technologies,[51] blockchain implementation may need more education and buy-in among stakeholders and may require adjustments to the business model.[50,52,53]

For blockchain consortia, technical and operational decisions should be addressed early. Participating organizations should plan for how to manage malicious users, how to apply controls, and whether to apply limits to the nature of data that will be placed on the blockchain.[14] There should also be legal discussions about policy, maintenance, engagement of stakeholders for decision-making, and liability.[53]

Challenges

Uncertainties With an Immature Technology

Healthcare organizations tend to be risk averse when introducing new technologies and don't usually want to be early adopters.[54] Because blockchain is novel, healthcare organizations are concerned about uncertain privacy and security risks.[7] Lazar et al.[44] noted that blockchain has "potential to revolutionize the way data are stored,"[(p4)] but more technical issues need to be addressed before it can be adopted with confidence. Because of its immaturity, there is little public or expert knowledge about blockchain, creating challenges for forecasting clear strategies or visions for future uses in healthcare.

While there is great hype about blockchain as "immutable" or "unhackable," Sulkowski reminds that blockchains are "unhackable like the Titanic was unsinkable." [53p10] Blockchains, and particularly smart contracts, have already been hacked in highly publicized failures.[55-57] Destafanis et al.[58] described the concept of error-free code as a "utopia" and noted that blockchain coding is a very new science. Performing extensive testing of smart contracts, in particular, is critical because once smart contracts are added to the blockchain, they cannot be modified.[58]

There should also be planning about potential legal responsibility for oversight of smart contracts when used to manage mental health. If using smart contracts to alert providers about worsening symptoms or potential harms, who is responsible (or liable) if the smart contract fails to trigger an alert?[40] Would it be the person who wrote the smart contract or the care provider?

Regulatory Considerations

To use blockchain for healthcare, it may be necessary to obtain or create documentation of testing and validation for regulatory compliance. While new digital health technologies had been regulated by the U.S. Food and Drug Administration, many forms of digital health technologies are no longer subject to regulation.[59] The 21st Century Cures Act[60] amended the Food and Drug Administration Amendments Act[61] by removing Food and Drug Administration's regulatory jurisdiction over certain technologies. The act also reconciled policy, legal, and scientific conflicts.[59]

When storing protected health information on a blockchain, covered entities (healthcare providers, health plans, and health clearinghouses) must address Health Information Privacy and Portability Act (HIPAA) regulatory requirements. In my role on the Health Information Management and Systems Society Blockchain Task Force, we encouraged covered entities to wait to add protected health information directly on chain until they gain more experience with blockchain.[62] This may be a short wait as some blockchain hosts have already been certified as meeting HIPAA technical safeguards[63] and could assist covered entities with documentation of their administrative and physical safeguards. For the addition of mental health records on a blockchain, there may be additional state statutes to ensure privacy of those sensitive records.[64]

Research Needed

More research should be conducted to understand the effectiveness of using blockchain to advance mental healthcare and record management. Currently, adoption is being hindered by lack of evidence-based data. Many mental health professionals request documentation of evidence-based practice about novel technologies to make informed decisions.[54] Kazgan[54] argues that validation studies that link uses of digital technologies to clinical outcomes are particularly desirable—especially by enrolling research participants who have experienced the mental health condition being studied. These participants should provide critical feedback about the ways in which the technology could enhance the success of the intervention.[65]

Conclusion

Blockchain-based applications for mental health are still in their infancy. When considering blockchain solutions for mental health, mental health professionals are encouraged to learn about blockchain technology to the degree that they could explain basic principles to wary patients and administrators. Blockchain should not be considered a "black box" but a promising new technology. With recognition that mental healthcare is based on interpersonal connections to improve mental well-being, blockchain must advance—or at least not detract—from this critical goal.[65] To make advances in blockchain, it will be important to create partnerships between various stakeholders in many transsectional fields of study. As more evidence is collected to demonstrate its effectiveness, blockchain-based solutions will likely become more widely accepted for uses in mental health.

References

1. Nakamoto S. Bitcoin: a peer-to-peer electronic cash system. https://bitcoin.org/bitcoin.pdf. Published 2008. Updated March 24, 2009. Accessed May 18, 2018.

2. Vaughn Bailey E. Enterprise, history, and change. In: Metcalf D, Bass J, Hooper M, Cahana A, Dhillon V, eds. *Blockchain in Healthcare: Innovations That Empower Patients, Connect Professionals and Improve Care*. Orlando, FL: Merging Traffic; 2019:151–166.

3. Ornes S. Core concept: blockchain offers applications well beyond Bitcoin but faces its own limitations. *Proc Natl Acad Sci USA*. 2019;116(42):20800–20803 https://doi.org/10.1073/pnas.1914849116.

4. Crosby M, Nachiappan, Pattanayak P, Verma S, Kalyanaraman V. Blockchain technology: beyond bitcoin. *Appl Innov Rev*. 2016;2(June):6–10.

5. Richardson M, Gomez U, Wisner T, Abdelkawi A, Salinas W, Santos R. Global blockchain glossary of terms 2.0. Blockchain Training Alliance. https://blockchaintrainingalliance.com/blogs/news/global-blockchain-glossary-of-terms-2-0. Published 2019. Updated April 17, 2019. Accessed Apr 18, 2019.

6. Conte de Leon D, Stalick AQ, Jillepalli AA, Haney MA, Sheldon FT. Blockchain: properties and misconceptions. *Asia Pacific J Innov Entrep*. 2017;11(3):286–300 https://doi.org/10.1108/apjie-12-2017-034.

7. Gebremedhin TA. *Blockchain as a Technology to Facilitate Privacy and Better Health Record Management*. Bergen, Norway: The University of Bergen: Department of Informatics, Western Norway University of Applied Science; 2018.

8. Bennett K, Decker C. Certified Blockchain Business Foundations (CBBF): Official Exam Study Guide, Vol 1.1. *Blockchain Training Alliance*. https://blockchaintrainingalliance.com/collections/blockchain-exam-prep-guides/products/cbbf-official-exam-study-guide. Published 2019. Accessed January 22, 2019.

9. Bookkeeping. *Encyclopaedia Britannica*. https://www.britannica.com/topic/bookkeeping. Published 1998. Updated July 20, 1998. Accessed November 30, 2019.

10. Li H, Zhu L, Shen M, Gao F, Tao X, Liu S. Blockchain-based data preservation system for medical data. *J Med Syst*. 2018;42(8):141. https://doi.org/10.1007/s10916-018-0997-3.

11. Funk E, Riddell J, Ankel F, Cabrera D. Blockchain technology: a data framework to improve validity, trust, and accountability of information exchange in health professions education. *Acad Med*. 2018;93(12):1791–1794 https://doi.org/10.1097/acm.0000000000002326.

12. Hosch WL. Cryptography. *Encyclopaedia Brittanica*. https://www.britannica.com/topic/cryptography. Published 2017. Updated April 13, 2017. Accessed November 30, 2019.

13. Zhao H, Bai P, Peng Y, Xu R. Efficient key management scheme for health blockchain. *CAAI Trans Intell Technol*. 2018;3(2):114–118 https://doi.org/10.1049/trit.2018.0014.

14. Yaga D, Mell P, Roby N, Scarfone K. Blockchain technology overview (NISTIR 8202). Gaithersburg, MD: National Institute of Standards and Technology; October 3 2018.

15. Yeow A. Bitnodes: an estimate of the size of the Bitcoin network by finding all the reachable nodes in the network. *Earn.com.* https://bitnodes.earn.com/dashboard/?days=365. Published *2019*. Updated October 7, 2019. Accessed November 28, 2019.

16. Shahaab A, Lidgey B, Hewage C, Khan I. Applicability and appropriateness of distributed ledgers consensus protocols in public and private sectors: a systematic review. *IEEE Access.* 2019;7:43622–43636 https://doi.org/10.1109/access.2019.2904181.

17. Sato T, Himura Y. *Smart-contract based system operations for permissioned blockchain.* Paper presented at 2018 9th IFIP International Conference on New Technologies, Mobility and Security (NTMS); February 26–28, 2018; Paris, France.

18. Ma C, Kong X, Lan Q, Zhou Z. The privacy protection mechanism of Hyperledger Fabric and its application in supply chain finance. *Cybersecurity.* 2019;2(1):5. https://doi.org/10.1186/s42400–019-0022-2.

19. Tosh DK, Shetty S, Liang X, Kamhoua C, Njilla L. *Consensus protocols for blockchain-based data provenance: challenges and opportunities.* Paper presented at 2017 IEEE 8th Annual Ubiquitous Computing, Electronics and Mobile Communication Conference (UEMCON); October 19–21, 2017; New York, NY https://doi.org/10.1186/s42400-019-0022-2.

20. Chamber of Digital Commerce. "Smart contracts" legal primer. https://digitalchamber.org/wp-content/uploads/2018/02/Smart-Contracts-Legal-Primer-02.01.2018.pdf. Published February 22 2018.

21. Griggs KN, Ossipova O, Kohlios CP, Baccarini AN, Howson EA, Hayajneh T. Healthcare blockchain system using smart contracts for secure automated remote patient monitoring. *J Med Syst.* 2018;42(7):130. https://doi.org/10.1007/s10916-018-0982-x.

22. McKinney SA, Landy R, Wilka R. Smart contracts, blockchain, and the next frontier of transactional law. *Wash J L Tech & Arts.* 2018;13(3):313–347 https://doi.org/10.1007/s10916-018-0982-x.

23. Gupta M. *Blockchain for Dummies.* 2nd ed. Hoboken, NJ: Wiley; 2018: https://www.ibm.com/downloads/cas/36KBMBOG.

24. Heston T. A case study in blockchain healthcare innovation. *Int J Curr Res.* 2017;9(11):60587–60588.

25. Gemalto. Estonian eHealth and the blockchain. https://www.gemalto.com/review/Pages/Estonian-eHealth-and-the-blockchain.aspx. Published 2017. Updated June 21, 2017. Accessed April 30, 2018.

26. Priisalu J, Ottis R. Personal control of privacy and data: Estonian experience. *Health Technol (Berl).* 2017;7(4):441–451 https://doi.org/10.1007/s12553-017-0195-1.

27. Walch K. Adoption of AI and blockchain at HHS: interview with Jose Arrieta, U.S. Department of Health and Human Services (HHS). Forbes. https://www.forbes.com/sites/cognitiveworld/2019/11/04/adoption-of-ai-and-blockchain-at-hhs-interview-with-jose-arrieta-us-department-of-health--human-services-hhs/#5fe3bd4d385d. Published 2019. Updated November 4, 2019. Accessed November 29, 2019.

28. Friedman S. HHS expects ATO for blockchain acquisition solution this month. *FCW.* https://fcw.com/Articles/2018/12/05/hhs-blockchain-ato-friedman.aspx?p=1. Published 2018. Updated December 5, 2018. Accessed November 29, 2019.

29. Mensch J. How can blockchain be used for data sharing? *CORHIO.* https://www.corhio.org/blogs/expertise/2018/9/25/how-can-blockchain-be-used-for-data-sharing. Published 2018. Updated September 25, 2018. Accessed October 8, 2019.

30. Dodson A. How a Denver blockchain firm is making sense of health-care data. *Denver Business Journal.* https://www.bizjournals.com/denver/news/2018/08/20/burstiq-

blockchain-firm-health-care.html Published 2018. Updated August 20, 2018. Accessed October 9, 2019.

31. CORHIO. State innovation model funds first blockchain-enabled data aggregation and reporting collaboration in Colorado. https://www.corhio.org/news/2018/8/27/993-state-innovation-model-funds-first-blockchain-enabled-data-aggregation-and-reporting-collaboration-in-colorado. Published 2018. Updated August 27, 2018. Accessed October 9, 2019.

32. Corkery M, Popper N. From farm to blockchain: Walmart tracks its lettuce. *The New York Times*, September 24, 2018: B1(L).

33. Kamath R. Food traceability on blockchain: Walmart's pork and mango pilots with IBM. *J Br Blockchain Assoc*. 2018;1(1). https://doi.org/10.31585/jbba-1-1-(10)2018.

34. Clark S. Walmart combines blockchain and QR codes to let Chinese consumers verify source of fresh produce in stores. *NFC World*. https://www.nfcworld.com/2019/07/02/363418/walmart-combines-blockchain-and-qr-codes-to-let-chinese-consumers-verify-source-of-fresh-produce-in-stores/. Published 2019. Updated July 2, 2019. Accessed August 3, 2019.

35. Eyre HA, Lavretsky H, Insel TR. Convergence science: shaping 21st century psychiatry. *Psychiatric Times*. https://www.psychiatrictimes.com/schizophrenia/convergence-science-shaping-21st-century-psychiatry/. Published 2015. Updated November 13, 2019. Accessed July 10, 2019.

36. Eyre HA, Lavretsky H, Forbes M, et al. Convergence science arrives: how does it relate to psychiatry? *Acad Psychiatry*. 2017;41(1):91–99 https://doi.org/10.1007/s40596-016-0496-0.

37. Khurshid A, Gadnis A. Using blockchain to create transaction identity for persons experiencing homelessness in America: policy proposal. *JMIR Res Protoc*. 2019;8(3):e10654. https://doi.org/10.2196/10654.

38. Barak A, Klein B, Proudfoot JG. Defining internet-supported therapeutic interventions. 2009;38(1):4–17 https://doi.org/10.1007/s12160-009-9130-7.

39. Topol EJ. High-performance medicine: the convergence of human and artificial intelligence. *Nat Med*. 2019;25(1):44–56 https://doi.org/10.1038/s41591-018-0300-7.

40. Hariman K, Ventriglio A, Bhugra D. The future of digital psychiatry. *Curr Psychiatry Rep*. 2019;21(9):88. https://doi.org/10.1007/s11920-019-1074-4.

41. Global Future Council on Neurotechnologies. Empowering 8 billion minds: enabling better mental health for all via the ethical adoption of technologies. *World Economic Forum*. https://www.weforum.org/whitepapers/empowering-8-billion-minds-enabling-better-mental-health-for-all-via-the-ethical-adoption-of-technologies. Published 2019. Updated July 1, 2019. Accessed August 27, 2019 https://doi.org/10.1007/s11920-019-1074-4.

42. Lopez D, Brown AW, Plans D. Developing opportunities in digital health: the case of BioBeats Ltd. *J Bus Ventur Insights*. 2019;11:e00110. https://doi.org/10.1016/j.jbvi.2019.e00110.

43. Islam N, Faheem Y, Din IU, Talha M, Guizani M, Khalil M. A blockchain-based fog computing framework for activity recognition as an application to e-healthcare services. *Futur Gener Comput Syst*. 2019;100:569–578 https://doi.org/10.1016/j.future.2019.05.059.

44. Lazar MA, Pan Z, Ragguett RM, et al. Digital revolution in depression: a technologies update for clinicians. *Pers Med Psychiatry*. 2017;4:6:1–6 https://doi.org/10.1016/j.pmip.2017.09.001.

45. Sanyal V. Blockchain technology and mental health care in India. *Yourstory.com*. https://yourstory.com/2018/09/blockchain-impact-mental-health-care-india. Published September 3, 2018.

46. Huynh C. VitalHub Corp brings blockchain technology to mental health. *Coinsquare*. https://news.coinsquare.com/blockchain/vitalhub-blockchain-technology-mental-health/. Published 2018. Updated February 17, 2018. Accessed July 7, 2019.

47. VitalHub. Blockchain as a service. https://vitalhub.com/products-and-solutions/blockchain/. Published 2019. Accessed Nov 29, 2019.

48. Goldwater JC. *The Use of a Blockchain to FOSTER the development of Patient-Reported Outcome Measures*. Washington, DC: National Quality Forum; August 8 2016.

49. Ichikawa D, Kashiyama M, Ueno T. Tamper-resistant mobile health using blockchain technology. *JMIR Mhealth Uhealth*. 2017;5(7):e111. https://doi.org/10.2196/mhealth.7938.

50. Mulligan C, Zhu Scott J, Warren S, Rangaswami JP. *Blockchain Beyond the Hype: A Practical Framework for Business Leaders*. Geneva, Switzerland: World Economic Forum; April 23 2018 https://doi.org/10.2196/mhealth.7938.

51. Haugen A, Fred CL. In: Stansfield T, Vuletich IC, eds. *Beyond Implementation: a Prescription for the Adoption of Healthcare Technology*. 2nd ed. Denver, CO: Magnusson-Skor; 2016.

52. Morkunas VJ, Paschen J, Boon E. How blockchain technologies impact your business model. *Bus Horiz*. 2019;62(3):295–306 https://doi.org/10.1016/j.bushor.2019.01.009.

53. Sulkowski AJ. Blockchain, business supply chains, sustainability, and law: the future of governance, legal frameworks, and lawyers? *Del J Corp L*. 2018;43:25. https://doi.org/10.2139/ssrn.3262291.

54. Kazgan M. Real challenge in digital health entrepreneurship: changing human behavior. In: Wulfovich S, Meyers A, eds. *Digital Health Entrepreneurship*. Cham, Switzerland: Springer Nature Switzerland; 2019:7–16.

55. Werbach K, Cornell N. Contracts ex machina. *Duke Law J*. 2017;67:313–382.

56. Xu JJ. Are blockchains immune to all malicious attacks? *Financ Innov*. 2016;2(25):1–9 https://doi.org/10.1186/s40854-016-0046-5.

57. Orcutt M. Once hailed as unhackable, blockchains are now getting hacked. *MIT Technology Review*. https://www.technologyreview.com/s/612974/once-hailed-as-unhackable-blockchains-are-now-getting-hacked/. Published 2019. Updated February 19, 2018. Accessed February 20, 2019.

58. Destefanis G, Marchesi M, Ortu M, Tonelli R, Bracciali A, Hierons R. *Smart contracts vulnerabilities: a call for blockchain software engineering?* Paper presented at the 2018 International Workshop on Blockchain Oriented Software Engineering (IWBOSE); March 20, 2018; Campobasso, Italy.

59. Sapsin J. FDA and digital health. In: Wulfovich S, Meyers A, eds. *Digital Health Entrepreneurship*. Cham, Switzerland: Springer Nature Switzerland; 2019:119–142.

60. 21st Century Cures Act. Pub L.114–225, 130 Stat. 1033 (December 13, 2016).

61. Food and Drug Administration Amendments Act of 2007. Pub L.110–85, 121 Stat. 823 (September 27, 2007).

62. HIMSS Blockchain Task Force. Health Information and Management Systems Society. https://www.himss.org/regulatory-and-compliance. Published 2019. Accessed November 30, 2019.

63. Bennett B. BurstIQ: blockchain platform for securing, analyzing and monetizing all of your PHI. *Blockchain Healthcare Review*. https://blockchainhealthcarereview.com/burstiq-blockchain-platform-for-securing-analyzing-and-monetizing-all-of-your-phi/. Published 2017. Updated July 31, 2017. Accessed November 30, 2019.

64. Stoltzfus Jost T. Contraints on sharing mental health and substance-use treatment information imposed by federal and state medical records privacy laws. In: Institute of Medicine, ed. *Improving the Quality of Health Care for Mental and Substance-Abuse Conditions*. Washington, DC: National Academy of Sciences; 2006.

65. Fortuna KL, Walker R, Fisher DB, Mois G, Allan S, Deegan PE. Enhancing standards and principles in digital mental health with recovery-focused guidelines for mobile, online, and remote monitoring technologies. *Psychiatr Serv*. 2019;70. https://doi.org/10.1176/appi.ps.201900166.

SECTION V

OPERATIONAL ORGANIZATIONS CULTIVATING CONVERGENCE MENTAL HEALTH

24

Global Mental Health and Technology

Examples of the Asia-Pacific Economic Cooperation Digital Hub for Mental Health and the Enhanced Measurement-Based Care Effectiveness in Depression

Chee H. Ng, Victor Li, David Gratzer, and Raymond W. Lam

Introduction

Mental health is an increasingly prioritized area in healthcare. Over 450 million people globally suffer from mental or neurological disorders with widespread impact on families, communities, schools, workplaces, and businesses. Depression, which currently affects over a quarter of a billion people, is already a leading cause of disability.[1] In a decade, the projected total impact of depression, anxiety, and schizophrenia is likely to be the leading cause of mortality and morbidity in the world.[2]

As a response, developed economies in the last several decades have been increasing resource allocation, public awareness, and research to address the growing need. However, developing economies, especially those of low- to middle-income countries (LMICs), face unique barriers to implementing effective mental health systems and continue to have large treatment gaps.

The major barrier for accessing mental health services in LMICs is inadequate human resource. There is a significant shortage of mental healthcare workers globally, especially in LMICs. According to the World Health Organization (WHO), there is about one psychiatrist per 1 million people and three psychiatric nurses per 1 million people in LMICs.[3] What limited resources are available tend to exist in centralized institutions that cannot adequately cover rural communities, and community providers lack capacity to provide adequate mental healthcare.[4] Increasing funding and the number of healthcare workers is necessary, but this is limited by low gross domestic product and low political priority in many LMICs. Expansion of existing healthcare services has been explored[4,5] but remains challenging on an urgent timescale. There is a need for new directions with scalable and efficient solutions to help address the unmet need.

Another significant barrier to mental health is stigma. Negative perceptions toward being mentally unwell act as a barrier to mental health literacy and interfere with an individual's ability to recognize mental health problems and to seek appropriate help.[6] Policymakers are also less likely to prioritize mental health for resource allocation, especially when the stigmatized are unable to adequately advocate for themselves.[4] There have been public health campaigns and initiatives in high-income countries

(HICs) that have curbed some of the stigma toward mental illness, but in LMICs where similar activities have not occurred, significant stigma that impedes care remains. There is a critical need to promote mental health education and awareness in a culturally sensitive and appropriate way, while also being practical in tackling the unique set of challenges in each economy.

Recently, the mental health crisis has been recognized by the WHO, World Bank, and the United Nations' Sustained Development Goals as a top priority, which has invigorated the field of global mental health.[7-9] In this landscape, convergent approaches bringing together policy, technology, and medicine are poised to offer new, nontraditional solutions to long-standing unsolved problems. This chapter will explore new developments in the intersection between technology and global mental health, specifically focusing on two initiatives in the Pacific Rim, Asia-Pacific Economic Cooperation forum (APEC) and Enhanced Measurement-Based care Effectiveness in Depression (EMBED), to illustrate some lessons from convergent approaches for targeting the treatment gap of mental illness in LMICs.

Overview of APEC Digital Hub in the Context of Global Mental Health

The convergence between mental health and economics is exemplified by APEC's new prioritization of mental health and how economic prosperity and mental health can be framed as a common objective to advance both fields synergistically. APEC is the premier regional economic forum in the Asia-Pacific. It aims to support sustainable economic growth, advocate free trade, promote economic integration, enhance human security, and encourage technical cooperation across the Asia-Pacific. This diverse region is characterized by rapid changes in economic and technological development, social demographics, population growth, and migration. The 21 APEC member economies comprise around 2.8 billion people and represent about 59% of world gross domestic product and 49% of world trade in 2015.[10] In merely two decades, its vibrant economies have increased the population per capita income by 74%, lifting millions out of poverty and creating a burgeoning middle class.

To achieve sustainability and social equity across the APEC communities, mental well-being is now recognized to be of critical importance to the APEC economies, with explicit economic cost. According to the World Economic Forum, mental disorders are expected to cost the global economy more than US$16 trillion between 2010 and 2030, accounting for one-third of the global economic cost of all chronic diseases.[11] In the Asia-Pacific region, mental illness causes a significant health and socioeconomic burden, which on average accounts for more than 20% of total years lost due to disability and 9.3% of all disability adjusted life years.[12]

As a result, APEC has joined the call to address global mental health as outlined in the WHO's Mental Health Action Plan (2013–2020)[9] and the Commonwealth of Nations' focus on the economic and social inclusion of mental health.[13] In 2014, APEC formed a technical working group and developed the APEC Roadmap to Promote Mental Wellness in a Healthy Asia Pacific (2014–2020), which strives for overall health, social, and economic participation; workplace productivity; and public–private engagement to promote innovations, best practices, and collaborations in mental health in the Asia-Pacific region.[14] Supporting the implementation of the APEC's roadmap is consistent with the United Nations' Sustainable Development Goals to ensure healthy lives and promote well-being for all at all ages, specifically Goal 3.4 (to reduce by one-third premature mortality from non-communicable diseases through prevention and treatment and promote mental health and well-being by 2030).[7] As with any aspirational global plans and targets, each member economy in the Asia-Pacific need to set its own national targets taking into account situations and realities within the member economy and decide how best to incorporate them into national planning processes, policies and strategies.

In April 2016, the World Bank Group and the WHO formed a strategic partnership to bring mental health into the center of the global development agenda. APEC Executive Director Alan Bollard together with World Bank Group President Jim Yong Kim and WHO Director-General Margaret Chan jointly called for mental wellness to be a global development priority at the World Bank Headquarters in Washington, DC. Multisectoral strategies were identified to respond to this global challenge as well as leveraging technologies, civil society participation, and innovative financing mechanisms.[8] APEC is putting the spotlight particularly on the reduced productivity related to chronic diseases and mental health, given that the annual global cost of mental health (US$2.5 trillion) is almost equivalent to a global financial crisis. However, numerous challenges remained to be tackled for each economy, notably the inadequate mental health policies, legislations, strategies, and funding at the national level.

APEC launched the APEC Digital Hub for Mental Health in November 2016 to enhance awareness, share information and experiences, develop customized curricula, and identify and implement evidence-based models in multilateral and diverse public–private partnerships.[8] The Digital Hub has served as a regional incubator for creating fresh ideas, scaling up innovations, sharing information, facilitating partnerships, and mapping all involved stakeholders. Additionally, the Digital Hub has acted as a digital portal of best and innovative practices to prevent and treat mental illness, as well as research and training activities. Through establishing regional and global academic networks to advance collaboration in mental health policy and research, the APEC Digital Hub will continue to serve as the Asia-Pacific region's platform for intergovernmental and public–private collaboration to implement the APEC roadmap. The Digital Hub has contributed to the implementation of global partnerships for Sustainable Development, specifically as in Goal 17.6 (to enhance North–South, South–South and triangular regional and international cooperation on and access to science, technology and innovation, and enhance knowledge sharing on mutually agreed terms, including through improved coordination among existing mechanisms, and through a global technology facilitation mechanism).[7]

APEC has further focused attention on the common priority areas identified by member economies and collaborating institutions through a strategic needs assessment. The assessment of the priorities, challenges, and potential areas of regional and multi-stakeholder cooperation in the APEC region resulted in a consensus to work in seven common priority areas on which the economies could focus their collaborative efforts. The common priority areas of mental health development include: workplace wellness and resilience; integration with primary care and community settings; advocacy and public awareness; mental wellness for indigenous communities, vulnerable communities and children; data collection and standardization; and disaster resilience and trauma.[15] Moreover, the strategic needs assessment has facilitated the development of new partnerships and projects within the relevant focus areas, involving multi-sectoral stakeholders. The Digital Hub have to this point facilitated interactive exchanges, mapped mental health stakeholders, and implemented a working strategy for three of key focus areas (i.e., workplace wellness, data standardization, and integration with primary care and community).[15]

Takeaways From APEC

Government prioritization of mental health has been an ongoing major challenge for global mental health, but by engaging governments with the concept of explicit economic cost of mental ill health, APEC bypassed much of the stigma impeding mental health funding and directly refuted the common misconception that mental health measures are cost ineffective. Furthermore, it brought together member economies, some HICs and some LMICs, into healthcare collaborations with each other and the industry and private sectors via the Digital Hub. The workplace best-practices guidelines developed via Digital Hub for better prevention and detection of mental illness is a key example of what positive outcomes can emerge from overlapping fields.

The top-down approach by APEC for increased global mental health prioritization and convergent collaboration is remarkable in that it did not require policy makers to have expertise in psychiatric conditions and the mental healthcare systems, but still resulted in significant engagement and investment by economy leaders toward mental health. Here we see that convergence between fields can find new ways of enacting change by finding motivators more accessible to a large number of stakeholders.

EMBED as Convergence in Global Mental Health

A project affiliated with the APEC Digital Hub, EMBED, is a good example of convergence science in global mental health. EMBED is a Canada–China collaborative study using technology to improve depression care in Shanghai, China. Funded jointly by the Canadian Institutes of Health Research and the National Natural Sciences Foundation of China, EMBED uses an implementation science framework to address complex systems issues that affect the routine use of measurement in clinical treatment of psychiatric disorders. Implementation science is the study of how evidence-based practices are best implemented into healthcare systems.[16] As a branch of knowledge translation, implementation science is itself multi- and transdisciplinary, as it involves patients, healthcare providers, behavioral scientists, economists, and policy analysts within complex hospital and community healthcare systems.

Measurement-based care (MBC) is an evidence-based approach for providing effective clinical care to patients with major depressive disorder. MBC utilizes validated rating scales to assess symptom severity, functional impairments, treatment adherence, and side-effect burden to personalize clinical decision-making based on measured outcomes and clinical algorithms.[17] However, despite evidence demonstrating improved outcomes,[18] MBC is still not routinely used by doctors.[19] Barriers to the use of MBC include lack of knowledge of which scales to use, the perceived extra time and effort needed for repeated assessments, and difficulty incorporating measurements into clinical charting systems.[20]

Much of the research on implementation of MBC has focused on clinicians using paper–pen versions of scales or electronic data entry located within a clinic. Although MBC seeks to support clinical decision-making and the physician-patient dyad is very important to MBC implementation, the patient has been a neglected factor in MBC research. EMBED seeks to address this by having patients track their own outcomes using technology enhancements such as smartphone apps. By leveraging mobile technology, the "enhanced" MBC directly involves the patient in a collaborative venture with their doctors and untethers MBC from the hospital or clinic setting. We now describe some of these mobile technologies for MBC.

Mobile Apps for Measurement-Based Care

MoodFx (pronounced *mood effects*) is a mobile-optimized web app that was designed by a partnership between the UBC Mood Disorders Centre (Raymond Lam), the UBC eHealth Strategy Office (Kendall Ho), and the Canadian Network for Mood and Anxiety Treatments to engage patients in collaborative MBC for depression. The

Table 24.1. MoodFx Scales

Assessment	Scale	Number of Items	Notes
Depression	Patient Health Questionnaire (PHQ-9)	9	• Sensitivity and specificity for diagnosis of major depressive disorder = 83% and 83%.
Anxiety	Generalized Anxiety Disorder scale (GAD-7)	7	• Sensitivity and specificity for diagnosis of GAD = 89% and 82% • Sensitivity and specificity for diagnosis of other anxiety disorders = 66%–74% and 80%–81%.
Cognition	Perceived Deficits Questionnaire for Depression (PDQ-D-5)	5	• A brief measure of subjective cognitive deficits that are commonly found in depression.
Work functioning	Lam Employment Absence and Productivity Scale (LEAPS)	7	• A measure of work functioning validated in patients with depression.
Medication side effects	Frequency, Intensity and Burden of Side Effects Rating (FIBSER)	3	• Created for use in the U.S. STAR*D effectiveness study.

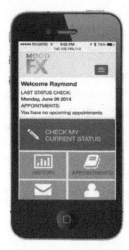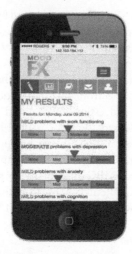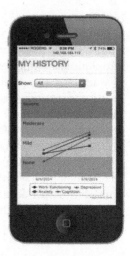

Figure 24.1 Screenshots from MoodFx.

objective of MoodFx is to enable patients to track their own outcomes using brief, standardized, and validated rating scales (Table 24.1).

MoodFx is simple, free, easy to use and available in English and French (see www. MoodFx.ca). It takes only five minutes to complete the online scales, and the results are immediately available to users in a graphical format (Figure 24.1), along with explanations about the scores. MoodFx can be used as a screening tool, but users can also track their scores longitudinally while being treated for depression. If medications are used, side effects can be assessed using the Frequency, Intensity, and Burden of Side Effects Ratings (FIBSER) scale. Users are encouraged to print their results to bring in to their clinician or to directly show them the results on their smartphone or tablet device during their appointment. Although direct linkage to electronic health records is not available, clinicians can scan the written reports into the electronic health record.

Given that people with depression are often unmotivated and have cognitive deficits, MoodFx includes reminder systems. Users can elect to have a reminder alerts sent by email or SMS to complete their MoodFx ratings regularly. They can also enter their next clinician appointment to have reminder alerts sent the day before to complete MoodFx. Finally, users can also access links to online resources and/or subscribe to weekly self-management tips sent via email or SMS link.

We conducted a preliminary online satisfaction survey of the first 500 MoodFx users with a response rate of 13% ($n = 64$). This group of users were predominantly female (78%) and computer literate: 95% either agreed or strongly agreed that they were "generally pretty comfortable using technology like computers, mobile phones, tablets, and the Internet," and 67% endorsed using "interactive websites and apps for [their] health." Most had previously seen a mental health clinician (92%) and were in current treatment (87%).

The majority of users usually accessed MoodFx via desktop computer (53%) but smartphones (43%) and tablets (16%) were also used. Many users used MoodFx regularly (e.g., monthly, 28%) or somewhat regularly (18%), but others had only used the app occasionally but irregularly (29%) and only once or twice (25%). MoodFx

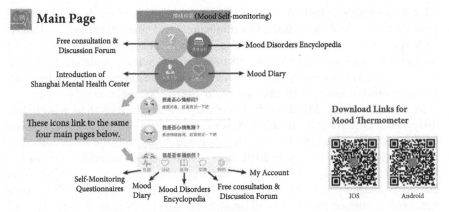

Figure 24.2. Features of Mood Thermometer.

was endorsed by most users as overall useful (strongly agree, 18%; agree, 53%; neutral, 18%; disagree, 8%; strongly disagree, 4%). Most users had also accessed several features of MoodFx, including self-management tips (68%), reminder alerts (55%), symptom tracking (52%), and online resources (33%). Our survey also included the System Usability Scale, an industry standard scale that has been used to evaluate thousands of websites and other online applications. MoodFx scored in the 75th percentile for usability according to the System Usability Scale. In summary, we found that MoodFx was both useful and useable for most users.

In the EMBED study, we are using an adapted Chinese version of MoodFx called Mood Thermometer, which is a fully functional iOS or Android smartphone app. Like MoodFx, it includes the same standardized outcome scales (Patient Health Questionnaire-9, Generalized Anxiety Disorder-7, FIBSER) and has many online resources for depression education and care (Figure 24.2). We conducted a preliminary patient survey in Shanghai ($n = 300$) and found that 96% of respondents had a smartphone with data access and were very familiar (53%) or somewhat familiar (39%) with mobile apps. In addition, 80% of respondents agreed with the statement, "I would be willing to track my symptoms with a mobile app if my doctor recommended it." Hence, we believe that Mood Thermometer would be easily implemented within the Shanghai healthcare system.

Supported Self-Management via WeChat

We are also adapting a Canadian depression program, Bounce Back, for the Shanghai context. Bounce Back is a guided self-management program.[21] developed by the Canadian Mental Health Association British Columbia Division as an evidence-based, low-cost, low-intensity psychological treatment. In Canada, Bounce Back is offered as an online or print-based modular program supplemented by videos and a telephone coaching service. Telephone coaches are lay people (often with lived experience), trained and monitored by a registered psychologist, who support patients to work through the self-management program. MBC is embedded within Bounce Back by use of validated scales including the Patient Health Questionnaire-9 and other assessments, with feedback to the referring doctor by fax and mailed reports at beginning and end of coach contact. Since its implementation in 2008 in British Columbia (population 4.6 million, dispersed over a huge geographic area with many rural and remote areas), Bounce Back has significantly improved patient outcomes for over 40,000 patients.[22]

In Shanghai for the EMBED study, we are adapting Bounce Back to be delivered entirely through the WeChat (in China, Weixin) mobile platform. WeChat is a combination of Facebook, Instagram, Twitter, WhatsApp, and Apple Pay that is firmly embedded into everyday Chinese society. In 2019, there were 1.13 billion monthly active users of WeChat, with an average daily use of 77 minutes.[23] The penetrance of WeChat is not limited to younger people—as of 2018, over 63 million WeChat users were 55 years of age or older, representing 98.5% of all smartphone users in China aged 50 to 80 years.[23] Patients will be able to register on WeChat and have access to all Bounce Back materials and videos, as well as access to the Bounce Back coach via preferred method of communication (videoconference, audio call, or asynchronous SMS messaging).

Takeaways From EMBED

The use of mobile technology for healthcare may be easier to implement in LMICs by "leap frogging" some of the ingrained but outdated technology that act as structural barriers in higher income countries. For MBC, leveraging the ubiquity, convenience, and advanced processing power of smartphones and mobile apps like MoodFx and Mood Thermometer enables measurement of symptoms and impairments in real time, anytime and anywhere, providing instant visual summaries that also track treatment progress (or lack thereof) over the long term. Since results can be easily displayed or printed to share with clinicians, these apps offer a simple and cost-effective means to integrate MBC into standard practice at the point of care, without needing additional materials, equipment, or staffing.

Although economic resources are available in China, there is still a significant equity gap in the provision of evidence-based psychological treatments, especially in rural and remote areas. To train enough mental health professionals for the high population demand is a daunting task that is likely impossible to achieve. The use of technology such as WeChat programs for guided self-management can address this equity gap by providing low-intensity, low-cost services to people with milder severity of illness, thereby streaming more intensive and costly treatments to more severe or complex cases.

Future Directions in Technology for LMIC Mental Health

We are in an exciting time of technological development. There are 4.7 billion mobile phone users globally,[24] of which 3.5 billion are smartphone users.[25] Furthermore, the number of smartphone users is projected to increase by 300 million a year.[25] Connectivity for these cellphones is also expanding at a rapid pace; 5G cell networks are rolling out around the world and SpaceX is in the midst of launching Starlink, a satellite network to offer globally available high-speed internet. Easy accessibility to a smart platform with internet has been revolutionary for social media, e-commerce, and media consumption, and is now increasingly leveraged as a way to augment healthcare. For LMICs, increasing ubiquity and accessibility to digital resources has allowed for highly scalable solutions such as phone apps, chatbots, and artificial intelligence (AI) to emerge as potential tools to address the immense mental health need. As the fields converge over the next several years, we anticipate large charges for global mental health, and next we identify some areas that show the most promise.

Telehealth

The internet is ideally suited for removing barriers to mental health resources for low-access communities, and its spread globally is connecting more people to mental health resources. People now have unprecedented access to mental health information and a means to learn about their local resources. Video conferencing for psychiatric assessments and follow-ups would be possible in places such as rural China or Indonesia, perhaps modeled after those that already established for rural HIC communities.[26,27] Access to online resources also benefits providers, especially given that community providers in LMICs have found guidance and support for mental health an ongoing challenge. Programs such as internet-delivered cognitive-behavioral therapy, which delivers web-based modules supported by a real-life therapist, have shown moderate to large effect sizes for generalized anxiety disorder, posttraumatic stress disorder, and major depressive disorder in a recent large meta-analysis and could be adapted for community settings in LMICs.[28]

Mobile Apps

Mobile health apps have become a burgeoning new market, with over 315,000 available from global app stores. Many of these are targeted toward mental health, including those that optimize sleeping, journal mood, or even remind patients to take medication.[29] Other categories of apps include self-help psychoeducation resources, peer support, chatbots, and mindfulness or medication apps.[30] Despite their wide differences in scope, mobile apps have the advantage of being much more accessible compared to traditional psychiatric services. For some, help could literally be available from the palm of their hand, rather than hours and an expensive commute to the closest clinic. Others may even prefer to interact with their mobile phone rather than having a face-to-face discussion, especially where avoiding stigma is a concern.

At present, the mental health app market is a place of ongoing innovation and experimentation. Despite their many advantages for access, the quality of apps still vary considerably. A recent study found that only 25% of apps passed basic quality standards, such as citing their sources.[31] Market forces do allow for community cura-tion of the best apps, but the process may be lacking in health expert oversight. Other factors to consider are difficulties of localization for language and culture of a prima-rily Western- and English-centric healthcare app market for global consumption, as well as ways to integrate these digital tools into existing healthcare resources in their respective countries. Further development is required to optimize delivery of services via mobile platforms, but apps remain a very promising resource for LMIC mental health.

Chatbots

With improvement in machine learning for natural speech recognition and artifi-cial intelligence, chatbots as a scalable way to deliver mental healthcare is emerging. Chatbots are already integrated into many customer service websites and speaking variants are becoming commonplace and powerful in the forms of Alexa, Cortana, and Siri. A recent review covers current applications of chatbots in mental health, including delivering cognitive-behavioral therapy, encouraging medication adher-ence, and offering psychoeducation, all of which have high user satisfaction with little risk of harm.[32] However, most research in chatbots occurs outside of medicine, and studies that do apply chatbots to mental health do not follow any consensus for evalu-ation or reporting.[32] As a result, there is yet to be a systematic path for implementation despite the very promising capabilities of the technology.

In the future, more complex chatbots may even take on therapist roles, which could help address the mental health worker shortage in many countries. Already, some re-search has shown that it is possible for bots to produce empathic responses with a fair degree of acceptability,[33] a domain typically thought to be outside the realm of ma-chines. With further improvements to processing power and AI, chatbots may even-tually become a viable mode of care for low-access communities.

AI and Digital Phenotyping

Neural net models first emerged in the mid-20th century but fell out of vogue due to lack of sufficiently powerful hardware that could run them for useful applications. Over the last decade, they experienced a resurgence in popularity as improved par-allel processing enabled powerful neural nets to accomplish impressive deep learning tasks for the first time. Whereas Deep Blue beat Kasparov two and a half decades ago with a heavily human-supervised "intelligence," deep learning algorithms such as Deep Mind's AlphaZero can reach pinnacle levels of ability in different games such as chess, shogi, go, or even the real-time strategy game StarCraft within hours to days of self-training with minimal human guidance.[34,35]

AI in healthcare is still in early stages but has already shown considerable promise, especially in visually based diagnostics such as medical imaging, dermatology, and pathology.[36-38] In mental healthcare, ventures such as Mindstrong are pairing AI with digital phenotyping. Digital phenotyping is the concept that a person's digital behaviors, such as geographic movement, sleep patterns, and even keystroke speed and latency inform on his or her mental health,[39] much like a more fundamental form of MBC. This phenotype, which are data too large and unwieldy for human interpretation, can be fed as an input into a deep learning network to track mood over time and respond by contacting emergency services or referring resources as appropriate.[40] Not only do such implementations of AI potentially reduce the burden on human workers, they also increase the fidelity of assessing patient mental status through long-term objective measures.

Similar to apps and chatbots, AI and digital phenotyping has the advantage of being much more scalable than a human workforce with no need for years of training to produce cycles of expert providers. For LMICs, AI systems, either on smart phones or in the workplace, capable of monitoring the mental state of opted-in participants would be a powerful aid for primary care workers who may neither have sufficient time nor training to screen people for mental health issues otherwise.

Potential Pitfalls

As technological advancements illuminate new possibilities in mental healthcare, so too do the needs of healthcare inform new precautions and limitations for new technologies.

Privacy

With greater integration of technology in mental healthcare comes a higher risk to user privacy. Where does all the patient information get stored, and what safeguards would be in place to protect them? How would a tech company address the need to process sensitive information domestically while serving an international client base? Does the local government have protections for data privacy, or conversely, have policies for monitoring its citizens? With digital phenotyping, how much tracking is too invasive? These are all ethical and legal questions to consider when evaluating for appropriateness and potential for implementation.

Potential Harm of Overenthusiasm

At present, much of the discussed technology is in an immature state. Careful application is required to avoid ineffectual or even harmful uses of technology in LMICs. For example, the apps and chatbots of today are still limited in ability and sometimes provide unhelpful responses when told suicidal thoughts.[41] Overeager investment in immature technology may lead to loss of faith as well, as demonstrated by the failure of IBM's Watson for Oncology[42]; if a digital service promises large benefits but severely underdelivers, it hinders willingness for adoption of similar services in the future. As such, a considered and realistic approach is best for implementation of available technologies in LMICs.

Balancing Innovation With Evidence

The digital world is defined by rapid change. Apps or tools can roll out weekly updates and feature pushes to meet new demands, contrasting against traditional mental healthcare standards of largely unchanging drug formulations and psychotherapy schools. Traditional research methodology, which has found robustness with years-long study of fixed interventions, is incompatible with constantly evolving digital interventions. New paradigms are needed that balance free-market innovation with scientific rigor, while simultaneously ensuring that patient care takes priority over profits.

Conclusions

This chapter has highlighted the need for the convergence of multisectors including public, private, academic, economic, digital health, and other sectors to address the challenges of global mental health burden, especially in LMICs. In response, APEC's endorsement of the importance mental health in economic development have led to greater engagement of diverse stakeholders and the establishment of the APEC Digital Hub for Mental Health. The chapter has also emphasized the use of digital technology for mental healthcare to overcome barriers to closing treatment gaps and has outlined the EMBED project as a feasible and cost-effective means to integrate MBC into standard clinical practice in low-resources settings. Finally, the chapter has presented highly scalable digital health solutions such as phone apps, chatbots, and AI that can maximize mental health treatment availability and quality. Consideration is also given to limitations for new technologies such as issues of privacy, underdelivery, and need for evidence-based practice.

References

1. World Health Organization. *Depression.* 2019; https://www.who.int/news-room/fact-sheets/detail/depression. Accessed January 24, 2020.
2. World Health Organization. *Mental health statistics: global and nationwide costs.* 2020; https://www.mentalhealth.org.uk/statistics/mental-health-statistics-global-and-nationwide-costs. Accessed January 24, 2020.
3. World Health Organization. *Global Health Observatory (GHO) data 2016;* https://www.who.int/gho/mental_health/human_resources/psychiatrists_nurses/en/. Accessed January 24, 2020.
4. Eaton J, McCay L, Semrau M, et al. Scale up of services for mental health in low-income and middle-income countries. *Lancet.* 2011;378(9802):1592–1603 https://doi.org/10.1016/s0140-6736(11)60891-x.

5. Wainberg ML, Scorza P, Shultz JM, et al. Challenges and opportunities in global mental health: a research-to-practice perspective. *Curr Psychiatry Rep.* 2017;19(5):28 https://doi.org/10.1007/s11920-017-0780-z.

6. Henderson C, Evans-Lacko S, Thornicroft G. Mental illness stigma, help seeking, and public health programs. *Am J Public Health.* 2013;103(5):777–780 https://doi.org/10.2105/ajph.2012.301056.

7. United Nations. *The global goals for sustainable development.* 2015; https://www.globalgoals.org/. Accessed January 24, 2020.

8. Marquez PV, Saxena S. *Making Mental Health a Global Priority.* Cerebrum, 2016;2016:cer-10-16.

9. World Health Organization. *Comprehensive mental health action plan 2013–2020.* 2013; https://www.who.int/mental_health/action_plan_2013/en/. Accessed January 24, 2020.

10. Asia-Pacific Economic Cooperation. *About APEC.* 2019; https://www.apec.org/About-Us/About-APEC/. Accessed January 24, 2020.

11. Bloom DE, Cafiero ET, Jané-Llopis E, et al. *The Global Economic Burden of Noncommunicable Diseases.* Geneva: World Economic Forum; 2011.

12. Ng CH. Mental health and integration in Asia Pacific. *BJPsych Int.* 2018;15(4):76–79 https://doi.org/10.1192/bji.2017.28.

13. Ng CH. *Mental health: towards economic and social inclusion: a report to the commonwealth secretariat.* London: Commonwealth Secretariat; 2013.

14. Asia-Pacific Economic Cooperation. *APEC roadmap to promote mental wellness in a healthy Asia Pacific (2014–2020).* 2014; http://mddb.apec.org/Documents/2014/MM/AMM/14_amm_014.pdf. Accessed January 24, 2020.

15. Ng CH, Goodenow MM, Greenshaw AJ, Upshall P, Lam RW. Inclusion of mental health in global economic development. *BJPsych Int.* 2018;15(4):74–76 https://doi.org/10.1192/bji.2017.23.

16. King KM, Pullmann MD, Lyon AR, Dorsey S, Lewis CC. Using implementation science to close the gap between the optimal and typical practice of quantitative methods in clinical science. *J Abnorm Psychol.* 2019;128(6):547–562.

17. Culpepper L, Trivedi MH. Using measurement-based care with patient involvement to improve outcomes in depression. *Prim Care Companion CNS Disord.* 2013;15(6).

18. Guo T, Xiang YT, Xiao L, et al. Measurement-based care versus standard care for major depression: a randomized controlled trial with blind raters. *Am J Psychiatry.* 2015;172(10):1004–1013 https://doi.org/10.1176/appi.ajp.2015.14050652.

19. Harding KJ, Rush AJ, Arbuckle M, Trivedi MH, Pincus HA. Measurement-based care in psychiatric practice: a policy framework for implementation. *J Clin Psychiatry.* 2011;72(8):1136–1143 https://doi.org/10.4088/jcp.10r06282whi.

20. Lewis CC, Boyd M, Puspitasari A, et al. Implementing measurement-based care in behavioral health: a review. *JAMA Psychiatry.* 2019;76(3):324–335 https://doi.org/10.1001/jamapsychiatry.2018.3329.

21. Houle J, Gascon-Depatie M, Belanger-Dumontier G, Cardinal C. Depression self-management support: a systematic review. *Patient Educ Couns.* 2013;91(3):271–279 https://doi.org/10.1016/j.pec.2013.01.012.

22. CMHA-BC. *Bounce back: reclaim your health: Annual Report 2015–2016.* Vancouver, BC: Canadian Mental Health Association; 2016.

23. Smith C. *110 amazing WeChat statistics and facts (2019): by the numbers.* 2019; https://expandedramblings.com/index.php/wechat-statistics/ Accessed January 26, 2020.

24. Statistica. *Number of mobile phone users worldwide from 2015 to 2020.* 2018; https://www.statista.com/statistics/274774/forecast-of-mobile-phone-users-worldwide/. Accessed January 24, 2020.

25. Statistica. *Number of smartphone users worldwide from 2016 to 2021.* 2019; https://www.statista.com/statistics/330695/number-of-smartphone-users-worldwide/. Accessed January 24, 2020.

26. Jong M, Mendez I, Jong R. Enhancing access to care in northern rural communities via telehealth. *Int J Circumpolar Health.* 2019;78(2):1554174 https://doi.org/10.1080/22423982.2018.1554174.

27. O'Gorman LD, Hogenbirk JC, Warry W. Clinical telemedicine utilization in Ontario over the Ontario Telemedicine Network. *Telemed J E Health.* 2016;22(6):473–479 https://doi.org/10.1089/tmj.2015.0166.

28. Andersson G, Carlbring P, Titov N, Lindefors N. Internet interventions for adults with anxiety and mood disorders: a narrative umbrella review of recent meta-analyses. *Can J Psychiatry.* 2019;64(7):465–470.

29. Byambasuren O, Sanders S, Beller E, Glasziou P. Prescribable mHealth apps identified from an overview of systematic reviews. *NPJ Digit Med.* 2018;1:12 https://doi.org/10.1038/s41746-018-0021-9.

30. Chan S, Li L, Torous J, Gratzer D, Yellowlees PM. Review and implementation of self-help and automated tools in mental health care. *Psychiatr Clin North Am.* 2019;42(4):597–609 https://doi.org/10.1016/j.psc.2019.07.001.

31. Shen N, Levitan MJ, Johnson A, et al. Finding a depression app: a review and content analysis of the depression app marketplace. *JMIR Mhealth Uhealth.* 2015;3(1):e16 https://doi.org/10.2196/mhealth.3713.

32. Vaidyam AN, Wisniewski H, Halamka JD, Kashavan MS, Torous JB. Chatbots and conversational agents in mental health: a review of the psychiatric landscape. *Can J Psychiatry.* 2019;64(7):456–464.

33. Morris RR, Kouddous K, Kshirsagar R, Schueller SM. Towards an artificially empathic conversational agent for mental health applications: system design and user perceptions. *J Med Internet Res.* 2018;20(6):e10148 https://doi.org/10.2196/10148.

34. Silver D, Hubert T, Schrittwieser J, et al. A general reinforcement learning algorithm that masters chess, shogi, and Go through self-play. *Science.* 2018;362(6419):1140–1144 https://doi.org/10.1126/science.aar6404.

35. Vinyals O, Babuschkin I, Czarnecki WM, et al. Grandmaster level in StarCraft II using multi-agent reinforcement learning. *Nature.* 2019;575(7782):350–354 https://doi.org/10.1038/s41586-019-1724-z.

36. Lee JG, Jun S, Cho YW, et al. Deep Learning in medical imaging: general overview. *Korean J Radiol.* 2017;18(4):570–584 https://doi.org/10.3348/kjr.2017.18.4.570.

37. Du-Harpur X, Watt FM, Luscombe NM, Lynch MD. What is AI? Applications of artificial intelligence to dermatology. *Br J Dermatol.* 2020. [Epub ahead of print] https://doi.org10.1111/bjd.18880

38. Wang S, Yang DM, Rong R, Zhan X, Xiao G. Pathology image analysis using segmentation deep learning algorithms. *Am J Pathol.* 2019;189(9):1686–1698 https://doi.org/10.1016/j.ajpath.2019.05.007.

39. Bhugra D, Tasman A, Pathare S, et al. The WPA–Lancet Psychiatry Commission on the Future of Psychiatry. *Lancet Psychiatry.* 2017;4(10):775–818.

40. Insel TR. Digital phenotyping: technology for a new science of behavior. *JAMA.* 2017;318(13):1215–1216 https://doi.org/10.1001/jama.2017.11295.

41. Torous J, Larsen ME, Depp C, et al. Smartphones, sensors, and machine learning to advance real-time prediction and interventions for suicide prevention: a review of current progress and next steps. *Curr Psychiatry Rep.* 2018;20(7):51 https://doi.org/10.1007/s11920-018-0914-y.

42. Artificial intelligence in health care: within touching distance. *Lancet.* 2018;390(10114):2739.

25

Digital Health Entrepreneurship

A Convergent Discipline for Mental Health

Wendy Charles, Sharon Wulfovich, and Arlen Meyers

Introduction

In the past decade, there have been considerable advances in health technology that impact human communication, cognition, and quality of life.[1] The importance of continuing improvement in healthcare was summarized by the Institute for Healthcare Improvement in 2008: "to improve the patient care experience, improve the health of a population, and reduce per capita healthcare costs."[2p760] These aims were augmented into the quadruple aim by Sikka et al[3] in 2015 to include workforce engagement and safety; and one of us (AM)[4] recently proposed a quintuple aim to address "sick care" business processes and revenue cycle technology. To specifically advance digital health technologies into the quadruple aim, the American Medical Association[5] created a Digital Health Implementation Playbook that instructs healthcare facilities on strategies and methodology.

Digital technologies are used by nearly all patients in their everyday lives, and the younger generations that are native to digital skills are driving the penetration of digital health into many treatment areas.[6] Digital health can be defined as the "use of information and communications technologies to exchange medical information"[7p1] where intended uses include education, information, prevention, diagnosis, treatment, and rehabilitation.[7] For mental health, digital health innovation is increasingly used for addressing mental health diagnostic and treatments,[8,9] and methods include telemental health, digital medication management,[10] wearable sensors to assess mobility,[11] novel uses of artificial intelligence to diagnose or treat mental health conditions,[12] personalized medicine,[13] and smartphone apps for monitoring symptoms for patients with mental illness.[14] There is even a movement to use digital health to address the social determinants of mental health,[15] such as providing support for addictions, food insecurity, and community care.[15] Detailed examples of digital health innovations in mental health are covered in detail in other chapters of this book.

The processes and motivations of creating innovation in digital health are often referred to as digital health entrepreneurship. Digital health entrepreneurship involves the pursuit of opportunity under volatile, uncertain, complex, ambiguous conditions[16] with the goal of creating user-defined value through the deployment of digital health innovation using a viable business model. Digital health entrepreneurship also supports organizational structures and care delivery models conducive to innovation,[17] such as empowering individuals' creativity and convergence: collaborating across disciplines to develop new perspectives.[16,18] Digital health convergence for innovation is not just among healthcare providers, but may also include engineers, scientists, payers, industry partners in industries, and sometimes even patients.[6] This convergence of knowledge creates an environment for entrepreneurship and the ability to recognize opportunities at the transdisciplinary boundaries.[19] Therefore, convergence is a vital requirement for entrepreneurship.[18]

As evidence of large scale acceptance for convergence science in digital health technologies, U.S. federal agencies, such as the Department of Defense, Department of Energy, Department of Health and Human Services, National Institutes of Health, and the National Science Foundation (NSF) have publicized that they are involved in aspects of innovative convergence research.[20] In fact, the National Science Foundation has described a focus on convergence research as one of its priorities.[20] With specific regard to mental health innovations, the Department of Health and Human Services engaged in a partnership with Indian Health Services (HIS) to deliver telehealth to IHS's remote and geographically diverse patient population.[21] Further, the Health Research Service Administration partnered with the Centers for Medicare and Medicaid Services to include remote behavioral health in rural populations.[21]

Strategies for Advancing Digital Health Entrepreneurship in Mental Health

Digital health technologies could transform the medical field by improving patient outcomes, increasing quality of healthcare and reducing costs that the U.S. healthcare system faces.[16] However, to capitalize on these opportunities, entrepreneurs not only have to solve a technological problem but also the interrelated clinical and business problems.[4] This section provides an overview of individual and organizational approaches, as well as digital health technology development strategies, to foster digital health entrepreneurship for digital mental health technologies.

Individual and Organizational Approaches

Individual Approaches

To successfully implement digital health technologies into mental health practices, clinicians need broader education and training about how to translate innovative ideas to patient care.[22] In a report titled "Strengthening Academic Psychiatry," the Academy of Medical Sciences[23] recommended expanding educational training programs to allow psychiatrists-in-training the opportunity to study neurology, immunology, pediatrics, and other related disciplines. El-Awad et al[24] demonstrated that higher levels of individual "boundary-crossing" increased new combinations of knowledge and increased the likelihood of technology-based innovation. Even while in medical school, there are entrepreneurial characteristics and behaviors that students can acquire, such as people skills and creative vision.[25]

To prepare psychiatrists and other mental health professionals for the ability to understand and adopt convergent approaches to digital health innovations, providers should be trained in digital health delivery methods to understand their strengths and limitations.[26] Gossman et al[27] even recommend competency assessments in clinical digital health to demonstrate proficiencies in technologies and applications. New biomedical entrepreneurship education programs offer interdisciplinary courses in data science and digital health entrepreneurship.[6] The University of Hawaii,[28] for example, developed a psychiatry telemental health remote training curriculum in collaboration with the Mayo Clinic. This collaborative training program meets the requirements for the Accreditation Council for Graduate Medical Education for psychiatry[28] and has demonstrated success in advancing virtual methods of providing mental healthcare. The University of Rochester[26] incorporates education about telemedicine and remote patient care into its psychiatric nursing curricula from undergraduate coursework through to doctoral programs. To educate mental health professionals who provide American Indian/Alaska Native populations with telemental health, IHS's Telebehavioral Health Center of Excellence[29] (mentioned earlier) created a tele-education program. This program not only teaches best practices for delivering mental health services remotely, but also educates mental health professionals about culturally sensitive approaches.[29] While education about digital health for clinical care is improving, aspiring physician entrepreneurs still need education about the core areas of business innovation, such as the legal environment, regulatory affairs, intellectual property, and reimbursement.[22]

Introduction of digital mental health innovations into clinical care also requires changes in mindset and behaviors. Psychiatrists and other mental health professionals should be open to adding digital mental health tools to their clinical routines. While clinicians are taught that one-to-one sessions typically offer the best method of care, digital mental health tools can facilitate effective therapy for less intensive needs and can be delivered at an expanded scale.[30] A report by the Global Future Council on Neurotechnologies, "Empowering 8 Billion Minds: Enabling Better Mental Health for All via the Ethical Adoption of Technologies,"[30] cautions, however, implementation of digital technologies for mental health, as with any other health field, requires trust by both patients and practitioners. Without trust, the technologies that contain sensitive information will be abandoned.

Organizational Approaches

The core of digital health entrepreneurship involves innovation, which starts with leadership. The Center for Creative Leadership[31] describes the need for (i) innovative leaders to bring creative thinking and approaches for how they lead and for (ii) leadership for innovation. Leadership for innovation involves creating a culture and environment that fosters innovation in others: promoting diversity of ideas, freedom to experiment, and developing team members' aspirations.[31] Moreover, leaders should develop strong convergence ecosystems, which may include venture capital investors, to provide additional ideas and financial support.[19] Considering that there have already been high-profile digital health failures and consolidations, digital health leaders, and investors may be cautious about risk as the industry and markets continue to mature.[6]

When developing new digital health technologies that involve mental health, leaders should also advocate responsible business and technology practices[30]— mindful that this population may be more vulnerable. Specifically, there are many ethical considerations involving digital health, such as ownership of personal data, collection of biometrics, and using patient or practice data to further the interests of the business.[32] Meyers,[32] in his role as the president of the Society of Physician Entrepreneurs, recognizes that there are many reasons why physician entrepreneurs are not trusted and emphasizes that digital health entrepreneurs need to reconcile the ethics of business and medicine by practicing "compassionate capitalism."[32p2]

In technology-based ventures, convergent thinking drives entrepreneurial teams. Santos et al[33] identified dynamic learning processes in technology companies. The workforce may start with team members viewing themselves as individuals with their own training and conditioning, but evolving into teams and eventually adopting organizational routines and behaviors.[33] Team members learn from each other and demonstrate a different mindset[34] resulting in a collective unit of collaboration and entrepreneurial capabilities.[33] If leaders are not integrated in this coalition, team members feel compelled to work around the leaders.[35] Perez-Vaisvidovsky and Aviram[35] found that entrepreneurship coalitions involving mental health are complicated because there are often more policy and regulatory constraints. They recommend developing channels of communication to encourage regular interaction for integrating leaders and other stakeholders in the coalition.[35]

As academic medical centers are transitioning their research from drug discovery toward digital health development,[6] these institutions have recently rebranded their tech transfer offices into convergence-focused research institutes[6] to foster clinical innovation and team development toward convergence medicine.[36] As examples, the Wyss Institute for Biologically Inspired Engineering at Harvard University[37] brings together experts with experience in industrial product development, engineering, clinical care, intellectual property, and entrepreneurship. Faculty members are evaluated not only on customary publication metrics, but also on development of licensing agreements, intellectual property, and corporate alliances. The University of California's Institute for Quantitative Biosciences[38] converges more than 250 researchers in physics, chemistry, engineering, and applied math to create new diagnostic tools and innovation. This partnership between three University of California campuses, private industry, and venture capital also provides training to graduate students and fellows on how to start new companies with a "startup in a box."[19p39] The University of California–Irvine Beall Applied Innovation[39] advances entrepreneurship by connecting campus-based inventions to the Orange County business community. These are only a few examples of convergence-focused academic centers designed to facilitate start-up companies and pursue entrepreneurial opportunities.

When not working in a research incubator, there are still mechanisms that academic institutions can utilize to encourage cross-disciplinary research and entrepreneurship. To advance digital health entrepreneurship, inventors should be offered equitable ownership options with the institution's technology transfer office.[40] Last, the National Academy of Sciences[41] recommends modifying department ranking criteria to include factors that recognize an entrepreneurial start-up culture, such as rewarding cross institutional collaborations and giving more weight to generation of patents.

Digital Health Technology Product Development

As there are now thousands of apps intended to address mental health conditions,[42] psychiatrists and other mental health professionals regularly receive questions about the effectiveness and risks of new digital technologies. The American Psychiatric Association has developed an app evaluation model with resources to help mental health professionals and patients evaluate effectiveness and security of apps prior to use in clinical practice.[43] This framework is targeted toward apps but includes practical advice for evaluating many types of connected digital technologies. The four areas in the model include evaluations of privacy, evidence of effectiveness, ease of use, and interoperability[43] to help clinicians make judgments on their patient's (or patients') behalf about the benefits and risks of digital mental health.[40]

Security and Privacy
Among the top challenges for adoption of digital health technologies in healthcare remain security and privacy.[44] The 8th Annual Industry Pulse Survey[45] from Change Healthcare and Healthcare Executive Group found that for about half of the organizations surveyed, privacy and security concerns were the leading factor on why adoption of these technologies was not more extensive. For digital health technologies developed for mental health, the security and privacy are heightened due to the sensitive nature of mental health information collected.[30]

To advance digital health technologies for mental health, psychiatrists and other mental health practitioners must focus on transparency and security to build their patients' trust around new digital tools. For example, there should be clear discussions about how and why data are used, who has control of information, who can access information, and the nature of security.[30,46] Likewise, technology developers and cloud-based data hosts must clearly document ethical practices about data protections, use, and control. Gaps in communication or protections jeopardize the advancement of technology adoption.[30] Organizations should actively manage data breaches, security threats, risk assessments for any digital product implemented.[47]

Effectiveness
Instead of finding a fit for a new technology or the focus on trying something new,[30] mental health providers should identity their patients' or clients' needs and priorities.[4,48] Ideally, digital health entrepreneurs should use continuous testing, validations, and verifications of value[13,49] with prospective patients and their providers.

Regardless of the digital innovations proposed for mental health, use of the innovations must remain evidence-based.[34] While new digital health technologies are being promoted to address mental health issues, marketing hype and unvalidated claims create confusion for patient/consumers, providers, and regulators who seek an accurate risk-benefit assessment.[30] Researchers and practitioners should incorporate evidence-based practices drawn from medical, social, behavioral, and economic sciences as well as strategic planning and program management.[19]

Usability

When considering innovative digital mental health tools, testing the usability by the target patient population is equally important[50] and often under-represented in mental health.[51-53] The International Organization for Standardization defines usability as "the extent to which a product can be used by specified users to achieve specified goals with effectiveness, efficiency and satisfaction in a specified context of use."[54p2] The domain of effectiveness is defined as "the accuracy and completeness with which users achieve specified goals," efficiency as the "resources expended in relation to the accuracy and completeness with which users achieve specified goals," and satisfaction as the "freedom from discomfort and positive attitudes towards the use of the product."[54p2]

Unfortunately, most digital tools for mental health, such as smartphone apps, evidence poor usability. These apps try to package together too many complex activities[8] and/are not designed using user-centric best practices.[26] There is a tendency for digital health developers to forego usability testing on patients with mental illness even though individuals with mental illness-related conditions may have related cognitive limitations that constrain their ability to use complicated digital technologies.[14] The needs and abilities of individuals with severe mental illness are different and require technologies that reduce their cognitive efforts.[55] Sauro[56] has determined that (even for the general population), 90% of new technology products fail—partly due to insufficient usability.[8]

Developers of new digital health technologies for mental health are cautioned to carefully study populations with the mental condition that the technology is intended to address. Common design features from gamification, such as bright colors, reinforcing sounds, and challenge tasks, can be added to nearly any digital health intervention to improve usability.[8] Additionally, apps should be more personalized and context-aware of an individual's routine, state and healthcare needs, supporting self-management and self-efficacy of an individual's health condition.[57] Without such design and testing for usability, the technology may not be sufficiently usable to be adopted.

Interoperability

The evolution of connected digital health has also prompted concern about interoperability. If digital health technologies are intended to augment care, psychiatrists and other mental health professionals should be able to access the information and discuss findings with their patients.[43] Thus far, most digital health technologies cannot link to existing electronic health records (EHRs).[58] With the goal of achieving eventual interoperability,[59] the Office of the National Coordinator for Health Information Technology[60] released a 2018 report specifying that interoperability of health information is one of its top t priorities with the focus on opening app and EHR architecture.[61] Until there is more acceptance of this initiative, it may be difficult for digital health entrepreneurs to gain access to the API architecture in EHR systems to design interoperable solutions.[6]

Regulatory

To innovate in healthcare, regulatory requirements must be taken into account early in the process.[6] With regard to health record privacy, data-driven digital health technologies involving covered entities (healthcare providers, health plans, and health clearinghouses) must follow the Health Information Privacy and Portability Act (HIPAA)[62] and there are often more restrictive state statutes for privacy of mental health records.[63] Within covered entities, there are strict privacy regulations for authorization of PHI for research (45 CFR § 164.508 and 512) and storing and transmitting to portable devices (45 CFR § 164, Subpart C).

Digital health entrepreneurs are advised that use of digital tools and technologies for mental health may require review and approval by the U.S. Food and Drug Administration (FDA) and/or the European Medicines Agency. Specifically, some mental health software, including mobile medical apps, could be categorized as "software as a medical device."[30] For determining best practices for regulating devices used in the United States, the FDA participates in the International Medical Device Regulators Forum,[64] which has increasingly focused on refining a framework to "accelerate international medical device regulatory harmonization and convergence."[65p1]

While many digital health entrepreneurs may view regulatory requirements as a major obstacle, the federal regulatory climate is becoming more accommodating to innovation, and certain types of digital health technologies are no longer regulated.[66] Congress modified the Food and Drug Administration Amendments Act[67] via the 21st Century Cures Act[68] by moving common consumer-facing technologies out of the FDA's regulatory jurisdiction. This legislation also reconciled scientific, policy, and legal conflicts.[66]

Even though regulations seem to offer more flexibility, digital health entrepreneurs would be wise to consult with the FDA and other pertinent regulatory authorities at the early stages of developing digital tools for mental health to understand whether pre-market approval would be required. In September 2019, the FDA published new guidance regarding how medical software and apps should be regulated and which types of software as a medical device would be subject to regulatory oversight.[69] While the FDA does not provide examples of mental health technologies in its digital health guidance, the Global Future Council on Neurotechnologies advises that technologies or software intended to diagnose or treat a mental disorder (e.g., diagnostic and treatment planning tools for bipolar disorder) should conduct rigorous efficacy studies and submit for FDA premarket approval.[30]

Future Directions

To secure a promising future of digital health entrepreneurship in mental health, it will be valuable to address certain gaps in provider reimbursement and evidence-based practices.

Provider Reimbursement

An ongoing challenge to digital health entrepreneurship involves obtaining provider reimbursement for clinical care involving new digital health technologies. Most providers don't get reimbursed for providing care using digital health technologies.[6,27] In 2018, new legislation was introduced through Public Law 115-271: Support for Patients and Communities Act.[70] This act expanded use of telehealth services for treatment of opioid use disorder—including co-occurring behavioral health needs—and described state-based approaches to Medicaid payments for these services. It was also promising to note that 20% of new Common Procedural Technology codes for reimbursement could be considered as having a digital health component.[71] With the importance of ensuring reimbursement for services, digital health entrepreneurs should design their products and product research for reimbursement proposals. Davis[71] cautions that too many digital health technologies are abandoned because they cannot secure reimbursement.

Gaps in Evidence

As digital health innovations are expanding access to mental health services and creating new treatment modalities, digital health entrepreneurs should determine the degree to which their claims will make health-related claims. Most digital health technologies no longer require clinical validation with the FDA prior to marketing but may require evidence to meet truth in advertising expectations from the Federal Trade Commission or the Consumer Products Safety Commission.[6]

Even if research-based evidence is not required from federal agencies, many clinicians request validation from rigorous clinical trials because they may not perceive data collected from novel digital health technologies to be accurate enough or significant enough to make informed decisions.[47] Therefore, we encourage digital health entrepreneurs to consider validation studies to assess the relationships between different types of digital data and their relationships to mental health conditions.[72] Ideally, clinicians would prefer to see research that establishes the validity of digital health technologies to clinical outcomes.[47]

Because digital health innovations, such as telemental health, can extend mental health services to patients in rural areas who lack access to psychiatric care or those that perceive too much stigma when obtaining care in a psychiatrist's office,[26] research should establish the value of this care. Currently, data about the benefits of telemental health are not routinely and systematically collected.[26] This research may establish the benefits of these services and help to counter the lower reimbursement fees when compared to in-person visits.[26]

Conclusion

Digital health entrepreneurship creates an environment conducive to converging expertise to create innovation in mental health. We are entering the new digital era of psychiatry where digital technological advancements are becoming part of regular healthcare practices. These practices offer potential to transform mental health by improving patient outcomes, increasing quality of healthcare, and reducing costs. However, digital health innovations in mental health will succeed only if the innovations add value and improve healthcare.[1] Efforts to address current gaps and promote value need to be well-integrated and systematic to counter risk-averse providers and healthcare organizations.[22] We encourage digital health entrepreneurs to address the privacy, interoperability and regulatory requirements while conducting research to establish the effectiveness, usability, and reimbursement needs of new digital health technologies to increase the likelihood of successful adoption.

References

1. Roco MC, Bainbridge WS, Tonn B, Whitesides G, eds. *Converging Knowledge, Technology, and Society: Beyond Convergence of Nano-Bio-Info-Cognitive Technologies.* New York, NY: Springer; 2013.
2. Berwick DM, Nolan TW, Whittington J. The triple aim: care, health, and cost. *Health Aff (Millwood).* 2008;27(3):759–769 https://doi.org/10.1377/hlthaff.27.3.759.
3. Sikka R, Morath JM, Leape L. The quadruple aim: care, health, cost and meaning in work. *BMJ Qual Saf.* 2015;24(10):608. https://doi.org/10.1136/bmjqs-2015-004160.
4. Meyers A. *The forgotten quintuple aim.* 2019; https://www.linkedin.com/pulse/forgotten-quintuple-aim-arlen-meyers-md-mba/. Updated June 24, 2019. Accessed November 1, 2019.
5. *Digital Health Implementation Playbook.* Chicago, IL: American Medical Association; 2018. https://www.ama-assn.org/system/files/2018-12/digital-health-implementation-playbook-REV1.pdf. Accessed Oct 29, 2019.
6. Zajicek H, Meyers A. Digital health entrepreneurship. In: Rivas H, Wac K, eds. *Digital Health: Scaling Healthcare to the World.* Cham, Switzerland: Springer International; 2018:271–287.
7. Meyers A. The status of physician digital health use. July 15, 2017; https://www.cliexa.com/2017/07/status-physician-digital-health-use/. Updated July 15, 2017. Accessed November 1, 2019.
8. Tuerk PW, Schaeffer CM, McGuire JF, Adams Larsen M, Capobianco N, Piacentini J. Adapting evidence-based treatments for digital technologies: a critical review of functions, tools, and the use of branded solutions. *Curr Psychiatry Rep.* 2019;21(10):106. doi:10.1007/s11920-019-1092-2.
9. Williams PA, Lovelock B, Cabarrus T, Harvey M. Improving digital hospital transformation: development of an outcomes-based infrastructure maturity assessment framework. *JMIR Med Inform.* 2019;7(1):e12465. doi:10.2196/12465.
10. Peters-Strickland T, Pestreich L, Hatch A, et al. Usability of a novel digital medicine system in adults with schizophrenia treated with sensor-embedded tablets of aripiprazole. *Neuropsychiatr Dis Treat.* 2016;12:2587–2594 https://doi.org/10.2147/ndt.s116029.
11. Osipov M, Behzadi Y, Kane JM, Petrides G, Clifford GD. Objective identification and analysis of physiological and behavioral signs of schizophrenia. *J Ment Health.* 2015;24(5):276–282 https://doi.org/10.3109/09638237.2015.1019048.
12. Price WN, Cohen IG. Privacy in the age of medical big data. *Nat Med.* 2019;25(1):37–43 https://doi.org/10.1038/s41591-018-0272-7.
13. Lopez D, Brown AW, Plans D. Developing opportunities in digital health: The case of BioBeats Ltd. *J Bus Ventur Insights.* 2019;11:e00110. https://doi.org/10.1016/j.jbvi.2019.e00110.

14. Batra S, Baker RA, Wang T, Forma F, DiBiasi F, Peters-Strickland T. Digital health technology for use in patients with serious mental illness: a systematic review of the literature. *Med Devices (Auckl)*. 2017;10:237–251 https://doi.org/10.2147/mder.s144158.

15. Allen J, Balfour R, Bell R, Marmot M. Social determinants of mental health. *Int Rev Psychiatry*. 2014;26(4):392–407 https://doi.org/10.3109/09540261.2014.928270.

16. Wulfovich S, Meyers A, eds. *Digital Health Entrepreneurship*. Cham, Switzerland: Springer Nature Switzerland AG; 2019.

17. Meyers A. *How is digital health entrepreneurship different?* 2016; https://www.linkedin.com/pulse/how-digital-health-entrepreneurship-different-arlen-meyers-md-mba/. Updated June 22, 2016. Accessed November 2, 2019.

18. Lee C, Park G, Kang J. The impact of convergence between science and technology on innovation. *J Technol Transf*. 2018;43(2):522–544 https://doi.org/10.1007/s10961-016-9480-9.

19. National Research Council. *Convergence: Facilitating Transdisciplinary Integration of Life Sciences, Physical Sciences, Engineering, and Beyond*. Washington, DC: The National Academies Press; 2014. https://www.nap.edu/download/18722#. Accessed July 12, 2019.

20. Sharp P, Hockfield S. Convergence: the future of health. *Science*. 2017;355(6325):589. https://doi.org/10.1126/science.aam8563.

21. Institute of Medicine. The role of telehealth in an evolving health care environment: workshop summary. Washington, DC: The National Academies Press; 2012. https://www.ncbi.nlm.nih.gov/books/NBK207133/. Accessed October 5, 2019.

22. Meyers A. *Barriers to physician entrepreneurship*. 2017; https://www.linkedin.com/pulse/barriers-physician-entrepreneurship-arlen-meyers-md-mba. Updated November 13, 2017. Accessed October 5, 2019.

23. Kmietowicz Z. Cross specialty training would improve academic psychiatry. *BMJ*. 2013;346(7902):2 https://doi.org/10.1136/bmj.f2080.

24. El-Awad Z, Gabrielsson J, Politis D. Entrepreneurial learning and innovation. *Int J Entrepreneurial Behav Res*. 2017;23(3):381–405 https://doi.org/10.1108/ijebr-06-2016-0177.

25. Murphy B. Effective med student-entrepreneurs have these 5 traits. 2019; https://www.ama-assn.org/residents-students/medical-school-life/effective-med-student-entrepreneurs-have-these-5-traits. Updated July 15, 2019. Accessed October 29, 2019.

26. Hasselberg MJ. The digital revolution in behavioral health. *J Am Psychiatr Nurses Assoc*. 2019. doi:10.1177/1078390319879750.

27. Gossman W, Meyers A, Korvek S. *Digital Health. Treasure Island*, FL: StatPearls Publishing; 2019. https://www.ncbi.nlm.nih.gov/books/NBK470260/. Accessed October 29, 2019.

28. Kaonga NN, Morgan J. Common themes and emerging trends for the use of technology to support mental health and psychosocial well-being in limited resource settings: a review of the literature. *Psychiatry Res*. 2019;281:112594. https://doi.org/10.1016/j.psychres.2019.112594.

29. Indian Health Service. Tele-education. 2019; https://www.ihs.gov/teleeducation/. Accessed October 27, 2019.

30. Global Future Council on Neurotechnologies. *Empowering 8 billion minds: enabling better mental health for all via the ethical adoption of technologies*. 2019; https://www.weforum.org/whitepapers/empowering-8-billion-minds-enabling-better-mental-health-for-all-via-the-ethical-adoption-of-technologies. Updated July 1, 2019. Accessed August 27, 2019.

31. World Economic Forum. *Leading through the fourth industrial revolution: putting people at the centre*. 2019; https://www.weforum.org/whitepapers/leading-through-the-fourth-industrial-revolution-putting-people-at-the-centre. Updated January 11, 2019. Accessed August 27, 2019.

32. Meyers A. Digital health ethics. 2019; https://www.linkedin.com/pulse/digital-health-ethics-arlen-meyers-md-mba/. Updated July 29, 2019. Accessed November 1, 2019.

33. Santos SC, Morris MH, Caetano A, Costa SF, Neumeyer X. Team entrepreneurial competence: multilevel effects on individual cognitive strategies. *Int J Entrepreneurial Behav Res.* 2019;25(6):1259–1282 https://doi.org/10.1108/ijebr-03-2018-0126.

34. Wilson N. On the road to convergence research. *Bioscience.* 2019;69(8):587–593 https://doi.org/10.1093/biosci/biz066.

35. Perez-Vaisvidovsky N, Aviram U. The rehabilitation of the mentally disabled in the community act in Israel: entrepreneurship, leadership, and capitalizing on opportunities in policy making. *Int J Law Psychiatry.* 2019;66:101457. https://doi.org/10.1016/j.ijlp.2019.101457

36. Eyre HA, Forbes M, Raji C, et al. Strengthening the role of convergence science in medicine. *Converg Sci Phys Oncol.* 2015;1(2):026001. https://doi.org/10.1088/2057-1739/1/2/026001.

37. Wyss Institute Team. 2019; https://wyss.harvard.edu/team/. Accessed October 27, 2019.

38. Berkeley Research. California Institute for Quantitative Biosciences. 2019; https://vcresearch.berkeley.edu/research-unit/california-institute-quantitative-biosciences. Accessed October 27, 2019.

39. UCI Beall Applied Innovation. Connecting UCI and the business community. 2019; http://innovation.uci.edu/. Accessed October 27, 2019.

40. Fortuna KL, Walker R, Fisher DB, Mois G, Allan S, Deegan PE. Enhancing standards and principles in digital mental health with recovery-focused guidelines for mobile, online, and remote monitoring technologies. *Psychiatr Serv.* 2019;70. doi:10.1176/appi.ps.201900166.

41. National Academies of Sciences Engineering and Medicine. *Fostering the Culture of Convergence in Research: Proceedings of a Workshop.* Washington, DC: The National Academies Press; 2019. https://www.nap.edu/catalog/25271/fostering-the-culture-of-convergence-in-research-proceedings-of-a. Accessed July 29, 2019.

42. American Psychiatric Association. Mental health apps. 2019; https://www.psychiatry.org/psychiatrists/practice/mental-health-apps. Accessed October 26, 2019.

43. American Psychiatric Association. App evaluation model. 2019; https://www.psychiatry.org/psychiatrists/practice/mental-health-apps/app-evaluation-model. Accessed October 26, 2019.

44. Morgan SA, Agee NH. Mobile healthcare. *Front Health Serv Manage.* 2012;29(2):3–10 https://doi.org/10.1097/01974520-201210000-00002.

45. Change Healthcare. The 8th annual industry pulse report: a national survey of leading health plans and other healthcare stakeholders commissioned and conducted by the HealthCare Executive Group and Change Healthcare. 2018; http://discover.changehealthcare.com/2018-Industry-Pulse-Results. Updated February 2, 2018. Accessed October 5, 2019.

46. Bennett K, Bennett AJ, Griffiths KM. Security considerations for e-mental health interventions. *J Med Internet Res.* 2010;12(5):e61. https://doi.org/10.2196/jmir.1468.

47. Kazgan M. Real challenge in digital health entrepreneurship: changing human behavior. In: Wulfovich S, Meyers A, eds. *Digital Health Entrepreneurship.* Cham, Switzerland: Springer Nature Switzerland; 2019:7–16 https://doi.org/10.2196/jmir.1468.

48. Almario CV. The effect of digital health technology on patient care and research. *Gastroenterol Hepatol (NY).* 2017;13(7):437–439.

49. Meyers A. *Fundamentals of digital health entrepreneurship.* 2016; https://www.linkedin.com/pulse/fundamentals-digital-health-entrepreneurship-arlen-meyers-md-mba-1/. Updated June 23, 2016. Accessed November 2, 2019.

50. Sauro J, Lewis JR. *Quantifying the User Experience: Practical Statistics for User Research.* Waltham, MA: Morgan Kaufman; 2012.

51. Brown W, 3rd, Yen PY, Rojas M, Schnall R. Assessment of the health IT usability evaluation model for evaluating mobile health (mHealth) technology. *J Biomed Inform.* 2013;46(6):1080–1087 https://doi.org/10.1016/j.jbi.2013.08.001.

52. Luxton DD, McCann RA, Bush NE, Mishkind MC, Reger GM. Mhealth for mental health: integrating smartphone technology in behavioral healthcare. *Prof Psychol Res Pr.* 2011;42(6):505–512 https://doi.org/10.1037/a0024485.

53. Yeager CM, Benight CC. If we build it, will they come? Issues of engagement with digital health interventions for trauma recovery. *mHealth.* 2018;4:37 https://doi.org/10.21037/mhealth.2018.08.04.

54. *Ergonomic Requirements for Office Work with Visual Display Terminals (VDTs): Part 11 Guidance on Usability, International Standard 9241-11.* Geneva, Switzerland: International Organization for Standardization; 1998.

55. Rotondi AJ, Eack SM, Hanusa BH, Spring MB, Haas GL. Critical design elements of e-health applications for users with severe mental illness: singular focus, simple architecture, prominent contents, explicit navigation, and inclusive hyperlinks. *Schizophr Bull.* 2015;41(2):440–448 https://doi.org/10.1093/schbul/sbt194.

56. Sauro J. *A Practical Guide to the System Usability Scale: Background, Benchmarks and Best Practices.* Denver, CO: Measuring Usability; 2011.

57. Wulfovich S, Fiordelli M, Rivas H, Concepcion W, Wac K. "I must try harder": design implications for mobile apps and wearables contributing to self-efficacy of patients with chronic conditions. *Front Psychol.* 2019;10(2388). doi:10.3389/fpsyg.2019.02388.

58. Becker S, Miron-Shatz T, Schumacher N, Krocza J, Diamantidis C, Albrecht U-V. mHealth 2.0: experiences, possibilities, and perspectives. *JMIR Mhealth Uhealth.* 2014;2(2):e24. doi:10.2196/mhealth.3328.

59. Zhong D, Kirwan MJ, Duan X. Regulatory barriers blocking standardization of interoperability. *JMIR Mhealth Uhealth.* 2013;1(2):e13. https://doi.org/10. 10.2196/mhealth.2654.

60. Office of the National Coordinator for Health Information Technology. Justifications of estimates for appropriations committee. 2018; https://www.hhs.gov/sites/default/files/combined-onc.pdf. Updated May 28, 2018. Accessed February 18, 2019.

61. Estrin D, Sim I. Health care delivery. Open mHealth architecture: an engine for health care innovation. *Science.* 2010;330(6005):759–760 https://doi.org/10.1126/science.1196187.

62. Price WN. Drug approval in a learning health system. *Minn L Rev.* 2018;102:2413–2462.

63. Stoltzfus Jost T. Contraints on sharing mental health and substance-use treatment information imposed by federal and state medical records privacy laws. In: Institute of Medicine, ed. *Improving the Quality of Health care for Mental and Substance-Abuse Conditions.* Washington, DC: National Academy of Sciences; 2006.

64. U.S. Food and Drug Administration. International Medical Device Regulators Forum (IMDRF). 2019; https://www.fda.gov/medical-devices/cdrh-international-programs/international-medical-device-regulators-forum-imdrf. Updated August 27, 2019. Accessed October 26, 2019.

65. International Medical Device Regulators Forum. 2019; http://www.imdrf.org/index.asp. Accessed October 26, 2019.

66. Sapsin J. FDA and digital health. In: Wulfovich S, Meyers A, eds. *Digital Health Entrepreneurship.* Cham, Switzerland: Springer Nature; 2019:119–142.

67. Food and Drug Administration Amendments Act of 2007. Pub L.110-85, 121 Stat. 823 (September 27, 2007).

68. 21st Century Cures Act. Pub L.114-225, *130 Stat.* 1033 (December 13, 2016).

69. U.S. Food and Drug Administration. *Changes to existing medical software policies resulting from Section 3060 of the 21st Century Cures Act. 2019;* https://www.fda.gov/regulatory-information/search-fda-guidance-documents/changes-existing-medical-software-policies-resulting-section-3060-21st-century-cures-act. Updated September 26, 2019. Accessed October 26, 2019.

70. Substance Use-Disorder Prevention that Promotes Opioid Recovery and Treatment (SUPPORT) for Patients and Communities Act. *Pub L. 2018;*115–271, 132 Stat. 3894 (October 24, 2018).

71. Davis DD. Getting reimbursed for digital health. In: Wulfovich S, Meyers A, eds. *Digital Health Entrepreneurship.* Cham, Switzerland: Springer Nature Switzerland AG; 2019:143–156.

72. Reilly T, Mechelli A, McGuire P, Fusar-Poli P, Uhlhaas PJ. E-clinical high risk for psychosis: viewpoint on potential of digital innovations for preventive psychiatry. *JMIR Ment Health.* 2019;6(10):e14581. doi:10.2196/14581.

26

Stanford's Brainstorm Lab for Mental Health Innovation

Anjali Albuquerque, Neha P. Chaudhary, Gowri G. Aragam, and Nina Vasan

> *You have lived my dream. ... Innovation is going to be a cornerstone of the future of psychiatry. And you folks who have been working in this space are going to be the leaders of that movement.*
> —Altha Stewart, MD, President of the American
> Psychiatric Association, May 2019[1]

At the 2019 American Psychiatric Association's (APA) Annual Meeting, the biggest gathering of psychiatrists in the country, Altha Stewart, the association's president, addressed a topic that a few years prior would have been a rarity. The APA—and psychiatry as a field—had for years been considered by many to be overly traditional and slow to adopt change.[2] Yet Stewart took to the stage to celebrate the work of the Psychiatry Innovation Lab, an initiative started in 2015 by Nina Vasan, currently chair of the APA's Committee on Innovation. "When I met you, I knew you were onto something special," Stewart told Vasan in front of the captivated audience. "I didn't know what it was, but I knew with time I'd find out." As the first African American to hold the title of president of the APA, Stewart was herself a pioneer and trailblazer, and in Vasan she saw a kindred spirit. "You have lived my dream," Stewart continued. "Innovation is going to be a cornerstone of the future of psychiatry. And you folks who have been working in this space are going to be the leaders of that movement."[3]

The Psychiatry Innovation Lab, founded by Vasan, had grown year after year into becoming the signature event of the APA's Innovation Zone at the Annual Meeting. As it grew, it brought Vasan together with young psychiatrists and visionaries from around the country—in particular Neha Chaudhary and Gowri Aragam—who would go on to become leaders and partners in the effort to transform the future of mental health through innovation. This next generation of psychiatrists would unite from around the country to build what Stewart had called "the future of psychiatry" by founding Stanford Brainstorm, the world's first academic lab dedicated to using technology and entrepreneurship to redesign the way the world views, diagnoses, and treats mental illness.

Just as Stewart perceived a mysterious potential in Vasan's disruptive vision and leadership, Brainstorm's leadership team—Vasan, Chaudhary, Aragam, and a handful of other young professionals who came in and out to shape Brainstorm's evolution—intuited "something special" in the field of mental health innovation.[4] While they did not know exactly how technology would transform mental health access, they became the early adopters of technology's potential to provide mental healthcare to people in need. Technology offered a new way for psychiatry to address the burgeoning crisis of global mental illness. A beacon of hope for the field, Stewart embraced both the rapid current of innovation within psychiatry and the innovators themselves. Her message galvanized a diverse audience of young professionals—spanning disciplines, geographies, expertise, and demographics—to brandish 21st-century weapons of technology and innovation in the battle against mental illness.

"Mirrors of Distorting Glass": Systemic Barriers to Mental Health

I am invisible, understand, simply because people refuse to see me. Like the bodiless heads you see sometimes in circus sideshows, it is as though I have been surrounded by mirrors of hard, distorting glass. When they approach me they see only my surroundings, themselves or figments of their imagination, indeed, everything and anything except me.

—Ralph Ellison, *Invisible Man*[5]

For health professionals, the startling image of human isolation presented in Ralph Ellison's *Invisible Man* serves as a metaphor for the challenges mental health systems face worldwide to observe, diagnose, and treat the two billion people who struggle daily with brain and behavioral health disorders. In the United States alone, 50% of all Americans will experience a mental illness at some point during their lifetime.[6] Globally, depression presents as the number one cause of ill health and disability.[7] Not surprisingly, grappling with mental illness comes at a tremendous cost—in dollars, output, potential, and community.[8] In fact, the United States spends more money treating mental illness than on diabetes and heart disease combined.[9]

This crisis of mental illness is daunting to solve, primarily because so many people lack access to mental health care. When people do seek out mental health treatment, they struggle to find a doctor due to the great supply-and-demand mismatch.[10] Seventy percent of the world's population lives in a country with fewer than one psychiatrist per 100,000 people.[11] Despite this enormous demand, mental health workers make up only 1% of the global health workforce.[12] Additionally, access appears most unattainable for people who suffer the worst based on their age, disease state, geographical location, and ethnicity, yet these people are often the ones most in need of help. Having an untreated mental illness often entrenches already existent social and health disparities; the most vulnerable are the highest at risk.[13] In the end, all of this neglect comes at a deadly cost: those suffering from severe mental illness die 25 years earlier than the general population, making mental illness a brazen thief of human potential.[14]

Unfortunately, current mental health care systems use outdated approaches to deliver treatment and as a result cannot respond effectively to the crisis. The biggest limitation of the current model hinges on its inability to bring person-to-person care to those who suffer from mental illness.[15] With so few providers per capita, combined with the growing spectrum and severity of mental disorders as well as the stigma attached to seeking out care, it would seem impossible to bolster the workforce with competent professionals quickly enough to reach those in need, let alone convince all those who suffer to seek professional help.[16]

The Promise of Innovation

Stanford Brainstorm believes these elements of the mental health crisis—a huge impacted population, stigma, and supply–demand mismatch with providers—make it ideally suited to solutions leveraging innovation, technology, and entrepreneurship. Many others agree.[17] In response to this crisis, tech companies have begun stepping in to fill in the void.[18] Over the last few years, tech start-ups such as Lyra Health, Ginger, and Mindstrong Health have sprung up, offering those with mental health challenges technological options with which to monitor and address their disorders. Scalable technology has dealt with crises of supply and demand across fields in creative ways; for example, inventing mobile apps and programs to improve access to a diversity of social resources, from education to healthy food.[19] Vasan, Chaudhary, Aragam, and the rest of the Brainstorm team view these technologies as offering tremendous potential for patients, loved ones, and future generations to achieve good mental health and well-being.[20]

From 2011 to 2018, venture capital funding designated for mental health tech start-ups exploded from $50 million to $700–$800 million annually.[21] The increase in investment was a promising step toward developing the new field of mental health innovation. However, those funds had still not resulted in substantial improvements to either the system or to individual patients. The field of mental health innovation seemed trapped in market inefficiency. In part, because many innovative problemsolvers in the psychiatric field who aren't operating in start-ups don't receive the necessary funds designated for research and development.[22] Additionally, product designers often lack the clinical knowledge they need to make an effective product. In a similar vein, clinicians don't often have experience with building and scaling products. What is missing is the culture of innovative collaboration—marked by interdisciplinarity and convergence—needed to drive product design tailored to the nuanced problems they aim to solve.[23]

When Brainstorm's team began to engage around mental health technology and innovation, the field consisted primarily of smaller start-up companies leveraging mobile tech to deliver mental health treatment. The treatments they offered were ones that had already proven to work in person and the companies were those that understood how to use technology to deliver the same benefit on a much bigger scale than one-to-one. For example, several companies (e.g., Lantern, Joyable) popped up offering online cognitive behavioral therapy—a popular and well-evidenced therapy done in individual and group therapy sessions—as it translates well from face-to-face to computerized settings.[24] Similarly, dozens of companies—the most popular being Calm and Headspace—provided wellness interventions such as mindfulness meditation through mobile apps. Others, such as 7 Cups, BetterHelp, and TalkSpace connected users to therapists and coaches via text or phone therapy.[25] Of note, larger entities such as tech giants, national organizations, and big employers had yet to address mental health in a meaningful way, but that was about to change.[26]

As these companies were evolving, Brainstorm was also evolving. From 2015 to 2019, the Brainstorm team was building credibility as leaders in mental health innovation while building the connective tissue among academia, technological innovators, and policy experts. Brainstorm's progression can be understood as evolving from a 1.0 focus on education to a 3.0 focus on product development. In Brainstorm 1.0, the organization's goal was to incubate the ideas, people, and tools—mainly through teaching innovation principles and workshops to students and professionals—needed for scaling the mental health innovations poised for greatest impact. Brainstorm 2.0 was about building an organization across disciplines, states, and technological focus areas. All this evolution culminated in Brainstorm 3.0. By 2018, it was becoming clear that tech leaders needed the support of psychiatrists to design products to support the mental health of their users. The historical moment was ripe for industry and academia to converge, and Brainstorm was catapulted into the role of protagonists in this movement, invested with the authority and opportunity to collaborate with partners like Silicon Valley's tech giants to design tech products to reach millions. When the right people with the right ideas and expertise converge, they form a crucible for the discipline's most revolutionary ideas. Brainstorm: The Stanford Lab for Mental Health Innovation is one such crucible, and an important organizational case study of convergence mental health. Brainstorm reflects the convergence of disciplinary approaches within the field of psychiatry, and the group itself leverages convergence science to advance mental health innovation.

Birth of Stanford Brainstorm

No one in the world is doing what you are doing.
—Walter Greenleaf, Chief Science Officer at Pear Therapeutics,
speaking about Stanford Brainstorm[27]

It was 2:30 AM at the Rosewood Hotel on Menlo Park's famous Sand Hill Road, site of the after-party for the Brainstorm Lab Launch, and the room was still buzzing with activity. While most of those gathered had just met for the first-time hours earlier, they were celebrating as if they'd known each other for years. "I just could have stayed there all night," one participant said. "I've never had the experience of meeting so many different people with the passion to bring our talents together to create mental health products that could change the world."[28]

Brainstorm's Launch event gathered together a diverse group of professionals and students at Stanford's School of Engineering. The event's purpose was to introduce the Brainstorm team—which had been growing steadily over the past year—to the public, as well as to create a knowledge-sharing network through which social capital—norms, resources, ideas, and power—could be activated to drive innovation within the mental health field. "The energy was contagious and magical," said

Vasan, Stanford Brainstorm's founder and executive director. "And at the after-party, we closed down the Rosewood. I think many of us felt like we had finally found our village, our people."[29]

Rewind to 2015. Nina Vasan was a Leadership Fellow with the American Psychiatric Organization, living in Silicon Valley while in the midst of her psychiatric residency at Stanford and about to start her MBA at the Stanford Graduate School of Business. Having lived in Boston for a decade as a college and medical school student at Harvard, she was eager to immerse herself in the spirit of innovation for which Silicon Valley was famous. She had worked at the consulting firm McKinsey & Co.'s Silicon Valley office, followed by what was then a new tech start-up, Lyra Health. "When I was at McKinsey and Lyra," says Vasan, "I felt like an ambassador for the world of psychiatry. I was surrounded by brilliant people in business and tech and was sharing with them the needs and culture of psychiatry. Being at the convergence of industries helped me see that there was a huge opportunity and potential for something formalized that could unite these different worlds and help them work together."[30]

Vasan had observed the start-up boom firsthand and attended numerous health-related hackathons. So, when confronted by the pressing question of bringing psychiatrists to the forefront of mental health solutions, it was only natural that Vasan would try to build innovation into psychiatric education, networks, and problem-solving. Energized by the proliferation of tech start-ups attempting to address health-care needs, Vasan pitched the concept of a mental health "hackathon" as an innovative possibility for the APA's Annual Meeting in Atlanta in May of 2016. In traditional hackathons, people get together to create a minimally viable product for a start-up over the course of a day or two. However, the energy often dissipates in the weeks following the event, and meaningful action fails to materialize. Vasan wondered, "How do we do something that gets the energy going, gets people motivated, interested, and learning ... but also leads to something concrete?"[31] She tweaked the idea of the hackathon and morphed it into the Psychiatry Innovation Lab, a Shark Tank-style pitch contest geared to serve as an incubator for mental health start-ups. The first Innovation Lab occurred at the 2016 APA Annual Meeting. The Lab issued a call for submissions from around the country and selected the top seven to present their pitches to a multidisciplinary panel of expert judges including doctors, CEOs, and the president of the National Alliance on Mental Illness. Vasan secured a $2500 donation from Doctor on Demand, a telemedicine start-up, which became the grand prize award.[32]

In addition to helping catalyze the start-up ideas themselves, the Lab was critical in bringing together young psychiatrists from across the country who shared the same vision for the potential of technology and innovation. The first was Cody Rall, a psychiatry resident in the US Navy who was a semifinalist in the inaugural Innovation Lab, and the founder of TechforPsych, a YouTube channel for sharing technologies aimed at improving mental health. Rall was eager to interview Innovation Lab finalists and share their stories via You Tube. Swathi Krishna was a finalist in the 2nd Innovation Lab in Washington, DC, where she pitched a start-up idea for kids with autism (after winning the Lab's Impact Award, she wanted to use her background in investing and business to help the initiative grow and scale). Neha Chaudhary was an

APA Child Psychiatry Fellow in the audience of the 2nd Innovation Lab, where she helped finalist teams improve their ideas during the event. She was inspired by the energy of this event and realized it could help bring about new ideas for kids and schools. Gowri Aragam, then a psychiatry resident at Harvard's MGH/McLean training program, saw the Innovation Lab not only as a place to address the inequalities in healthcare that her patients faced but also to change negative messaging around mental health and connect with others to create a shared language. These young psychiatrists reached out to Vasan and contributed their time and talent to help grow the Innovation Lab; each year, the lab grew in size, structure, and sophistication.[33] This group of seven became the Lab's leadership board, with each member being responsible for tasks from fundraising to mentoring to ensure the event's success.[34]

Today, the Innovation Lab has grown into the signature event of the Innovation Zone, a section of the Annual Meeting dedicated to technology and start-ups.[35] It continues to incubate ideas and, as of March 2020, has helped over 60 start-ups get off the ground. One finalist start-up, Spring Health, utilizes Precision Mental Healthcare to "predict the right treatment to the right person at the right time" to "accelerate recovery." Their unique personalized approach to mental healthcare has been shown to lower employers' behavioral costs by up to 10%, with a net promoter score, which is a metric for assessing customer loyalty, of +72.[36] The Innovation Lab brought company CEO April Koh together with a psychiatrist, who then performed clinical trials with Spring to help validate their work. The Innovation Lab demonstrated to tech innovators and psychiatrists the great enthusiasm, need, and opportunity that existed for interdisciplinary collaboration.[37] "The Innovation Lab became my community and supported all of us to develop as mental health clinicians and as innovators," says Chaudhary.[38]

Since Vasan had launched the Innovation Lab, she became known as the Stanford Department of Psychiatry's innovation expert. As a result, the department called on her to educate and advise students who had ideas for start-ups and mobile apps. She also found herself mentoring and developing entrepreneurs in a variety of contexts through the Psychiatry Department and the social entrepreneurship community throughout the country. She identified three needs within the newly emergent space of mental health tech. First, that start-up companies needed to develop an understanding for the clinical context of mental health and the mental health system. Second, they needed top–down support to design and build products that could address mental illness in a sustainable, responsible, and effective manner. Finally, the field of mental health innovation needed an institutional gatekeeper to vet the best-in-field people, companies, and products that were indeed equipped to improve patient outcomes. No current organization or company was providing this guidance, so it would be critical for stakeholders to come together and form a cohesive field of mental health innovation, as well as for the field to flourish.[39]

Vasan studied the growth of other new fields and noted the benefit of a player that could see the big picture opportunities and challenges, as well as have the credibility and buy-in from other players to be able to build a coalition. The field of mental health innovation needed a neutral third-party leader who could assess the ebbs and flows of trends from a macro perspective and address the dynamic synergies that accelerate the demand for mental healthcare. She envisioned an organization that could marry psychiatry with technology to provide forward guidance and moral vision to the fledgling, inchoate mental health innovation field. Well-networked in the Graduate School of Business at Stanford and the Stanford Medical School, Vasan turned to Silicon Valley's vibrant culture of technology and entrepreneurship for inspiration.[40]

Silicon Valley's culture helped create the conditions that made Brainstorm's birth possible. Stanford's own academic culture did not just appreciate innovation; it actually "celebrates the ethos of entrepreneurship," as Vasan observed. Part of this welcoming culture is intrinsic to Stanford's location in the heart of Silicon Valley. Since the mid-20th century, Silicon Valley has been a hub for scientific and technological advancement with such companies as Google, Hewlett Packard, and Facebook laying claim to the once-agrarian region. Vasan took it upon herself to integrate all the innovations she had originated at Stanford—the first course created on mental health innovation, workshops, and trainings around *Do Good Well*, and budding partnerships with other institutions and organizations—to drive mental health innovation with intentionality and focus.

While other mental health institutions conducted research on a granular level, Vasan's new lab would examine the ecosystem of mental health innovation in multiple directions: from a top–down perspective with a cross-disciplinary lens and realized through a bottom–up movement. After considering multiple business models, including an investment fund, a third-party start-up incubator, a business, and a nonprofit, Vasan decided to build an academic lab to serve as a space where intellectual collaboration and scientific rigor could thrive. "Collaboration and partnership are core values and I saw that all stakeholders from the federal government to a scrappy start-up would want to partner with an academic lab, though that wouldn't necessarily be the case with other business structures," said Vasan. [41] So, in 2016 Vasan pitched the idea for an academic lab, Brainstorm (a name thought up by Vasan's brother, Neil Vasan, a medical oncologist at Memorial Sloan Kettering Cancer Center) to Laura Roberts, Chair of the Stanford Psychiatry Department. Roberts approved and designated it as a special initiative of the chair within the department of psychiatry and School of Medicine. Finally, Brainstorm, Silicon Valley's latest agent for change and the world's first academic lab for mental health innovation, was born.

Vasan's discussions with academic stakeholders at Stanford informed her strategy and vision for how Brainstorm could revolutionize psychiatry. Her conversations with Roberts, Chair of the Department of Psychiatry, helped Vasan realize that Brainstorm needed to embed mental health innovation within societal nodes of influence (such as schools, sports associations, and technology communities) to precipitate the trickle down of mental health access throughout society. Vasan consulted with other Stanford faculty, including Director of Community Partnerships Steve Adelsheim and Director of Education Alan Louie, to help shape Brainstorm's strategic focus. Adelsheim had a background in telepsychiatry and reaching underserved populations through technology, and Louie had started a special initiative called Reimagining Mental Healthcare that taught design thinking to clinicians as a way to foster innovation. Roberts, Adelsheim, and Louie served as mentors to Vasan as she navigated the behind-the-scenes work of starting an organization at Stanford and building the political, financial, and structural backbone of Brainstorm.

Into this gap of mental health innovation came a group of seven psychiatry residents who had initially met through the APA and the Psychiatry Innovation Lab. These physicians were Chaudhary and Aragam from Harvard, Rall from the US Navy, Krishna from Morehouse and Emory, Kenechi Ejebe and Linda Drozdowicz from Mt. Sinai School of Medicine, and Reza Hosseini Ghomi from the University of Washington.[42] Treating patients and observing the systemic causes of mental illness, this group of young psychiatrists had grown frustrated with the mental health system's inefficiencies while becoming fascinated with technology's potential to solve mental health problems. Over the years of growing the Innovation Lab, they had conversations with each other and as a group about what mental health innovations could be pursued beyond the parameters of the APA and, together, brainstormed myriad ideas. After Brainstorm was approved by Roberts, Vasan invited the seven psychiatrists to work together as Founding Partners for Brainstorm, with each heading up a particular element of the organization's programming. The seven enthusiasts were hungry to do something revolutionary within psychiatry. Innovation spoke to their hearts, providing the energy they needed to disrupt traditional and ineffective mental health treatments. "I came to believe that Brainstorm was onto something special when work didn't feel like work anymore," says Chaudhary. "I felt a creative energy and excitement and had fun working toward our cause. Once we started gaining the support of our board members and early clients, it started to feel real."[43]

Aragam and Chaudhary both helped design and execute Brainstorm's early programs. The energy of these early days carried a captivating allure. Aragam said,

> It excited me to be a part of a group where people's skill sets complement one another in a way that had the potential to move initiative and projects forward. I felt like I would be encouraged and motivated by this group of people, which to me was necessary in any work environment. The growth of Brainstorm felt so organic and well-timed. After discussing the decision heavily with my mentors at residency, I decided that given the timing of the public's growing interest in mental health, this would be a window of opportunity to be involved in something new from the ground up. To give it best chance for success, I had to fully commit.[44]

Vasan, Aragam and Chaudhary discerned "a special call within a call" to mental health innovation as their professional and career focus within the field of psychiatry. While Aragam and Chaudhary were at Harvard, they sought out communities centered around mental health innovation. "My adviser motivated me by saying that I was getting lost-in-translation in my current environment," says Aragam. "She motivated me to keep sharing my interests with new people. I believed firmly that I would find similar minds."[45] The residents supported one another, and through numerous conversations, developed a language to conceptualize this new field.

While each of the doctors tried to build an ecosystem for mental health innovation at their home institution, they realized there was a special alchemy at Stanford, and in Vasan's collaborative leadership style, that convinced them to pool their energies into building Brainstorm. Chaudhary explained:

> I talked to people at my home institution about starting an initiative around mental health innovation, and it wasn't in their lexicon at that moment in time. It now is, but

the go-to place for interdisciplinary innovation for any field was Stanford, with the design school as an established space. It just strategically made a lot of sense to build out that kind of initiative at Stanford, which had a precedent for facilitating and encouraging cross-disciplinary and cross-school collaboration. The activation energy would be lower to get buy-in and projects like the class off the ground.[46]

Aragam was captivated by Brainstorm's mission, especially its emphasis on convergence. She said:

> Remembering that as physicians, entrepreneurs, millennials, and South Asian women, we are ultimately trying to serve individuals (patients, families, users) in whatever role we play, and pay respect to the influence each world has had on our perspective, and pay respect to the views and positions of others who also inhabit those world and roles. We do this while knowing that none of these worlds defines us, but rather it is our identity that positions us to understand and reach certain populations, able to see what they have in common, not only how they differ.[47]

She felt she belonged with Vasan and Chaudhary because the team was committed to recognizing that a convergence of backgrounds and identities is necessary and instrumental to drive the innovation needed in the mental health field.

While Vasan galvanized the vision and community that gave rise to Brainstorm, Chaudhary brought her creativity and operational excellence to execute that strategy. Her background in consulting and media helped Brainstorm not only organize but also develop into a public and media-facing organization, rare for most academic labs. Aragam brought her commitment to tackling the social and economic disparities that perpetuate health inequalities. Her keen understanding of what makes communities function has helped Brainstorm to design culturally sensitive solutions to mental illness. As they were determining their next professional step after finishing their residency and fellowship at Harvard, Aragam and Chaudhary were both convinced that the Brainstorm team contained great potential and was worth moving across the country to support. "We were excited to finish our training commitments so that we could move to the Bay Area and dive in fully," said Chaudhary.

Brainstorm's Impact: "Breathing Life Into the Mental Health Ecosystem"

> Brainstorm is breathing life into the mental health ecosystem to tackle the complexities of mental health that extend beyond our traditional algorithms. Brainstorm provides opportunity and space for all these diverse components within the mental health innovation to converge, driving innovation, driving access, and creating a unique disruption.
> —Jon Sole, Brainstorm Fellow and Stanford Medical Student[48]

As of this writing, it is 2020, and Brainstorm's female-founded, physician-led lab is built on the premise that solving the mental health crisis in an ethical and socially responsible manner requires solutions based on scientific evidence and interdisciplinary collaboration, integrated inside and outside the traditional healthcare system, and scalable to millions at a time. The lab strives to [t]ake the best insights from academic research and practice and apply them in [its] partnerships with leading entities to work toward ... more effective, accessible, and engaging technologies and innovations that improve health and unlock human potential.

While working to reach the millions of people who suffer from mental illnesses with insufficient or no access to treatment, the Brainstorm solution recognizes the importance of building community at a historical moment when the social glue that binds communities has lost its stickiness. People are lonely or at least don't always get enough social interaction.[49] Creating social cohesion in particular to counteract the loneliness epidemic is part of Brainstorm's vision for social change. Brainstorm aspires to talk about community beyond the traditional definition. Rather than thinking of communities in ethnic, geographical, or class-based terms, Brainstorm re-imagines them to encompass "how people actually spend their time, and what they identify with—maybe belonging to a social media network, identifying as a Googler, participating in a sports community fan base, and following a rap YouTuber."[50]

Communities in today's technological age may be organized around these new categories and settings, but they still influence one's sense of belonging as deeply as do traditional, non-virtual communities. Nonconventional communities still act as social hubs with positive benefits, including validation and opportunities for growth. "Meeting people where they are" is not simply a therapeutic idiom to improve clinical outcomes. More fundamentally, it's literal; systemic solutions need to be designed for the broader context of mental illness, its root causes, and its relationship to where people actually spend their time in today's globalized and technological age. According to Vasan,

> the hypothesis is that if we are creating 'mental health' solutions that are tailored to the needs of communities and then helping communities own those solutions, then the likelihood of success for mental health innovation is much greater had the focus been solely on individuals. Members of a community are tightly bound. Those tight bonds help improve the community's receptivity to mental health products we are trying to deliver, and community members are invested in improving products so they can improve their herd.[51]

Brainstorm's leaders saw the collaboration between academia and industry as pivotal to reimagining the field of psychiatry and advancing the field as a whole. Brainstorm aspires to lay a sturdy foundation upon which can be built an entirely new structure for mental health innovation. This vision for Brainstorm stemmed from the leaders' understanding that technology allows professionals to reach people who might not otherwise seek treatment due to stigma, access, or myriad other issues. While technology can isolate individuals and worsen mental health, technology can also provide mental health education, support for referrals that lead to care, online communities, and even opportunities for sufferers to tell their own stories. Brainstorm's impact evolved as the organization evolved. While Brainstorm 1.0 was focused on building a foundation for the field, Brainstorm 3.0 was focused on designing mental healthcare products for the millions. Stewart's prophecy of Brainstorm being onto something special has become ever more prescient with time. In Chaudhary's words,

> I think Brainstorm is going to truly establish the area of mental health innovation as its own field to the point where on a societal level, we will start to see shifts. We will start to really meet people where they are when it comes to their mental health, and the stigma barriers will start to dissolve. I can see us empowering people with the right tools so that they can recapture what so far has been lost potential in terms of wasted resources or efforts.[52]

Fashioning "Swiss-Army-Knives": Brainstorm's Impact

> *A pattern I noticed is how it seems from a leadership perspective we lack "Swiss-army-knives" leadership in mental healthcare of people who can bridge business, academy, policy and the various incentives in the field. We, right here, are developing those kinds of leaders. I've also noticed that the different scientists involved [like the ones who helped create the thermometer] are so diverse and had such rich backgrounds. It's so evident that convergence is how innovators are formed.*
>
> —Erin Smith, Stanford University Freshman, student in
> Brainstorm's Stanford University course, "Designing for 2
> Billion: Leading Innovation in Mental Healthcare"[53]

By bringing together medicine, business, and technology, Brainstorm's cross-disciplinary approach aims to reach the masses of people suffering from the same mental illnesses at the same time. A cross-disciplinary approach made necessary a cross-disciplinary team. Comprised of a leadership team, an advisory board, fellows, and interns, Brainstorm's team spans a medley of disciplines, geographies, and demographics. The common denominator is a determination to drive the future of mental health through innovative collaboration.

Brainstorm works to accomplish the objectives outlined in its mission statement within four pillars: education, research, clinical practice, and product development. The four pillars converge to support a pipeline for future mental health innovation. The education pillar trains the next generation of leaders in mental health. The research pillar collects relevant data, conducts research, and shares knowledge pertinent to mental health innovation so that clinicians, industry, and community can all become more effective in designing solutions. The clinical practice pillar is building the first artificial intelligence and technology mental health clinic to beta test, implement, and analyze the impact of technologies in patient care. For the product development pillar, the Brainstorm leaders partner with companies and organizations to design new products that can support mental health for millions of people. Finally, their community presence focuses on driving collaboration across disciplines, geographies, industries, and demographics to share knowledge and support innovation.

Pillar 1: Education

Brainstorm aims to transform the ways people attack the problem of mental illness by training students, clinicians, and innovators from all disciplines to become foot soldiers in the battle against mental illness. The lab builds a community around mental health innovation, disseminates clinical knowledge on mental health, and utilizes design thinking and consulting modalities to drive action planning for mental health innovation. One of the primary ways that Brainstorm's leaders hope to train current and future innovators is through a class they teach called "Designing for 2 Billion: Leading Innovation in Mental Healthcare." The course was first designed and taught in 2017 by Vasan and Belinda Bandstra, a clinical associate professor and Assistant Director of Residency Training at Stanford. When launched in 2017, it was the country's first university-level course on mental health innovation. It taught students about the realities of the mental healthcare system and gave them a path to creating innovation in mental health, through the social innovation framework described in the book *Do Good Well*, written by Vasan and Jennifer Przybylo.[54]

"It is an understatement to say that Innovation in Mental Health changed my life," said Ariela Safira. Safira was a senior at Stanford in 2017 when she was a student in the course.[55] Less than two years later, she had founded Real, a first-of-its-kind mental health studio, designed to improve the quality of mental healthcare and make it an essential part of wellness. Safira has raised $2.5 million in funding and is the CEO of Real. She said,

> An amazing element of Stanford is that it is filled with professors encouraging students into entrepreneurship. Throughout my time at Stanford, as a Math and Computer Science student deeply passionate about mental healthcare, I was consistently encouraged by professors and peers to build technology that enhances mental health. But it wasn't until 'Innovation in Mental Healthcare' that the vision to build something much larger than an app became a reality. I spent most of the course learning about Stanford's inpatient mental health facility, learning about the gaps, decision makers and workflows in the system that I would later change. I was introduced to decision makers in the hospital I couldn't access on my own and exposed to information an undergrad like me wouldn't have been in the know of. Previous professors who encouraged me to build a company were math and computer science professors—people I admire greatly, but who didn't quite flip the switch in me like Vasan did. Of course I knew I·could build a technology company or app—all that took was coding—but what Vasan inspired in me was the realization that, despite not being a doctor myself, I could evolve mental healthcare by building therapy spaces, hiring clinicians, reinventing training, and building something with more impact than an Apple Watch feature can dream of. Vasan spent the entirety of the class pulling me aside, insisting I should bring my ideas to life.[56]

The second iteration of the course was delivered in 2020 with Vasan, Aragam, and Chaudhary, along with Steve Chan, serving as teaching faculty. In this second iteration, the course was redesigned around Stanford Brainstorm's eight-part framework for designing products in mental health innovation, with each week of the course dedicated to one of the eight parts. Aragam and Brainstorm Fellow Madison McCall spent nearly a year studying best practices in education and implementing changes in the course to better facilitate collaborative learning. They completed a multidisciplinary literature review to add to the course's readings and resources. Aragam mapped clinical content onto the Brainstorm framework to determine the most strategic places for teaching medicine and public health to a diverse group of students.

The year 2020 also saw the launch of Brainstorm's second course, PSYC 242: Mental Health Innovation Studio: Entrepreneurship, Technology, and Policy. This hands-on, highly interactive course allowed students the space to work in interdisciplinary teams to build out innovative projects. These two courses ran in tandem. Every week, world-renowned guest speakers joined the faculty in lecturing and introducing a case study for mental health innovation. Postclass dinner sessions allowed students to engage intimately with the faculty and guest speakers and work on the granular implementation of socially responsible technology to address mental illness.[57]

Thomas Insel, Founder of Mindstrong Health, former Director of the National Institute of Mental Health, member of Brainstorm's advisory board, joined the class during the week focused on "measurable devices" to lecture on the need for more measurement in clinical care and solutions that improve quality of care. His discussion with students during the postclass dinner covered varied grounds: healthcare incentives with insurance companies, the latest data on therapeutic alliances between doctor and patient, and the potential for natural language processing to uncover psychoses through one's text message history. "Thank you for including me," Insel wrote the faculty in an email after the course. "You are doing something really important."

The course attracts students and faculty from a wide variety of disciplines at Stanford and taps into the University's full bounty of resources, giving Designing for 2 Billion an uncommon energy. As head teaching assistant and Stanford medical student Jon Sole says, "The inherent beauty of Stanford and Silicon Valley in general that is unique is the capacity for interdisciplinary engagement. It's not just stated it's lived." Because of the welcoming course environment, business students, engineering students, law students, undergraduates, and more are able to take classes at the medical school and learn together, bringing their expertise to this field. Students have a wide range of stories, backgrounds, and desires, which converge to create high quality conversation and diversity. "When you ask students to answer the same question and leverage the same principles, you get a beautiful mix of knowledge, and that lends itself to a community of people whose diversity is as beautifully complex as the problem they are aiming to solve," says Sole.[58]

The Brainstorm class is connected to a lab component: The Mental Health Innovation Studio, where students build products, tools, and processes that uniquely address the interdisciplinary problem within mental health that they have chosen to solve for the course's duration. The Brainstorm faculty identify the most pressing mental health issues to tackle, such as circumventing stigma in medical care, increasing adoption of innovative tech in hospital systems, or promoting mental fitness in youth. Within these topical frameworks, students develop their own research projects to understand the convergent contexts that drive challenges and opportunities. Informed by their research, the students then work in teams to identify, design, and implement innovative solutions to address their topics and, by extension, develop effective communication, collaboration, and problem-solving skills. Vasan says, "The course has a bias towards action. Mental health is in a crisis state and we don't have time to waste. We want to equip students with the knowledge and tools to start making change today. We designed the course to turn their idealism into impact." [59]

Because most students in the class don't have a background in the mental health field, Brainstorm's faculty present digestible clinical information throughout the course. They rely on a diverse reading list to unify the subject for those who lack prior training in the field, a list that includes clinical studies, primary documents, thematic readings, and guidelines for product design of mental health tools and programs. From Sole's standpoint, having so many students enrolled who don't come in with prior knowledge about the mental health profession turns out to be a bonus: "Part of the beauty [of the course] is the students don't have exceptional knowledge so they aren't jaded by a ton of experience. Their naiveté lends itself to the creation of ideas that can be buffed and honed. These are ideas one may have never come up with 10 years into the field." [60] Their projects are a diverse selection; including the neurobiology of risk in mood disorders, building behavioral nudges into technology in the classroom to improve adolescents' mental health literacy, and integrating emotional sensors into social media programs to incentivize companies to track their mental health externalities. One student group is designing an app to circumvent the stigma mothers face as they confront the stress and anxiety of returning to the workforce.

The palpable energy of the course extends beyond the classroom to the different disciplines at Stanford University, creating a hub for action. "You can see the students leave with a buzz and a purpose. It's like a beehive. Warm, sweet, and there is buzz for action," says Sole. [61]

Pillar 2: Research

The lab's research endeavors to build the foundation for the study of mental health by fostering collaboration among faculty, business leaders, and global institutions while simultaneously publishing the expertise of Brainstorm's own staff. Inspired by Vasan and Przybylo's social innovation principles that they distilled in *Do Good Well*, Brainstorm developed a mental health framework for improvement that is uniquely tailored to address the challenges within the mental health ecosystem (Figure 26.1). Inspired by content analyses and examination into industry best practices, the framework's guiding principles and tools support the practitioners and communities working in the mental health space to spearhead innovation that can be scaled.

Chaudhary has been instrumental in publishing Brainstorm's research and sharing this work with the media. Having worked as a medical journalist at the ABC News Medical Unit, she is savvy in building relationships with editors and understanding the culture of media. She has written for multiple publications including *The Washington Post*, ABC News, and *Wire*, and she has been interviewed by journalists from Good Morning America and CNN. She has also been a featured expert on the Drew radio show. Chaudhary is quick to draw on her media training to help

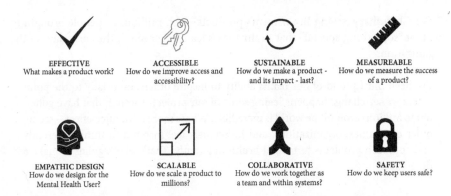

EFFECTIVE
What makes a product work?

ACCESSIBLE
How do we improve access and accessibility?

SUSTAINABLE
How do we make a product - and its impact - last?

MEASUREABLE
How do we measure the success of a product?

EMPATHIC DESIGN
How do we design for the Mental Health User?

SCALABLE
How do we scale a product to millions?

COLLABORATIVE
How do we work together as a team and within systems?

SAFETY
How do we keep users safe?

Figure 26.1 Stanford Brainstorm Framework for Mental Health Innovation.

Brainstorm disseminate its research with multiple audiences in tech, business, and the general public. Her interpersonal astuteness, aesthetic sensibility, and ability to penetrate the issues and define them for a broad audience have their origins as well in Chaudhary's background in management consulting. Having worked at Deloitte before attending medical school, she learned the "importance of communicating with your audience to drive impact."[62] From its inception, Brainstorm focused on the science, but it still had to concern itself with storytelling and marketing to clarify its mission. The Brainstorm team sought inspiration in campaigns set up to battle illness. Such campaigns have existed for decades. For example, back in 1948, the Jimmy Fund was set up as campaign to fight cancer at the Dana Farber Institute in Boston. The Jimmy Fund designed its campaign's "icons, mascots, images, and slogans" using the tools of business and political campaigning to transform the disease politically so that it could be transformed scientifically.[63] Brainstorm, in turn, has appropriated tactics from journalism and management consulting to make mental health innovation appealing beyond the world of academia. Mentoring students from all walks of life is another important way Brainstorm's leaders continue to support the next generation of mental health innovators. Starting with the lab staff itself, Brainstorm has trained nearly 30 interns and fellows from different academic backgrounds, and the lab's leaders commit significant time and energy toward mentoring students and trainees. They also have instituted a culture of mentorship, facilitating a system for older fellows to mentor younger interns as well as encouraging all members of the team to connect with each other in-person or online. This has created a closeness among the members of the lab that is unique and continues to be a draw for the members to feel emotionally connected to the team beyond the passion for the work itself. Mental health start-up founder Dan Seider reflects on Vasan's mentorship in his own life: "Vasan is the most charismatic person I know. When spending time with Vasan, it feels like I'm seen and heard, and that there is a primary validation for my own entrepreneurial work . . . She has an aura to her that I can't put into words."[64] Mentorship helps advance the field of mental health innovation by supporting entrepreneurs with community, and helping them refine their passions, products, and principles.

For Chaudhary, seeing Brainstorm's products reach millions of people brought to life that "something special" that Brainstorm's leaders sensed in the early days of the organization:

> I've been most proud of our team's ability to inspire others, especially to the point where we see change happen. Seeing some of our projects through that have gotten out to millions around the world is incredible. What's more is the after-effect—seeing other companies, organizations, and individuals feel inspired to think differently and approach problems to mental health differently. That's what's going to make a difference.[65]

Pillar 3: Clinical Practice

Brainstorm is also committed to training the next generation of clinicians. Brainstorm Fellow Sara Johansen is creating a formal "Innovation Pathway" in Stanford's Psychiatry Residency Training Program, which will provide residents with the training and exposure they need to work at the intersection of medicine and entrepreneurship. That pathway has three components: education, research, and clinical. In addition, residents will serve as clinical advisors to start-up companies, learning how to build and share clinical knowledge in an interdisciplinary setting. Through project-based learning, residents will apply their clinical knowledge to a problem in the community. Per Johansen, psychiatry residents want to understand the world of innovation so they can be attentive to forging tools and solutions that address the scourge and scale of mental illness. Residents perceive that building convergent approaches into psychiatric education will equip future generation of psychiatrists with the skills they need to innovate sustainably. Johansen hopes that the downstream repercussions of interdisciplinary psychiatric training will include better psychiatrists, better quality of care, and greater access.

The clinical component of the pathway will see residents rotate through a newly created Technology and Artificial Intelligence Patient Clinic. It is expected to launch in Stanford School of Medicine's Department of Psychiatry in early 2021 and will be the first clinic of its kind for practical implementation of artificial intelligence and tech in an academic psychiatric clinic. Brainstorm is laying the foundation for this clinic, in which physicians can implement new technological solutions in their practice, to understand not only the opportunities and challenges for clinicians and patients using these tools, but also to create a space to explore the legal, ethical, economic, and policy impact of the new technologies. Psychiatry faculty and residents will treat patients in the clinic, who will experience the technologies of the future in the clinical setting. This will allow feedback and insights from patients and clinicians alike. Brainstorm also plans to collaborate with faculty in other departments such as Stanford Law School, School of Engineering, and Graduate School of Business, as well as centers such as Stanford's Human-Centered Artificial Intelligence and Design School to study this clinic and the ramifications from the perspective of these other disciplines. The clinic embraces convergence in its structure, execution, and purpose.

Pillar 4: Product Development

Independent from Stanford, Vasan, Chaudhary and Aragam work through an independent company to consult for technology companies and other organizations. The team aims to apply insights from clinical practice and research to design products for organizations that reach at least 100 million people. For example, Brainstorm designed a compassionate search option for Pinterest that offers mental health resources and support to people who search anxiety and stress-related terms. with resources and support for their mental health. Pinterest, with over 330 million monthly active users as of March 2020, "is known for being a place where users, known as 'Pinners,' can collect images to 'pin' onto a board. This board can serve as a catalogue of products, a display of inspirational images, or creative ideas and tutorials that users can try out in the real world."[66] The doctors, along with Pinterest engineers and product developers, designed "compassionate search" so that "when someone's search includes keywords, such as 'anxiety' and 'stress,' users receive a prompt to engage in one of multiple evidence-based exercises such as relaxation techniques and activities that might improve their mood. Pinterest CEO Ben Silberman worked with Stanford Brainstorm's team to design Compassionate Search "to normalize emotions but not the behavior of self-harm." [67] Before "compassionate search," Pinterest users struggling with their mental health found themselves in echo chambers that amplified their negative experiences and emotions, worsening their mental health, and missing an important opportunity for critical intervention. In addition to creating these exercises for stress and anxiety, the doctors worked with Pinterest to address self-harm and suicide on the platform.

Community

Finally, Brainstorm leverages the power of in-person and virtual communities to support mental health innovation. Loneliness is a lubricant for already existing and multifaceted social problems. Intervening to decrease loneliness requires prosocial venues that encourage engagement and friendship. Since 2013, Vasan has been teaching workshops on mental health innovation, bringing together clinicians, researchers, entrepreneurs, and students from different backgrounds to promote cross-disciplinary dialogue. These workshops have been delivered to over 1,000 people from six countries including China, Australia, India, Hong Kong, and Israel.

Brainstorm launched Stanford's first Augmented Reality and Virtual Reality Innovation Lab for Mental Health in 2017. Aragam, Rall, and Vasan partnered with Alan Louie, Director of Education for the Department of Psychiatry and Kim Bullock, founder and director of Stanford's Virtual Reality and Immersive Technologies Clinic and Lab at Stanford, to pair experts and designers in augmented reality (AR)/virtual reality (VR) technology to advance brain and behavioral health. Drawing on their experience running the Psychiatry Innovation Lab for the APA, they created this program to bring together and nurture start-ups that were using AR and VR technologies to address mental health. Aragam and Rall hosted the event, which brought together five finalist teams tackling a range of topics from using VR to help with addiction recovery to a VR game that simulated the experience of schizophrenia. Five final-ists pitched their ideas to a panel of expert judges and audience members during the Brainstorm VR/AR Innovation Lab at the Stanford Innovations in Psychiatry and Behavioral Health Conference. After the success of this program, Aragam was in-spired to create other collaborations and launched a partnership between Brainstorm and MIT's Solve, an MIT-sponsored competition for tech entrepreneurs to address the causes of mental health problems in their communities, develop ideas to address outstanding issues and design creative solutions.

To further build community worldwide, Brainstorm created a Facebook group to foster collaboration within the mental health innovation community, encouraging people to use the network as a tool to learn, teach, develop, and share ideas. The group has reached more than 1,200 members and has given rise to innovation pitch contests, surveys to improve cutting edge mental health products, and avenues for funding for budding entrepreneurs. Says mental health CEO Dan Seider: "Brainstorm has put to-gether the best online group of any mental health community. There are a number of great discussions and opportunities that come up that make it seem like this is a group of high signal people in the mental health space who care about making an impact and doing good work."[68]

The impact of this has been to catalyze conversation outside the university con-text by using Facebook, an innovative tool for community creation, to reach people from all walks of life. The Facebook group also serves as an antidote for virulent isola-tion: "Being part of the Brainstorm Facebook group and knowing a community exists to support the work I'm doing helps my own mental health," says one participant.[69] The Facebook group drives interdisciplinary conversation beyond academia and in-dustry to galvanize a mass movement around the potential for technology to reach people who struggle with their mental health.

The community-building has extended to younger members as well. Hillsborough high school senior and Brainstorm intern Anika Nayak has been making connections on the Facebook group to support entrepreneurs' efforts to develop new products and industries:

> The Facebook group has contributed to the growth of the mental health innovation field by bringing people together and developing strategic connections that position ideas for greatest impact. Joining such a diverse community has opened my eyes to mental health issues in the community. The collaboration and connection-making have empowered me to write articles in publications such as *Washington Post*'s Lily, *Thrive Global*, and *Harvard Technology Review* that display what the community vocalizes.[70]

Brainstorm's team is also an example of cross-disciplinary community-building, as the team brings together expertise from different industries, demographics, and age groups to brainstorm creative ways to move the mental health innovation field for-ward. Fellows include private equity associates, health policy experts, medical stu-dents, management consultants, and graduate students in neuroscience. Fellows have engaged in cutting edge research and programming to address systemic barriers to mental health. One such barrier is the lack of political will and support for mental healthcare among elected officials. To address this barrier, fellows Victor Agbafe and Angela Li have been tracking the American political candidates' mental health policies to raise visibility into how various candidates' platforms will affect mental health nationally. Fellows Sara Johanson and Tony Olmert created a survey to identify barriers to technology uptake among mental health clinicians; their hope is that identifying pain points for tech usage will enable targeted interventions to improve mental health clinicians' ability to use technology for impact. Equity and social justice are core values to the Brainstorm team; this led to fellows Madison McCall, Ope Okerele, and Aauyshi Jain researching the gap between the mental health needs of minority communities and current innovations.

To further build community, Brainstorm's interns have galvanized to post news articles about mental health innovation daily on social media platforms Twitter, Facebook, and Linked In, creating a conversation around mental health innovation and scaling that conversation so that it reaches thousands of people online. They have researched important topics in mental health innovation and taken to the media to share their perspectives. For example, intern Kaavya Pichai examined the controversy around whether social media "likes" are worsening online social pressure, and whether they should be removed.

What captured me most about Brainstorm is Brainstorm works to raise awareness and make mental health more accessible. It brings care to people in need rather than relying on them to seek access, which can make a big difference. Brainstorm's internship helped me realize firsthand the impact you can have in mental health by driving awareness and reducing barriers to access.[71]

Brainstorm's community presence has created a culture shift in the field of psychiatry: changing the conversation to include convergent approaches, empowering foot soldiers to advance innovation, and mobilizing stakeholders from all walks of life to join the movement for mental health innovation and make it their own through their talents, expertise, and graces.

Conclusion

At the 2019 APA annual meeting, prior to Stewart's celebration of innovation, Vasan gave an introduction of President Altha Stewart. Vasan referenced Issac Newton's poignant ode to those who have come before: "If I have seen further, it is by standing upon the shoulders of giants. Altha Stewart is that giant."[72] Stewart saw the future of mental health innovation in the convergence of medicine and industry. While mental illness siphons off potential, Brainstorm's innovative leaders, business model, and activities aim to restore that potential, build a movement upon it, and catalyze the creative, sustainable innovation desperately needed to protect our potential, today and for the future. Brainstorm's future work will continue to build on the strong foundation established by Stewart, Vasan, and others in the field. Catalyzed by the spirit of convergence, Brainstorm hopes to take psychiatry in a revolutionary direction.

Notes

1. Rall C, "Psychiatry Innovation Lab" Video. June 10, 2019 ("A pattern").
2. "How do we," Vasan N, personal interview, November 2019.
3. Rall C. "Psychiatry Innovation Lab" Video. June 10, 2019 ("A pattern").
4. "The Innovation Lab," Chaudhary N, personal interview, November 2019.
5. Ellison, Ralph. *Invisible Man.* New York, NY: Vintage Books; 1995.
6. Kessler KC, Angermeyer M, Anthony JC, et al. Lifetime prevalence and age-of-onset distributions of mental disorders in the World Health Organization's World Mental Health Survey Initiative. *World Psychiatry.* 2007 Oct; 6(3): 168–176.
7. Kessler KC, Angermeyer M, Anthony JC, et al. Lifetime prevalence and age-of-onset distributions of mental disorders in the World Health Organization's World Mental Health Survey Initiative. *World Psychiatry.* 2007 Oct; 6(3): 168–176.
8. Chaib F. Global health workforce, finances remain low for mental health. World Health Organization Web site. https://www.who.int/mediacentre/news/notes/2015/finances-mental-health/en/ July 14, 2015.
9. Raphelson S. Severe shortage of psychiatrists exacerbated by lack of federal funding. NPR Web site. https://www.npr.org/2018/03/09/592333771/. March 9, 2018.
10. Chaudhary N, Vasan N. Why mental-health tech must ally with academia. VentureBeat Web site. https://venturebeat.com/2019/05/25/why-mental-health-tech-must-ally-with-academia/. March 25, 2019.
11. Raphelson S. Severe shortage of psychiatrists exacerbated by lack of federal funding. NPR Web site. https://www.npr.org/2018/03/09/592333771/. March 9, 2018.
12. Chaib F. Global health workforce, finances remain low for mental health. World Health Organization Web site. https://www.who.int/mediacentre/news/notes/2015/finances-mental-health/en/ July 14, 2015.
13. Myers HF, Wyatt GE, Ullman JB, Loeb TB, Chin D, Prause N, Zhang M, Williams JK, Slavich GM, Liu H. (2015). Cumulative burden of lifetime adversities: Trauma and mental health in low-SES African Americans and Latino/as. *Psychological Trauma: Theory, Research, Practice, and Policy, 7*(3), 243–251.
14. Raphelson S. Severe shortage of psychiatrists exacerbated by lack of federal funding. NPR Web site. https://www.npr.org/2018/03/09/592333771/. March 9, 2018.
15. "How do we," Vasan N, personal interview, November 2019.
16. Chaudhary N, Vasan N, Why mental-health tech must ally with academia. VentureBeat Web site. https://venturebeat.com/2019/05/25/why-mental-health-tech-must-ally-with-academia/. March 25, 2019.
17. "How do we," Vasan N, personal interview, November 2019.
18. Olsen D. A look at the boom in VC funding for mental health start-ups. PitchBook Web site. https://pitchbook.com/news/articles/a-look-at-the-boom-in-vc-funding-for-mental-health-startups. June 20, 2018.
19. "The Innovation Lab," Chaudhary N, personal interview, November 2019.
20. "The Innovation Lab," Chaudhary N, personal interview, November 2019.
21. Gaussen Edouard. Mapping out the mental health startup ecosystem. *Medium.* July 13, 2018.

22. Chaudhary N, Vasan N. Why mental-health tech must ally with academia. VentureBeat Web site. https://venturebeat.com/2019/05/25/why-mental-health-tech-must-ally-with-academia/. March 25, 2019.

23. Patel V, Saxena S. Transforming lives, enhancing communities—innovations in global mental health. *N Engl J Med*. 2014;370(6):498–501.

24. Olsen D. A look at the boom in VC funding for mental health start-ups. PitchBook Web site. https://pitchbook.com/news/articles/a-look-at-the-boom-in-vc-funding-for-mental-health-startups. June 20, 2018.

25. "How do we," Vasan N, personal interview, November 2019.

26. "Stanford's culture," Vasan N, personal interview, December 2019.

27. "No one in the world," Walter Greenleaf, CEO at Pear Therapeutics. Business development meeting prep with Vasan and Greenleaf, 2019.

28. "I've never had," anonymous event participant, personal interview, December 2019.

29. "How do we," Vasan N, personal interview, November 2019.

30. "Stanford's culture," Vasan N, personal interview, December 2019.

31. "Stanford's culture," Vasan N, personal interview, December 2019.

32. Gorrindo T. 2020 Psychiatry Innovation Lab. American Psychiatric Association Web site. https://www.psychiatry.org/psychiatrists/education/mental-health-innovation-zone/psychiatry-innovation-lab.

33. "How do we," Vasan N, personal interview, November 2019.

34. "How do we," Vasan N, personal interview, November 2019.

35. Gorrindo T. 2020 Psychiatry Innovation Lab. American Psychiatric Association Web site. https://www.psychiatry.org/psychiatrists/education/mental-health-innovation-zone/psychiatry-innovation-lab.

36. "The Innovation Lab," Chaudhary N, personal interview, November 2019.

37. "How do we," Vasan N, personal interview, November 2019.

38. "The Innovation Lab," Chaudhary N, personal interview, November 2019.

39. "Stanford's culture," Vasan N, personal interview, December 2019.

40. "Rather than," Vasan N, personal interview, November 2019.

41. "Rather than," Vasan N, personal interview, November 2019.

42. "Stanford's culture," Vasan N, personal interview, December 2019.

43. "The Innovation Lab," Chaudhary N, personal interview, November 2019.

44. "It excited me," Aragam G, personal interview, November 2019.

45. "My adviser motivated me," Aragam G, personal interview, November 2019.

46. "The Innovation Lab," Chaudhary N, personal interview, November 2019.

47. "My adviser motivated me," Aragam G, personal interview, November 2019.

48. "The inherent beauty," Jon Sole, Brainstorm Fellow and Stanford Medical Student, personal interview, January 2020.

49. "The Innovation Lab," Chaudhary N, personal interview, November 2019.

50. "Stanford's culture," Vasan N, personal interview, December 2019.

51. "Stanford's culture," Vasan N, personal interview, December 2019.

52. "The Innovation Lab," Chaudhary N, personal interview, November 2019.

53. "A pattern," Smith E, Stanford University student, during discussion with speaker Thomas Insel at Brainstorm's Stanford University course, "Designing for 2 Billion: Leading Innovation in Mental Healthcare," February 2019.

54. Syllabus for Stanford University undergraduate course Psych 240, Designing for the 2 Billion: Leading Innovation in Mental Health, Winter 2019.

55. Class comments, Psych 240 and Psych 242, Designing for the 2 Billion: Leading Innovation in Mental Health, Winter 2019.

56. Class comments, Psych 240 and Psych 242, Designing for the 2 Billion: Leading Innovation in Mental Health, Winter 2019.

57. Syllabus for Stanford University undergraduate course Psych 240, Designing for the 2 Billion: Leading Innovation in Mental Health, Winter 2019.

58. "Brainstorm is," Sole J, Brainstorm fellow and Stanford medical student, personal interview, January 2020.

59. "Stanford's culture," Vasan N, personal interview, December 2019.

60. "Brainstorm is," Sole J, Brainstorm fellow and Stanford medical student, personal interview, January 2020.

61. "Brainstorm is," Sole J, Brainstorm fellow and Stanford medical student, personal interview, January 2020.

62. "The Innovation Lab," Chaudhary N, personal interview, November 2019.

63. Mukherjee, Siddhartha. *The emperor of all maladies: A biography of cancer.* New York: Toronto: Scribner, 2010.

64. "Brainstorm's impact," Seider D, personal interview, March 2020.

65. "I've been proud," Chaudhary N, personal interview, November 2019.

66. Pardes A. Feeling stressed out? Pinterest wants to help. Wired Magazine Web site. https://www.wired.com/story/pinterest-compassionate-search/. July 22, 2019.

67. Ta A. Introducing a more compassionate search experience for people in distress. Pinterest.com Web site. https://newsroom.pinterest.com/en/post/introducing-a-more-compassionate-search-experience-for-people-in-distress. July 22, 2019.

68. "Brainstorm's impact," Seider D, personal interview, March 2020.

69. Brainstorm Holiday party, personal interview, December 2019.

70. "Facebook group," Nayak A., personal interview, March 2020.

71. "Internship," Pichaii K, personal interview, March 2020.

72. Rall, R, "Psychiatry Innovation Lab " Video. June 10, 2019.

27

Innovating Dementia Care Through Convergence Science in Brain Health

UCSF Memory Aging Center as a Case Example

Laís Fajersztajn, Maira Okada de Oliveira, and Bruce L. Miller

Introduction

Thanks to medical and social development, life expectancy has been rising over the past decades. Projections indicate that longevity will continue to increase during coming years and female life expectancy will break the 90-year barrier in several industrialized countries (Kontis et al. 2017). Unfortunately, the risk of developing a neurodegenerative disorder increase with age, and 4 out of every 10 persons 85+ has some type of cognitive impairment (Yaffe et al. 2011). Without a medical breakthrough, by 2030, over 74 million people will be living with dementia globally, at a cost of US$2 trillion (Alzheimer's Disease International 2015). Sixty-eight percent of the dementia cases will occur in low-and middle-income countries (Alzheimer's Disease International 2015), where resources to face the problem are scarce.

Dementia is a complex problem from the population perspective and from the individual perspective. Notably, the diagnosis of dementia in clinics usually represents very bad news for the individual and the family. Despite significant differences in the types and etiologies for neurodegenerative dementias, there is no cure for these diseases. The diagnosis of dementia is accompanied by high caregiver burden, high financial costs for the family, and few therapeutic alternatives. However, there are ways to help relieve some of the symptoms with strategies to improve an individual's quality of life, to ease the burden on caregivers and to delay admission to a nursing home. To face the global burden of dementia, we need to pursue these strategies at the individual level. At the same time, we should concentrate efforts to find innovative ways to understand, find treatments and ultimately cures for Alzheimer's disease, frontotemporal dementia, and other conditions that cause dementia. It is also important to acknowledge that we already know of multiple risk factors for dementia that can be ameliorated or prevented including diabetes mellitus, hypertension, obesity, depression, physical inactivity, smoking, and cognitive inactivity. A 10% to 25% reduction in these risks could prevent as many as 1.1 to 3.0 million cases of dementia worldwide and between 184,000–492,000 cases in the United States (Barnes and Yaffe 2011).

If we are to understand convergence science in mental health or brain health as the integration of diverse disciplines to solve complex problems (Eyre et al. 2017, Sharp et al. 2017), dementia would be a good fit to test if convergence science in brain health can in fact lead to medical and technological breakthroughs. If we add the integration of different stakeholders, such as science, industry, government, health practitioners, and patients as partners of the convergence brain health enterprise (Eyre et al. 2017), then dementia is a perfect case to test convergence science in brain health feasibility.

In fact, convergence science in brain health is a major reason for the successes of the University of California–San Francisco (UCSF) Memory and Aging Center (MAC) and the Global Brain Health Institute (GBHI), two programs that we discuss in this chapter.

The UCSF MAC grew from a single faculty member in 1998, into a recognized national and international leader in dementia care, research, and education with approximately 300 employees. The UCSF MAC has grown in a wide variety of directions through the pursuit of funding from philanthropy, the National Institutes of Health (NIH), private foundations, the pharmaceutical industry, and patient billing. It has embraced art and artists and is in contact with journalists and filmmakers to spread the message of brain health. Further, its outreach programs for care, research and education influence local community. The UCSF MAC also influences global community as a reference center for patients and receives international visitors through the GBHI, a program that which goal is to reduce the burden of dementia globally. By telling the history of the UCSF MAC and the GBHI, we expect to present a successful case of convergence science in brain health. For a graphical overview of the core themes of the MAC, see Figure 27.1.

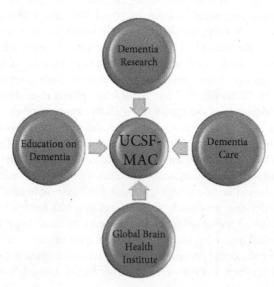

Figure 27.1 UCSF-Memory and Aging Center (MAC) as an example of convergence science in brain health.

The Memory and Aging Center

The UCSF MAC envisions a positive future for society's elders. The center exists to provide model care for individuals with cognitive problems and their families, conduct research on causes and cures for degenerative brain diseases, and to educate health professionals, patients and their families.

Dementia Care

To provide highest quality care, the UCSF MAC relies on the multidisciplinary work of neurologists, geriatricians, neuropsychologists, neuroscientists, neuropathologists, speech pathologists, psychiatrists, genetic counselors, nurses, pharmacists, social workers, research coordinators, technologists, and administrators. The UCSF MAC houses 38 faculty members from these fields, employs over 300 talented faculty and staff and enlists the support of more than 40 volunteers. It fulfills three missions: research, education, and care.

Care is personalized and centered on individual and families, whether they reach the program through research, education, or care pathways. The program takes a holistic view of his or her work, communicating and coordinating with experts across disciplines to support the needs of each unique patient with a cognitive disorder. There are approximately 6,000 outpatient visits yearly, and many patients are seen in the clinic longitudinally, while others are referred back to their primary physicians. While the majority of patients are seen in outpatient clinics, the program touches patients in the hospital and through home visits. A program that supports patients and their caregivers that was designed by psychologist Katherine Possin and nurse Jennifer Merrilees, Care ecosystem, has a care team navigator help the patient–caregiver dyad navigate through a maze of critical social and legal services, and end-of life care. The care ecosystem is being implemented at six sites around the United States, with more locations coming soon. The UCSF MAC has established outreach programs to provide care to underserved Asian and Latinx communities in the San Francisco Bay Area.

Dementia Research

In the research arm, clinical trials are available for patients with mild cognitive impairment, Alzheimer's disease, frontotemporal dementia, progressive supranuclear palsy, corticobasal degeneration, and chronic traumatic encephalopathy. Other studies being developed by the trials team. Innovation has been a hallmark of the clinical trials developed at the UCSF MAC. In 2005 led by Michael Geschwind, MD, PhD, UCSF MAC led the first randomized, double-blind, placebo-controlled treatment trial in patients with sporadic Creutzfeldt–Jakob disease. The primary outcome of this trial was survival. Geschwind and his clinical research team continue to work with Stanley Prusiner, MD, on other potential treatments. In 2007, led by Adam Boxer, MD, PhD, the UCSF MAC ran the first randomized, multicenter, double-blind, placebo-controlled treatment trial of memantine for patients with frontotemporal dementia. In 2009, the leader of the trials team, Boxer and his team implemented the first Phase 2 trials for tau-related therapies for frontotemporal dementia. In 2013, Boxer initiated the first clinical trial of a compound purported to raise progranulin levels in patients with progranulin mutations leading to frontotemporal dementia. This trial arose from a close collaboration between Li Gan, PhD, at the Gladstone Institutes and the UCSF MAC.

Boxer and his team continue to perform cutting-edge clinical trials and biomarkers research and are bringing biomarkers like neurofilament into clinical trials.

From 2015 to 2018, Gil Rabinovici led the Imaging Dementia–Evidence for Amyloid Scanning (IDEAS) study. Now he co-leads the Longitudinal Early-Onset Alzheimer's Disease Study (LEADS), a two-year observational study designed to look at disease progression in adults with early-onset Alzheimer's disease that will enroll 600 participants at 20 sites.

The UCSF MAC is the hub of two unique cure-focused philanthropy-based consortia: the Consortium for Frontotemporal Dementia and the Tau Consortium. Initial funding from private donors allowed the creation of these interdependent, nimble teams of basic, translational and clinical scientists from around the world to sharply focus on a specific problem—finding a cure for molecular subtypes of frontotemporal dementia. With the leadership Boxer and Howard Rosen, MD, UCSF MAC has played an important role in multicenter studies such as ARTFL (the Advancing Research and Treatment for Frontotemporal Lobar Degeneration) and LEFFTDS (Longitudinal Evaluation of Familial Frontotemporal Dementia Subjects). These two studies are the largest NIH grants ever for frontotemporal dementia and now been merged into the ARTFL–LEFFTDS Longitudinal Frontotemporal Lobar Degeneration (ALLFTD) research consortium. Investigators at the UCSF MAC collaborate with researchers across the world, establishing links with major research centers in Asia, Europe and Latin America.

Notably, the UCSF MAC has made important discoveries in the field of neurodegenerative diseases. In 2013 alone, William Seeley, MD, revealed that neurodegenerative diseases spread across brain networks in predictable patterns based on the neurons' shared vulnerability to disease. Second, Zachary Miller, MD, discovered a link between systemic inflammation due to autoimmune disease and forms of frontotemporal dementia that involve the protein TDP43, opening up new avenues for diagnosis, prognosis and treatment. Third, in collaboration with Yadong Huang, PhD, at the Gladstone Institutes, the UCSF MAC created the first cellular model of tauopathy from adult human stem cells with a rare mutation that increases susceptibility to Alzheimer's disease, progressive supranuclear palsy, and frontotemporal dementia. These models provide a unique way to study the mechanisms that break down in human disease.

UCSF MAC multidisciplinary research to understand the brain also encompasses dyslexia. The UCSF–UC Berkeley Schwab Dyslexia and Cognitive Diversity Center is a new $20-million two-campus multidisciplinary clinical and research alliance to deepen the understanding of dyslexia and other specific neurodevelopmental differences that impact learning, with Marilu Gorno Tempini serving as the inaugural co-director.

Education on Dementia

Believing that education of health professionals in the early stages of their careers is critical for the long-term needs of our society, the UCSF MAC is committed to training individuals from many disciplines, ranging from neurology, psychiatry, geriatric medicine, nursing, social work, and psychology to basic neuroscience and welcomes trainees from around the globe. Every year more than 200 students, from high school undergraduates to tenured professors, participate in the UCSF MAC's onsite training, while many thousands attend lectures offered by the faculty. The center provides seven different professional training programs, including the Behavioral Neurology and the Neuropsychology Training programs, and different formats for visiting students from and outside the United States.

The UCSF MAC offer community lectures, conferences, and support groups aiming to spread knowledge about dementia for those who seek it and for the society. The center has a website and YouTube channel, launched more than 10 years ago with informative videos about dementia for a general audience and interacts with media to increase their educational reach. For example, in 2019, Bruce Miller was featured on the US television show *60 Minutes* in a segment on frontotemporal dementia.

Beyond biomedical science, the UCSF MAC embraces art and artists, through exhibitions and by a residence program for an artist. Each year, an accomplished artist (visual artist, musician, writer, comedian, performer, or other creative individual) spends a year at the center in a creative exchange with scientists, clinicians, patients, and families, inspiring original public art and science that raises awareness about neurodegenerative disorders. The UCSF MAC also examines the importance of creativity to people suffering from neurodegenerative disorders and had hosted for several years a small monthly arts group as new outlet for expression and communication for the patients.

In 2016, the UCSF began a collaboration with Voice of Witness through the hear/say project, shedding light on the personal and rarely heard day-to-day experiences of aging and dementia and, through the oral history process, reduce the stigma and othering that occurs by perpetuating a "single story." The project has already published two books, and a documentary film will be released soon. The UCSF MAC also established a new partnership with the San Francisco Conservatory of Music to continue to build on the links between the arts and science.

Global Brain Health Institute

Since 2015, UCSF MAC has hosted the US site of the Global Brain Health Institute (GBHI), a groundbreaking initiative that aims to tackle the looming dementia epidemic and improve brain health and dementia care worldwide. This enterprise brings individuals from different disciplines, stakeholders and countries, fueled by a partnership between UCSF and Trinity College Dublin and funded from the Atlantic Philanthropies for 15 years.

Hosted by UCSF MAC and Trinity College Dublin (Trinity), GBHI is a strong example of how convergence science in brain health has the potential to change the world. Funded in 2015, with significant fund from the Atlantic Philanthropies, GBHI works to reduce the scale and impact of dementia globally, through a program named Atlantic Fellows for Equity in Brain Health. There are other six interconnected Atlantic Fellows programs across the world concerned with other levels of equity, such as racial, socioeconomic, and health equity. Together, the seven Atlantic Fellows programs create a global community to advance fairer, healthier, and more inclusive societies that enhance the reach and the strength of GBHI. In other words, the Atlantic Fellows programs provide another level to the convergence science in brain health of GBHI, supporting the goal of reducing the burden of dementia. Virtual meetings and technology allow USCF MAC and the Trinity College Dublin to connect with each other and with the communities around them.

GBHI itself operates in three ways: (i) by training and connecting the next generation of leaders in brain health; (ii) by collaborating in and expanding preventions and interventions; and (iii) by sharing knowledge and engaging in advocacy. By training a new generation of leaders, GBHI goal is to truly transform our societies. Eighty leaders in brain health from 28 countries have completed training, and another 32 are current under training. Together with the Alzheimer's Association and the UK-based Alzheimer's Society, GBHI provides a competitive funding program to support the work of these leaders in their communities. In 2019 the total amount of $675,000 will support 27 pilot projects to address global challenges related to dementia in 14 countries across five continents, including Argentina, Botswana, Brazil, Colombia, Costa Rica, Egypt, Ireland, Israel, Mexico, Peru, Romania, South Africa, the United Kingdom, and the United States. The projects include areas of advocacy, systems change, applied research, and others. Together these projects will address disparities in dementia diagnosis, treatment, and care for vulnerable populations and their families worldwide.

An Atlantic Senior Fellow from Argentina, Agustín Ibáñez, in collaboration with other leaders in South American from Brazil, Colombia, Peru, and Argentina and faculty from the UCSF MAC, was awarded with a $2.5 million grant from the NIH to develop the first digital platform of shared data on dementia in South America. Data will be compared with individuals from the United States seen at the MAC.

This unique proposal tackles problems that could not be completed without collaboration across the Americas. An example of the convergence started inside GBHI, inside the MAC, extrapolating barriers to tackle challenges of increasing incidence of dementia across South America. The ambitious project aims to evaluate the genetic, social/environmental, and neurocognitive determinants of dementia in more than 3,000 individuals from Colombia, Peru, Brazil, and Argentina and has recently been expanded to Mexico and Chile with support from the Alzheimer's Association and the Tau Consortium.

Among the projects current ongoing, Phaedra Bell, PhD, leads the Multimodal Intergenerational Social Contact Intervention (MISCI). The project matches two younger people with each older person screened for loneliness living in San Francisco, California. These "triads" develop a creative project together at six weekend meetings. Everyone shares their work at a showcase.

Elisa Resende, a neurologist from Brazil, is studying how teaching literacy to adults in Brazil has a high potential to lower their risk of dementia. Another fellow from Brazil, Maira Okada de Oliveira, is a neuropsychologist also studying dementia in populations with low education. However, her goal is to improve diagnosis of dementia among illiterate groups in Brazil. The convergence of these two projects will guide shape a more equitable brain health world in Brazil and beyond. Maira leads an interest group in GBHI to facilitate spreading the knowledge about better diagnosis in people with low education to other parts of the world.

Convergence is also occurring between Atlantic Fellows from other programs, not only those focused in brain health. An example is a group of 19 Atlantic Fellows from around the world, including activists, academics, artists, change-makers, 15 not from the brain health program, who are concerned with displacement and health. The group got together in Jordan in a forum where they visited a university near the Jordanian–Syrian border and refugee camps and participated in creative activities such as cooking and connecting with refugees and the local community. Now they are planning how to promote health for population of refugees.

Characteristics for Success of Convergence Science in Brain Health

As described above, the UCSF MAC worked in different levels of convergence science to become a nationally and internationally leader in dementia care, research, and education. A crucial tool for all these achievements is a successful history of funding and an impressive capability of attracting talents. All these together was just possible because of the creative vision and leadership of faculty at the MAC. Core values of the UCSF MAC emphasize empathy and equality.

The UCSF MAC has a successful history of funding from government and philanthropy that was crucial to the center become the leader it is now. This history started back in the 1998, when Miller first arrived at UCSF to establish a clinical dementia program within the Department of Neurology with Joel Kramer, Rosalie Gearhart, and Howie Rosen. One of program's first efforts was to secure the center's role as a state-funded Alzheimer's Disease Research Center of California. In 2000, the UCSF MAC received a gift from the Koret Foundation that was instrumental establish initial fiscal stability to build infrastructure for a brand new program. It allowed for investments in personnel, technology and clinical trials. With a small clinic and several clinical trials for Alzheimer's patients, MAC began to recruit trainee Next MAC continued to successfully raise new research funding. In 2002 Miller was the first NIH investigator to receive grants to evaluate frontotemporal dementia. In the same year, Joel Kramer, PsyD, the MAC received a grant to stablish the Hillblom Aging Network to learn more about how healthy people age and what changes in the brain occur with aging. Next, in 2004, the UCSF MAC was designated a national Alzheimer's Disease Research Center with funding from the National Institute on Aging and the center serves the San Francisco Bay Area.

After that, the center has successfully raised funds from many types of grants from NIH, including the program project U, individual research, training grants, and fellowship awards. The MAC has also built new partnerships with several private foundations and individuals. These funds are critical for supporting non-reimbursable patient care, technology improvements, educational programs, and the pursuit of promising research not funded by highly restricted research grants. An example is the program funded by The Hellman Family Foundation supports the visit of one artist every year to the UCSF MAC. The program resulted in art installations, poetry collections, short films, caregiver story collection, and live performances for our communities. Some of the private foundations that have supported the MAC include Clausen Family Foundation, Hellman Family Foundation, John Douglas French Alzheimer's Foundation, Joseph and Vera Long Foundation, Koret Family Foundation, Rainwater Charitable Foundation, Richard Barker Family Fund, Marty & Anne Rohrer, the Bluefield Project, The Larry L. Hillblom Foundation, the McBean Family Foundation, the McKenzie Foundation, and Ed & Mona Zander, as well as anonymous gifts. As of 2018, GBHI has received over $US177 million from the Atlantic Philanthropies to run its program for 12 more years.

The talents of MAC UCSF include many others such as William W. Seeley, MD, who became the first neurologist to receive a MacArthur "Genius" award in 2011 and received the 2008 Larry L. Hillblom Distinguished Scholar Award and a 2009 Hellman Foundation Scientist Award.

The Role of Technology

The Care Ecosystem is a care program developed at UCSF MAC and led by neuropsychologist, Kate Possin, PhD, and nurse-scientist Jennifer Merrilees, RN, PhD, that exemplifies how technology is being used to improve health care services for patients with dementia and to increase access and communication with and for patients and families. The Care Ecosystem leverages technology and precision medicine to customize care provided to each individual and family member across all stages of dementia, from early detection and diagnosis, through the end of life. This network of care services improve the everyday lives of patients and their families with better support through the many health transitions experienced with dementia. It also links UCSF MAC experts with the multiple people involved in a patient's care management, benefiting the patient.

The Care Ecosystem includes extensive access to the clinical team, self-paced education modules, and guidance in reaching important milestones in care. Patient information is safely stored, via the internet, with accurate information about medications and current symptoms and problems. As symptoms are reported, advice is promptly disseminated to caregivers from physicians, nurses and social workers from the UCSF MAC. A care team navigator works with patients and their caregivers as they navigate the complexities of caring for a loved one through each stage of the disease. Interactive tools include small discussion groups or one-on-one exchanges targeted to specific stages of the illness. The program is being replicated in other settings.

The Global Neurology Forum is another format developed at UCSF MAC to address neurological disease globally. Sponsored by UCSF Global Teleneurology Service and Global Brain Health Institute, the series of periodic meetings provides an opportunity for learning and dialogue about the diagnosis and management of neurological conditions. The proposal is to help participants from different countries and cultures, including from rural and remote areas, to think holistically about responding to challenges in brain health in different realities. The forum also aims to influence the perception of neurological disease worldwide. The sessions last for 90 minutes, including presentation and discussion. Participation can be either in person at University of California, San Francisco, or by videoconference and translation to other languages is available whenever necessary. Examples of topics already addresses by the forum are "Where There Is No Multiple Sclerosis? Absence of Disease or Absence of expertise?"; "Who Is Protecting the Elderly?"' and "Epilepsy Care in Resource-Limited Settings: Challenges and Opportunities".

Conclusion

UCSF MAC is a an example of a successful case in convergence science in brain health involving the transdisciplinary integration as an approach to solve complex problems in health, in this case, dementia.

References

Barnes, D. E. and K. Yaffe (2011). "The projected effect of risk factor reduction on Alzheimer's disease prevalence." *Lancet Neurol* 10(9): 819-828 https://doi.org/10.1016/s1474-4422(11)70072-2.

Eyre, H. A., H. Lavretsky, M. Forbes, C. Raji, G. Small, P. McGorry, B. T. Baune and C. Reynolds, 3rd (2017). "Convergence science arrives: how does it relate to psychiatry?" *Acad Psychiatry* 41(1): 91-99 https://doi.org/10.1007/s40596-016-0496-0.

Alzheimer's Disease International. (2015). *World Alzheimer Report 2015. The Global Impact of Dementia: an Analysis of Prevalence, Incidence, Costs and Trends.* London: Alzheimer's Disease International.

Kontis, V., J. E. Bennett, C. D. Mathers, G. Li, K. Foreman and M. Ezzati (2017). "Future life expectancy in 35 industrialised countries: projections with a Bayesian model ensemble." *Lancet* 389(10076): 1323-1335 https://doi.org/10.1016/s0140-6736(16)32381-9.

Sharp, P., S. Hockfield and J. Sills (2017). "Convergence: The future of health." *Science* 355(6325): 589 https://doi.org/10.1126/science.aam8563.

Yaffe, K., L. E. Middleton, L. Y. Lui, A. P. Spira, K. Stone, C. Racine, K. E. Ensrud and J. H. Kramer (2011). "Mild cognitive impairment, dementia, and their subtypes in oldest old women." *Arch Neurol* 68(5): 631-636.

28

NODE.Health Algorithm to Support Digital Mental Health Validation

Amy Sheon, Steven Chan, Brian Van Winkle, and Benjamin Rosner

A version of the following article was originally published in Digital Biomarkers, 2018 Sep–Dec;2(3):139–154, a publication of S. Karger AG, Basel, Switzerland. The algorithm and related text are reproduced here with permission. Where necessary, the original text is augmented with special considerations that apply to digital mental health tools.

NODE.Health Foundation is a 501(c)(3) non-profit organization dedicated to education, validation and dissemination of evidence based digital medicine. As the largest professional association in digital medicine, NODE.Health empowers societies, executives and NODES from health systems, payers, life sciences, venture capital, startups and the public sector involved in healthcare digital transformation.

Introduction

Over the last 15 years, convergence research and convergence science have emerged as movements that have drawn insights and expertise from disciplines as diverse as life sciences, biomedicine, engineering, computer science, mathematics, earth sciences, and astronomy, generating a wealth of new knowledge. As new technologies and the opportunities associated with them evolve, so too do new questions that challenge our societal, ethical, technical, and regulatory frameworks. The implications of convergence science are particularly notable in healthcare, posing novel challenges in validating the safety, efficacy, real world effectiveness, and privacy associated with these new products. With digitization of healthcare in the United States following the passage of the Health Information Technology for Economic and Clinical Health (HITECH) Act in 2009,[1] digital technologies such as telemedicine, mobile health devices, and artificial intelligence, among others, have developed at a rapid pace and are prevalent in nearly every corner of the consumer marketplace and the healthcare ecosystem.

Unlike traditional sources of evidence that have typically preceded, and been instrumental for regulatory approval for medical devices and drugs, the evidence base for digital health tools has largely emerged in a post-market context after such tools have been put into clinical use. The leapfrog effect seen with such tools making their way to the marketplace before validation has been due, in part, to the speed with which these applications can be built, deployed, and iterated upon, coupled with a rapid go-to-market misperception that such tools may offer benefit with little risk of harm. Convergence science is especially promising not only as a potential ongoing source of new tools and insights, but as a means by which we may be able to better scale validation efforts to keep pace with innovation.

Across the full spectrum of healthcare, mental health is uniquely positioned at the intersection of physical, emotional, and behavioral well-being, affording prime opportunities for breakthroughs in convergence science. But like so many other areas touched by convergence science, the opportunities in mental health come with their own challenges including stigma; data security concerns in the context of the large number of stakeholders involved in the medical, social, emotional, educational, and legal aspects of life for those with mental illness; and the collision of the availability of consumer grade mobile health applications with the unique standards for healthcare privacy that govern mental health information.[2]

To navigate this complexity, this chapter describes an algorithm (Figure 28.1) to help health systems determine the appropriate pathway to digital medicine validation or adoption. The algorithm was developed based on the collective experiences of over 20 health systems and academic institutions who have established the Network of Digital Evidence for Health, NODE.Health (nodehealth.org), a 501c(3) nonprofit organization dedicated to education, validation, and dissemination of evidence based digital medicine. In addition, evidence-based clinical research taxonomies, syntheses, or frameworks for assessing technology or for improving reporting of clinical trials identified from a literature review framed this work. Informed by Realist Synthesis methods,[3,4] the immersion/crystallization method[5] was used to understand how a product works by looking at the relationships among the product, the context, the user population, and outcomes. This approach is especially relevant to digital technology where complex interventions are continuously updated to reflect the user and context.[6] Concepts emerging from our literature review of contextual issues include classification of users,[7-9] use of technology for collecting outcomes,[10] and factors associated with scale-up.[11,12] Concepts related to understanding outcomes were found in the literature related to methods of usability testing,[13,14] research design,[15-19] product evaluation or efficacy testing,[20-23] and reporting of research.[21,24-27] To better understand the mechanism of action, we considered classification of technology,[28-32] patient engagement or technology adoption,[33-39] and reasons for nonuse of technology.[40]

The Digital Medicine Testing Algorithm

To make effective use of the algorithm, some key features of digital medicine products and their development ecosystems are discussed in the following text. The user-task context framework provides a lens for considering choices or plans for technology testing and adoption.[41] First, the institution should define its use case(s) for the product—know the target population (users), the required functions (tasks), and understand what is required for successful adoption within a specific setting. In assessing the fit of a technology under consideration, one should consider whether a product

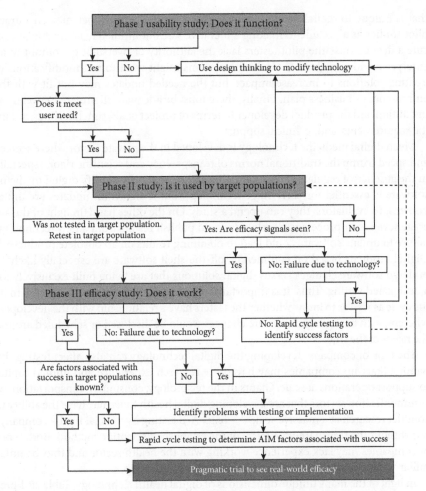

Figure 28.1 The NODE.Health digital medicine testing algorithm.

has been shown to work in the target user population. User dimensions especially important to health technology adoption include age, language, education, technology skills, and access to underlying necessary equipment and connectivity (e.g., smartphones or computers and broadband or mobile data). Similarly, one must ensure that a technology successfully used in one setting was used for the same tasks as are needed in the target situation. For example, reports may show that a program performed well with scheduling in a comparable setting but that no evidence was provided about its use for referrals, the task required by the target setting. Finally, numerous dimensions of the setting could affect the likelihood of success; consider, for example, the physical location, the urgency of the situation[41] and the social context (e.g., whether researchers or clinicians are involved, and their motivations for doing so).[42]

The potential for a misalignment of goals and incentives of institutional customers and technology developers and vendors is a dimension of the social context that is unique to digital health products. For example, a developer may encourage pilot studies as a prelude to making a lucrative sale but ultimately be unable to execute a deal because the pilot testers lack the authority or oversight to commit to an enterprise-wide purchase.[43] Or, health systems might want to test modifications of existing solutions to increase impact, but the needed updates may not fit with the entrepreneur's business plan. Finally, there must be adequate alignment between the institution and the product developer in terms of project goals, timeline, budget, capital requirements, and technical support.

Much digital medicine technology is developed in the private sector where secrecy and speed trump the traditional norms of transparency and scientific rigor, especially in the absence of regulatory oversight. The ability to rapidly modify digital medicine software is essential for early-stage technology, but if algorithm updates are unbeknownst to evaluators, they can upend a study. On the other hand, in light of the average seven-year process to develop, test and publish results from a new technology, failure to update software could lead to obtaining results on an obsolete product[18,44] Digital products based on commercial off-the-shelf software are especially likely to undergo software changes versus digital solutions that are being built exclusively for a designated setting. Thus, it is important to understand where a technology is in its life cycle as well as to know whether the testers have a relationship with the developers whereby such background software changes would be disclosed or scheduled around the needs of the trial.

The type of company developing the digital technology can also affect testing dynamics. Start-up companies may have little research experience and limited capital to support operations at scale. Giants in the technology, consumer, transportation, or communication sectors that are developing digital health tools may have the ability to conduct research at a massive scale[45,46] (e.g., A/B testing by a social media company) but without the transparency typical of the established scientific method. Both types of companies may lack experience working with the health sector and thus be unfamiliar with bifurcated clinical and administrative leadership.

In light of the many unique dimensions of digital health technology, Table 28.1 presents questions to consider when initiating or progressing with a phased trial process. These questions have been informed by the experience of NODE.Health in validating digital medicine technologies,[47–51] and by industry-sponsored surveys of digital health founders, health systems leaders, or technology developers;[52,53] or other industry commentary.[43,54]

Testing Drugs and Devices Versus Digital Solutions

Table 28.2 proposes a pathway for testing digital health products that addresses their unique characteristics and dynamics. The testing pathway used for regulated products is shown on the left with parallel digital testing phases shown on the right half of Table 28.2.

Preclinical studies, often performed in animals, are meant to explore the safety of a drug or devices prior to administration in humans.[55] The digital medicine analog

Table 28.1. Special Considerations for Working with Start-Ups and Nontraditional Firms

Topic	Questions to Ask
Company and product maturity	How consistent is the proposed activity with the priorities of a company (ideally including founders, investors and other players who may influence the long-term relationship with the company)? Can product development survive key personnel transitions? How mature is the product? Can it remain stable for study duration? Does the company have expect that the healthcare system will become a paying customer after the pilot phase? Who will pay for the product during and after a study? Will the company be able to support implementation if the testing progress to adoption and scale-up? How many paying customers does the company currently have and have they undergone any type of studies already?
Fit with healthcare	Can the company provide the secure environment required to protect patient data ad follow current regulations? Does the company understand the timeline, cost and cultural norms involved in working with healthcare institutions?
Research experience	Does the company understand requirements associated with undergoing an institutional review board review? Does the company understand the need to adhere to a protocol? Does the company understand requirements regarding human subject protection in research studies and health data privacy? Does the company understand issues with actual or appearance of conflict of interest in research?

is either absent or perhaps limited to determination of whether or not a product uses regulated technology such as cell phones that emit radiation.

Traditional and digital Phase I studies may be the first studies of a drug or a technology in humans, are generally nonrandomized, and typically include a small number of healthy volunteers, or individuals with a defined condition. Whereas the purpose of traditional Phase I studies is to test the agent's safety and find the highest dose that can be tolerated by humans,[55] the digital equivalent usually begins with a prototype product that may not be fully functioning. These early digital Phase I studies increasingly use "design thinking"[13,56] to identify relevant use cases and rapidly prototype solutions. Through focus group discussions, interviews, and surveys, developers find out what features people with the target condition want and conduct usability testing to see how initial designs work.

Table 28.2. Crosswalk of Clinical and Digital Medicine Testing Phases

	Drug and Device Trials			Digital Medicine Studies		
	Therapeutic and Device Testing Phases			Digital Health (Nonregulated) Product Testing Phase		
Phase	Phase	Population	Purpose	Phase	Purpose	Population
Preclinical		Animals	Test drug safety and pharmacodynamics; Required to test new drug in humans	Premarketing	Classify device accessories into levels of risk (e.g., class I or class II); Ensure safety of radiation-emitting devices	Animals or lab only
Phase I: in vivo		Healthy or sick volunteers (n = very small)	Safety and toxicity	Phase I: in silico	Identify likely use cases; Rapidly determine whether and how a product is used; Identify desired and missing features	Healthy or sick volunteers (n = small)
Phase II: therapeutic exploratory		Sick volunteers	Safety, pharmacokinetics, optimal dosing, frequency and rout of administration, and endpoints; Generate initial indication of efficacy to determine sample size needed for phase III	Phase II: feasibility	Develop/refine clinical work flow; Assess usability; Generate initial indication of efficacy to determine sample size needed for phase III	Volunteers reflecting intended users (n = medium)
Phase III: Pivotal or efficacy		Diverse target population (n = medium)	Experimental study to demonstrate efficacy; Estimate incidence of common adverse events	Phase III: pivotal or efficacy	Experimental study to demonstrate clinical effectiveness and/or financial return on investment	Intended users, defined settings and context (n = medium/large)

Phase IV: therapeutic use or post marketing	Observational study to identify uncommon adverse events Evaluate cost effectiveness in populations	Reports collected from universe of real-world users (n = census)	Implementations	Observational or experimental design Uses implementation science including change management and rapid cycle testing to deploy a tested intervention at scale Assess effectiveness and unintended consequence in specific or real-world settings ability, staffing and staff training requirement for widespread adoption	Intended users, real-world setting and context (n = universe in a specific setting)
Pragmatic (effectiveness trail)	Understand effectiveness of drugs or device in real-world settings	May use electronic health record or other "big data" sources Diverse settings and patient population	Pragmatic (effectiveness trial)	Understand effectiveness of technology in real-world settings	May use electronic health record or other big data sources Diverse settings and patients population May be conducted completely independently from healthcare setting

Traditional Phase II studies look at how a drug works in the body of individuals with the disease or condition of interest. By using historical controls or randomization, investigators can get a preliminary indication of a drug's effectiveness so that endpoints and the sample size needed for an efficacy trial can be identified.[55] These techniques may require that study volunteers be homogenous, limiting understanding of product use among the full range of target product users. The digital analogue could be a feasibility study in which an application is tested with individuals or in settings reflecting the targeted end users. Because nonregulated digital products are by definition at low or no risk of harm, Phase II studies of digital products may involve larger numbers of subjects than traditional trials.

Phase III trials of traditional and digital products are typically randomized studies to determine the efficacy of the drug or digital intervention. Ideally, volunteers reflect the full range of individuals with the condition, but, at least with therapeutic and device trials, the study population is likely to be homogeneous with respect to variation in disease severity, comorbidities and age to control main sources of bias and maximize the ability to observe a significant difference between the treatment and control arms.[57] Digital studies may have fewer eligibility criteria resulting in studies that could be more broadly generalizable.

Because traditional efficacy trials are not likely large enough to detect rare adverse events, the US Food and Drug Administration (FDA) may require postmarketing (Phase IV) studies to detect such events once a drug or device is in widespread use.[57] For low-risk applications, postmarketing surveillance studies may be unnecessary. Instead, we propose a class of studies that apply implementation science methods such as rapid cycle testing to generate new knowledge about technology dissemination beyond the efficacy testing environment and identification of unintended consequences in specific real-world settings. The trial may involve assessing requirements needed to integrate the novel product with existing technology and determine staffing requirements, training, and workflow changes. In this category, we also include strategies that allow for testing multiple questions in a short period of time, such as "n of 1" and factorial studies.[18] Again, the realist synthesis perspective points to using these studies to best understand how and why a product does or does not work in specific settings.[6]

Pragmatic trials are a next step common to both traditional and digital interventions; they seek to understand effectiveness in a real-world setting and with diverse populations.[19,58] Pragmatic studies of digital technology could be undertaken completely outside of the context of healthcare settings such as with studies that recruit participants and deliver interventions through social media,[59] that deliver interventions and collect data from biometric sensors and smartphone apps,[60] or that market health-related services such as genetic testing directly to consumers.[61] The FDA's move toward the use of real-world evidence and real-world data suggests that digital health tools used by consumers may assume greater importance for testing drugs and devices[57] as well as unregulated products.

Focus on External Validity

Many digital solutions can be widely adopted because they lack regulatory oversight and are commercially available to consumers. However, the specter of widespread utilization may magnify shortcomings of a testing process that may not have been conducted adequately in diverse settings and/or with desired groups of end users. The RE-AIM framework has been used since the late 1990s to evaluate the extent to which an intervention reaches, and is representative of, the affected population.[62] More recently, the framework has been used to plan and implement research studies[63] and to assess adoption of community-based healthcare initiatives.[64] Therefore, application of the RE-AIM framework to digital medicine testing can be especially valuable for those seeking to understand the likelihood that a specific digital health solution will work in a specific setting. Table 28.3 summarizes the original RE-AIM domains and

Table 28.3. RE-AIM Dimension and Key Questions for Testing Decisions

RE-AIM Dimension and Efficacy/Effectiveness Criteria	Original RE-AIM Conception[a]	Digital Health Application
Reach	Percentage and risk characteristics of individuals who receive or are touched by an intervention compared with an overall population How do participants differ from nonparticipants?	Who participated in testing a product versus who is the product intended for? Important population characteristics to consider include: Health condition (e.g., chronic vs. acute) Demographics (age, race, gender, education) Language and literacy (English, other, health literacy) Technology access (smartphone, computer, mobile data, fixed broadband, Wi-Fi) Technology skills
Efficacy	Assess positive and negative outcomes; include behavioral, quality of the and satisfaction in addition to health outcomes	How effective was the product overall? Were the intended benefits seen across various subgroups as previously defined?
Adoption	The proportion and representativeness of settings that adopt a program. Reasons for nonadaption should also be assessed.	In what setting (e.g., ambulatory care, in patient, emergency department) was the product tested? How was it received by institutional user? Who (e.g., clinical, marketing IT staff) needs to be involved in decisions to adopt the new technology?

(continued)

Table 28.3. Continued

RE-AIM Dimension and Efficacy/Effectiveness Criteria	Original RE-AIM Conception[a]	Digital Health Application
Implementation	The extent to which a program is delivered as intended. Outcomes should be assessed in terms of organizational delivery and individual use	How was the intervention delivered in trials? How was it received by end users? How long will it take to implement? How important is fidelity to the conditions seen in prior tests versus real-world use? What staff and training are required? How much will it cost end users?
Maintenance	The extent to which organizations routinize implementation of the program, and to which individuals maintain their use of the program or continue to experience benefits from the program	Is the intervention one-time, ad hoc or for ongoing use? Are effects expected to grow, plateau or diminish? How long are the results sustained? Are boosters and updates needed? Is staff onboarding and retraining needed?

[a]Adapted from Glasgow et al.[70]

then applies them to illuminate reliability and validity issues that could arise in testing digital medicine technologies.

The RE-AIM Dimensions and Key Questions

"Reach" concerns the extent to which populations involved in the testing reflect populations intended to use the product. "Effectiveness" concerns whether the product was effective overall or in subgroups typically defined by health status or age. Based on standards that have been articulated to improve the reporting of web-based and mobile health interventions[25] and reporting of health equity,[26] we extend the traditional reach and effectiveness dimensions to highlight specific populations in whom digital medicine technologies might exhibit heterogeneity of effect due to "social disadvantage." Traditional social determinants of health (education, race, income) plus age are highly associated with access to and use of the internet and smartphones. Digital skills are, in turn, highly associated with having and using computers and smartphones, as such skills develop from use,[65] and usage grows with access to equipment and connectivity.[66] Digital skills, computers or smartphone, and mobile data or fixed broadband are essential for almost all consumer-facing health technology such as remote monitors and activity tracking devices. Given the covariance of digital skills and access with age, education, and income,[67-72] and the likelihood that those with low digital skills may resist adoption of a digital technology or may have challenges using it.[48,73-76] It is especially important to determine whether such individuals were included in prior testing of a product and whether prior studies examined heterogeneity in response by such categories.

For products that have proven effectiveness, "adoption" concerns the incorporation of the intervention into a given context after pilot testing. Stellefson's application of the RE-AIM model to assess the use of Web 2.0 interventions for chronic disease self-management in older adults is especially instructive for assessing how a healthcare institution moves to adoption after a trial.[77] To what extent does the current setting replicate the context of previous trials? If a product was tested in an inpatient setting but is being considered for use in an ambulatory setting, for example, it is vital to understand who would need to be involved in a decision to move to adoption after efficacy testing. Do current staff have the skills and authority needed to integrate new technology? Where will funds for the technology adoption project come from?

"Implementation" refers to the types of support needed for the intervention to be administered and how well it was accepted by end users. "Maintenance" addresses the sustainability of the intervention in a setting and the duration of effect in the individual user.

We next apply the RE-AIM framework to help health systems assess evidence gaps and identify the most appropriate testing to use in a specific situation. For a product at an early stage of development, as shown in Table 28.4, questions of "reach" are most relevant. Since early testing focuses on how well a device or application functions, there may be limited information available about how well the device functions among individuals or settings similar to those under consideration. For a technology that has completed an efficacy trial, it is important to understand the extent to which the test results would apply in different populations and settings. It is also crucial to understand features of the study such as whether careful instruction and close monitoring were necessary for the technology to function optimally. For a technology with ample evidence of efficacy in relevant populations and settings, those considering moving to widespread adoption must understand institutional factors associated with successful deployment such as engagement of marketing and IT departments to integrate data systems.

Application of NODE.Health Algorithm for Mental Health Use Cases

We apply the algorithm to three use cases to help elucidate how it may be put to use in a mental health context to help health systems determine whether or how to incorporate digital medicine solutions in their environments. These use cases are composites developed in part from published literature or by first-hand knowledge of emerging technologies gleaned by the authors. The use cases span a range of digital medicine technology, delivery modes, functions, and settings.

Table 28.4. Application of RE-AIM Framework to Digital Medicine Testing by Phase

Digital Medicine Testing Phase	RE-AIM Dimensions	Questions to Ask Existing Evidence Base	When to Use
Phase I: Use case identifications	Reach	In which populations was technology tested? How similar were testers to current target population?	Developing a new product. Using an existing product for a new indication or with a different population
Phase II: Feasibility	Reach Effectiveness Implementation	In which setting was technology tested? How similar was study setting to target setting? How usable was the technology to the target population? To what extent were invited users interested in participating? What sort of support was needed from administrators, clinical staff and technology groups for the product to be tested?	Earlier tests were in populations or settings dissimilar to current target
Phase III: Pivotal or efficacy	Reach Effectiveness Adoption Implementation	Was technology efficacious overall? Did study look for heterogeneity of results? Was technology effective in subgroups of interest? Was adherence adequate? Was testing of sufficient duration to know what will be needed for implementation, if efficacious? Are there study conditions (such as staff or patient training or executive championship) needed for the technology to be effective in real world adoption? Does the study document financial outcomes that confirm a business case for product adoption?	Efficacy has not been proven in the population of interest. Return on investment needs to be demonstrated for enterprise-wide adoption to be considered. A target setting lacks characteristics that were necessary for efficacy in prior studies

Implementation	Reach	How well was technology accepted by the institution?	There are no successful real-world adoption examples
	Effectiveness	What factors were associated with successful and failed implementation?	Target institution lacks success scaling up new technologies
	Adoption	Did real-world efficacy match that seen in trials?	Target institution has settings and populations that are heterogeneous in factors connected with successful technology adoption
	Implementation	Was adoption and efficacy consistent across settings and populations?	
	Maintenance	Did usage improve and expand over time?	
		Did technology adapt as needed over time?	
Pragmatic	Implementation	What level of support is needed from the company to support implementation?	Factors needed for successful implementation are known from other settings and replicable in the target setting
	Adoption	How does the technology interact with existing systems?	Factors associated with successful adoption of other technologies in this setting are known and replicable
	Maintenance	What support is needed to sustain and use and keep the technology updated?	

Use Case 1: Real-Time, Synchronous Video Conferencing for Telepsychiatry

Case Summary

Rural Hospital (RH) decides to adopt Widget Company's video-conferencing system to increase the access of their patients to specialists. The Widget platform had been chosen by RH after the RH CMIO had seen a demonstration at a medical innovation conference. The system had been tested in and adopted by Large Hospital System (LHS) where it enabled patients to access specialists throughout that hospital system. RH agreed to be the first system to test use of Widget's video-conferencing to enable patients to have video visits with specialists at community-based institutions across the state. RH initiated a Phase I study to test the connection with 10 different community-based facilities across the state. They then established Business Associate Agreements with 5 of the 10 institutions for which the video connection was most reliable. RH then invited all of their patients who saw specialists at those five institutions to participate in a Phase II test of having specialist visits via video from the RH primary care clinic. Most patients enthusiastically consented to scheduling upcoming specialist appointments via video. After checking in at the RH primary care clinic, a medical assistant escorted patients to a video-equipped exam room and established the video link with the provider. The medical assistant remained in the exam room to facilitate procedures requested by the specialist such as obtaining a peak flow test. Because of poor internet speeds, connections sometimes dropped, so the medical assistant re-established the video connection when needed. Most patients were understanding and willing to tolerate the disruption as an adequate tradeoff for not having to travel to their appointments. However, two of the five community institutions dropped out due to specialist frustration with the dropped connections. For privacy reasons, and since the visits did not involve any physical exam or procedures, the medical assistants exited the exam room for patients whose consultations were with their psychiatrists. Eight of ten psychiatry patients experienced dropped calls, which were very disruptive because there was no one present who could re-establish the connection. The remaining two patients were enthusiastic about continuing their psychiatry consultations via video, but the others were unwilling to do so.

Analysis

The Digital Medicine Testing Algorithm (Figure 28.1) can be used to ascertain whether RH's decision to participate in that pilot was reasonable and to identify potential next steps for Widget in further product development and testing and for RH in considering further deployment of Widget video conferencing.

The algorithm first asks whether the product had been shown to function and to meet user needs. The vendor had provided numerous case studies confirming that the Widget system satisfied both of these Phase I testing questions. Based on published literature showing that video consultation-based collaborative care systems in general decreased costs and improved access to mental healthcare, especially in rural areas, by reducing travel time.[78,79] Widget encouraged RH leaders to deploy Widget system-wide and to progress directly to a pragmatic trial. Widget offered to make the system available to RH at no cost for two years, hoping to gain a foothold in a rapidly growing market. However, in line with questions of reach, effectiveness, and implementation (Table 28.4), RH leaders recognized that Widget had only been tested with provider–provider communications and at clinics belonging to the same institution. RH recognized that patient–provider connections might raise novel implementation issues and that connecting with multiple community-based institutions might raise novel technology issues. They therefore started with Phase I testing to make sure connections worked and then embarked on a Phase II study to assess usability and determine optimal work flow.

RH IT officials contacted their counterparts at LHS and learned that LHS had implemented Widget with their high-speed secure intranet that enabled seamless, secure, and reliable video communications. Second, they learned that the Widget system was more bandwidth-intensive than its competitors, an especially crippling limitation for a rural facility with much lower bandwidth than was available at LHC. Thus, while Widget was successful for patients seeing specialists other than psychiatrists at 3 of the original 10 community-based institutions, the overall test at RH could be seen as having had a technology failure at Phase II testing.

RH was able to determine the minimum bandwidth and connection speeds necessary for reliable connectivity, allowing them to expand deployment to institutions meeting that minimum threshold. In the meantime, the Widget company worked on modifying the programming to be less bandwidth intensive. Through rapid cycle testing as the system was reprogrammed, RH was able to lower the required connectivity threshold, eventually re-engaging with a total of 8 of the original 10 clinics, plus adding others. They also tested methods of enabling psychiatry patients to rapidly summon a medical assistant for the now rare times when connections were dropped. Thinking that they had learned the factors required for successful deployment of the Widget system, RH proceeded to full scale adoption. Early on, RH recognized, consistent with other reports,[80] that patients opting for video visits were more likely to be white, younger, and less sick than those refusing invitations to use Widget. RH conducted rapid cycle testing of methods to engage the disparate patient groups. In exchange for receiving two years of free service, RH agreed to conduct the full deployment as a pragmatic trial, providing and publishing data on the experience over the next year of adoption.

Use Case 2: Mobile App-Based Platforms for Diagnosing and Managing Mental Health

Case Summary

Counselors at outpatient Public Addiction Treatment Program (PATP) sought to improve outcomes by enabling patients to complete the post-acute phase of treatment from home. Because addiction clinic services are sparse in their state, many patients live over 100 miles away. Since many are low income, a considerable number do not have automobiles. PATP sought a smartphone app that would enable patients to complete treatment using asynchronous psychotherapy exercises with optional synchronous live support. They selected a start-up vendor whose KWT+NOW app had been reported on in a major online journal. KWT+NOW combines self-guided educational material with weekly check-ins to both an automated chatbot and a live connection to a counselor in the clinic. Content includes goal setting and general health and wellness tips. Through a cloud-based platform, counselors, physicians, and other providers can log in to KWT+NOW to check on the progress of their patients, and administrators can assess overall progress of patients for each provider.

Published results of a single arm pre–post intervention design study showed that KWT+NOW increased time to alcohol relapse among patients at Alcohol Treatment Clinic (ATP) after introduction of the app. Speaking to the ATP medical director, the PATP medical director satisfied herself that the results were due to the introduction of the app and not to other factors.

Analysis

Based on questions suggested in Table 28.4, the PATP director felt that Phase I testing was not needed because the alcohol treatment use case was thought to be quite similar to the substance use treatment use case. In addition, the director informally polled patients and found they seemed very enthusiastic about the product. However, several patients expressed concern about the amount of data that the program would consume, since many had no home broadband, and most had mobile plans with very limited data. Upon passing these concerns along, the vendor suggested that patients could use the app at a library or other places with public WiFi. Patients rejected this option due to lack of privacy and concerns about data security. The vendor then told the director that the app could operate offline and with low-bandwidth data connections and that users could connect via telephone in case low-quality data transmission interrupted video connections.

With patients and the director now satisfied with these responses, PATP thus initiated a Phase II study to look at adoption rates and for initial signs of efficacy. The staff were very split with about half being very enthusiastic and half refusing to use it. About 20% of patients downloaded the app but only 5% of patients used the app more than once. However, more than half of this small group used the app at least once per week and were wildly enthusiastic about it. Their outcomes seemed very positive over a 12 week period. At the end of the trial, exploratory analysis revealed that successful users (staff and patients) had diverse socioeconomic characteristics but *all were iPhone users*. Upon scrutinizing the published paper, the PATP director realized that ATP patients were private and self-pay patients with high income and education. Not only did they have strong digital skills and data plans but they also tended to have late model iPhones for which the app had been optimized. Although training was provided to both PATP staff and patients, the user interface shown was for recent phones models that few had. In fact, the company had abandoned development of the product for Android phones, so most patients and providers had downloaded an outdated, unsupported version of the app. Thus, although efficacy signals were seen in a small subset of patients, the product was considered a technology failure at Phase II (Figure 28.1).

The PATP clinic director looked into purchasing iPhones for patients and staff since few would have been able to afford them on their own. However, the patients themselves said that they frequently lost phones and that high-end phones would elevate their already high risk of robbery and theft. Instead, the clinic partnered with a local organization that helped low income staff and patients to get low cost or free unlimited data plans. The clinic ultimately sought a vendor whose product was optimized for low end, android phones.

Use Case 3: Virtual Reality for Treating Mental Health Conditions

Virtual reality (VR) applications have been developed to help treat a variety of mental health conditions.[81] These products commonly immerse the user in a simulated environment viewed through a visor or headset. Patients can move through and interact with the environment and/or have experiences that are responsive to their actions.

Case Summary

The medical director of outpatient psychiatry at suburban health system (SHS) is considering purchasing the posttraumatic stress disorder (PTSD) virtual reality (VR) application as a scalable means of delivering interventions at two suburban ambulatory care clinics to patients who have PTSD. The medical director carefully examined the demographic characteristics and outcomes of patients in known studies of PTSD-VR. In one randomized study of 200 patients, the application was well accepted by patients. The demographic mix in terms of age, gender, race/ethnicity, and insurance coverage was diverse and similar to that in the SHS clinics. On average, patients in the treatment arm experienced a modest positive benefit relative to patients in the control arm that persisted six months after treatment ended. Not wanting to base her decision on a single study, the medical director also found results of a feasibility study that had been conducted earlier with patients who tried the application at a community health fair. Presented at a credible scientific meeting, the feasibility study results indicated that a diverse patient group enjoyed the initial testing experience, the majority of whom expressed interest in continuing treatment, and nearly all of whom completed the entire treatment phase. Six month outcomes were positive, although they did not reach statistical significance due to the small sample size. Although the feasibility study had been conducted in an urban rather than suburban setting, the patient demographics were similar to those in SHS. As the medical director believed the application had shown high acceptability and usability in comparable populations, with reasonable efficacy signals, she decided to implement PTSD-VR at the SHS suburban clinics and conduct a pragmatic trial.

Deployment of the application went smoothly, but after completing the full treatment regimen, the medical director realized that her patient population did not realize the clinical benefit reported in the studies.

Analysis

Upon a deeper examination, the medical director learned that patients in the published study had had limited prior encounters with the mental healthcare system. On the other hand, the average SHS patient had been receiving conventional PTSD treatment for at least one year. Although the medical director had done her diligence to assure that the application met criteria for Phase III in the algorithm (Figure 28.1), she had not realized that factors associated with success in the previous studies—patients who were new to the mental healthcare system—may not have aligned with her own patient population. Not seeing a clear path to success with PTSD-VR in her patient population, the medical director sought other options to scale care delivery.

Conclusion

Digital solutions developed by technology companies and start-ups pose unique challenges for healthcare settings due to potential for lack of alignment of goals between a health system and a technology company, the potential for unmeasured heterogeneity of effectiveness, and the need to understand institutional factors that may be crucial for successful adoption. Taxonomies and frameworks from public health and from efforts to improve the quality of clinical research publications lead to a set of questions that can be used to assess existing data and choose a testing pathway designed to ensure that products will be safe and effective with the target populations and in target settings.

Although far from complete, the digital medicine testing algorithm attempts to provide some structure and common terminology to help health systems efficiently and effectively test and adopt digital health solutions. In addition, a framework analogous to clinical trials.gov is needed to track and learn from the evaluation of digital health solutions that do not require FDA oversight.

Convergence science has brought many changes in a short amount of time to healthcare and particularly to the mental health space. Many of these changes offer scalable alternatives to resource constrained healthcare systems but have leapfrogged standard regulatory processes that have historically been in place for validating their safety and efficacy. While evaluation models such as the NODE.Health algorithm are available as frameworks for testing digital health tools, convergence science may play a future role in scaling the pace at which validations can be done.

At the federal level in the United States, there remains interest in the safety of higher-risk software. The FDA, for example, approved the first digital mental health tool in December of 2018.[82] While formal regulatory approval of digital mental health apps is still in its infancy, we can expect to see more in this space. Furthermore, evolving regulatory policies are also on the horizon, including the Beneficiary Education Tools Telehealth Extender Reauthorization (BETTER) Act, which expands Medicare telehealth benefits to improve access to mental health services,[83] and Cures 2.0 with a focus on digital health and real world evidence.[84] Furthermore, the National Institute of Mental Health has signaled its commitment to validation by investing in "research projects to test strategies to increase the ... effectiveness, and quality of digital mental health interventions ... to rapidly refine and optimize existing evidence-based digital health interventions and to conduct clinical trials testing digital mental health interventions that are statistically powered to provide a definitive answer regarding the intervention's effectiveness."[85]

Keeping pace with and validating digital health tools will always present challenges, but as convergence science catalyzed the emergence of these tools, so too may we find that it will catalyze scalable modalities for validating them so that as a society, we will continue to assure the safety, efficacy, and real-world effectiveness of these innovations.

References

1. Adler-Milstein J, Jha AK. HITECH Act drove large gains in hospital electronic health record adoption. *Health Aff Proj Hope.* 2017;36(8):1416–1422. doi:10.1377/hlthaff.2016.1651
2. U.S. Department of Health and Human Services, Office for Civil Rights. HIPAA Privacy Rule and Sharing Information Related to Mental Health. December 2017. https://www.hhs.gov/sites/default/files/hipaa-privacy-rule-and-sharing-info-related-to-mental-health.pdf. Accessed November 4, 2019.
3. Pawson R. *Evidence-Based Policy.* London: SAGE; 2006. doi:10.4135/9781849209120
4. Pawson R, Greenhalgh T, Harvey G, Walshe K. Realist review: a new method of systematic review designed for complex policy interventions. *J Health Serv Res Policy.* 2005;10(Suppl 1):21–34. doi:10.1258/1355819054308530
5. Borkan J. Immersion/crystallization. In: Crabtree BF, Miller WL, eds. *Doing Qualitative Research.* 2nd ed., pp. 179–194. Newbury Park, NJ: SAGE; 1999.
6. Otte-Trojel T, de Bont A, Rundall TG, van de Klundert J. How outcomes are achieved through patient portals: a realist review. *JAMIA.* 2014;21(4):751–757. doi:10.1136/amiajnl-2013-002501
7. Parasuraman A, Colby CL. An updated and streamlined Technology Readiness Index: TRI 2.0. *J Serv Res.* 2015;18(1):59–74. doi:10.1177/1094670514539730
8. Najaftorkaman M, Ghapanchi AH, Talaei-Khoei A, Ray P. A taxonomy of antecedents to user adoption of health information systems: a synthesis of thirty years of research: a taxonomy of antecedents to user adoption of health information systems: a synthesis of thirty years of research. *J Assoc Inf Sci Technol.* 2015;66(3):576–598. doi:10.1002/asi.23181
9. Kayser L, Kushniruk A, Osborne RH, Norgaard O, Turner P. Enhancing the effectiveness of consumer-focused health information technology systems through eHealth literacy: a framework for understanding users' needs. *JMIR Hum Factors.* 2015;2(1):e9. doi:10.2196/humanfactors.3696
10. Perry B, Herrington W, Goldsack JC, et al. Use of mobile devices to measure outcomes in clinical research, 2010–2016: a systematic literature review. *Digit Biomark.* 2018;2(1):11–30. doi:10.1159/000486347
11. Van Dyk L. A review of telehealth service implementation frameworks. *Int J Environ Res Public Health.* 2014;11(2):1279–1298. doi:10.3390/ijerph110201279
12. Granja C, Janssen W, Johansen MA. Factors determining the success and failure of eHealth interventions: systematic review of the literature. *J Med Internet Res.* 2018;20(5):e10235. doi:10.2196/10235
13. Mummah SA, Robinson TN, King AC, Gardner CD, Sutton S. IDEAS (integrate, design, assess, and share): a framework and toolkit of strategies for the development of more effective digital interventions to change health behavior. *J Med Internet Res.* 2016;18(12):e317. doi:10.2196/jmir.5927

14. Heffernan KJ, Chang S, Maclean ST, et al. Guidelines and recommendations for developing interactive ehealth apps for complex messaging in health promotion. *JMIR MHealth UHealth*. 2016;4(1):e14. doi:10.2196/mhealth.4423

15. Bradway M, Carrion C, Vallespin B, et al. mHealth assessment: conceptualization of a global framework. *JMIR MHealth UHealth*. 2017;5(5):e60. doi:10.2196/mhealth.7291

16. Mason V. Innovation for medically vulnerable populations, part 3: experiment design. https://tincture.io/innovation-for-medically-vulnerable-populations-part-3-experiment-design-47c8c7b00919#.r6wt2gwlb. Accessed February 27, 2018.

17. Malikova MA. Optimization of protocol design: a path to efficient, lower cost clinical trial execution. *Future Sci OA*. 2016;2(1):FSO89. doi:10.4155/fso.15.89

18. Baker TB, Gustafson DH, Shah D. How can research keep up with eHealth? Ten strategies for increasing the timeliness and usefulness of eHealth research. *J Med Internet Res*. 2014;16(2):e36. doi:10.2196/jmir.2925

19. Porzsolt F, Rocha NG, Toledo-Arruda AC, et al. Efficacy and effectiveness trials have different goals, use different tools, and generate different messages. *Pragmatic Obs Res*. 2015;6:47–54. doi:10.2147/POR.S89946

20. Philpott D, Guergachi A, Keshavjee K. Design and validation of a platform to evaluate mhealth apps. *Stud Health Technol Inform*. 2017;235:3–7 doi:10.2196/jmir.2925.

21. van Gemert-Pijnen JEWC, Nijland N, van Limburg M, et al. A holistic framework to improve the uptake and impact of eHealth technologies. *J Med Internet Res*. 2011;13(4):e111. doi:10.2196/jmir.1672

22. World Health Organization. *Monitoring and Evaluating Digital Health Interventions: A Practical Guide to Conducting Research and Assessment*. Geneva. World Health Organization; 2016:144. https://apps.who.int/iris/bitstream/handle/10665/252183/9789241511766-eng.pdf. Accessed February 5, 2018.

23. Fanning J, Mullen SP, McAuley E. Increasing physical activity with mobile devices: a meta-analysis. *J Med Internet Res*. 2012;14(6):e161. doi:10.2196/jmir.2171

24. Agarwal S, LeFevre AE, Lee J, et al. Guidelines for reporting of health interventions using mobile phones: mobile health (mHealth) evidence reporting and assessment (mERA) checklist. *BMJ*. March 2016:i1174. doi:10.1136/bmj.i1174

25. Eysenbach G, CONSORT-EHEALTH Group. CONSORT-EHEALTH: improving and standardizing evaluation reports of web-based and mobile health interventions. *J Med Internet Res*. 2011;13(4):e126. doi:10.2196/jmir.1923

26. Welch VA, Norheim OF, Jull J, et al. CONSORT-Equity 2017 extension and elaboration for better reporting of health equity in randomised trials. *BMJ*. 2017;359:j5085. doi:10.1136/bmj.j5085

27. Eldridge SM, Chan CL, Campbell MJ, et al. CONSORT 2010 statement: extension to randomised pilot and feasibility trials. *BMJ*. 2016;355:i5239. doi:10.1136/bmj.i5239

28. Hors-Fraile S, Rivera-Romero O, Schneider F, et al. Analyzing recommender systems for health promotion using a multidisciplinary taxonomy: a scoping review. *Int J Med Inf*. 2018;114:143–155. doi:10.1016/j.ijmedinf.2017.12.018

29. Basher KM, Nieto-Hipolito J-I, Leon MDLAC, Vazquez-Briseno M, López J de DS, Mariscal RB. Major existing classification matrices and future directions for internet of things. *Adv Internet Things*. 2017;07(04):112–120. doi:10.4236/ait.2017.74008

30. World Health Organization. Classification of Digital Health Interventions v1.0: a shared language to describe the uses of digital technology for health. 2018. https://apps.who.int/iris/bitstream/handle/10665/260480/WHO-RHR-18.06-eng.pdf. Accessed September 25, 2019.

31. Donnelly JE, Jacobsen DJ, Whatley JE, et al. Nutrition and physical activity program to attenuate obesity and promote physical and metabolic fitness in elementary school children. *Obes Res*. 1996;4(3):229–243. doi:10.1002/j.1550-8528.1996.tb00541.x

32. Wang A, An N, Lu X, Chen H, Li C, Levkoff S. A classification scheme for analyzing mobile apps used to prevent and manage disease in late life. *JMIR MHealth UHealth*. 2014;2(1):e6. doi:10.2196/mhealth.2877

33. Singh K, Bates D. Developing a framework for evaluating the patient engagement, quality, and safety of mobile health applications. Commonwealth Fund. https://www. commonwealthfund.org/publications/issue-briefs/2016/feb/developing-framework-evaluating-patient-engagement-quality-and. Accessed March 27, 2018.

34. Barello S, Triberti S, Graffigna G, et al. eHealth for patient engagement: a systematic review. *Front Psychol*. 2015;6:2013. doi:10.3389/fpsyg.2015.02013

35. Abelson J, Wagner F, DeJean D, et al. Public and patient involvement in health technology assessment: a framework for action. *Int J Technol Assess Health Care*. 2016;32(4):256–264. doi:10.1017/S0266462316000362

36. Or CKL, Karsh B-T. A systematic review of patient acceptance of consumer health information technology. *JAMIA*. 2009;16(4):550–560. doi:10.1197/jamia.M2888

37. Kruse CS, DeShazo J, Kim F, Fulton L. Factors associated with adoption of health information technology: a conceptual model based on a systematic review. *JMIR Med Inform*. 2014;2(1):e9. doi:10.2196/medinform.3106

38. Karnoe A, Furstrand D, Christensen KB, Norgaard O, Kayser L. Assessing competencies needed to engage with digital health services: development of the ehealth literacy assessment toolkit. *J Med Internet Res*. 2018;20(5):e178. doi:10.2196/jmir.8347

39. Sawesi S, Rashrash M, Phalakornkule K, Carpenter JS, Jones JF. The impact of information technology on patient engagement and health behavior change: a systematic review of the literature. *JMIR Med Inform*. 2016;4(1):e1. doi:10.2196/medinform.4514

40. Greenhalgh T, Wherton J, Papoutsi C, et al. Beyond adoption: a new framework for theorizing and evaluating nonadoption, abandonment, and challenges to the scale-up, spread, and sustainability of health and care technologies. *J Med Internet Res*. 2017;19(11):e367. doi:10.2196/jmir.8775

41. Kushniruk A, Turner P. A framework for user involvement and context in the design and development of safe e-Health systems. *Stud Health Technol Inform*. 2012;180:353–357.

42. Trivedi MC. Role of context in usability evaluations: a review. *Adv Comput Int J*. 2012;3(2):69–78. doi:10.5121/acij.2012.3208

43. Baum S. How can digital health startups steer clear of pilot study pitfalls? *MedCity News*. https://medcitynews.com/2018/03/how-can-digital-health-startups-steer-clear-of-pilot-study-pitfalls/?rf=1. Accessed August 17, 2018.

44. Kumar S, Nilsen WJ, Abernethy A, et al. Mobile health technology evaluation: the mHealth evidence workshop. *Am J Prev Med*. 2013;45(2):228–236. doi:10.1016/j.amepre.2013.03.017

45. Kramer ADI, Guillory JE, Hancock JT. Experimental evidence of massive-scale emotional contagion through social networks. *Proc Natl Acad Sci U S A*. 2014;111(24):8788–8790. doi:10.1073/pnas.1320040111

46. Cobb NK, Graham AL. Health behavior interventions in the age of Facebook. *Am J Prev Med*. 2012;43(5):571–572. doi:10.1016/j.amepre.2012.08.001

47. Makhni S, Atreja A, Sheon A, Van Winkle B, Sharp J, Carpenter N. The broken health information technology innovation pipeline: a perspective from the NODE Health Consortium. *Digit Biomark*. 2017;1(1):64–72. doi:10.1159/000479017

48. Sheon AR, Bolen SD, Callahan B, Shick S, Perzynski AT. Addressing disparities in diabetes management through novel approaches to encourage technology adoption and use. *JMIR Diabetes*. 2017;2(2):e16. doi:10.2196/diabetes.6751

49. Winkle BV, Carpenter N, Moscucci M. Why aren't our digital solutions working for everyone? *AMA J Ethics.* 2017;19(11):1116–1124. doi:10.1001/journalofethics.2017.19.11. stas2-1711

50. Atreja A, Khan S, Otobo E, et al. Impact of real world home-based remote monitoring on quality of care and quality of life in IBD patients: interim results of pragmatic randomized trial. *Gastroenterology.* 2017;152(5):S600–S601. doi:10.1016/S0016-5085(17)32145-5

51. Atreja A, Daga N, Patel NP, et al. Sa1426 validating an automated system to identify patients with high risk lesions requiring surveillance colonoscopies: implications for accountable care and colonoscopy bundle payment. *Gastrointest Endosc.* 2015;81(5):AB210. doi:10.1016/j.gie.2015.03.197

52. Evans B, Shiao S. Streamlining enterprise sales in digital health. *Rock Health.* https://rockhealth.com/reports/streamlining-enterprise-sales-in-digital-health/. Accessed August 19, 2018.

53. Validic Report: How digital health devices and data impact clinical trials. September 2016. https://hitconsultant.net/2016/09/19/validic-digital-health-devices-report/. Accessed August 19, 2018.

54. Surve S. How to survive IRBs and have successful digital health pilots. *MedCity News.* November 2017; https://medcitynews.com/2017/11/survive-irbs-successful-digital-health-pilots/?rf=1. Accessed August 19, 2018.

55. Umscheid CA, Margolis DJ, Grossman CE. Key concepts of clinical trials: a narrative review. *Postgrad Med.* 2011;123(5):194–204. doi:10.3810/pgm.2011.09.2475

56. Dorst K. The core of "design thinkin" and its application. *Des Stud.* 2011;32(6):521–532. doi:10.1016/j.destud.2011.07.006

57. Corrigan-Curay J, Sacks L, Woodcock J. Real-world evidence and real-world data for evaluating drug safety and effectiveness. *JAMA.* 2018;320(9):867–868. doi:10.1001/jama.2018.10136

58. Ford I, Norrie J. Pragmatic trials. Drazen JM, Harrington DP, McMurray JJV, Ware JH, Woodcock J, eds. *N Engl J Med.* 2016;375(5):454–463. doi:10.1056/NEJMra1510059

59. Napolitano MA, Whiteley JA, Mavredes MN, et al. Using social media to deliver weight loss programming to young adults: design and rationale for the Healthy Body Healthy U (HBHU) trial. *Contemp Clin Trials.* 2017;60:1–13. doi:10.1016/j.cct.2017.06.007

60. Chen T, Zhang X, Jiang H, et al. Are you smoking? Automatic alert system helping people keep away from cigarettes. *Smart Health.* 2018;9–10:158–169. doi:10.1016/j.smhl.2018.07.008

61. Tung JY, Shaw RJ, Hagenkord JM, et al. Accelerating precision health by applying the lessons learned from direct-to-consumer genomics to digital health technologies. *NAM Perspect.* 2018;8(3). doi:10.31478/201803c

62. Glasgow RE, Vogt TM, Boles SM. Evaluating the public health impact of health promotion interventions: the RE-AIM framework. *Am J Public Health.* 1999;89(9):1322–1327. doi:10.2105/ajph.89.9.1322

63. Carlfjord S, Andersson A, Bendtsen P, Nilsen P, Lindberg M. Applying the RE-AIM framework to evaluate two implementation strategies used to introduce a tool for lifestyle intervention in Swedish primary health care. *Health Promot Int.* 2012;27(2):167–176. doi:10.1093/heapro/dar016

64. Glasgow RE, Estabrooks PE. Pragmatic applications of RE-AIM for health care initiatives in community and clinical settings. *Prev Chronic Dis.* 2018;15:E02. doi:10.5888/pcd15.170271

65. McCloud RF, Okechukwu CA, Sorensen G, Viswanath K. Entertainment or health? Exploring the internet usage patterns of the urban poor: a secondary analysis of a randomized controlled trial. *J Med Internet Res.* 2016;18(3):e46. doi:10.2196/jmir.4375

66. Schartman-Cycyk S, Meissier K. Bridging the gap: what affordable, uncapped internet means for digital inclusion. *Mobile Beacon*; 2017. https://www.mobilebeacon.org/wp-content/uploads/2017/05/MB_ResearchPaper_FINAL_WEB.pdf. Accessed May 20, 2017.

67. Anderson M, Perrin A, Jiang J, Kumar M. 10% of Americans don't use the internet. Who are they? *Pew Research Center*. 2018; https://www.pewresearch.org/fact-tank/2019/04/22/some-americans-dont-use-the-internet-who-are-they/. Accessed April 13, 2018.

68. Internet/broadband fact sheet. *Pew Research Center, Internet and Technology*. 2019; https://www.pewresearch.org/internet/fact-sheet/internet-broadband/. Accessed December 4, 2019.

69. Anderson M, Perrin A. Tech adoption climbs among older adults. *Pew Research Center Internet and Technology*. May 2017; https://www.pewresearch.org/internet/2017/05/17/technology-use-among-seniors/. Accessed May 20, 2017.

70. Anderson M, Kumar M. Digital divide persists even as lower-income Americans make gains in tech adoption. *Pew Research Center*. May 2019. https://www.pewresearch.org/fact-tank/2019/05/07/digital-divide-persists-even-as-lower-income-americans-make-gains-in-tech-adoption/. Accessed December 4, 2019.

71. Horrigan J. Digital readiness gaps. *Pew Research Center Internet and Technology*. September 2016; https://www.pewresearch.org/internet/2016/09/20/digital-readiness-gaps/. Accessed February 14, 2017.

72. Anderson M, Horrigan J. Smartphones may not bridge digital divide for all. *Pew Research Center*. October 2016; https://www.pewresearch.org/fact-tank/2016/10/03/smartphones-help-those-without-broadband-get-online-but-dont-necessarily-bridge-the-digital-divide/. Accessed November 8, 2016.

73. Perzynski AT, Roach MJ, Shick S, et al. Patient portals and broadband internet inequality. *JAMIA*. 2017;24(5):927–932. doi:10.1093/jamia/ocx020

74. Ackerman SL, Sarkar U, Tieu L, et al. Meaningful use in the safety net: a rapid ethnography of patient portal implementation at five community health centers in California. *JAMIA*. 2017;24(5):903–912. doi:10.1093/jamia/ocx015

75. Tieu L, Schillinger D, Sarkar U, et al. Online patient websites for electronic health record access among vulnerable populations: portals to nowhere? *JAMIA*. 2017;24(e1):e47–e54. doi:10.1093/jamia/ocw098

76. Lyles C, Schillinger D, Sarkar U. Connecting the dots: health information technology expansion and health disparities. *PLoS Med*. 2015;12(7):e1001852. doi:10.1371/journal.pmed.1001852

77. Stellefson M, Chaney B, Barry AE, et al. Web 2.0 chronic disease self-management for older adults: a systematic review. *J Med Internet Res*. 2013;15(2):e35. doi:10.2196/jmir.2439

78. Backhaus A, Agha Z, Maglione ML, et al. Videoconferencing psychotherapy: a systematic review. *Psychol Serv*. 2012;9(2):111–131. doi:10.1037/a0027924

79. Richardson LK, Frueh BC, Grubaugh AL, Egede L, Elhai JD. Current directions in video-conferencing tele-mental health research. *Clin Psychol Publ Div Clin Psychol Am Psychol Assoc*. 2009;16(3):323–338. doi:10.1111/j.1468-2850.2009.01170.x

80. Abel EA, Shimada SL, Wang K, et al. Dual use of a patient portal and clinical video telehealth by veterans with mental health diagnoses: retrospective, cross-sectional analysis. *J Med Internet Res*. 2018;20(11):e11350. doi:10.2196/11350

81. Bouchard S, Dumoulin S, Robillard G, et al. Virtual reality compared with in vivo exposure in the treatment of social anxiety disorder: a three-arm randomised controlled trial. *Br J Psychiatry*. 2017;210(4):276–283. doi:10.1192/bjp.bp.116.184234

82. FDA Office of the Commissioner. FDA clears mobile medical app to help those with opioid use disorder stay in recovery programs. September 11, 2019; http://www.fda.gov/

news-events/press-announcements/fda-clears-mobile-medical-app-help-those-opioid-use-disorder-stay-recovery-programs. Accessed November 30, 2019.

83. Neal, Brady introduce legislation to improve and expand Medicare. Ways and Means Committee, Democrats. June 24, 2019; https://waysandmeans.house.gov/media-center/press-releases/neal-brady-introduce-legislation-improve-and-expand-medicare. Accessed November 30, 2019.

84. DeGette, Upton call for ideas on Cures 2.0. November 22, 2019; https://degette.house.gov/media-center/press-releases/degette-upton-call-for-ideas-on-cures-20.   Accessed November 30, 2019.

85. RFA-MH-20-510: Laboratories to Optimize Digital Health (R01 Clinical Trial Required). https://grants.nih.gov/grants/guide/rfa-files/RFA-MH-20-510.html. Accessed December 1, 2019.

29

Key Considerations for Developing Digital Health Accelerators

Grace Lethlean

Acknowledgment

Bronwyn Le Grice, Founder of ANDHealth, has been instrumental in the hypotheses and approaches to digital health acceleration which are reflected in this chapter. Without her sector leadership and expertise, this chapter would not have been possible, and programs providing valuable digital health support would not have been designed.

Accelerators: What Are They, How Do They Work, and Do They Work?

What Are They and How Do They Work?

Accelerator programs typically support early-stage, growth-driven companies through education, mentorship, and financing. Over the past decade there has been a rapid global boom in the number of accelerator and incubator programs. The International Business Innovation Association indicates that there are more than 7,000 business incubators and accelerators, and the *Harvard Business Review* notes that the number of accelerators in the United States increased by an average of 50% each year between 2008 and 2014.[1]

Terms such as *incubator, accelerator, co-working space,* and *maker space,* among others, are often used interchangeably. These terms are well defined by the Impact Index, which measures the impact of entrepreneurial support programs in the United States.[2] They can be quite different in execution, with a notable distinction between for-profit and not-for-profit models.

Broadly, accelerators typically offer fixed-term support, are cohort based and culminate in a graduation.[3] Often, but not always, accelerators focus on earlier stage

---

[1] Hathaway I. What startup accelerators really do. *Harvard Business Review.* https://hbr.org/2016/03/what-startup-accelerators-really-do. Published March 1, 2016. Accessed October 10, 2019.

[2] InBia. Operational definitions: entrepreneurship centers. https://inbia.org/wp-content/uploads/2016/09/Terms_4.pdf?x84587. Published September, 2017. Accessed October 3, 2019.

[3] Cohen S. Accelerating startups: the seed accelerator phenomenon. *Seed Accelerators Ranking Project.* http://seedrankings.com/pdf/seed-accelerator-phenomenon.pdf. Published March, 2019. Accessed October 10, 2019.

"start-up" companies. (By contrast, incubators may provide years of support, often have no "graduation," and tend to focus on later-stage companies.[4])

Accelerators also often offer seed money in exchange for equity in the company. This may range from tens of thousands to hundreds of thousands of dollars.

A typical accelerator process recruits, screens, and accepts (or rejects) companies, potentially provides financing, and puts the companies through a focused learning period, including a set curriculum, workshops, seminars, mentorship and networking opportunities. The final graduation is likely to take the form of a "Demo Day," during which companies demonstrate their capabilities and new-found maturity, with an ultimate focus often on securing investment.[5] A notable accelerator, and one of the first globally, is Silicon Valley-based Y Combinator, which was established by Paul Graham in 2005.

While attending an accelerator is by no means an essential step toward commercialization, many well-known technology companies have come through accelerators, including AirBnB, Dropbox, and Stripe.

Do They Work?

The accelerator sector globally has received a great deal of attention, but little scrutiny. There is a lack of established, harmonized regulation on the quality of the information and networks they provide, and there is a lack of established mechanisms for measuring the quality and success of accelerator programs.

Systematic research is beginning to emerge on the effects of accelerator participation on companies themselves and the broader ecosystem in which they operate. A study comparing 164 accelerator-backed new ventures over eight US accelerators with a matched set of 164 nonaccelerated new ventures found that the former group was quicker to raise venture capital and gain customer traction[6]. However, the study showed that this effect was uneven across accelerators, which highlights the discrepancy between accelerators and the difficulty of configuring an effective accelerator and calls into question the necessity for widespread and rapid growth of accelerators.[7] It also illustrates the challenges faced by companies as they try to find the accelerator that will be best for them. Interestingly, the authors concluded that a company founder's prior experience (whether entrepreneurial or academic) was no substitute for accelerator participation—suggesting that top accelerators

[4] Hathaway I. What startup accelerators really do. *Harvard Business Review*. https://hbr.org/2016/03/what-startup-accelerators-really-do. Published March 1, 2016. Accessed October 10, 2019.

[5] Cohen S. What do accelerators do? Insights from incubators and angels. *Innovations*. 2013;8:19-25. https://www.mitpressjournals.org/doi/pdf/10.1162/INOV_a_00184. Accessed October 10, 2019.

[6] Hallen BL, Bingham CB, Cohen S. Do accelerators accelerate? A study of venture accelerators as a path to success? *Acad Manage Proc*. 2014;2014(1). https://journals.aom.org/doi/10.5465/ambpp.2014.185#. Accessed October 6, 2019.

[7] Hallen BL, Bingham CB, Cohen S. Do accelerators accelerate? A study of venture accelerators as a path to success? *Acad Manage Proc*. 2014;2014(1). https://journals.aom.org/doi/10.5465/ambpp.2014.185#. Accessed October 6, 2019.

do indeed provide a unique form of entrepreneurial teaching and networking opportunity.[8]

Another study compared 619 companies that had participated in the Y Combinator and Tech Stars accelerators from 2005 to 2011 to a matched sample of 619 who did not participate in an accelerator but instead raised funding from angel investor groups. Results showed substantial differences between the two sets. Participation in a top accelerator program did indeed increase the likelihood and speed of exit by acquisition, as well as exit by quitting; however, the angel investment set were quicker to attract follow-on venture funding.[9]

A study aiming to demonstrate accelerator performance in aiding venture development, above factors such as credential signaling to future investors or previous founder experience at top companies, established that the value of accelerators is real and replicable and likely comes from the intensive learning environment provided by accelerators.[10]

Beyond the individual outcomes of the companies, accelerators also have a positive impact on regional entrepreneurial ecosystems, especially with regard to the financing ecosystem.[11] Metropolitan areas where an accelerator is established subsequently attract more seed and early-stage entrepreneurial financing activity, which appears not to be restricted to accelerated start-ups themselves but spills over to nonaccelerated companies as well, occurring primarily from an increase in investors' exposure to start-up companies.[12]

What Is Digital Health?

Digital health represents a technological change that cuts across every aspect of healthcare, spanning delivery, prevention, diagnosis, management, and treatment, transforming the way in which frontline healthcare services are created, delivered, and measured.[13] Originally coined to represent the digitization of health records and administrative systems, the definition is now much broader. As Paul Sonnier describes it in his book *The Fourth Wave: Digital Health*,

[8] Hallen BL, Bingham CB, Cohen S. Do accelerators accelerate? A study of venture accelerators as a path to success? *Acad Manage Proc.* 2014;2014(1). https://journals.aom.org/doi/10.5465/ambpp.2014.185#. Accessed October 6, 2019.

[9] Smith S, Hannigan TJ. Home run, strike out, or base hit: how do accelerators impact exit and VC financing in new firms? *Acad Manage Proc.* 2014;2014(1). https://journals.aom.org/doi/10.5465/ambpp.2014.1381labstract. Accessed October 10, 2019.

[10] Hallen BL, Cohen S, Bingham CB. Do accelerators work? If so, How? *SSRN.* https://papers.ssrn.com/sol3/papers.cfm?abstract_id=2719810. Updated April 5, 2019. Accessed October 6, 2019.

[11] Fehder DC, Hochberg YV. Accelerators and the regional supply of venture capital investment. *Seed Accelerators Ranking Project.* http://www.seedrankings.com/pdf/accelerators-and-regional-suppy-of-vc-investment.pdf. Published September 19, 2014. Accessed October 10, 2019.

[12] Fehder DC, Hochberg YV. Accelerators and the regional supply of venture capital investment. *Seed Accelerators Ranking Project.* http://www.seedrankings.com/pdf/accelerators-and-regional-suppy-of-vc-investment.pdf. Published September 19, 2014. Accessed October 10, 2019.

[13] ANDHealth. Digital health: Creating a new growth industry for Australia. https://andhealth.com.au/wp-content/uploads/2019/04/Digital-Health_Creating-a-New-Growth-Industry-for-Australia.pdf. Published 2018. Accessed October 6, 2019.

the convergence of the digital and genomic revolutions with health, healthcare, living, and society—is empowering us to better track, manage, and improve our own and our family's health, live better, more productive lives, and improve society. It's also helping to reduce inefficiencies in healthcare delivery, improve access, reduce costs, increase quality, and make medicine more personalised and precise.[14]

Sonnier's sentiments are echoed by the US Food and Drug Administration, which states:

"The broad scope of digital health includes categories such as mobile health (mHealth), health information technology (IT), wearable devices, telehealth and telemedicine, and personalized medicine. Patients and consumers can use digital health to better manage and track their health and wellness related activities. The use of technologies such as smart phones, social networks and internet applications is not only changing the way we communicate, but is also providing innovative ways for us to monitor our health and well-being and giving us greater access to information. Together these advancements are leading to a convergence of people, information, technology and connectivity to improve healthcare and health outcomes.[15]

Several industry groups—the Digital Medicine Society, Digital Therapeutics Alliance, HealthXL, and NODE.Health—have collaborated to propose a framework to define and differentiate digital health products from digital medicine and digital therapeutics[16] as outlined in Table 29.1. This is a helpful distinction as there are different claims, levels of health impact, and evidence requirements depending whether the product simply displays general health information to a patient, remotely monitors and diagnoses a patient, or directly treats their disease or disorder.

Mental health is a key area for digital therapeutics.[17] One example is Pear Therapeutics' reSET-O app, a prescription cognitive behavioral therapy to support outpatient treatment programs for individuals with opioid use disorder.[18] But barriers to widespread adoption of digital therapeutics remain high. A meta-analysis published in December 2019 concluded that "although some trials showed potential of apps targeting mental health symptoms, using smartphone apps as standalone psychological interventions cannot be recommended based on the current level of

---

[14] Sonnier P. *The Fourth Wave: Digital Health*. [Kindle edition]. https://www.amazon.com.au/Fourth-Wave-Digital-Health-ebook/dp/B077H67J6T. Accessed October 6, 2019.

[15] US Food & Drug Administration. Digital health. https://www.fda.gov/medicaldevices/digitalhealth/. Updated May 12, 2019. Accessed November 4, 2019.

[16] Goldsack J, Coder M, Fitzgerald C, Navar-Mattingly N, Coravos A, Atreja, A. Digital health, digital medicine, digital therapeutics (DTx): What's the difference? *HealthXL*. https://www.healthxl.com/blog/digital-health-digital-medicine-digital-therapeutics-dtx-whats-the-difference. Published November 11, 2019. Accessed November 15, 2019.

[17] Chandrashekar P. Do mental health mobile apps work: evidence and recommendations for designing high-efficacy mental health mobile apps. *Mhealth*. 2018;4:6. doi:10.21037/mhealth.2018.03.02.

[18] US Food and Drug Administration. FDA clears mobile medical app to help those with opioid use disorder stay in recovery programs. https://www.fda.gov/news-events/press-announcements/fda-clears-mobile-medical-app-help-those-opioid-use-disorder-stay-recovery-programs. Published December 10, 2018. Accessed November 19, 2019.

Table 29.1 Definitions in Digital Health

	Digital Health	Digital Medicine	Digital Therapeutics
Definition	Digital health includes technologies, platforms, and systems that engage consumers for lifestyle, wellness, and health-related purposes; capture, store or transmit health data; and/or support life science and clinical operations.	Digital medicine includes evidence-based software and/or hardware products that measure and/or intervene in the service of human health.[1]	Digital therapeutic (DTx) products deliver evidence-based therapeutic interventions to prevent, manage, or treat a medical disorder or disease.[2]
Clinical evidence	Typically do not require clinical evidence.	Clinical evidence is required for all digital medicine products.	Clinical evidence and real world outcomes are required for all DTx products.
Regulatory oversight	These products do not meet the regulatory definition of a medical device[3] and do not require regulatory oversight.	Requirements for regulatory oversight vary. Digital medicine products that are classified as medical devices require clearance or approval. Digital medicine products used as a tool to develop other drugs, devices, or medical products require regulatory acceptance by the appropriate review division.	DTx products must be reviewed and cleared or certified by regulatory bodies as required to support product claims of risk, efficacy, and intended use.

[1]https://www.dimesociety.org/index.php/defining-digital-medicine

[2]https://www.dtxalliance.org/dtxproducts/

[3]It is important to check with local regulatory requirements in each jurisdiction the product is manufactured, registered, or used on.

Source: Goldsack J, Coder M, Fitzgerald C, Navar-Mattingly N, Coravos A, Atreja A. (2019). Digital Health, Digital Medicine, Digital Therapeutics (DTx): What's the difference? *HealthXL*. https://www.healthxl.com/blog/digital-health-digital-medicine-digital-therapeutics-dtx-whats-the-difference. Published November 7, 2019. Accessed November 8, 2019.

evidence."[19] While there has been rapid growth in the development of digital therapeutics for mental health in recent years,[20] further evidence and support for the emerging companies is required for widespread success of digital therapeutics in mental health.[21]

Why Digital Health Requires Specialized Business Accelerator Programs

The delivery of healthcare is inherently complex. Healthcare systems everywhere involve a matrix of public and private sector entities and are highly regulated, risk-aware environments. The inherent complexity limits their ability to quickly adopt new technologies and innovations, no matter how potentially beneficial they might seem to be. However, most health systems recognize that embracing new types of digital health tools will be key to ensuring the future well-being of the population.

Typical consumer technology accelerator approaches are not well suited to digital health. In fact, principles that work in the consumer technology sector can either be false or detrimental when applied to healthcare. For example, advice from a consumer technology accelerator to "put your minimum viable product in the hands of the end user, and earn some early revenue to fund future development" can be foolhardy or even illegal if applied to a health setting.[22] The "fail fast, fail often" mantra espoused by technology accelerators is impeded by the complex regulatory landscape of healthcare. This cultural clash is further exacerbated by the cautious, stage-gated, and time-consuming process of healthcare innovation that is grounded in the risk-averse clinical principle of "First, do no harm."[23]

Successfully developing any product for healthcare means having a clear understanding of healthcare systems' complex chains of funding and payment, long sales cycles, and the need for buy-in from clinicians and/or payers along with investors, as well as the strong distinctions between the product's user, such as a patient or nurse, and its buyer, such as a hospital system or health insurer.[24] Understanding and

---

[19] Weisel KK, Fuhrmann LM, Berking M, Baumeister H, Cuijpers P, Ebert DD. Standalone smartphone apps for mental health—a systematic review and meta-analysis. *npj Digit Med.* 2019;2;118. doi:10.1038/s41746-019-0188-8.

[20] Hill C, Martin J, Thomson S, Scott-Ram N, Penfold H, Creswell C. Navigating the challenges of digital health innovation: considerations and solutions in developing online and smartphone-application-based interventions for mental health disorders. *Br J Psychiatry.* 2017;8;211(2):65-69. doi:10.1192/bjp.bp.115.180372.

[21] Hollis C, Morriss R, Martin J, Amani S, Cotton R, Denis M, Lewis S. Technological innovations in mental healthcare: harnessing the digital revolution. *Br J Psychiatry.* 2015;206(4):263–265. doi:10.1192/bjp.bp.113.142612.

[22] Yock P. Why do digital health startups keep failing? *Fast Company.* https://www.fastcompany.com/90251795/why-do-digital-health-startups-keep-failing. Published October 17, 2018. Accessed November 19, 2019.

[23] Smith CM. Origin and uses of primum non nocer—above all, do no harm! *J Clin Pharmacol.* 2015;45:371–377.

[24] Baum S. What can digital health startups learn about commercialization from Medtech And Life Science companies? *Medcity News.* https://medcitynews.com/2018/10/digital-health-startups-and-commercialization/?rf=1. Published October 9, 2018. Accessed November 19, 2019.

teaching these interactions, incentives, and pathways is critical to a program aiming to add value to digital health companies to support them in building a sustainable business in healthcare. As summarized in the report *Digital Health: Creating a New Growth Industry for Australia*, "evidence-based digital health products face a significantly different commercialization pathway, an evolving regulatory landscape and limited reimbursement potential. In addition, these digital health products require novel commercial models to penetrate risk-averse and budget constrained procurement systems."[25]

To add to this complexity, the regulatory systems and pathways for navigating digital health regulation are specialized and evolving. For example, the FDA has adjusted the way it regulates some types of digital health technology and has launched a precertification pilot program to streamline what can be a lengthy approval process.[26] On the other side of the regulation divide, organizations which protect consumers from false and misleading claims such as the US Federal Trade Commission, can enforce substantial fines on companies which it decides are making misleading marketing claims using unsupported medical claims, such as a teledermatology app that claimed it could help identify skin cancer earlier,[27] a blood pressure monitoring app developer[28] and a business that developed an app claiming brain training properties.[29] The same is true in the EU, where a study of 2,830 companies that claimed to use artificial intelligence found that artificial intelligence was not material to 40% of the businesses.[30] No matter the jurisdiction, companies must be able to back up their claims if they want to avoid prosecution for misleading their customers.

Even the protection of intellectual property (IP) during digital health commercialization is distinct from traditional medical device or pharmaceutical industries. Health entrepreneurs are often familiar with these more established commercialization pathways, where the need to publish clinical trial data to gain regulatory approval makes early patent filings and aggressive IP enforcement policies an essential part of the business strategy. However, the nuances of the law around protection of computer-implemented innovations can mean that an IP strategy built around securing a blockbuster patent can be risky for some digital health businesses.[31] The true invention and

[25] ANDHealth. Digital health: creating a new growth industry for Australia. https://andhealth.com.au/wp-content/uploads/2019/04/Digital-Health_Creating-a-New-Growth-Industry-for-Australia.pdf. Published 2018. Accessed October 6, 2019.

[26] Shuren J, Patel B, Gottlieb S. FDA regulation of mobile medical apps. *JAMA*. 2018;320:337–338.

[27] US Federal Trade Commission. FTC cracks down on marketers of "melanoma detection" apps. https://www.ftc.gov/news-events/press-releases/2015/02/ftc-cracks-down-marketers-melanoma-detection-apps. Published February 23, 2015 Accessed November 19, 2019.

[28] US Federal Trade Commission. Marketers of blood-pressure app settle FTC charges regarding accuracy of app readings. https://www.ftc.gov/news-events/press-releases/2016/12/marketers-blood-pressure-app-settle-ftc-charges-regarding. Published December 12, 2016. Accessed December 19, 2019.

[29] US Federal Trade Commission. Lumosity to pay $2 million to settle FTC deceptive advertising charges for its "brain training" program. https://www.ftc.gov/news-events/press-releases/2016/01/lumosity-pay-2-million-settle-ftc-deceptive-advertising-charges. Published January 5, 2016. Accessed November 19, 2019.

[30] Kelnar D.. The state of AI divergence, 2019. *MMC Ventures*. https://www.mmcventures.com/wp-content/uploads/2019/02/The-State-of-AI-2019-Divergence.pdf. Published 2019. Accessed November 19, 2019.

[31] Wright R. Talking tech: from Digital Health to Medtech. *Medical Plastics News*. https://www.medicalplasticsnews.com/news/opinion/talking-tech/. Published August 10, 2017. Accessed November 19, 2019.

novelty may reside within software or an algorithm, which may or may not be eligible for patent protection. Other mechanisms, such as know-how protection through confidentiality clauses in employment contacts, coupled with a focus on establishing a trusted brand and protecting it using trademarks, may be more commercially useful than a patent. From a commercial perspective, strategies around evidence of clinical efficacy and strategic commercial partnerships may prove the best defense against competitive products and businesses.

Ultimately, digital health is emerging as a separate investment class, with dedicated investment teams and firms. Start-Up Health, a US-based company that invests, accelerates, and collects and shares market insights in digital health, has tracked US$13.7 billion of investments into digital health companies in 2019.[32] Other groups such as Rock Health and HealthXL have also built global digital health data sets. As such, it is recommended that any program that aims to support digital health commercialization now needs to understand the criteria for digital health investment, which is substantially distinct from consumer technology, medical device, and biotechnology assets.

Mental health is recognized as a subgroup within digital health with its own opportunities and constraints, with key barriers to people not getting help widely accepted as stigma, cost, and access. Reflecting this, digital health investment publications such as Start-Up Health, Rock Health, Health XL, and Galen Growth, among others, track investment in mental health as a distinct subset of digital health. Specific investment interests and accelerator programs have also sprung up to support, and profit from, the growing awareness of the importance of monitoring, diagnosing, and treating mental health conditions.

Start-Up Health's 2019 Insights report tracked 135 deals across their Mental Health and Happiness and Brain Health categories, with the vast majority of deals in the Seed and Series A stage,[33] reflecting the increasing number of early stage companies in this space. Looking toward Asia Pacific, Galen Growth also notes a similar trend in their 2019 report when looking at the 29 deals tracked in Mental Health and Neurology.[34] An early 2020 review of 1,000 digital health mental health focused start-ups found that although a quarter were in the less regulated Wellness category, Measurement and Testing accounted for a sixth, as did Telehealth, and Digital Therapeutics account for just under a tenth.[35] This shows that while starts ups are addressing wellness and access, companies are also tackling the more complex issues of measurement, diagnosis, and treatment. Additionally, many workplaces are heeding the World Health Organization's advice that investing in employee mental wellness yields a fourfold increase in productivity,[36] which is driving employers to increasingly implement digital mental health programs for their employees.

[32] Laster L, Hanin P, Powers B. StartUp health insights 2019 year-end report. *StartUp Health Insights*. 2020.

[33] Plaster L, Hanin P, Powers B. StartUp health insights 2019 year-end report. *StartUp Health Insights*. 2020. p. 16.

[34] De Salaberry, J. AsiaPac Healthtech Investment Landscape—Year End 2019. *Galen Growth*. 2020. p. 15.

[35] What If Ventures. Approaching 1,000 mental health startups in 2020 [Blog post]. https://whatif.vc/blog/approaching-1000-mental-health-startups-in%C2%A02020. Updated January 10 2020. Accessed February 22, 2020.

[36] World Health Organization. Mental health in the workplace: information sheet. https://www.who.int/mental_health/in_the_workplace/en/. Updated May 2019. Accessed February 22, 2020.

The mental health digital start-up ecosystem is still nascent, with a handful of accelerators globally specifically focused on digital mental health start-ups, but none has emerged as clear leaders yet, although established accelerators, such as Y-Combinator, are increasingly active in the mental health sector and are one of the most active seed stage investors in mental health start-ups.[37,38]

As mental health issues are global, they are a system wide issue for consideration from the individual level to the institutional and government level. Accelerators themselves must consider the mental health of their participants, as Michael Freeman revealed in an extensive study of 242 entrepreneurs,[39] entrepreneurs are 50% more likely to report having a mental health condition, with some specific conditions being distinctly prevalent. Entrepreneurs are

- Twice as likely to suffer from depression;
- Six times more likely to suffer from ADHD;
- Three times more likely to suffer from substance abuse;
- 10 times more likely to suffer from bipolar disorder;
- Twice as likely to have a psychiatric hospitalization; and
- Twice as likely to have suicidal thoughts.

Accelerators are increasingly implementing internal programs to support founder mental health, which must continue to be an additional key consideration when establishing a digital health accelerator.

Key Considerations in Developing Accelerators for Digital Health Commercialization

Any successful digital health accelerator whose aim is to advise companies on growth should consider a solid understanding of several key tenets. The following section will discuss some key considerations for establishing a digital health accelerator with the overall aim of providing quality advice to sustainably scale digital health companies so that they can reach selected impact milestones.

Metrics for Success

The importance of careful selection of metrics for success upfront in accelerator program development cannot be overemphasized. Careful metric selection will inform

[37] Plaster L, Hanin P, Powers B. StartUp health insights 2019 year-end report. *StartUp Health Insights.* 2020. p. 6.

[38] CB Insights. Psych 101: the most active investors in mental health tech. *CB Information Services.* https://www.cbinsights.com/research/active-investors-mental-health-tech-startups/. Published September 1, 2017. Accessed March 2, 2020.

[39] Freeman M, Johnson S, Staudenmaier P, Zisser, M. Are entrepreneurs "touched with fire"? http://www.michaelafreemanmd.com/Research_files/Are%20Entrepreneurs%20Touched%20with%20Fire-summary.pdf. Updated April 17, 2015. Accessed February 22, 2020.

many other important considerations, including mentor selection, company selection, and the accelerator's funding model. In an accelerator's early stages, clearly articulated metrics sends a message to potential applicants and the broader ecosystem about what the program will deliver. In the longer term, clear metrics and objectives for success and good data are crucial to demonstrate the continued efficacy of the program.

Whether one is designing an early-stage, research institute–based accelerator looking to support applied research or an industry backed later-stage accelerator, it is essential to be clear inwardly and externally on the metrics for success. The former may have success metrics around numbers of patients impacted, numbers of clinical studies commenced, or numbers of technologies supported. The latter may include metrics around numbers of partnership deals, revenue generation, or securing new capital.

As the management adage goes, "What gets measured, gets done." The following is a list of 10 key metrics used in digital health accelerators globally, and some key considerations:

- *Number of companies supported.* It is often best to pursue quality over quantity. A very large cohort is no recipe for success—more bespoke or concentrated cohorts tend to have stronger long-term success.
- *Capital raised.* Typically, securing funding for further development or scale is an immediate requirement of companies in accelerator programs. Theoretically, a well-supported company should be stronger and more attractive to investors following accelerator completion.
- *Patients impacted.* For some accelerators this is a "feel good" metric, but for others it is at the core, especially for those that are not-for-profit, funded through philanthropy or are especially patient-centric. This metric will be harder to measure for some companies (e.g., innovations in nurse rostering) than those who specialize in direct-to-consumer intervention.
- *Revenue generated.* As it is sometimes said, "the cheapest capital you can get is customer revenue," and generating revenue is indeed an indication that a customer is willing to pay for a product or service. But sales cycles in healthcare are long, which means revenue can take a long time to generate. Too much focus on securing early revenue can ultimately damage efforts to build a sustainable digital health business, especially if pursued at the expense of creating genuine clinical evidence.
- *Jobs created.* Many government and ecosystem growth-driving accelerators focus on creating jobs as a direct outcome and as a reflection of the impact of the accelerator. Typically, the ability to hire more team members is an indication of business growth.
- *Pilots.* Due to the nature of sales cycles, established business practice, and the generally risk adverse nature of healthcare systems, pilots are a common first step for digital health customers. But it can be important to differentiate between paid and unpaid pilots. Too many pilots at once, paid or unpaid, can be difficult for an early-stage company to sustain and can put extreme pressure on their resources, leading to "death by pilot."[40]

[40] Tecco H. A caution for would-be digital health entrepreneurs. *KQED Science.* https://www.kqed.org/futureofyou/3027/a-caution-for-would-be-digital-health-entrepreneurs. Published March 19, 2019. Accessed November 19, 2019.

- *Corporate partners secured.* Success in digital health is likely to require partnering with larger players in the healthcare ecosystem, including hospitals, health insurers, pharmaceutical companies, and more tangential providers such as employee wellness or technology companies. For some accelerators, successfully creating sustainable corporate partnerships is a key purpose for their existence.
- *Gender and cultural diversity.* Supporting underrepresented groups is key to creating true change across all industries and is an import metric to measure to identify risk areas, prioritize initiatives, set targets and other program goals, assign accountability, and measure the impact of initiatives.
- *Customer acquisition.* Securing customers is an undeniably crucial aspect of company maturity. It is important to note that in digital health, the number of customers may be a misnomer—a direct to consumer company will rapidly advance their customer numbers, whereas a company selling to large healthcare providers or government systems may still be successful with single-digit numbers of customers.
- *Clinical trials and studies commenced.* Clinical evidence is essential for regulation and to avoid making false claims and can be an important differentiator between like products. While the level of clinical evidence required will vary with the claims of the product and from market to market, it is essential to encourage and measure the clinical evidence proportional to the product claims.

Importantly, the number of technologies terminated as a metric is an often overlooked but very critical metric. Alongside providing support to companies, it must be acknowledged that not every idea is a commercially successful or clinically relevant one, and celebrating the lessons learned and early termination of companies are essential to a healthy support ecosystem.

It is essential to note the effect of the support provided by an accelerator may not be felt immediately and may take months or even years. As such, setting up methods for continued data gathering on the supported companies is key.

As well as selecting the metrics and gathering ongoing data against them, it is also recommended to measure the genuine impact of a technology and ensure that the accelerator program is having a measurable uplift on the defined success of the companies. A relatively easy and effective way to do this is to collect information on unsuccessful applicants and comparable companies in your ecosystem and measure their milestones and outcomes against the companies that have been supported, thereby demonstrating the impact of the program. To do this it is essential to collect a baseline measurement at the start of the program that you can measure against. For a successful accelerator, companies should move through maturity stages faster than the average unaccelerated company and also should fail faster than the average.

Health technology accelerators have proliferated, but data and research measuring their performance are disappointingly limited. This needs to be addressed—to properly gauge their impact, accelerator programs need to improve the ways in which they collect data. These data can help to manage companies' expectations of the kinds of support they need, as well as create credibility for the accelerator—an increasingly important currency.

Which Business Areas to Support and Selecting Effective Mentors

It is essential that accelerators provide digital health company participants with clear end goals and methods to plan their path to market or exit. For instance, if they are aiming to sell into the UK National Health Service, they should understand the criteria of the NHS Apps Library[41] and, as healthcare adoption methodologies become more uniform, ensure that they will comply with relevant evaluation criteria.[42]

Broadly, to be successful, a digital health solution must be clinically and commercially verified and validated, and an accelerator should support this. The usual definitions are

- *Validation*: Are we building the right system? In digital health, this applies to technology, commercial viability and clinical efficacy. Will the system meet customers' needs? Will it also be attractive and able to raise the required investment? Does it address a clinical need?
- *Verification*: Are we building the system right? This also applies technically, commercially and clinically. Is it error free, complying with regulations, protecting the health data correctly, able to integrate into the required systems, and clinically proven to be effective?

Expertise to address these considerations must be available and will all be reinforced with a mentoring culture of frank and fair feedback, both positive and negative, from mentors.

Unsurprisingly, the quality of the mentorship and information provided by an accelerator program has been shown to be proportional to the value inflection of the companies through the accelerator program.[43] Mentors must have directly relevant experience in the aspect of digital health commercialization in which they are mentoring and must be able to demonstrate this experience. Enthusiasm and generosity of time is no substitute for genuine expertise and mentors should be carefully vetted.

One method of vetting is to consider the proven experiences and expertise of potential mentors with regards to the metrics of success that have been determined for the accelerator. For digital health, it is important to consider a multidisciplinary mentor pool, drawing from the many stakeholders in digital health and ensuring that mentors stick to their area of expertise.

[41] United Kingdom National Health Service. NHS Apps Library. https://apps.beta.nhs.uk/. Established April 2017.

[42] Boudreaux ED, Waring ME, Hayes RB, et al. Evaluating and selecting mobile health apps: strategies for healthcare providers and healthcare organizations. *Transl Behav Med.* 2014;12;4(4):363–371.

[43] Dushnitsky G, Sarkar S. Variance decomposing of accelerator and cohort effects among london startups. *Acad Manage Proceed.* 2018;2018(1). https://doi.org/10.5465/AMBPP.2018.80

Stakeholders of digital health are many and varied and can include the patient, medical staff, regulators, healthcare providers, pharmaceutical companies, insurers, government systems, and carers.[44] Multidisciplinary perspectives are indispensable in determining whether or not a certain digital health product will succeed.

The areas supported in the accelerator should reflect the selected metrics of the accelerator. Areas to consider supporting through the accelerator include

- Clinical validation.
- Intellectual property.
- Commercial validation, including true voice of customer.
- Health economics.
- Business models.
- Data privacy and security.
- Access to investment.
- Corporate structure and strategy.
- Product development and user-informed design.
- Revenue and reimbursement.
- Regulation.

One reason digital health commercialization programs often fail is that they consider the business model too late, instead of upfront, as part of an initial commercial feasibility. It is critical for digital health start-ups to do a thorough analysis and assessment of the proposed business model, including an extensive dive into who the customers are, who captures the value on the customer side, and who will ultimately pay for the services.[45] A strong digital health accelerator program will have the expertise onboard to address this up-front. Because patients and consumers are only part of the stakeholder landscape in digital health, even in the consumer-centric healthcare system of the United States, nearly two-thirds of digital health companies end up selling products to "insurance companies, employers, hospitals or other healthcare providers," as opposed to consumers.[46]

How Is the Accelerator Funded?

Accelerator programs are funded in a variety of ways, often linked to their proposed outcomes. An accelerator inside a health research institute, for example, may be funded by the institute's innovation budget with an aim to train research staff in commercial skills. An accelerator inside a large health provider may be funded by the marketing or training budget to increase the organization's reputation as innovative and to train staff in upcoming technologies. Often governments fund accelerators to attract

[44] Van Velthoven MH, Cordon C. Sustainable adoption of digital health innovations: perspectives from a stakeholder workshop. *J Med Internet Res*. 2019;21(3):e11922. doi:10.2196/11922

[45] Rivas H, Wac K. *Digital Health: Scaling Healthcare to the World*. Switzerland: Springer International; 2018.

[46] Evans B, Shiao S. Streamlining enterprise sales in digital health. *Rock Health*. https://rockhealth.com/reports/streamlining-enterprise-sales-in-digital-health/. Published 2019. Accessed December 19, 2019.

businesses to their area and to support local businesses to create jobs. Privately funded commercial accelerators support companies with a view to eventually profiting off their success via equity positions in cohort companies.

It is common for an accelerator to take equity in cohort companies, typically ranging from 5% to 30% in exchange for cash and services provided to the start-up. Generalist acceleratornY Combinator, for example, has a standard deal to take around 7% equity for approximately US$100,000 to $120,000 of funding,[47] and the accelerator 500 Startups invests US$150,000 in exchange for 6%.[48] Taking equity can pay off for the accelerator in the long run but there may be drawbacks. Taking equity can deter founders, especially if the value of the program is not well established, and may therefore limit the pipeline of quality applicants.

In addition, due to long company maturity cycles in health when compared to the tech sector, it is likely to take up to a decade and multiple potentially dilutive capital rounds before a company can exit and the accelerator can realize its equity, if the companies are indeed successful. Taking equity can also make cohort companies less attractive to investors in the next rounds of investment, which will hamper the success of the companies the accelerator is designed to help.

There is also the matter of conflict of interest to consider. Some argue that when an accelerator takes equity in the companies they support, they have more incentive to help those companies succeed. But an equity position also means that there are disincentives for the companies to fail, which could lead to a lack of frank and firm feedback and encourage accelerators to keep failing companies alive to ensure that the accelerator's equity holdings are intact. In addition, equity alone is not a revenue stream to cover accelerator operations, so an accelerator program will require some form of funding or income to allow it to cover its own operating costs.

Selecting Companies for the Accelerator

One can broadly determine the success of an accelerator program in creating genuine and measurable value by how well they screen applicants for selection and the value add of the program content itself. The design of the screening process should reflect the desired outcomes and also reflect the nature of the program content (e.g., multi-disciplinary approach, clear metrics, removal of and acknowledgement of bias). The process should be performed by and informed by experts selected from the key stakeholders from the sector. Logically, a larger pool of quality applicants and greater accuracy of the selection capabilities should result in increased venture success.

Broad elements to consider in the screening process for digital health companies include

- *Product, problem and solution.* Understanding of the problem to be addressed and the value of the proposed solution. Demonstrated understanding of

---

[47] Nathoo K. The Y combinator deal. *Y Combinator.* https://www.ycombinator.com/deal/. Published September 2019. Accessed November 18, 2019.

[48] 500.co. Seed program. https://500.co/seed-program/. Accessed November 19, 2019.

end-users and how they will interact with the product, and their needs overall. Identification and differentiation of users and customers and the extent of the value proposition to each.

- *Business model.* Understanding customer requirements and the product's unique value proposition to the customer and revenue model. Clear articulation of what they are selling, or plan to sell, and who will pay and how. Identification of a market, investment or business case, including value proposition, size of market and pathway to market, barriers to market entry, competitive position, and product advantage.

- *Maturity.* As well as the developmental maturity of the product, consideration of the maturity of the commercial aspects, including use of the product in a clinical or market setting, level of product evidence including clinical trials and technical certification where applicable, any consideration of regulatory certification strategy, and IP strategy and position.

- *Team.* An assessment of the team's strength, including business skills, technical skills, ability to achieve market uptake, knowledge of the problem space, and an assessment of their coachability.

- *Is this program a good fit?* This will be a reflection back on the desired outcomes of the program and the elements that will be supported in it. It may be that the product is excellent against many of the criteria, but it is too early or too late to truly benefit from the program.

Case Study: ANDHealth, a Novel Model for Digital Health Commercialization Support

ANDHealth, Australia's national digital health initiative, is an Australian industry-led, nonprofit collaborative model, was founded by Bronwyn Le Grice, with a clear objective from the outset. As Le Grice explained in a 2019 interview with *Bioworld Medtech*, "When we set out to create ANDHealth, we had the hypothesis that there were quite a lot of Australian digital health companies, some of which were quite evolved but were unable to find high-quality advice, support and access to industry people who had done this before in digital health."[49] Notably, the focus was primarily on high potential scale-up companies with proof of principle, not early ideation stage start-ups:

ANDHealth was founded to address an identified gap in investible, scalable, evidence based digital health companies in Australia whilst removing common deterrents to accelerator participation around equity participation, standardised content and conflicts of interest. Having taken this model to conferences in the UK and the US we are pleased but surprised to hear that it is unique, as to us it seemed a logical solution. (Personal Communication, November 18, 2019)

[49] Sami, T. ANDHealth makes strides developing a robust digital health ecosystem in Australia. *BioWorld MedTech.* 2018;22(203):7–9.

The flagship ANDHealth program, ANDHealth+, supports five evidence-based digital health companies in each yearly cohort toward institutional investment and international market entry. Each company is assessed by more than a dozen C-suite judges from a diverse background of industries, ensuring that the perspectives of multiple stakeholders in digital health are represented including: pharmaceutical, medical product development, health user experience and software, global digital health, medical research, university, heath delivery, legal, and people and culture.

The selected companies work with a subset of the judging panel for six to nine months, meeting regularly, to create a bespoke project plan. The project plan's objectives are informed by a multidisciplinary due diligence processes, which identifies specific elements of the cohort company's business strategy that would deter enterprise customers or professional investors. AUD$60,000 is made available fund third parties to deliver on the mutually agreed project outcomes. The program also leverages industry in-kind so that on average companies receive AUD$350,000 of direct value. The resulting impact is highly tailored to each company and involves no formal curriculum.

Robert McLeay, founder of DoseMe, a company supported in the FY2018 ANDHealth+ cohort and acquired by Tabula Rasa Healthcare (NASDAQ), upon exiting explains in a 2019 interview with *Healthcare IT News Australia*,

> If you're at that inflection point in your business where your product is clinically validated and has reached commercial viability, the ANDHealth+ program will help you move away from just thinking about the technology to getting the business aspect of it right. The program not only helped us in terms of funding, but we also received in-kind support across a range of business areas from the additional members of the program. A lot of people underestimate the value of this but for us, it proved to be very valuable. It moved us from not having the ability to get into the US market to rapidly expanding, and make sure that as we do so, we globally protected our IP. These were all critical milestones for our company to reach.[50]

The accelerator takes no equity, does not make any claim on the IP, and uses a nonprofit membership model to leverage industry participation beyond financial contribution into hands-on participation. This is enabled by the support of government funding alongside industry.

Le Grice highlights that not taking equity is the key to attracting quality companies and the ability to deliver genuine commercialization outcomes.

> There is no conflict of interest for us to tell companies that, after working deep in their business with them for a few months, they are not suitable for investment in a

---

[50] Osman H. Here's how one digital health company commercialised its business. *Healthcare IT.* https://www.healthcareit.com.au/article/heres-how-one-digital-health-company-commercialised-its-business. Published January 25, 2019. Accessed November 17, 2019.

global market. We have delivered this insight and the companies have been appreciative of the advice and the ultimate time and money savings of licensing their technology instead of commercialising themselves. If we had taken equity, I would need to write this asset down and inform my board; an equity-taking accelerator may be incentivised to not pass on impartial advice. Not everyone can succeed and we need fail fast and consider other models such as licencing or, where appropriate, philanthropy. (Personal Communication, November 18, 2019)

ANDHealth directly measures the impact of the involvement in ANDHealth+, with cohort companies reporting quarterly against metrics of money raised, revenue, jobs, pilots, clinical trials and studies, international market launches, commercial customs, patients served, operational sites, partnerships, and product releases for a period of three years from involvement.

According to Le Grice, the key to the success of ANDHealth+ is the quality and multidisciplinary nature of the personnel supporting the companies to ensure high-quality, experienced and tailored support: "In my view the real power of ANDHealth lies in its by industry, for industry' origins, the diversity and leadership of its corporate members and the central philosophy that people with genuine, demonstrable expertise who are active in the sector are best placed to support emerging companies" (Personal Communication, November 18, 2019). ANDHealth partners, advisors, and key operational staff all meet strict criteria, demonstrating hands-on experience in either

- Product development of a market-ready product, which is evidence-based and has a sustainable business model;
- Negotiation of a significant (preferably international) commercial agreement between two or more parties, where at least one party is from industry; and/or
- Raising a significant amount of capital for one or more digital health companies.

Le Grice says:

ANDHealth was established to solve a key problem in bridging key gaps for companies in a new and fast emerging sector which required cross-sectoral understanding and networks, and a sophisticated understanding of global market trends and opportunities. It's also an industry that attracts lots of "hype" but in which it can be hard to identify industry experts with genuine expertise. (Personal Communication, November 18, 2019)

Prior to ANDHealth Le Grice held the role of investment director with leading Australian healthcare venture capital firm, BioScience Managers. Here she was responsible for managing significant transactions in the health technology and digital health sectors, resulting in more than AUD$65 million of private and public equity raisings. As a result, Le Grice understands first-hand the criteria for investment in digital health and how it is distinct from consumer technology, medical device and biotechnology assets.

Her advice to creating a successful digital health support program centers on surrounding the innovator with quality people:

> My recommendation to any innovator seeking to commercialize is to seek out people with proven, demonstrable and independently verifiable experience in the innovator's chosen area, and to do as much due diligence on their advisors and investors as they would a core staff member (noting that innovators may have to look globally for the right people). Good investors and advisors are priceless; those that are not a good fit can cost time, money and resources. (Personal Communication, November 18, 2019)

SECTION VI
SPECIAL CONSIDERATIONS FOR OPERATIONALIZING CONVERGENCE MENTAL HEALTH

30

Screening for Convergent Practitioners in Health Research and Innovation

The Role of a High Potential Personality

Ian MacRae and Adrian Furnham

Introduction

One of the most significant investments for any company, organization, or team is on people. The salaries, socialization, and development of people is major cost. Hiring, developing, and retaining the right people is an ongoing challenge and opportunity for all organizations. Although considerable progress has been made in the science of how to identify, develop, and retain high potential employees,[1] many organizations still use unscientific, unproven, and unreliable methods to select employees. These methods are often intuitive, based on personal opinions or hunches, and can often be both unscientific and amateurish.

Getting the right people into the right roles must be a key consideration for selecting and developing convergence teams. It is important to identify individuals who are most likely to be successful and effective in that role. Moving toward a convergence model in health research and innovation should draw on the most effective tools and methods from occupational psychology to identify, manage, and develop convergence practitioners.

One of the challenges of integrating knowledge and different ways of thinking between different practitioners, teams, departments, organizations, and sectors is that individuals who are likely to be effective in their own fields as sole practitioners, researchers, innovators, or technicians are not guaranteed to be effective in a convergence research environment with different requirements, responsibilities, and job demands.

Past research on transdisciplinary practice provides some general outlines for transdisciplinary practice and even has developed inventories for assessing suitability for transdisciplinary roles.[2] Other research has set about cataloguing the various skills, attributes, values, personality traits, and virtues associated with success in transdisciplinary practice.[3] While this initial research is valuable in exploring the potential relationships between individual difference factors and transdisciplinary practice, it would be extremely valuable for future research to test hypotheses related to specific traits and tangible, measurable outcomes in transdisciplinary practice.

This chapter builds on previous conceptualizations of transdisciplinary practice and embeds convergence roles with a clear model of workplace potential. The chapter will first outline potential and explain how potential can be understood and defined in the context of workplace success.

Then, using the model of potential, this chapter will define and characterize a profile for the effective convergence practitioner with a particular emphasis on personality traits as predictors of success in convergence practice.

Building on previous research to define potential predictors of success in a convergence environment will help to build at this testable model of potential in a convergence role. The model will then provide useful insight and guidelines into how to identify and select those most likely to be successful as convergent practitioners. Later in this chapter, we define personality traits linked to success in the workplace and hypothesize their links to success in convergence practice.

With a clear definition of what is required in a convergence role, it can then be possible to identify individuals who are most likely to be successful in a convergence role. The most important question to ask when discussing potential is, "The potential to do what?" Without asking this question, the concept of potential is too vague and nonspecific to have any real meaning. If we want to develop a model of convergence practice that represents a certain type of job role, type of work, or set of responsibilities, then it is possible to identify individuals who are the most likely to be successful in that role and to develop skills and abilities that are important for convergence roles. The potential to be successful and the criteria for success are different for different roles, so when the definition of a convergence practitioner is clearly defined, it is then possible to identify the traits of a high potential convergence practitioner.

What Potential Is

Potential is the upper (and lower and middle) possible trajectory of what a person can do.[1] While someone's past behavior could be defined as success, potential is the capacity for what someone could achieve in the future. This is an important distinction because while past performance can be a useful indicator of potential, it is not always a reliable predictor.

When past behavior is to be repeated in similar social structures, physical environments, and with similar job resources and demands, then it is a fairly good indicator of future performance. However, when a role is significantly different, past performance may not always be a good indicator of potential. If someone has been extremely effective, with a record of high performance in a role that focuses on individual performance, that is not necessarily a good indicator that they have a high potential to succeed as a convergence practitioner.

Potential is not a guarantee of success but can be understood as a probability of success in a clearly specified domain. When we can clarify the desired outcomes along with the predictors of those outcomes, it is then feasible to estimate someone's potential based on a set of factors.

Potential is variable, contextual, and an interaction between factors that are internal to the individual and external factors such as the environment, management, job demands, and resources. A list of behaviors that a affect the success of convergence practitioners is discussed later in this chapter.

The important point to remember is that potential is a range of possible trajectories. If we can clearly define the predictors of potential in a certain domain, it will help to estimate an individual's likelihood of success. An uppermost limit of potential always exists, when an optimal combination of the right traits mix with the right environment and opportunities. A potential "floor" exists—where even very intelligent, talented people may end up if deprived of education or opportunities to develop and hone skills.

Key Points About Potential

The lessons of talent and potential[1] can be used to understand the potential of convergence practitioners:

Potential reflects cultural and organizational values.[4] Individuals who are high potential convergence practitioners are based on value judgements about what types of performance and behavior is useful and desirable. In the case of convergence practice, that includes qualities like self-awareness and awareness of others, the ability to understand language across disciplines, and setting shared outcomes to name a few. These are described in greater detail later in this chapter.

The value judgements also reflect that which is undesirable, in the case of convergence practice this would include behaviors like sequestering knowledge, building up silos, hindering communication, and violating trust between people.

High potential leads to specific outcomes. A fundamental aspect of defining potential means that it will lead to specific, desirable outcomes. Clearly defining potential means clearly operationalized and well-defined outcomes.

Potential is specific to certain jobs and domains. Defining potential means defining the job and the domain. While there can be overlap between high potential in different domains, potential to be successful in one area does not translate directly into potential to be successful in another. Thus someone who has a high potential to be effective as an individual performer should not be assumed to be high potential in convergence practice.

Multiple factors influence potential including biology, psychology, social, and cultural groups. There is no single measure or one predictor of potential. Individual differences such as personality and intelligence will affect potential, as will social and cultural factors. Even practitioners with individual difference traits that predispose them to be high potential in convergence practice may not be effective without the appropriate resources (organizational and managerial supports, tools and technology, etc.) to facilitate their success.

Potential is relative. High potential is relative because as a range of possible trajectories it exists only relative to moderate and low potential. Potential is high when it indicates the greatest probability of success or the uppermost levels of achievement. Levels of performance and potential are normally distributed so, by definition, the highest and lowest echelons of potential are rare.

Defining Types of Potential

The best framework for understanding potential has been provided by Silzer and Church.[5] They developed a clear and useful framework of definition potential that can be applied to any job or type of work and thus is extremely useful for understanding potential in the context of convergent practice. Silver and Church's framework is broad enough that is can be used and translated for understanding potential in any type of work while being flexible enough to incorporate different types of performance and the broad range of knowledge, experience, and roles involved in convergent practice. The three dimensions are defined well enough to be testable, while being broad and adaptable enough to be practical for convergence practice. See Figure 30.1 for further details.

Foundational Dimensions

Certain individual differences are stable across the individual lifespan and consistent predictors of performance and potential across the various domains of work, job roles, and practice areas.

Foundational dimensions of potential are those stable characteristics that predict success across the range of careers and types of work. Foundational dimensions are consistent across time so are excellent at predicting short- and long-term potential. Foundational dimensions are attributes that contribute to success in any career, job,

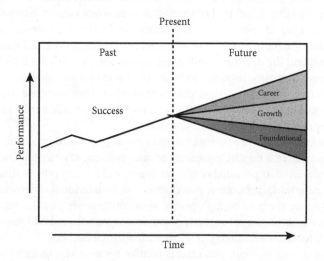

Figure 30.1 A model of past performance and potential future trajectories.
Adapted from MacRae and Furnham, 2018.

or time. Intelligence is the prime example of a foundational dimensions of potential because it is highly stable across the lifespan and is consistently found to be a predictor of work performance.[6] The personality traits conscientiousness and adjustment[1,7] are excellent examples foundational dimensions because they predict potential across nearly all types of work and job function.

Situational and environmental factors will only have limited effects on foundational potential. Foundational dimensions are quite stable across the adult lifespan and can only be changed with serious intervention.[8]

Foundational dimensions are exceptionally useful for screening those who have high potential to be successful in convergent practice because the individual differences traits of intelligence and personality are highly stable across the adult lifespan and therefore can be used to predict long-term potential.

Growth Dimensions

Growth dimensions are the components of potential that are related to development and improvement over time. These can be influenced by stable traits like the personality trait curiosity or by self-awareness and emotional intelligence. These tend to be attributes that are relatively consistent over the adult lifespan and that help people learn an adapt to new environments, situations, and types of work.

Growth dimensions are an important component of potential in convergence practice because the nature of the convergence environment requires continually learning and adaptation. The convergence practice environment is one of complexity, various stakeholders, potentially conflicting objectives, and learning from others. Growth potential can at least partially be identified early on by assessing personality and emotional intelligence. Yet an individual's growth potential necessarily interacts with the environment and team dynamics. Therefore, an individual with significant growth potential may have their potential inhibited by poor leadership, a lack of communication, or lack of the appropriate resources or support to learn from their colleagues.

Growth dimensions of potential can either improve or inhibit an individual or a team's overall potential. For example, those who learn quickly from training have higher growth potential.

Whereas those who are suspicious of others, distrustful of new information or approaches, and have poor awareness of themselves and others are less likely to learn and adapt within a convergence environment. Growth potential can be a combination of internal characteristics and can also be situational factors.

Situational factors can also have a significant effect here, when a team of convergence practitioners have a culture of open communication, trust, and collaboration; develop strong and constructive interpersonal relationships with their colleagues; and have processes for managing conflict, all members of the convergence team are likely to have higher growth potential.

Growth potential is important for identifying potential and predicting likelihood for future success because a significant gap between current performance and future potential is bolstered or held back by growth potential.

Career Dimensions

Career dimensions of potential are characteristics that lead to success in a specific occupations, jobs, or types of work. A career dimension of potential is any unique or specific skills that is necessary for success in a certain endeavor. A convergence team may bring together people from a broad range of work backgrounds such as entrepreneurs, a medical technicians, coders, psychologists, and even marketing experts in pursuit of a particular objective. Each individual will have unique skills, training, and experience that is essential for success in their work, but the skills or knowledge may not be prerequisites for success in any other member of the team.

Any type of work has specific career dimensions of potential that are absolutely essential for that work, but may also be unique to that type of work. For example, mechanical knowledge is specific to being a mechanic. Accountancy training is specific to being an accountant. Knowledge of the human anatomy is a skill that is specifically useful for being a surgeon but may not be necessary for other jobs.

Career dimensions of potential are also the most plastic. Career dimensions can be learned, trained, developed, and improved over time and therefore are not stable. It can be more challenging to use career dimensions to predict an individual's potential, especially in the long-term, because the absence of a particular skills, knowledge, or experience does not preclude that person from developing those skills, knowledge, or experience in the future. Career dimensions can be learned and taught, and many employers find it most useful to select people based on foundational and growth dimensions of potential and then train people in the career dimensions.

Career dimensions of potential vary in complexity and difficulty. In the case of convergent practice, different members of a team will bring extremely difficult and complex fields together. This means that the skills and knowledge that can take years or even a lifetime accumulate. Therefore, one of the valuable components of a convergence team is bringing together a broad range of different career dimensions of potential that may not be realistic or feasible to develop in one person alone.

Potential to Do What?

The model of potential initially described by Silzer and Church[5] is an excellent methods for analyzing potential and developing models of potential in different types of work. It is universally applicable to any job or type of work or task. It is also flexible enough to be useful for defining and predicting potential in any clearly defined job or task.

However, the role and responsibilities of a convergence practitioner may be substantially different from a sole practitioner. It should not be assumed that past performance as an individual practitioner will necessarily translate into potential as a convergence practitioner. The attributes that make someone successful as a specialist or technician for example are not always the same set of attributes that lead to success working in the complex and dynamic environment of a convergence team.

A Model of Convergence Potential

Using Silver and Church's[5] model of potential, we can develop a clear framework for identifying and developing potential in convergence practice. While some of the attributes of each dimension of potential have been mentioned in the previous section, this section provides a greater level of detail about how intelligence, each of the personality traits and convergence team characteristics contribute to potential.

	Foundational Potential	Growth Potential	Career Potential
Personality Traits	Conscientiousness	Curiosity	Ambiguity acceptance
	Adjustment	Risk approach	Competitiveness (low)
	Intelligence	Self-awareness	Specific skills, abilities, qualifications

Intelligence

Although there is still some discussion and debate about the exact definition of intelligence, there is consensus about its' general components. The research surrounding intelligence also consistently and clearly demonstrates that higher intelligence is linked to success and potential in the workplace. The two key themes underlying all expert definitions of intelligence are[1]:

- *The ability to learn from experience.* Learning from experience is essential for success, as well as for basic survival.
- *The ability to adapt to the environment.* Adaptation to the physical and social environment is a fundamental component of intelligence.

In the workplace, people who learn quickly from training can use it to improve their performance at work. Those who can't seem to learn how to improve their performance at work based on past experience struggle to perform well at any task. Intelligence is both a valid and useful explanation of human survival, learning, and adaptation. It is equally useful in understanding performance and potential in the workplace.

Scientific research has shown that, quite consistently, cognitive ability accurately predicts job performance across all jobs and is an even stronger predictor in complex jobs or tasks. Intelligence is a better predictor of success in a CEO than in a line manager. However, intelligence is desirable for both and is related to improved performance in both. Much of the research demonstrates that intelligence is the single best predictor of work performance.

A meta-analysis of research from the United Kingdom investigating intelligence and performance.[6] They combined the results of 283 separate studies and results from over 80,000 people. The results show tests of intelligence are very strong predictors of success both in training and in work. The relative importance of intelligence varied between professions, but the more complex and challenging the position is, the more important intelligence is as a predictor of success. Intelligence is a better predictor of success for more highly skilled professions, but the research also clearly shows that intelligence is a strong component of success for most professions and success in professional development and training.

Intelligent people learn faster. They quickly notice patterns and analyze issues well. They make fewer errors and have a higher rate of recall. It is hardly surprising then that intelligence is seen as a fundamental component of potential. But intelligence alone is not enough to explain the full picture of potential.

Intelligence is *necessary but not sufficient* when explaining what makes a high potential convergence practitioner. And it also appears that the level of intelligence that predicts success peak at a certain level: it is more important to be "intelligent enough" than to have the highest intelligence. Studies that track thousands of children across generations show exceptional intelligence is not necessary to succeed; above-average intelligence is usually enough.[9]

Personality

Personality traits help to select high potential in all types of work. But understanding personality traits is particularly important for convergence teams because different levels of traits can be desirable than in other types of work. Research[1,10,11] has found that personality, as measured by the High Potential Trait Indicator, strongly predicts both objective and subjective measures of career success.

Personality traits can be used to predict potential because linking the concepts of high potential and personality are challenging but, based on what we know about personality, can be done.

1. *Personality is relatively stable from early adulthood onward.* Personality develops as part of the maturation process. It cannot be learned or taught and thus is not primarily a career dimension of potential. It is an important constant, so it is a useful early indicator of potential.

2. *Personality is rooted in neurological structures.* Brain structure and biochemistry are linked to personality. Although it is not as simple as specific personality traits existing in specific areas of the brain, personality is rooted in biology and brain structure.

3. *Personality traits interact to influence thinking, feeling, and behaving.* Although behavior, thoughts, and emotions can be separated, they are all directly influenced by personality. When considering two personality combinations, a high conscientiousness/high adjustment profile and a high conscientiousness/low adjustment profile can manifest very differently in the workplace. Although the two are similar in conscientiousness and different in adjustment, there are significant differences between personality traits and how they interact at different levels. Interactions create unique patterns of thoughts and behaviors.

4. *Some personality traits are better suited to certain careers.* Certain personality traits and profiles interact with certain roles are types of work to improve performance. However, no personality traits is exclusively required for a job, task, or career in the same way as knowledge or experience.
5. *Personality and job fit are based on optimality, not maximality.* Higher scores on personality traits do not necessarily predict performance. Personality traits have optimal levels of effectiveness for certain types of work. In other words, there is a curvilinear relationship between personality traits and work performance.[12]

There are six High Potential Trait Indicator traits, each of which is helpful for predicting potential, but again it is important to ask the question, Potential to do what? And while previous research has shown clear links between personality and a range of workplace performance metrics, there has been less research conducted examining the personality traits of workplace performance in a transdisciplinary setting.

Some recent research has demonstrate links between attributes like values, attitudes, and beliefs in relation to achievement in transdisciplinary work.[4,6]

We explain each of the traits in detail and map the personality traits onto Silzer and Church's model of potential. We also discuss the thoughts, emotions, and behavior that are components of each trait. This will help to inform future research investigating personality traits in the context of transdisciplinary work. While we will hypothesize that the traits will have curvilinear relationships with work outcomes in transdisciplinary work, future research must be done to test these hypotheses in transdisciplinary workplaces.

Conscientiousness

Conscientiousness is highly stable and predictable over the course of the adult lifespan, and conscientiousness tends to increase slightly over the course of the a person's life.[14] Unless there are extreme psychological interventions or severe physical trauma to the brain, conscientiousness is very unlikely to change. A consistent trait such as conscientiousness is an excellent predictor of performance and potential in almost any type of work.

People who are conscientious tend to be better at making commitments to a team or group, which will be linked to achievement in a convergence team. Those with high conscientiousness like to have goals and objectives to work toward both in the short- and long-term. This helps them work toward individual goals as well as team or group objectives. They usually can motivate themselves to start, continue, and complete the goals they set. Conscientiousness employees tend to be more organized, more punctual, and better at meeting deadlines than their colleagues with lower conscientiousness.

Adjustment

Adjustment is a person's emotional regulation and resilience to stressors.[14,15] People with lower levels of adjustment feel negative emotional responses more keenly and frequently than those with higher levels of adjustment. People who have very low levels of adjustment find relatively minor challenges more difficult than those with higher levels of adjustment.

Adjustment is a foundational element of potential. Those with higher levels of adjustment tend to perform better in any type of work. The more challenging, demanding, and stressful a job role is the more adjustment predicts success and potential in the workplace. Those with lower levels of adjustment may struggle to adapt to even modest stressors in the workplace.

Stress is a natural and adaptive response to threatening situations. Stress, as a response to threats can lead to adaptive physiological responses. However, the stress response can become overly sensitive and lead to maladaptive behaviors when people do not effective coping strategies to deal with stress.[1] Extremely low levels of adjustment or maladaptive copies strategies in response to stressors can turn a normal psychological responses and biological system into a major barrier to performance at work.

Convergence practice may involve complex, challenging, and often stressful interactions and environments, so higher levels of adjustment can be an asset for convergence practitioners. More demanding positions often present practitioners with more potential sources of stress from job demands.

Curiosity

Curiosity is a growth dimension of potential that describes whether or not people are open to new ideas, solutions to problems, and approaches to work. People who have high curiosity are more receptive to new ideas, more likely to adopt new tools and technologies, and are more interested in the experience and approaches of their colleagues. Curiosity is related to seeking out new experiences and ideas and a willingness to test out new approaches. Higher curiosity tends to be linked to improved performance, especially within teams and curiosity has been modestly associated with creativity and innovation.

Curiosity at work is focused on openness to new ideas, methods, or approaches of *doing the work*. It also represents interpersonal curiosity. That is, learning from others and being open to learning from the experience of others. This means those with higher curiosity tend to be more adaptable and flexible in the workplace to perform multiple tasks, explore new ideas, and continually learn.

Previous research would suggest that curiosity is essential for success in a transdisciplinary environment.[4,6]

The psychological research confirms that curiosity is linked with improved performance as well as improved learning outcomes.[16,17] Curiosity is moderately associated with training proficiency but was less related to performance than conscientiousness or adjustment.

Those with high curiosity are more likely to look for new information and be interested in training of development opportunities. Curiosity alone, though, is not sufficient to be successful in training. It is also useful to have colleagues in convergent teams who share higher levels of curiosity, so others within the team are open to sharing their own experiences and opinions and who value learning from new experiences, different people, and novel approaches.

Risk Approach

Risk approach indicates a capacity to consider and choose a range of potential options, even when challenged by negative emotions like fear, worry, or sadness. Risk approach can refer to challenges related to challenges in the job or interpersonal conflict in the context of the workplace. Those with high risk approach[18] use positive emotions to mitigate fear, confront risk, and react adaptively and proactively.

Risk approach comes from the research into positive psychology. Fredrickson's[19] *broaden and build theory* of positive psychology proposes that negative emotions restrict an individual's potential range of responses to stimuli. Negative emotions create overwhelming impulses to act in an instinctual way. For example, fear fuels a strong drive to avoid what is evoking the fear, which then restricts the perceived range of responses. These negative, instinctual responses are linked to the fight-or-flight response. Therefore, courage can be expressed in many situations including calculated risk-taking, interpersonal confrontation, or reasoned and proactive problem-solving.

Risk approach is particularly pertinent for teams of convergent practitioners who have competing interests, conflicting opinions, and a degree of interpersonal conflict is extraordinarily likely. Therefore, to work together effectively the convergence practitioners must approach the conflict constructively, manage the risk, and allow disagreements to take place without letting conflict run out of control. Therefore, for convergent practice, risk approach is a growth dimension of potential. Higher levels of risk approach allow the learning and development of different convergent practitioners and aid the performance of the team overall.

Ambiguity Acceptance

Ambiguity exists to a greater or lesser extent in almost any job or workplace. In convergence practice though, ambiguity is a fundamental part of the nature of the work. Complex, conflicting and mixed information, opinions, and ideas are a defining part of convergence practice. Larger and more diverse groups, complex organizational structures, different communication styles, and professional jargon are only a few of the factors that create ambiguity in convergence teams.

Most of us would like to live in a stable, orderly, predictable, and just world.[1,20] Many people struggle with ambiguity. Those with lower levels of trait ambiguity acceptance like to have stability, regularity, and consistency in their work.[21] They like to know exactly what has to be done and the correct way of doing it. However, in convergence practice, things are rarely so clear or simple.

Different practitioners with different experience and perspectives have different ideas about the best way of doing things. And a diverse team will have to synthesize different experience and expertise to come up with the most practical, the most suitable, or sometimes just the most realistic solution.

Those who have higher levels of ambiguity acceptance tend to perform well in complex or uncertain situations. They are also better at adapting to uncertain situations and environments. As with every other personality trait, differing levels of trait ambiguity acceptance may fit with different job roles. High ambiguity tolerance is useful for roles that involve large amounts of mixed information and complex solutions.

There are some jobs where low ambiguity tolerance is helpful. People with lower ambiguity tolerance like to have clear instructions, job descriptions, tasks with specific success criteria, and tangible outcomes. For the convergence practitioner, ambiguity is a fundamental feature that is inherent to the nature of the work. This means ambiguity acceptance is a career dimension of potential for the convergence practitioner.

Competitiveness

Adaptive levels of competitiveness vary more than any other trait for different types of work. High competitiveness is adaptive in roles than focus on individual performance.[22] For the convergence practitioner though, team outcomes are most important, and individual competitiveness can be detrimental to group performance for convergence teams.

For some personality traits, such as conscientiousness or adjustment, very high levels of the trait may be predictive of improved performance. Competitiveness, however, tends to be linked to improved performance at moderate or average levels. For work where team performance and cohesion is more important than individual achievement, lower levels of competitiveness is more adaptive.

This means for competitiveness there will be a negative, curvilinear relationship between performance and competitiveness for the convergence practitioner. Consequently, moderate to low levels of competitiveness will be a career dimension of potential in for convergence practitioners.

Career Dimensions of Convergence Potential

When we define convergence practice as a type of work, or a specific role, we can build a profile of potential based specifically on the requirements of convergence practice that involves working in a transdisciplinary team. Whereas individual practice, research, or another role will have a specific set of skills, required knowledge, experience, and abilities, it cannot be assumed that convergence practice will share the same qualities.[1,23]

Indeed, some attributes that make someone successful in their own individual work may not be useful attributes in convergence practice. Roles like sales, for example, often a high degree of competitiveness and performance is measured based on individual results. Some attributes that are useful for people who are measured based on individual performance may actually hinder an individual's potential in a convergent setting that requires collaboration and does not rely on individual performance metrics.

Based on previous convergence research and team science[23] we can add a list of 10 core behaviors of career dimensions of potential for the convergent practitioner:

1. *Practicing effective leadership and management skills.* Roles and responsibilities should include who, within the convergence team, is responsible for leadership, coordination, management, and administrative responsibilities. Bringing together a diverse team of convergence practitioners requires effective leadership to manage the team, develop the shared vision, and monitor and manage performance of the team.

2. *Maintaining awareness of self and others.* Working with a diverse convergence team requires understanding one's own skills and capabilities as well as the skills and capabilities of colleagues. Then, sharing the awareness across the team helps to develop respect and understanding for what different members of the team contribute to different functions and roles within the group.

3. *Establishing trust.* Sharing responsibility and relinquishing some of one's own individual control is a necessary part of the success for any convergence teams. Working with colleagues from a range of disciplines and specializations means team members need to trust in the experience and qualifications of others. The group must be proactive about establishing and maintaining trust.

4. *Practicing strategies for open communication.* Open communication and information flow among a diverse team is an important predictor of overall team performance. It can be challenging for practitioners with different backgrounds, from different fields, and sometimes with fundamentally different ways of working to communicate respectively and effectively. Maintaining open and effective communication is essential for team success.

5. *Understanding team development.* Convergent teams may be even more dynamic and fluid than the traditional conceptualization of teams as a fixed group of people within a department. Thus, it is important that convergence team members understand that their teams will be continually engaging in team development. This means continually demonstrating effective team building skills, setting shared expectations, and defining roles and responsibilities.

6. *Creating, sharing and revisiting a shared vision.* The team must develop and maintain a shared vision and purpose. Every team member must have a sense of the overarching goal, as well as a clear view of their roles and responsibilities within that vision and purpose.

7. *Providing appropriate recognition and credit.* It is necessary to clearly establish the roles and responsibilities of members of the team. Subsequently everyone in the team must be both accountable for their own actions within those roles and receive appropriate recognition and appreciation for a job well done.

8. *Promoting disagreement while containing conflict.* Any scientific endeavor will naturally lead to disagreement and healthy debate about discussions. Bringing together a diverse group of practitioners into a convergence team will naturally bring together different viewpoints, opinions, and approaches to the science and the work. The team must have appropriate and constructive mediums to communicate disagreement, along with the appropriate mediation and resolution channels or processes to ensure debate is encouraged and conflict will be resolved.

9. *Learning each other's languages.* Members of a convergence team will need to learn some of the language from their colleagues fields or disciplines. One of the most effective ways to bridge languages between fields is to set out clear performance expectations and evaluations. People must be evaluated based on their own contributions in a clearly defined and measured way. Regular communication as well as feedback and discussion about individual and group performance will help to bridge the gaps between language.

10. *Enjoying the science and the work together.* A shared vision and clear performance objectives should go a long way in helping people to thrive in their respective roles and to bring their own knowledge and expertise to good use in a convergence team. At its best a convergence team can bring a joy of the science, practice, and the work together to provide unexpected benefits to individuals as well as the team.

Conclusion

Using a clear, parsimonious, and valid model of potential is essential for identifying and selecting the right people for any role. This process is especially important in distinguishing high potential convergence practitioners. As has been reinforced throughout this chapter, it is always necessary to ask the question of potential: Potential to do what?

By using Silver and Church's[5] model of potential to understand the work of convergence practice, we can then clearly law out the three dimensions of potential to be successful in convergence teams.

Foundational dimensions: Intelligence and personality traits conscientiousness and adjustment are fundamental and stable individual differences that contribute to success in nearly any type of work. They are particularly important to complex, challenging, and demanding roles like that of the convergence practitioner.

Growth dimensions: Convergence practice requires continually learning and developing in the role, as well as proactively and effectively managing both communication and potential conflict within a diverse team. Therefore, the personality traits curiosity and risk approach are dimensions of potential as they relate to learning and improving in a convergence role. Self-awareness of one's own role and function within the team is also required for growth and development in a convergence role.

Career dimensions: Convergence practice requires collaboration, sublimating one's own objectives into the vision and the objectives of the team, as well as managing complexity. The traits of higher ambiguity acceptance and lower competitiveness are necessary career dimensions of potential in a convergence role. We also expanded on 10 behaviors that are related to career dimensions of potential in a convergence role in the previous section.

References

1. MacRae I, Furnham A. *High Potential: How to Spot, Manage and Develop Talented People at Work.* London, UK: Bloomsbury; 2018.
2. Misra S, Stokols D, Cheng, L. The Transdisciplinary Orientation Scale: factor structure in relation to the integrative quality and scope of scientific publications. *Journal of Translational Medicine & Epidemiology.* 2015; 3(2).
3. Augsburg T. Becoming transdisciplinary: the emergence of the transdisciplinary individual. *World Futures.* 2014; 70: 233-247 https://doi.org/10.1080/02604027.2014.934639.
4. MacRae I, Furnham A. *Motivation and performance: A guide to motivating a diverse workforce.* London, UK: Kogan Page; 2017.
5. Silzer R, Church AH. The pearls and perils of identifying potential. *Industrial and Organizational Psychology.* 2009; 2(4): 377-412 https://doi.org/10.1111/j.1754-9434.2009.01163.x.
6. Bertua C, Anderson N, Salgado JF. The predictive validity of cognitive ability tests: A UK meta-analysis. *Organizational Psychology.* 2011; 78(3): 387-409.

7. Furnham A. Personality and occupational success. In Zeigler-Hill V, Shackelford TK, eds. *The SAGE Handbook of Personality and Individual Differences*. London, UK: SAGE; 2018.

8. Edmonds GW, Jackson JJ, Fayard JV, Roberts BW. Is character fate, or is there hope to change my personality yet? *Social and Personality Psychology Compass.*, 2007; 2(1), 299-413.

9. Shurkin JN. *Terman's Kids: The Groundbreaking Study of How the Gifted Grow Up*. New York, NY: Little, Brown; 1992.

10. Teodorescu A, Furnham A, MacRae I. Trait correlates of success at work. *International Journal of Selection and Assessment.* 2017; *25*: 35-40 https://doi.org/10.1111/ijsa.12158.

11. Furnham A. Does it matter who we are? Personality at work. In Chmiel N, Fraccaroli F, Sverke M, eds. *An Introduction to Work and Organisational Psychology: An International Perspective*. 3rd ed. Hoboken, NJ: Wiley; 2017: 317-334.

12. Curseu PL, Ilies R, Vîrgă D., Maricutoiu L, Sava FA. Personality characteristics that are valued in teams: not always "more is better"? *International Journal of Psychology.* 2019; *54*(5): 638-649 https://doi.org/10.1002/ijop.12511.

13. Costa P, McCrae R. Four ways five factors are basic. *Personality and Individual Differences.* 1992; *13*: 357-372 https://doi.org/10.1016/0191-8869(92)90236-i.

14. Terrancciano A, McCrae RR, Costa PT. Personality traits: stability and change with age. *Psychology of Aging.* 2008; *11*(4): 474-478.

15. Willie B, Beyers W, De Fruyt F. A transactional approach to person-environment fit: reciprocal relations between personality development and career role growth across young to middle adulthood. *Journal of Vocational Behaviour.* 2012; *81*: 307-321 https://doi.org/10.1016/j.jvb.2012.06.004.

16. Linden D, Nijenhuis J, Bakker A. The general factor of personality: a meta-analysis of Big Five intercorrelations and a criterion-related validity study. *Journal of Research in Personality.* 2010; *44*(3): 315-327 https://doi.org/10.1016/j.jrp.2010.03.003.

17. Barrick MR, Mount MK, Gupta R. Meta-analysis of the relationship between the five factor model of personality and Holland's occupational types. *Personnel Psychology.* 2003; *56*(1): 45-74 https://doi.org/10.1111/j.1744-6570.2003.tb00143.x.

18. Hannah S, Sweeney PJ, Lester PB. Toward a courageous mindset: the subjective act and experience of courage. *Journal of Positive Psychology.* 2007; *2*(2): 129-135 https://doi.org/10.1080/17439760701228854.

19. Fredrickson BL. The role of positive emotions in positive psychology: the broaden-wand-build theory of positive emotions. *American Psychologist.* 2001; *56*, 218-226 https://doi.org/10.1037/0003-066x.56.3.218.

20. MacRae I, Furnham A. *Myths of Work: The Stereotypes and Assumptions Holding Your Organisation Back*. London, UK: Kogan Page; 2017.

21. Furnham A, Ribchester T. Tolerance of ambiguity: a review of the concept, its measurement and applications. *Current Psychology.* 1995; *14*(3): 179-199 https://doi.org/10.1007/bf02686907.

22. Wang G, Netemeyer RG. The effects of job autonomy, customer demandingness and trait competitiveness on salesperson learning, self-efficacy and performance. *Journal of the Academic Study of Marketing Science.* 2002; *30*: 217-227 https://doi.org/10.1177/0092070302303003.

23. Bennett LM, Gadlin H. Collaboration and team science: From theory to practice. *Journal of Investigative Medicine.* 2012; *60*(5): 768-775 https://doi.org/10.2310/jim.0b013e318250871d.

31

The Minds Behind the Technology

Lessons on Entrepreneurial Mental Health

Jessica Carson

Introduction

While the scope of this book is primarily focused on the mental health technologies created by entrepreneurs, the authors thought it relevant to examine the topic from a different angle: to explore the mental health of the entrepreneurs creating these technologies. Over the past few years, there has been a surge of interest in the mental health and well-being of entrepreneurs, with this sudden increase in attention likely due to a combination of factors: (i) provocative new research that has shed light on the state of entrepreneurial mental health,[1] (ii) a wave of notable venture capitalists and entrepreneurs coming forward about their mental health challenges,[2] and (iii) multiple suicides among entrepreneurs and creatives.[3] However, while this topic has finally received long-overdue attention, there remains a great deal of misinformation and confusion within the entrepreneurial ecosystem. Mental health issues are certainly not new to entrepreneurship, but the distress and disease within the entrepreneurial ecosystem has hit a crescendo that needs to be acknowledged and addressed, and solutions must be proposed that not only treat existing mental illness, but prevent the exacerbation of underlying mental and emotional vulnerabilities in entrepreneurs.

> **Overview of Core Themes**
>
> Research on Entrepreneur Mental Health
>
> Genetics of entrepreneurs
> Nature of entrepreneurial work
> Culture of the entrepreneurial ecosystem
>
> Potential Solutions
>
> Educating stakeholders
> Empowering entrepreneurs

While this chapter will shed light on the idea that entrepreneurs with mental health challenges may in fact have a competitive *advantage*, the consequence of not addressing the gratuitous burnout, emotional distress, and stress-related illness among entrepreneurs is dire: Entrepreneurs are key drivers of social and economic progress, responsible for creating new jobs and maintaining a viable economy, and if we do not insulate the individuals who are so valued for their creativity, productivity, and societal impact, we will surely begin to see negative ramifications trickle throughout society. The issue of entrepreneurial mental health and well-being is complex and demands nuanced and holistic solutions, and it could be argued that solutions *must* come from transdisciplinarians. In many ways, transdisciplinarians, like convergence mental health practitioners, are similar to entrepreneurs in their open-mindedness and passion for incorporating diverse and disparate perspectives, and I am confident the challenges in this chapter will resonate with those readers possessing an entrepreneurial spirit. With any luck, a new class of transdisciplinarians will emerge who develop conceptual, theoretical, methodological, and translational innovations that address this important issue facing our entrepreneurial ecosystem.

The State of Entrepreneurial Mental Health

In 2015, a gray cloud appeared in the seemingly ever-blue sky of entrepreneurship. In a now widely cited research article, it was revealed that self-reported mental health concerns are present across 72% of entrepreneurs, a statistic that far surpasses the prevalence of mental health issues in comparison subjects.[1] Specifically, this study found that entrepreneurs are more likely to struggle with depression (30%, 2× higher than comparison), attention-deficit/hyperactivity disorder (ADHD; 29%, ~6× higher than comparison), substance abuse (12%, 3× higher than comparison), and bipolar (11%, 11× higher than comparison). This research quickly escaped the confines of academic literature and began making its way into lay entrepreneurship articles published by Forbes, Inc., Business Insider, Fortune, and many others. Before long, it seemed nearly impossible to attend a pitch event or listen to a new venture podcast without hearing a whisper of this recently uncovered misfortune.

While these alarming findings undoubtedly elicited a call to action, they also triggered a reactionary response in the entrepreneurial ecosystem, as evidenced by articles with titles like, "Mental Illness May Plague Entrepreneurs More Than Other People."[4] As the words *crisis, epidemic,* and *plague* became commonplace at start-up panels and tech events without the rich context this article[1] offered, it made the halls of co-working spaces and incubators sound like infectious places to work. Seemingly overnight, entrepreneurs witnessed an increase in meditation and mindfulness sessions inside of start-up environments in a benevolent attempt to contain the outbreak, which left founders with a collection of techniques, but no real understanding of *why* they were struggling or *how* they could create a healthier ecosystem. Indeed, without context, these statistics sound rightfully fearsome and have left many entrepreneurs wondering how to best protect themselves and their employees. It is my intention to address these questions to encourage solutions that are not surface-level fixes, but offer entrepreneurs a pathway to develop greater self-awareness, self-acceptance, and sustainable self-care. I will attempt to explain the issue as holistically as possible to address entrepreneurial mental health as far from a personal failing, but as a self-selecting mechanism that underlies creativity, productivity, and dynamism.

The Reasons for This Mental Health "Crisis"

Perhaps the most common and most misinformed assumption about entrepreneurial mental health is that its prevalence is entirely related to the stresses of entrepreneurship. Based on this partially accurate assumption, many of the proposed solutions are based solely in stress-reduction techniques that have been met with limited success and adoption. While it is true that underlying vulnerabilities to mental illness (diathesis) can be activated by environmental triggers (stress), there is a much more complex web of variables at play in the genesis of illness. The following subsections will address the three key variables that contribute to entrepreneur mental health, all of which must be considered to understand and address the "crisis": (i) genetics of entrepreneurs, (ii) the nature of entrepreneurial work, and (iii) the culture of the entrepreneurial ecosystem.

Genetics of Entrepreneurs

Entrepreneurs may be wired with a susceptibility for mental, emotional, and physical challenges—and this may not be a truly terrible thing.[1] Indeed, researchers have proposed that individuals with certain mental health challenges may self-select into entrepreneurship because their diagnosis confers an adaptive advantage necessary for entrepreneurial success. Self-selection refers to the idea that individuals will opt into certain jobs, activities, or environments if they possess certain attributes or qualities that confer an adaptive advantage in that context.[5] For example, someone with a low risk tolerance might self-select into operational role in a large company that offers stability and security, while someone with a high risk tolerance may be more likely to self-select into an entrepreneurial role that offers dynamism and ambiguity. The likelihood of becoming an entrepreneur has been found to have genetic underpinnings, specifically related to dopamine receptor genes that modulate novelty seeking/sensation seeking,[6] and these polymorphisms—often associated with mental illness—may also offer an individual many of the most valued qualities of entrepreneurs, like risk tolerance, curiosity, and passion. In other words, entrepreneurs may not self-select into entrepreneurship *despite* the fact that they have a mental health diagnosis, but *because* they have a mental health diagnosis, thereby making the prevalence of these disorders particularly high in this population.

> *Depression:* Evolutionary psychologists believe that depression may be an adaptive state in which the individual conserves energy to focus on a critical issue at hand.[7] During a depressive episode, the individual slows down, observes their environment, and engages in realistic thinking and problem-solving.[8] While entrepreneurs may perceive a depressive episode as an unpleasant experience, many also report that it encourages them to slow down, reject unnecessary

engagements, and invest their energy in a more focused task, like coding an app, writing a book, or thinking realistically about a problem.[9] Entrepreneur and Moz founder, Rand Fishkin, touches on this depressive realism when he shared, "The weird part is, I think depressed Rand is actually a very authentic version of myself. When I felt depressed, I upheld ... the values of transparency and authenticity ... as the reasons why I could and should be such a raging, all-consuming, negative naysayer."[2]

ADHD: Dopamine receptor genes have been associated with ADHD,[10] and many entrepreneurs report having a distractible, energetic, and curious nature since childhood. While these tendencies may have been criticized or medicated in their youth, entrepreneurs often report enjoyable benefits from their ADHD diagnosis as an adult: An entrepreneur with ADHD may experience high energy, creativity, and the ability to hyperfocus on tasks that they are particularly engaged in.[11] Even though many struggle to engage with their environment and colleagues in a focused manner, they often value their diagnosis, like JetBlue founder David Neeleman, "If someone told me you could be normal or you could continue to have your ADD (the original name for what is now called ADHD), I would take ADD."[12]

Substance abuse: The same dopamine receptor that may be so advantageous to the entrepreneurial persona's novelty-seeking and sensation-seeking tendencies is also associated with substance abuse.[13] Therefore, while entrepreneurs may benefit from a higher risk tolerance, greater exploratory behaviors, and an intensified sense of passion, they may also be more likely to struggle with substance abuse.[14] This disposition for substance addiction may also explain why entrepreneurs are prone to "entrepreneurship addiction," which refers to the tendency to compulsively engage in entrepreneurial activities.[15] While these behaviors can certainly have harmful consequences, they can also make the persona of a fearless leader or impassioned founder.

Bipolar: A great many entrepreneurial minds throughout history have been characterized by manic–depressive tendencies.[16] Bipolar is a startling 11x higher in entrepreneurs than comparison subjects, and there is likely an adaptive reason behind this inflated diagnosis[1]: In manic episodes, the entrepreneur may benefit from enhanced risk tolerance, sociability, energy, optimism, confidence, and euphoria[17] which are essential for networking, selling, or launching a business. In depressive episodes, the entrepreneur may benefit from the "advantages" of depression as previously outlined. The highs and lows of bipolar are often further exacerbated by the "emotional rollercoaster" of start-up life, thereby making the manic and depressive tendencies even more pronounced.

Stress-related illness: Research has shown that a higher than average IQ predicts higher ratings on entrepreneurship indices,[18] and it makes sense that individuals with high IQs would self-select into a career that demands high creativity and cognitive capacity. But research has also found that individuals with high IQs have an increased risk of psychological and physiological disorders compared to national averages.[19] The hyper brain/hyper body theory of integration proposes that individuals with a high IQ display an overexcitable emotional and behavioral response to their environment, and while a hyperreactive central nervous system may offer an individual remarkable abilities in some domains, like perception, it can also render an individual in a fight, flight, or freeze state. If this response is prolonged, it can trigger a maladaptive series of changes in the brain and body.

Combined, findings on the genetics of entrepreneurs suggest that it may not be in the best interest of entrepreneurs or society to "fix" or "cure" them, as attempts to smother an entrepreneur's inborn vulnerabilities and sensitivities might simultaneously prevent them from accessing their innate and unique talents. Instead, it seems entrepreneurs would benefit from guidance that empowers them to harness their strengths while protecting themselves from mental, emotional, and physical depletion. It may not be realistic or advantageous to "prevent" mental illness in entrepreneurs, but it would most certainly be helpful to offer resources that support the nuanced personas who self-select into this special kind of work.

Nature of Entrepreneurial Work

While genetics play a large role in the manifestation of entrepreneurial mental illness, there is typically a stressor or series of stressors that "activate" the illness. The diathesis/stress model proposes that an individual's underlying genetic susceptibility for a mental or physical illness can be triggered by a stressor in their environment,[20] and this model explains why two people who are exposed to the same stressor may or may not develop the same physical or psychological pathology. While entrepreneurship is a rare career in that it offers entrepreneurs the opportunity to fulfill an assortment of needs—physiological, safety, belonging, esteem, and actualization—it also involves specific and potent stressors that can threaten these needs at every level. Indeed, the nature of entrepreneurial work poses stressors that can disrupt an entrepreneur's mental health and well-being in a variety of ways, and these stressors must be addressed as a dynamic web of interconnected variables:

Physiological: Entrepreneurs often report lack of sleep due to workload, insomnia, skipped or nonnutritious meals, excessive use of stimulants like caffeine, excessive use of sedatives like alcohol, and insufficient time to exercise.

Safety: Due to the competitive and rapidly changing innovation landscape, entrepreneurs face both acute and chronic threats to their sense of safety.[21] They experience chronic uncertainty and instability, like shifting team structure, product vision, and office environment and are often unable to predict their financial and professional future with any degree of accuracy. Largely beholden to the whims of investors and board-members who can withdraw support and at any moment, entrepreneurs often feel they have little control over their access to human or capital resources, and unlike employees who can enjoy the security of an employer's resources, like health insurance and steady income, entrepreneurs must often fend for themselves with a fight or flight mentality.

Love/belonging: Launching a venture not only requires a significant investment of monetary resources, but also of time and energy, which means that less time and energy can be allocated toward other activities, like friendships, family

486   SPECIAL CONSIDERATIONS FOR OPERATIONALIZING

time, and romantic relationships.[22] Entrepreneurs often report that starting a company is an isolating endeavor, requiring them to undergo long sprints of independent work and forcing them to make lifestyle sacrifices to accommodate the demands of their work. Once the venture has been launched, entrepreneurs often report that their status as a founder or leader can socially isolate themselves from the rest of the company, giving credence to the saying, "It's lonely at the top."

Esteem: Entrepreneurship can be a fickle career in which founders are celebrated and admired one moment and condemned and rejected the next. Perhaps more so than other type of career, entrepreneurs can derive lofty status and recognition through their work, often before any significant impact or profit has been made. As a result, many entrepreneurs report feelings of imposter syndrome and struggle to reconcile the drastic swings between confidence and capability and insecurity and self-doubt.

Self-actualization: Perhaps the most common goal among entrepreneurs—surpassing a desire for money or fame—is the desire to create something that supports the individual's pursuit of meaning, purpose, identity, and impact.[23] Entrepreneurship and other creative careers arguably offer a direct path toward self-actualization, as they allow the individual to realize their potential as a direct result of their own energy and efforts. However, many entrepreneurs intertwine their sense of purpose and identity with their work to such an extent that a failure, acquisition, change to management structure, or shift in company vision can create a direct threat to their self-actualization needs.

When the stressors of entrepreneurial work are examined with the framework of Maslow's hierarchy of needs, we see a myriad of interconnected threats to an entrepreneur's mental health and well-being. It's important to understand that the nature of entrepreneurial work is highly distinct from other types of careers, and solutions must be created accordingly. Indeed, what mitigates mental health concerns in a traditional employment setting may not translate as readily into the entrepreneurial workplace, and solutions must be realistic and easily adoptable within the uniquely demanding confines entrepreneurial work.

Culture of the Entrepreneurial Ecosystem

Historically, entrepreneurship has been a white, male-dominated profession.[24] It has only been recently that women and minorities have played a more active role in the innovation landscape, although women and minorities still represent just 2% and <1% of the venture capital deals, respectively.[25] Accordingly, entrepreneurship has largely been built upon the values and ideals of the masculine archetype like competition, aggression, and stoicism. While this has created a culture that values resilience, grit, and other admirable qualities of strength, it has also created a culture in which no amount of effort or success seems sufficient, and any weakness or sensitivity in the individual may be viewed as a liability. In many ways, entrepreneurial culture is a perfect storm for the genesis of distress: When an entrepreneur's personality—one which is frequently wired for the extremes—is combined with the tremendous pressures of entrepreneurial culture, burnout is often all but inevitable. It's the responsibility of every entrepreneur, venture capitalist, accelerator or incubator manager, and other key stakeholders to understand the impact that trends within entrepreneurial culture have on an entrepreneur's psyche:

Glorification of the hustle: Entrepreneurship has become synonymous with the colloquial word *hustle* or *hustling*. According to Gary Vaynerchuck, the celebrity entrepreneur who popularized the term, hustling is the key to entrepreneurial success.[26] In his words, "if you want bling-bling, if you want to buy the Jets, if you want to have fancy clothes, then you need to put in the work. It's the cost of entry. It's the only variable you can actually control. ... Stop crying and keep working. Hustle is the only activity of success." This term is now plastered across co-working spaces and venture firm websites and has in many ways become the anthem of entrepreneurship. But while hustle culture is intended to inspire and motivate entrepreneurs, it often does just the opposite, creating a culture in which burnout is glorified and sleepless nights are worn as a badge of honor. Indeed, many entrepreneurs view rest as self-indulgent, as evidenced by entrepreneurs like Bill Gates, "I never took a day off in my twenties. Not one."

Stoicism—the entrepreneur's religion: Stoicism is an ancient philosophy that was founded in Athens in the early third century BCE and was practiced by notable figures like Seneca and Marcus Aurelius.[27] This philosophy teaches its adherents that they cannot control the external world and must learn to control their own emotional responses to attain inner peace. This philosophy has been readily adopted by entrepreneurs who believe that Stoic principles can teach them to endure pain, hardship, and struggle without protest, complaint, or the display of feelings.[28] While Stoicism undoubtedly has benefits when practiced mindfully, its interpretation by many modern-day entrepreneurs does not teach resilience, but instead promotes emotional suppression. Not only does the Stoic culture of entrepreneurship perpetuate unrealistic expectations of resilience, but it also prevents entrepreneurs from acknowledging and resolving distress when it occurs.

An ecosystem of unicorns: In entrepreneurship, a "unicorn" refers to a privately held start-up that is valued at over $1 billion.[29] Coined in 2013 by venture capitalist Aileen Lee, the term *unicorn* was chosen because of its mystical nature and its rare and coveted status. This term has since infiltrated countless dialogues concerning entrepreneurs and has become a staple in the entrepreneurial vernacular. However, while the word *unicorn* was originally adopted to elicit awe and respect, this causal and frequent comparison to mythical status has introduced an unattainable expectation of success. Entrepreneurs are significantly more achievement-motivated than managers,[30] and when this achievement motivation is combined with the culture of entrepreneurship that celebrates unrealistic levels of achievement, it creates a culture in which no level of success is enough, and this mentality contributes to the culture of burnout and distress.

The culture in which entrepreneurs create should not be underestimated when proposing solutions to improve entrepreneurial mental health. Entrepreneurial culture is firmly couched in a masculine approach to work, communication, and leadership, and this single-noted culture can prove detrimental to both entrepreneurs of *all* genders. Indeed, many female entrepreneurs say that they feel they must hide or over-compensate for any sensitive qualities that could be perceived as weakness, creating a work culture in which many women experience imposter syndrome.

The Way Forward

In this chapter, we have discussed the current state of entrepreneurial mental health, and explored the three largest contributors to poor mental health and well-being: (i) genetics of entrepreneurs, (ii) the nature of entrepreneurial work, and (iii) the culture of entrepreneurial ecosystem. We now understand that, through a process of both self-selection *and* diathesis/stress, individuals with certain predispositions may be more likely to become entrepreneurs, and these individuals are faced with certain stressors and cultural variables that exacerbate underlying vulnerabilities. Some of these variables are controllable, like avoiding exposure to unhealthy motivational techniques, while other variables are less controllable, like the psychological and physiological wiring of entrepreneurs. But as we've explored, it seems that entrepreneurs do not need to be "fixed," as even their vulnerabilities may confer adaptive advantages for entrepreneurial success, but rather we must find long-term, sustainable solutions that support them on their path. For the remainder of the chapter, we will explore several avenues that can generate meaningful and sustainable solutions: (i) educating stakeholders and (ii) empowering entrepreneurs.

Educating Stakeholders

There is an increasing awareness of the importance of entrepreneur mental health and well-being among non-entrepreneur stakeholders, like investors, incubator managers, and board members. However, there remains a drastic misalignment between the vision, objectives, and incentives of entrepreneurs and those who profit from their successes, particularly investors. One of the most common protests I hear from entrepreneurs is, "You tell me to be more healthy and balanced, but I have a debt I owe to my stakeholders. I can't do both." While it may seem like an entrepreneur's health and well-being are at odds with productivity and profits, this is not necessarily the case: By intentionally shifting the dynamics of founder–stakeholder relationships, there are a number of ways that profits, productivity, and mental health can align to create meaningful value.

> *Creating aligned incentives:* Anecdotally, one of the most common triggers of anxiety and depression in entrepreneurs occurs when there are misaligned incentives between a founder and key stakeholders. This friction often comes in the form of discrepant vision, objectives, and key metrics for success. For example, many founders have a clear vision for their company, but after receiving significant support or investment, learn that their stakeholder has a very different

vision and set of values. Similarly, entrepreneurs often experience burnout or distress when undue pressures and unrealistic objectives are forced upon them by key stakeholders, often in the form of impractical expectations around profits, growth, or speed of execution. Indeed, when there is an insurmountable misalignment between the key metrics of success for a founder versus their stakeholders, it can be almost impossible to cultivate a healthy workplace. To prevent this dissonance, it may be important to ask questions like, Do we share the same vision, values, and virtues? Do we agree on key milestones? Do we share the same metrics of success?

Promoting a healthier culture: While many stakeholders intellectually appreciate the importance of entrepreneur mental health, they don't always see how they themselves contribute to a culture of burnout and distress. One of the clearest examples of this is the incubator or accelerator that wishes to create a healthy environment for their founders, but nonetheless manages a program that is intentionally designed to be a "pressure-cooker," encouraging founders to overwork, outcompete, and hyperimpress. Similarly, venture firms or co-working spaces may have an empathetic desire to support their founders as individuals, but nonetheless promote content that exacerbates the "hustle and grind" and "unicorn" mentality. It is important for every stakeholder to become accountable for their impact on entrepreneurial culture and understand how they are presenting discrepant messages. To address this, stakeholders can ask themselves questions like, Does my content/programming reflect my desire to improve the culture? Am I promoting a healthy approach to work? Am I making dissonant demands of my founders?

Supporting entrepreneurs as individuals: Many stakeholders assume they must adopt an all-or-nothing approach to supporting their entrepreneurs, choosing to invest in extensive offerings like custom content, coaching, therapy, and mindfulness support. While educational material and trainings can certainly empower entrepreneurs to better care for themselves, many stakeholders fail to pursue one of the easiest and most fruitful solutions: teaching themselves to be better coaches for their founders. Instead of outsourcing all support initiatives, it can be just as valuable for stakeholders to arm themselves with elevated communication tools like empathy, vulnerability, and self-awareness so they can work more effectively with their founders. Often, the greatest action a stakeholder can take is to simply listen. It may be relevant for stakeholders to ask themselves questions like, Should I participate in a coaching program? How could I become a more empathetic listening? How could I become a more vulnerable and authentic colleague?

Empowering Entrepreneurs

Surprisingly, one of the greatest obstacles I have witnessed in entrepreneurs who wish to improve their mental health and well-being is a simple misunderstanding of their own unique wiring and feelings of disempowerment around their own healing. The lack of visibility into their own inner workings can create distress and resistance, making the entrepreneur feel blocked, stuck, or ashamed of their own struggles. But once this misunderstanding remedied, the steps needed to attain sustainable health and well-being are much easier to grasp and maintain. Instead of focusing exclusively on stress-reduction or mindfulness techniques, it may be useful to take a multilayered approach when teaching entrepreneurs how to support their own mental health and well-being:

Elevating self-understanding: For many entrepreneurs, the path toward greater well-being starts as a journey of self-understanding. It is often an invaluable exercise for entrepreneurs—both personally and professionally—to engage in self-awareness practices, like therapy, coaching, journaling, peer groups, and reflection exercises. Through this process of self-discovery, entrepreneurs can cultivate a deeper understanding and appreciation of their inner workings, making their distress less "unknown" and empowering them to support themselves from a place of acceptance and self-compassion. It may be productive for the entrepreneur to ask themselves questions like, How am I wired as an individual and entrepreneur (mental, emotional, physical, etc.)? What are my strengths that—when not mindfully managed—are also my struggles? How can I reframe my challenges as my strengths?

Practicing mindfulness and self-care: This recommendation is aligned with much of the current thinking around stress-reduction and physical care regimens. By engaging in mindfulness practices (meditation, yoga, breathwork, etc.) and other forms of self-care (nutritious eating, technology-free days, etc.), entrepreneurs can better advocate for themselves and take their mental health into their own hands. It is important that entrepreneurs cultivate sustainable self-care practices that fit into their schedule and preferences, and are mindful to not engage with these practices in the same extreme way they engage in work. Indeed, when entrepreneurs first start caring for themselves, they often adopt quite rigorous diets or meditation regimens that are not sustainable. It may be important for the entrepreneur to ask themselves questions like, How can I create healthy boundaries (time, energy, emotions, etc.) with my company? What mindfulness practices do I enjoy? What are my needs around nutrition, exercise, and sleep?

Teaching and supporting others: Often times, the most healing experience is when an entrepreneur can use their personal experience—good or bad—as a tool to support others. Indeed, I have witnessed tremendous healing when entrepreneurs achieve a stable baseline from which they can support others and create a healthier ecosystem. At this step, they are able to act proactively—not just reactively—to change their company and culture, and benefit not just themselves, but the collective. It is often during these self-transcendent activities, like mentoring, teaching, and sharing, that entrepreneurs report the greatest feelings of mental and emotional stability. To engage with this kind of work, entrepreneurs may ask themselves, How can I use my experience to support and heal others? How can I improve the health of my employees and broader ecosystem? How can I lead from a place of greater authenticity and vulnerability?

Summary and Conclusions

An entrepreneur's mental health and well-being cannot healed in an echo chamber, and transdisciplinarians must appreciate that each creator is operating within a highly complex ecosystem that places an unusual set of demands and pressures upon them. Only when convergence mental health practitioners begin to look at entrepreneurial well-being *holistically* can they identify lasting and sustainable paths toward improved mental health and well-being. It is my hope that the insights in this chapter have sparked ideas in readers—a community of transdisciplinarians—on how we can transform entrepreneurial culture, make shifts to the nature of entrepreneurial work, create more alignment between entrepreneurs and stakeholders, and empower entrepreneurs to care for their sensitivities and vulnerabilities. By teaching the next generation entrepreneurs to have greater self-awareness and self-compassion, we as a society will inevitably benefit from the more conscious and enlightened innovations they bring into the world. Indeed, a creation often seems to have only as much integrity as its creator, and it should therefore be considered a societal imperative that we collectively ensure the health of future generations of entrepreneurs to come.

References

1. Freeman, M. A., Johnson, S. L., Staudenmaier, P. J., & Zisser, M. R. *Are entrepreneurs "touched with fire"?* Unpublished manuscript. 2015.
2. 12 quotes on entrepreneur burnout and depression, from those who've walked the path. *Medium.* July 3, 2017. https://medium.com/the-mission/12-quotes-on-entrepreneur-burnout-and-depression-from-those-whove-walked-the-path-a0d62a3ed389
3. Gourguechon, P. Entrepreneurs and suicide risk: A new perspective on entrapment provides hope. *Forbes.* 2018.
4. Harris, L. Mental illness may plague entrepreneurs more than other people: Here's why (and how to get help). *Entrepreneur.* 2018.
5. Rocha, V., Carneiro, A., & Varum, C. A. Serial entrepreneurship, learning by doing and self-selection. *International Journal of Industrial Organization*, 2015; 40, 91–106 https://doi.org/10.1016/j.ijindorg.2015.04.001.
6. Nicolaou, N., Shane, S., Adi, G. et al. A polymorphism associated with entrepreneurship: Evidence from dopamine receptor candidate genes. *Small Business Economics.* 2011; 36: 151 https://doi.org/10.1007/s11187-010-9308-1.
7. Henriques, G. Depression: Disease or behavioral shutdown mechanism. *Journal of Science and Health Policy.* 2000; 1: 152–165.
8. Andrews, P.W.; Thompson, J.A. The bright side of being blue: Depression as an adaptation for analyzing complex problems. *Psychological Review.* 2009; 116 (3): 620–654 https://doi.org/10.1037/a0016242.
9. Nesse, R. M. Is depression an adaptation? *Archives of General Psychiatry.* 2000; 57(1), 14–20 https://doi.org/10.1001/archpsyc.57.1.14.
10. Cornish, K. M., Manly, T., Savage, R., Swanson, J., Morisano, D. Association of the dopamine transporter (DAT1) 10/10-repeat genotype with ADHD symptoms and response inhibition in a general population sample. *Molecular Psychiatry.* 2005; 10(7), 686 https://doi.org/10.1038/sj.mp.4001641.

11. Williams J, Taylor E. The evolution of hyperactivity, impulsivity and cognitive diversity. *Journal of the Royal Society Interface.* 2006; 3(8): 399–413. doi:10.1098/rsif.2005.0102

12. Connolly, M. Just diagnosed with ADHD: next steps for adults. *ADDitude.* 2019 https://www.additudemag.com/just-diagnosed-with-adhd-next-steps-for-adults/.

13. Lusher, J. M., Chandler, C., & Ball, D. Dopamine D4 receptor gene (DRD4) is associated with novelty seeking (NS) and substance abuse: The saga continues. *Molecular Psychiatry.* 2001; 6(5), 497–499 https://doi.org/10.1038/sj.mp.4000918.

14. Keskin, G., Gümüşsoy, S., & Aktekin, E. Entrepreneurship: Is it an addiction?. *Procedia-Social and Behavioral Sciences.* 2015; 195, 1694–1697 https://doi.org/10.1016/j.sbspro.2015.06.259.

15. Spivack, A. J., & McKelvie, A. Entrepreneurship addiction: Shedding light on the manifestation of the "dark side" in work-behavior patterns. *Academy of Management Perspectives.* 2018; 32(3), 358–378 https://doi.org/10.5465/amp.2016.0185.

16. Furnham, A., Batey, M., Anand, K., & Manfield, J. Personality, hypomania, intelligence and creativity. *Personality and Individual Differences.* 2008; 44(5), 1060–1069 https://doi.org/10.1016/j.paid.2007.10.035.

17. Altman, E. G., Hedeker, D., Peterson, J. L., & Davis, J. M. The Altman self-rating mania scale. *Biological Psychiatry.* 1997; 42(10), 948–955 https://doi.org/10.1016/s0006-3223(96)00548-3.

18. Jones, G., & Hafer, R. W. IQ and entrepreneurship: International evidence. *SSRN Electronic Journal.* 2012. https://papers.ssrn.com/sol3/papers.cfm?abstract_id=2057396

19. Karpinski, R. I., Kolb, A. M. K., Tetreault, N. A., & Borowski, T. B. High intelligence: A risk factor for psychological and physiological overexcitabilities. *Intelligence.* 2018; 66, 8–23 https://doi.org/10.1016/j.intell.2017.09.001.

20. Ingram, R. E. & Luxton, D. D. *Development of psychopathology: A vulnerability stress perspective.* Thousand Oaks, CA: SAGE, 2005.

21. Grant, S., & Ferris, K. Identifying sources of occupational stress in entrepreneurs for measurement. *International Journal of Entrepreneurial Venturing.* 2012; 4(4), 351–373 https://doi.org/10.1504/ijev.2012.049828.

22. Sexton, D. L., & Bowman, N. The entrepreneur: A capable executive and more. *Journal of Business Venturing.* 1985; 1(1), 129–140 https://doi.org/10.1016/0883-9026(85)90012-6.

23. Carland Jr, J. W., Carland, J. A. C., & Carland III, J. W. T. Self-actualization: The zenith of entrepreneurship. *Journal of Small Business Strategy.* 1995; 6(1), 53–66.

24. Levine, R., & Rubinstein, Y. Smart and illicit: Who becomes an entrepreneur and do they earn more? *Quarterly Journal of Economics.* 2017; 132(2), 963–1018 https://doi.org/10.1093/qje/qjw044.

25. CB Insights, Pitchbook.

26. Vaynerchuk, G. Hustle: The cure for those who complain. 2017. https://www.garyvaynerchuk.com/hustle-cure-complain/.

27. Stoicism. https://en.wikipedia.org/wiki/Stoicism. Last edited July 17, 2020.

28. Stoicism for entrepreneurs: Practical philosophy for the 21st century [Blog post]. *99 Designs.* 2017. https://99designs.com/blog/business/stoicism/.

29. Lee, A. Welcome to the Unicorn Club. *TechCrunch.* November 11, 2013. https://techcrunch.com/2013/11/02/welcome-to-the-unicorn-club/.

30. Zhao, H. & S.E. Seibert. The big five personality dimensions and entrepreneurial status: A meta-analytical review. *Journal of Applied Psychology.* 2006; 91, 259–271 https://doi.org/10.1037/0021-9010.91.2.259.

32

Consumer Participation
in Personalized Psychiatry

Neha P. Chaudhary and Harris A. Eyre

Financial Disclosures

HAE owns shares in CNSdose. NPC has no relevant conflict of interest to declare.

Introduction

Novel discoveries are increasingly transitioning medicine from a "one size fits all" approach to one where diagnostic and therapeutic techniques are tailored to an individual's unique clinical, social, digital, and biological (e.g., genetic and epigenetic) profiles (1). This transformational approach seeks to enhance patient outcomes through more accurate screening, diagnosis, treatment, prevention, and patients' engagement in their own care (1). In psychiatry, the principles of personalized medicine are beginning to be applied, particularly in the research domain. One example of personalized psychiatry in action is the major National Institute of Mental Health campaign titled Research Domain Criteria—a global effort aimed at developing psychiatric diagnostic and treatment techniques that combine a matrix of biological, behavioral, and social factors (2). Examples of personalized psychiatry techniques include the collection of sensor, keyboard, voice, and speech data from smartphones, which have been correlated to behavior, cognition, and mood (3) and may be used to navigate the onset, course, and outcome of a psychiatric illness, such as onset of psychosis (4). Pharmacogenomics, the study of genomes in relation to psychotropic pharmacodynamics and pharmacokinetics, is also increasingly used to tailor pharmacologic therapy to individual patients (5).

Personalized medicine represents a paradigm shift—one in which the consumer, who is explicitly identified as the key stakeholder, is involved in informing, shaping, and driving change as it pertains to diagnostics and treatments. The central thesis of this shift is that the buy-in, participation, and engagement by the patient or consumer in their care is not just optional; it is the crux of the care itself as the care is only as good as the way in which it is received by the person who needs it and the outcomes as experienced by that end-user, consumer, or patient. In the field of bipolar disorder, for example, community-based participatory research leverages the lived-experience of bipolar disorder, inviting consumers to act as co-investigators rather than merely test subjects. Research priorities are dictated by the needs of the community, resulting

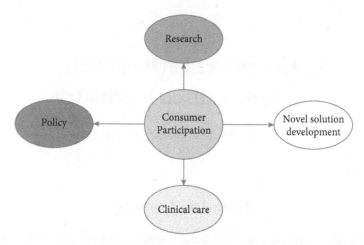

Figure 32.1 Consumer participation in personalized psychiatry. Consumer participation in the development of personalized psychiatry should occur via research, policy, ethics discussions, clinical care, or novel solution development.

in relevant, timely, and applicable findings that reciprocally benefit the community by improving mental health literacy, treatment planning, treatment adherence, and stigma reduction (6). Consumers are already involved in managing their own health through the use of smart devices, the internet as a source of information, and social networks to share ideas and organize (7).

This chapter outlines the rationale for consumer participation in research, policy, ethical issues, clinical care, and novel solution development, followed by examples and insights on ways to enhance this participation. See Figure 32.1 for a graphical representation.

Methods

Studies were identified for inclusion in this narrative review by searching PubMed, Google Scholar, PsychINFO, and Ovid Medicine from inception through May 2019 (HAE, RA). Articles were limited to those published in English. The literature search strategy was based on using combinations of the following keywords: *consumer, participation, personalized, precision, psychiatry, design thinking, research,* and *policy.*

Consumer Participation in Research

Traditional clinical research methods are based on the principle that outcomes of interventions applied to a representative cohort (by age, gender, ethnicity, etc.) can be extrapolated to the general population. Advances in technology allow us to appreciate the diversity in genotype, epigenetics, and phenotype psychometric and neurological testing, medical imaging, smartphone metadata, proteomics, genomics, microbiomes, and beyond. However, as we outline in this chapter, traditional research methodologies may not be adequately robust to account for this diversity (8). This has implications on the future directions in research.

Sociodemographic Considerations

The role of sex and gender diversity in disease prevalence, symptomology, risk and mediating factors, natural history and pathophysiology, and treatment are well recognized in psychiatry. There is increasing recognition of the role of gender in pathophysiology, behavior (including help-seeking behaviors), coping mechanisms, and adherence to therapy (9), alongside sex-specific considerations in psychopharmacology, hormonal effects, and gender-aware psychotherapy (10). Patient ethnicity is likewise important in personalized psychiatry. Many studies are either limited to Anglo-Saxon populations or rudimentary phenotype labels (and, indeed, controversial terminology) such as white, black, and Hispanic, which can make extrapolation of findings to a wider population difficult. Adequate representation of African American consumers, especially African American women, remains a challenge (11,12).

The use personalized medicine research methodologies may lead to more robust findings and improved outcomes on both single-patient and cohort-level. Human leukocyte antigen genotyping enables more robust understanding of cohort populations. For example, patients of Han-Chinese, Thai, and Malay heritage are more likely to carry the HLA-B*1502 allele, which may interact with carbamazepine to induce Steven–Johnson syndrome, a potentially fatal toxic epidermal necrolytic condition, and screening is highly recommended prior to treatment (13). Studies limited to a dominant ethnicity or mixed-ethnicity cohorts may miss such significant findings.

While genotyping represents an additional dimension in research that was previously limited to phenotype, the wealth of findings hinges on a broad representation of genetic material, which is underpinned by participation of consumers from a variety of sociodemographic backgrounds.

The Consumer as Scientist

Consumers can participate in the scientific process from the point of agenda-setting, study design, and recruitment all the way to data interpretation and dissemination. This manifests in both formal and informal ways (14). Many contemporary research units have consumer engagement forums. The Patient-Centered Outcomes Research Institute is a US-based independent, not-for-profit, nongovernment organization that evaluates clinical effectiveness of interventions. Consumers are not only identified as key stakeholders, and therefore represented on the board and advisory panels, but also participate in study design, peer review, and conduct and dissemination of results (15). By contrast, citizen science projects enable amateurs to conduct or participate in research by undertaking crowdsourcing, study design, data collection, analysis, distribution of results, and decisions regarding future directions (16). Studies can be formalized through the engagement of professionals on a collaborative or co-engagement basis.

Social media use is high among psychiatric patients and online patient communities are a rich network of patient peers and support networks (17,18). Forums such as PatientsLikeMe are a repository of health data shared by patients, enabling learning from shared experiences, unlike generalized and nonspecific information available on traditional health information websites. In 2017, more than 67,000 patients shared data about their mental health conditions (19). Online patient communities can facilitate screening and recruitment of patients into studies, transcending the conventional method that relies on treating clinicians. Not only is there a data set that can be readily accessed, this method may also offer greater study exposure and more diverse sample populations. The overarching message is that consumers can and do contribute to research and that existing platforms can be utilized to support the process.

Consumer Participation in Policy

Consumers are natural drivers of policy to improve outcomes that include the promotion, development and uptake of personalized psychiatry. These can be broadly divided into two areas: policy pertaining to research and policy pertaining to the implementation of novel technologies (i.e., translation from bench to bedside).

Policy-Facilitating Research

Evidence-based medicine relies on high-quality clinical trials, which are expensive to conduct and lacking for many promising technologies. Consumers must call for policies that require novel technologies, including personalized psychiatry, to demonstrate analytical validity, clinical validity, and clinical utility (20). The Oxford Evidence-Based Medicine Framework is a guide for researchers, clinicians, health services, policy makers, and consumers in evaluating evidence (21). The higher the level of evidence, the more conscientious and judicious the application of personalized psychiatry technologies.

Policy-Facilitating Implementation

Successful implementation can be described as the availability and use of personalized psychiatry technologies by patients across socioeconomic groups. Herein, the greatest challenges are believed to be economic and operational (22).

Patient access to new technology is often determined by finances. A study of oncology patients demonstrated a strong interest in personalized therapies and willingness to pay in the setting of survival benefit (23). However, many consumers rely on their health insurers, which typically require stringent criteria to be met to qualify for reimbursement, including a high level of evidence (24). Insurers frequently seek cost-effectiveness data to justify the economic impact of new technologies (25), but these data may not be available until it has been on the market for some time (22). Currently, the power ultimately lies with insurers, rather than consumers and clinicians. Yet, it seems that this trend is shifting; consumers are becoming increasingly aware of how their healthcare budget is spent, and the evolution of the financially aware consumer may lead insurers to offer more competitively priced or personalized products in the future (26).

Consumer groups can likewise be powerful advocates for policy change through lobbying healthcare providers and governments. Mental health is a politically charged policy area, and lessons can be drawn by reflecting on another major public health issue—that of HIV. The patient-led HIV movement was instrumental in bringing about changes in legislation, including the recognition of AIDS in the Americans with Disability Act, preventing discrimination of HIV-infected individuals through the Ryan White Care Act, and offering AIDS treatment as a federal benefit to all US citizens (27). The HIV movement continues to exert great influence on policymakers and is often referenced as a model of patient-led advocacy (28).

Consumer groups are keen to work closely with policymakers to facilitate implementation of novel solutions (29), and engaging these experts-by-experience can help foresee and troubleshoot challenges associated with implementation of novel technologies in personalized psychiatry.

Consumer Participation in Clinical Care

On a patient level, the use of personalized psychiatry may enrich the doctor–patient relationship. Whereas other medical diagnoses can be substantiated primarily by objective evidence (e.g., medical imaging), psychiatry currently relies more heavily on clinical judgement in diagnosis and treatment (30). The use of biological measurements or genetic information may validate the patient experience, support treatment decisions, and start to help quantify or qualify outcomes. It is, however, important to recognize there are limitations to these techniques; this is technology under development and therein lies a risk of placebo, as well as harm. These risks can be attenuated, in part, through shared-decision making, complemented by increased monitoring and clinical support (30).

Decision aids, such as pharmacogenetic-based decision support tools, are a relevant part of the concept of shared decision-making and appear useful in enhancing patient knowledge of their medication metabolism, medication efficacy, and side effects (30). In this example, patient investment and empowerment in their care may improve adherence to psychotropic medications and treatment effectiveness (30). The combination of greater patient involvement and the use of decision aids to inform clinical discussions between patients and doctors could markedly increase the real-world effectiveness of psychotropic medications.

Consumer Participation in Novel Solution Development

Engaging consumers in the development of novel clinical solutions that will be used by and ultimately benefit them is intuitive (31). This type of end-user engagement is an integral concept in the process of design thinking. Design thinking is a design methodology based on the principles of empathy, collectivism, and multidisciplinary teams to generate solutions focused on the end-user experience (31). Rapid proto-typing and concurrent testing, drawing upon feedback from continuous consulting with stakeholders, allows design thinkers to quickly develop and refine technologies that meet the needs of both users and academics (32). This process overcomes the notion that designers and academics are siloed in their field of research and lack real-world perspectives, by allowing patients to provide continuous feedback based on first-hand experience, which only they can uniquely offer. Indeed, this tends to result in an improved research process and outcomes with improved study designs, facili-tated recruitment, and more successfully disseminated results. There are a number of illustrative examples of this.

An illustrative example of the role of consumer participation in novel solution de-velopment can be seen in an e-health solution developed to assist patients undergoing weight loss treatment (33). This solution was developed via a workshop where health-care professionals and patients co-attended and mutually acknowledged the need for support in the typical treatment regimen via self-help (e.g., educational mater-ials, reminders, asynchronous communication between provider and patients, etc.). Therefore, an e-health portal was agreed to be developed. Once a prototype was built based on suggested user specifications, a number of iterations were completed to opti-mize the user quality and utility.

Novel Solutions for Ethical, Economic, and Data Protection Considerations

While many ethical issues encountered in personalized psychiatry exist in general psychiatry, with decision-making capacity in the setting of chronic psychiatric ill-ness being a clear example, personalized psychiatry presents additional challenges. As previously discussed, the ability to delve into a patient's unique genomic or internet data and medical records raises questions about privacy, confidentiality, and their weight in relation to research that may benefit the greater good (34,35). The misuse of sensitive medical data remains a particular concern among consumers, and pro-tections ought to exist at both legislative and organizational levels. The US Congress introduced the Genetic Information Nondiscrimination Act (GINA), with policies related to health coverage and employment (36). The European Union General Data Protection Directive governs the use of data across member nations, balancing the needs of research institutions with the rights of data subjects, including data porta-bility, mandatory data processing impact assessments, the mandatory appointment of a data protection officer, and the granting consumers the right to be forgotten (37).

The practicalities of personalized psychiatry need also be addressed. Direct-to-consumer genetic tests are already available on the market and offer consumers a wealth of genetic information, with varying degrees of interpretation and genetic counseling. While this highlights a shift toward patient autonomy, it is clear that there is a potential for harm; for example, where the presence of genetic traits is not diagnostic or prognostic and risk being misleading (38,39). Particular to psychiatry, interpretation of genetic testing is very complex as it typically involves disorders influenced by a highly polygenic environment so that even the most robust findings account for only a small amount of the variance in many disorders. Public impressions of genetics as singular or definitive is at odds with this reality.

There has also been discussion of cost and the presence of health disparities by socioeconomic status. There is concern that this bespoke brand of medicine may only be available in developed countries, and even there, to private or insured patients electing to use these technologies (40,41). However, novel solutions can increase access to psychiatric monitoring and treatment. For example, patient smartphone data can be used to assess stability and rhythmicity of bipolar disorder and deliver interventions, potentially preventing hospital admission (42,43). App development is relatively inexpensive, and should clinical validity be demonstrated, there is a persuasive fiscal argument for governments and insurers to make this technology widely available.

Data gathering is a labor intensive and costly task; however, these challenges may be attenuated through the use of shared databases. As owners of the information fed into databases, consumers have a role to play in advocating for their use, persuading other consumers to share their health information, and in calling for regulations around their use. In particular, the voice of consumer is critical to navigating the ethical concerns associated with the use of databases. These include issues of privacy, autonomy, informed consent, the delicate balance between beneficence to the patient and wider community, the potential maleficence of revealing sensitive genetic information, and insurance eligibility (44). Specific and comprehensive policies must exist to safeguard patients while maximizing the benefit from analyzing these vast repositories of data.

Conclusion

By engaging the end-user in the development of personalized psychiatry research studies, policies, and novel solutions, clinicians, researchers, health executives, technology developers, designers, and policymakers can benefit from the unique yet significant contribution that consumers offer. Such contributions are arguably necessary for success in today's changing landscape with the introduction of technological solutions in mental health, and their omission may come with risks. Involvement may range from improving study design to facilitating recruitment and retention to dissemination of results to stakeholders. Simply put, there is no substitute for the consumer voice.

Acknowledgments

We would like to thank the following experts for their inputs on our draft: Nina Vasan, Eric Storch, Arshya Vahabzadeh and Eric Lenze.

References

1. Ozomaro U, Wahlestedt C, Nemeroff CB. Personalized medicine in psychiatry: problems and promises. BMC Medicine. 2013;11:132 https://doi.org/10.1186/1741-7015-11-132.
2. National Institute for Mental Health. Research Domain Criteria (RDoC). https://www.nimh.nih.gov/research-priorities/rdoc/index.shtml. Accessed June 20, 2019.
3. Insel TR. Digital phenotyping: technology for a new science of behavior. JAMA. 2017;318(13):1215–1216 https://doi.org/10.1001/jama.2017.11295.
4. Bedi G, Carrillo F, Cecchi GA, Slezak DF, Sigman M, Mota NB, et al. Automated analysis of free speech predicts psychosis onset in high-risk youths. NPJ Schizophrenia. 2015;1:15030 https://doi.org/10.1038/npjschz.2015.30.
5. Bousman CA, Hopwood M. Commercial pharmacogenetic-based decision-support tools in psychiatry. Lancet Psychiatry. 2016;3(6):585–590 https://doi.org/10.1016/s2215-0366(16)00017-1.
6. Michalak EE, Jones S, Lobban F, Algorta GP, Barnes SJ, Berk L, et al. Harnessing the potential of community-based participatory research approaches in bipolar disorder. International Journal of Bipolar Disorders. 2016;4(1):4.
7. Sagner M, McNeil A, Puska P, Auffray C, Price ND, Hood L, et al. The P4 health spectrum—a predictive, preventive, personalized and participatory continuum for promoting healthspan. Progress in Cardiovascular Diseases. 2017;59(5):506–521 https://doi.org/10.1016/j.pcad.2016.08.002.
8. Fernandes BS, Williams LM, Steiner J, Leboyer M, Carvalho AF, Berk M. The new field of "precision psychiatry." BMC Medicine. 2017;15 https://doi.org/10.1186/s12916-017-0849-x.
9. Boyd A, Van de Velde S, Vilagut G, de Graaf R, O'Neill S, Florescu S, et al. Gender differences in mental disorders and suicidality in Europe: results from a large cross-sectional population-based study. Journal of Affective Disorders. 2015;173:245–254 https://doi.org/10.1016/j.jad.2014.11.002.
10. Riecher-Rossler A. Sex and gender differences in mental disorders. Lancet Psychiatry. 2017;4(1):8–9 https://doi.org/10.1016/s2215-0366(16)30348-0.
11. Halbert CH, McDonald J, Vadaparampil S, Rice L, Jefferson M. Conducting precision medicine research with African Americans. PloS One. 2016;11(7):e0154850 https://doi.org/10.1371/journal.pone.0154850.
12. Sheppard V, Zheng L, Graves KD, Hurtado-de-Mendoza A, Tadasse M. Opportunities for precision medicine: factors associated with participation in genetic research among breast cancer survivors. Journal of Clinical Oncology. 2016;34(3 Suppl):94. https://doi.org/10.1200/jco.2016.34.3_suppl.94.
13. Tangamornsuksan W, Chaiyakunapruk N, Somkrua R, Lohitnavy M, Tassaneeyakul W. Relationship between the HLA-B*1502 allele and carbamazepine-induced Stevens–Johnson syndrome and toxic epidermal necrolysis: a systematic review and meta-analysis. JAMA Dermatology. 2013;149(9):1025–1032 https://doi.org/10.1001/jamadermatol.2013.4114.

14. Abbott R. Governing medical research commons In: Strandburg KJ, Frischmann BM, Madison MJ, eds. *The Sentinel Initiative as a Cultural Commons*. Cambridge, UK: Cambridge University Press; 2017, p. 121–143.
15. Patient-Centered Outcomes Research Institute. [Home page]. https://www.pcori.org/. Accessed June 19, 2019.
16. Follett R, Strezov V. An analysis of citizen science based research: usage and publication patterns. PloS One. 2015;10(11):e0143687 https://doi.org/10.1371/journal.pone.0143687.
17. Kalckreuth S, Trefflich F, Rummel-Kluge C. Mental health related Internet use among psychiatric patients: a cross-sectional analysis. BMC Psychiatry. 2014;14:368 https://doi.org/10.1186/s12888-014-0368-7.
18. Chiauzzi E, Lowe M. PatientsLikeMe: crowdsourced patient health data as a clinical tool in psychiatry. Psychiatric Times, September 19, 2016 http://www.psychiatrictimes.com/telepsychiatry/patientslikeme-crowdsourced-patient-health-data-clinical-tool-psychiatry/page/0/3.
19. PatientsLikeMe. Patients Like Me [Home page]. https://www.patientslikeme.com/. Accessed June 19, 2019.
20. Haddow JE, Palomaki GE. ACCE : a model process for evaluating data on emerging genetic tests. In: Khoury M, Little J, Burke W, eds. *Human Genome Epidemiology: A Scientific Foundation for Using Genetic Information to Improve Health and Prevent Disease* Oxford University Press; 2003, p. 217–233.
21. Centre for Evidence-Based Medicine. *Oxford Centre for Evidence-Based Medicine—Levels of Evidence (March 2009)*. https://www.cebm.net/2009/06/oxford-centre-evidence-based-medicine-levels-evidence-march-2009/
22. Davis JC, Furstenthal L, Desai AA, Norris T, Sutaria S, Fleming E, et al. The microeconomics of personalized medicine: today's challenge and tomorrow's promise. Nature Reviews Drug Discovery. 2009;8(4):279–286 https://doi.org/10.1038/nrd2825.
23. Garfeld S, Douglas MP, MacDonald KV, Marshall DA, Phillips KA. Consumer familiarity, perspectives and expected value of personalized medicine with a focus on applications in oncology. Personalized Medicine. 2015;12(1):13–22 https://doi.org/10.2217/pme.14.74.
24. Robinson JC. Biomedical innovation in the era of health care spending constraints. Health Affairs (Project Hope). 2015;34(2):203–209 https://doi.org/10.1377/hlthaff.2014.0975.
25. Abbott R, Stevens C. Redefining medical necessity: a consumer-driven solution to the U.S. health care crisis. Loyola of Los Angeles Law Review. 2014;47(943):1–24.
26. Herzlinger RE. Let's put consumers in charge of health care. Harvard Business Review. 2002;80(7):44–50, 52–55, 123.
27. Volberding P. The impact of HIV research on health outcome and healthcare policy. Annals of Oncology. 2011;22(Suppl 7):vii50–vii53 https://doi.org/10.1093/annonc/mdr426.
28. Manganiello M, Anderson M. Back to basics: HIV/AIDS advocacy as a model for catalyzing change. Faster Cures, June 2011. https://www.fastercures.org/reports/view/13
29. Budin-Ljosne I, Harris JR. Patient and interest organizations' views on personalized medicine: a qualitative study. BMC Medical Ethics. 2016;17(1):28 https://doi.org/10.1186/s12910-016-0111-7.
30. Arandjelovic K, Eyre HA, Lenze E, Singh AB, Berk M, Bousman C. The role of depression pharmacogenetic decision support tools in shared decision making. Journal of Neural Transmission (Vienna, Austria: 1996). 2019;126:87–94 https://doi.org/10.1007/s00702-017-1806-8.
31. Orlowski S, Matthews B, Bidargaddi N, Jones G, Lawn S, Venning A, et al. Mental health technologies: designing with consumers. JMIR Human Factors. 2016;3(1):e4 https://doi.org/10.2196/humanfactors.4336.

32. Bhui K. Quality improvement and psychiatric research: can design thinking bridge the gap? British Journal of Psychiatry. 2018;210(5):377–378.

33. Das A, Svanaes D. Human-centred methods in the design of an e-health solution for patients undergoing weight loss treatment. International Journal of Medical Informatics. 2013;82(11):1075–1091 https://doi.org/10.1016/j.ijmedinf.2013.06.008.

34. Roberson M. An Overview of Psychiatric Ethics. Gladesville, Australia: Health Education and Training Institute; 2012.

35. Cosgrove V, Gliddon E, Berk L, Grimm D, Lauder S, Dodd S, et al. Online ethics: where will the interface of mental health and the internet lead us? International Journal of Bipolar Disorders. 2017;5(1):26 https://doi.org/10.1186/s40345-017-0095-3.

36. Shoaib M, Rameez MAM, Hussain SA, Madadin M, Menezes RG. Personalized medicine in a new genomic era: ethical and legal aspects. Science and Engineering Ethics. 2017;23(4):1207–1212 https://doi.org/10.1007/s11948-016-9828-4.

37. Ho C-H. Challenges of the EU general data protection regulation for biobanking and scientific research. Journal of Law, Information and Science. 2017;25(1):1–20.

38. Annas GJ, Elias S. 23andMe and the FDA. New England Journal of Medicine. 2014;370(23):2248–2249.

39. McPherson E. Genetic diagnosis and testing in clinical practice. Clinical Medicine & Research. 2006;4(2):123–129 https://doi.org/10.3121/cmr.4.2.123.

40. Chadwick R. The ethics of personalized medicine: a philosopher's perspective. Personalized Medicine. 2014;11(1):5–6 https://doi.org/10.2217/pme.13.98.

41. Daar AS, Singer PA. Pharmacogenetics and geographical ancestry: implications for drug development and global health. Nature Reviews Genetics. 2005;6(3):241–246 https://doi.org/10.1038/nrg1559.

42. Abdullah S, Matthews M, Frank E, Doherty G, Gay G, Choudhury T. Automatic detection of social rhythms in bipolar disorder. Journal of the American Medical Informatics Association. 2016;23(3):538–543 https://doi.org/10.1093/jamia/ocv200.

43. Hidalgo-Mazzei D, Reinares M, Mateu A, Juruena MF, Young AH, Perez-Sola V, et al. Is a SIMPLe smartphone application capable of improving biological rhythms in bipolar disorder? Journal of Affective Disorders. 2017;223:10–16 https://doi.org/10.1016/j.jad.2017.07.028.

44. Elger B. Ethical Issues of Human Genetic Databases: A Challenge to Classical Health Research Ethics? Abingdon, UK: Taylor and Francis; 2010.

SECTION VII

NOVEL FUNDING MODELS FOR CONVERGENCE MENTAL HEALTH

33

Collaborative Research and Investment to Secure "Healthy Brains for All"

A Selection of One Mind Projects

Garen K. Staglin

This chapter is adapted from a presentation at the 2019 Milken Institute Future of Health Summit. It was initially published online October 22, 2019, and the original version can be found here: http://milkeninstitute.org/articles/collaborative-research-path-healthy-brains-all

Introduction

It's no secret that mental illness is one of the greatest challenges of our time and the biggest unmet medical need. Physically, mentally, economically, and scientifically, the toll it takes is tremendous—and it strikes every population in the world, without regard for gender, race, nationality, or creed. One in four people worldwide suffers from at least one mental health disorder during their lifetime (Bloom et al., 2011), with over two-thirds of those people failing to receive the care they need (Ngui, Khasakhala, Ndetei, & Roberts, 2010). Each year, mental health conditions generate as much as $3 trillion in direct and indirect costs—and that number is projected to grow to $6 trillion by 2030 (Bloom et al., 2011). Stigma is still a major issue.

It doesn't help that many mental illnesses are still poorly understood. And mental health treatments are severely lacking: Research into new treatments is wildly underfunded worldwide, and existing treatments have left significant unmet need.

Fortunately, there's hope. Collaborative research practices to advance treatment development and care delivery have incredible potential to advance scientific knowledge—because, at the end of the day, we need answers, and we need cures if not new treatments. To achieve these goals, we must work together, not in silos. Convergence mental health clearly aims to break down siloes also (Eyre et al., 2017).

We already know that collaborative research works. In 1983, a study by the World Health Organization (WHO) concluded that cross-cultural collaborative research was effective in improving mental healthcare, particularly for those in greatest need (Harding et al., 1983). Collaborative research programs, wherein multiple organizations conduct research in service of a common goal, have successfully developed new treatments for depression (Elkin et al., 1989) and presented new and effective methods of care (University of Washington, 2017).

Other, more unconventional methods of collaboration have also proven effective at driving innovative, much-needed scientific research. Public–private partnerships capitalize on the strengths of both sectors, using basic science and funding from the public sector and more in-depth research from the private sector to make scientific inroads and develop new medications and treatments (WHO, n.d.). Such partnerships have enabled the National Association for Behavioral Healthcare (n.d.) in the United States to develop new clinical measures.

Public–private partnerships also work on the local level: A public–private partnership empowered the US metropolitan community of the Twin Cities, Minnesota, to improve care for people with mental illnesses, reduce the need for emergency psychiatric services, and lower overall costs related to psychiatric treatment (Health, 2018).

The mental health community is even now working to forge ever more creative methods of collaboration and advancement. The new model of benefit corporations can turn some pharmaceutical companies into mission-driven entities, bound both by fiduciary interests and a social mission (Eiser & Field, 2016). A number of pharmaceutical companies around the globe are already using this model to develop life-changing therapeutics at accessible prices.

Fortunately, the global leadership community has already taken initial steps toward engaging with the issue of mental illness. Heads of state and national leaders are recognizing the importance of mental health and calling for stronger, more urgent responses around the world; recently, at the 2018 G7 meeting, prime minister of Canada Justin Trudeau and other global leaders recognized mental illness as a top priority (Rinke, 2018). Mental health plenary and ancillary sessions were also prominent at the 50th Anniversary of the World Economic Forum in Davos in January 2020.

One Mind is a lived-experience–led mental health nonprofit focused on helping people with brain illness and injury to recover so that they can succeed in their lives (www.onemind.org). The guiding principles of One Mind include an emphasis on people with "lived experience" participation, strategy collaboration across sectors and institutions, open science, and recognizing mental health as disorders of the brain and not as character flaws. One Mind takes the approaches of funding via philanthropy, government, and industry, convening diverse groups of experts and advocating. One Mind has strategically provided seed funding for research resulting in follow-on grants from National Institutes of Health (NIH), the US Department of Defense, and other foundations of over $450 million over the last 20 years.

On the topic of public–private partnerships, One Mind itself has administered three major projects with the NIH and other federal agencies and the Department of Defense, bringing private philanthropy to advance translational outcomes, better diagnostics, and improved treatments. They include (i) Track II, a $80 million, 23-site, 3,000-person longitudinal study in traumatic brain injury that resulted in a US Food and Drug Administration letter of support for a blood and imaging biomarker; (ii) Project Aurora, a $40 million, 46-site, 5,000-person longitudinal study in post-traumatic stress; and (iii) the North American Prodrome Longitudinal Study, a $50 Million, 10-site, 1,500-person longitudinal study in early intervention and detection of youth at risk for psychosis, proving a 70% accuracy of detection.

In addition to the support of the Track II, Project Aurora, and the North American Prodrome Longitudinal Study public–private partnerships previously referenced, since 2005, One Mind has issued 35 Rising Star Awards, each for $250,000, to 35 of the most promising young scientists to accelerate their pursuit of cutting-edge research and neuroscience breakthroughs. Many of these seed-funding grants have resulted in importance breakthroughs and helped launch the careers of each of the awardees—the current head of the NIMH, Josh Gordon, was an early Rising Star Award recipient.

New science and new financing methods are being developed by a coalition of global leaders in neuroscience, finance, and policy and advocacy. With the support of the World Bank, WHO, and the World Economic Forum, One Mind and the National Academy of Medicine are leading the Healthy Brains Global Initiative (HBGI) with the goal of issuing $10 billion in a series of social impact like bonds or other financing instruments to fund accelerated global research on brain health (Bank, 2018). Independently verified metrics will prove the reduction in the $3 trillion annual global burden of mental illness sufficient to retire the bonds or additional return on investment measures to secure sovereign fund participation or philanthropic buydown. Four separate working groups have been formed within the HBGI involving more than 100 leaders in their respective fields. The working groups include Use of Proceeds, Finance Structure, Pay-for Metrics, and Governance. See Table 33.1 and Figure 33.1. This global collaboration is unprecedented in neuroscience and holds the potential of other chronic illnesses to follow this lead.

The HBGI has some precedent from the $3 billion California Institute for Regenerative Medicine (CIRM) financing issued in 2010. The primary mission of the CIRM's funding of stem cell research was to accelerate stem cell treatments to patients with unmet medical needs—but those funds also created tax income for the state. A 2019 independent Economic Impact Report conducted by the Schaeffer Center for Health Policy and Economics at the University of Southern California says that CIRM has had a major impact on California's economy, creating tens of thousands of new jobs, generating hundreds of millions of dollars in new taxes, and producing billions of dollars in additional revenue for the state (Wei & Rose, 2019). The report looked at the impacts of CIRM funding on both the state and national economy from the start of the Stem Cell Agency in 2004 to the end of 2018. The estimated impacts from the

Table 33.1 Current Working Group Members of the Healthy Brains Global Initiative

Finance Structure	Use of Proceeds	Pay-for Metrics	Governance
Charis	Charis	Chairs	Chairs
• David Chen, Equilibrium Capital	• Steve Hyman, Broad Institute of MIT and Harvard	• Chris Murray, University of Washington	• Tim Evans, McGill University
• Valerie Conn, Science Philanthropy Alliance	• Miranda Wolpert, Wellcome Trust	• Eliot Sorel, George Washington University	• Brad Herbert, Brad Herbert Associates
• Robert Klein, Klein Financial Corporation			

(*continued*)

Table 33.1 Continued

Finance Structure	Use of Proceeds	Pay-for Metrics	Governance
• Margaret Anadu, Goldman Sachs • Daniel Arbess, Xerion Investments • Karim Barrada, HSBC • Mukesh Chawla, World Bank Group • Norm Friedland, Fulsky Partners • Chris Lee, Milken Institute • Pierre Meulien, Innovative Medicines Initiative • Chris McCahan, IFC • Walter Ogier, Mending Minds Foundation/ Analexis Therapeutics • Tracy Palandjian, Social Finance • Russell Schofield-Bezer, HSBC • Mel Spigelman, TB Alliance, Word Bank	• Kimberly Allen, Big Blue Eye Consulting • Cara Altimus, Milken Institute • Robin Buckle, UK Medical Research Council • William Carson, Otsuka Pharmaceutical Development & Commercialization • Alon Chen, Weitzmann Institute • Murali Doraiswamy, Duke University • Howard Fillit, Alzheimer's Dementia Discovery Fund • Mona Hicks, One Mind • Richard Huganir, Johns Hopkins University • Tom Insel, Mindstrong Health • Danielle Kemmer, Graham Boeckh Foundation • Dévora Kestel, World Health Organization • Walter Koroshetz, National Institute for Neurological Disorders and Stroke • Husseini Manji, Janssen • Beverly Pringle, National Institute of Mental Health • Shekhar Saxena, T.H. Chan School of Public Health, Harvard University • Paul Stoffels, Johnson & Johnson • Katherine Switz, The Stability Network • Melissa Turgeon, Massachusetts General Hospital • Andrew Welchman, Wellcome Trust	• Francesca Colombo, Organisation for Economic Co-Operation and Development • Harris Eyre, CNSDose • Yueqin Huang, Institute of Mental Health/The Sixth Hospital, Peking University, Bejing • Mark McClellan, Duke University • Gerald McDougall, PwC • Mark Mynhier, PwC • Jennifer Payne, Johns Hopkins University	• Sarah Caddick, Thalamic • Sung Hee Choe, Milken Institute • Mickey Chopra, World Bank Group • Sadia Chowdhury, Freelance Global Public Health Consultant • Miyoung Chun, Alzheimer's X/MIT Sloan School of Management • Mark Feinberg, International AIDS Vaccine Initiative • Helen Hermann, University of Melbourne • Patrick Kennedy, The Kennedy Forum • Craig Kramer, Johnson & Johnson • Muhammad Pate, World Bank Group • Vikram Patel, T.H. Chan School of Public Health, Harvard University • Shekhar Saxena, T.H. Chan School of Public Health, Harvard University • Mointreyee Sinha, citiesRISE • Eliot Sorel, George Washington University • Nora Super, Milken Institute • Melissa Stevens, Milken Institute • Graham Thornicroft, Institute of Psychiatry, King's College London • George Vradenburg, UsAgainstAlzheimer's

One Mind and **NAM**, in collaboration with the **World Economic Forum, World Bank, and World Health Organization,** recruited global leaders across science, healthcare, finance, philanthropy, and governance who are donating time to this effort as well as individuals with lived experiences of mental and neurological disorders.

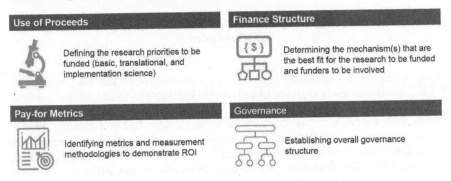

Use of Proceeds

Defining the research priorities to be funded (basic, translational, and implementation science)

Finance Structure

Determining the mechanism(s) that are the best fit for the research to be funded and funders to be involved

Pay-for Metrics

Identifying metrics and measurement methodologies to demonstrate ROI

Governance

Establishing overall governance structure

Figure 33.1 Healthy Brains Financing Initiative Working Group members.

report are $10.7 billion of additional gross output (sales revenue), $641.3 million of additional state/local tax revenues, $726.6 million of additional federal tax revenues, and 56,549 additional full-time equivalent jobs, half of which offer salaries considerably higher than the state average. Furthermore, an additional 2019 independent report conducted by the Schaeffer Center for Health Policy & Economics at University of Southern California says that developing stem cell treatments and cures for some of the most common and deadly diseases could produce multibillion dollar benefits for California in reduced healthcare costs and improved quality and quantity of life (Tysinger, Mulligan, Zhao, Cassil, & Goldman, 2019).

As another incentive mechanism in the United States, One Mind is developing congressional legislation seeking to provide tax credits for new neuroscience research to help "derisk" research and experimentation into new treatments. These credits will be competitively judged by the NIH and the US Treasury Department and are proposed at a level of $1 billion annually for 10 years. This bipartisan bill is in draft form and is targeted to pass before year-end 2020.

To address the shortfall in investment capital of early-stage brain health companies, or professional investors uncertainty about sufficiently high return on investment, we have also established the One Mind Catalyst Fund. The Fund intends to invest in mental and behavioral health research projects that have the potential to mature into small to large companies and that fill a gap between the discovery of promising diagnostic tools and treatments and the work needed to implement and evaluate them in real-world healthcare settings. In some cases, this may involve projects that leverage public-private partnerships and fill crucial gaps or support innovative, impactful enhancements. Several investments have been made already, including one in Mindstrong Health (www.mindstronghealth.com/) and Alto Neuroscience (www.altoneuroscience.com/).

These many efforts to address the global mental health crisis give us hope, but there's much work yet to be done. By funding and collaborating on scientific research and policy, we can begin to move toward the eradication of mental illness and toward better lives for a global citizenry. One day, our vision of "healthy brains for all" will be achieved.

References

Bank, W. (2018). Healthy brain bonds: Is this a feasible option Retrieved from http://documents.worldbank.org/curated/en/310661533223406666/Healthy-brain-bonds-is-this-a-feasible-option

Bloom, D. E., Cafiero, E. T., Jané-Llopis, E., Abrahams-Gessel, S. B., L.R., Fathima, S., Feigl, A. B., . . . Weinstein, C. (2011, September). The global economic burden of noncommunicable diseases. *World Economic Forum*. Retrieved from http://www3.weforum.org/docs/WEF_Harvard_HE_GlobalEconomicBurdenNonCommunicableDiseases_2011.pdf

Eiser, A. R., & Field, R. I. (2016). Can benefit corporations redeem the pharmaceutical industry? *American Journal of Medicine, 129*(7), 651–652 https://doi.org/10.1016/j.amjmed.2016.02.012.

Elkin, I., Shea, M. T., Watkins, J. T., Imber, S. D., Sotsky, S. M., Collins, J. F., . . . et al. (1989). National Institute of Mental Health Treatment of Depression Collaborative Research Program: General effectiveness of treatments. *Archives of General Psychiatry, 46*(11), 971–982; discussion 983. doi:10.1001/archpsyc.1989.01810110013002

Eyre, H. A., Lavretsky, H., Forbes, M., Raji, C., Small, G., McGorry, P., . . . Reynolds, C., III. (2017). Convergence science arrives: How does it relate to psychiatry? *Academy of Psychiatry, 41*(1), 91–99. doi:10.1007/s40596-016-0496-0

Harding, T. W., Climent, C. E., Diop, M., Giel, R., Ibrahim, H. H., Murthy, R. S., . . . Wig, N. N. (1983). The WHO collaborative study on strategies for extending mental health care, II: The development of new research methods. *American Journal of Psychiatry, 140*(11), 1474–1480. doi:10.1176/ajp.140.11.1474

Health, E. M. M. (2018). Mission: Mental health: East Metro Mental Health Roundtable: 10-year executive summary. Retrieved fromhttps://www.healthpartners.com/ucm/groups/public/@hp/@public/documents/documents/entry_202255.pdf

National Association of Behavioral Healthcare. (n.d.). Public–private partnership. Retrieved fromhttps://www.nabh.org/policy-issues/quality/public-private-partnership/

Ngui, E. M., Khasakhala, L., Ndetei, D., & Roberts, L. W. (2010). Mental disorders, health inequalities and ethics: A global perspective. *International Review of Psychiatry, 22*(3), 235–244. https://doi.org/10.3109/09540261.2010.485273

Rinke, A. (2018). The Charlevoix G7 Summit communique. Retrieved from https://www.reuters.com/article/us-g7-summit-communique-text/the-charlevoix-g7-summit-communique-idUSKCN1J5107

Tysinger, B., Mulligan, K., Zhao, H., Cassil, A., & Goldman, D. (2019). Future health dividends for California: Valuing medical innovations to fight cancer, diabetes, stroke, and dry age-related macular degeneration. *California Institute for Regenerative Medicine*. Retrieved from https://www.cirm.ca.gov/sites/default/files/files/about_cirm/Future%20Health%20Dividend_0.pdf

University of Washington, School of Social Work. (2017, September 20). New partnership creates innovative collaborate care model for people with mental illness.Retrievedfromhttps://socialwork.uw.edu/news/new-partnership-creates-innovative-collaborate-care-model-people-mental-illness

Wei, D., & Rose, A. (2019, October 3). Economic impacts of the California Institute for Regenerative Medicine (CIRM). *California Institute for Regenerative Medicine.* Retrieved from   https://www.cirm.ca.gov/sites/default/files/files/about_cirm/CIRM_Economic%20 Impact%20Report_10_3_19%20v.2.pdf

World Health Organization. (n.d.). Public–private partnerships (PPPs). Retrieved from https:// www.who.int/intellectualproperty/topics/ppp/en/

34

Unconventional Approaches to Investing in Mental Health Technology

Kunmi Sobowale

Burden of Illness and Treatment Gap

Over one billion people have mental illness and substance use disorders worldwide.[1] Mental illness and substance use disorders are among the leading causes of disease burden in high-, middle- and low-income countries.[2,3] Globally, these illnesses account for up to 13% of disease burden as measured by disability-adjusted life years, a measure of the years of life lived with disability and the years of life lost because of disease or injury.[2,3] Besides the distress of mental illness itself, mental illness is a risk factor for noncommunicable diseases (NCDs) including cardiovascular diabetes, obesity, and diabetes and can lead to poor disease management of these conditions.[4] In the United States, mental illness and substance use disorders contribute to decreased longevity[5] and are the costliest conditions at an estimated $201 billion annual cost.[6] Mental disorders are tied to several the Sustainable Development Goals, particularly SDG 3 (i.e., ensure health lives and well-being for all at all ages). Failure to address mental illness threatens the achievement of these goals and economic development.

Despite this large burden of disease and increased recognition of mental illness, most individuals with mental illness fail to receive appropriate, or any, treatment.[7] This lack of treatment is referred to as the "treatment gap."[8] In the United States, only one in four people with depression see a mental health clinician within a year.[9] For anxiety, the chances to see a clinician drop to less than one in five.[10] Because many mental illnesses are chronic, not receiving treatment negatively affects livelihood and well-being over the life course.[11,12]

Lack of mental health providers (psychiatrists, psychologists, nurses, etc.) is a primary reason for the large treatment gap for mental illness. Globally, the number of psychiatrists and psychologists per 100,000 people is 1.37 and 0.33, respectively.[13] Mental health providers are disproportionately concentrated in urban areas. As a result, access to care is limited, particularly in rural areas. Furthermore, many clinicians are inadequately trained to deal with complex psychiatric disease.[14]

In addition to low human resources, patient-related factors also contribute to lack of treatment. Patients may be unaware of their mental illness and may view their distress and abnormal behaviors as within the range of normalcy. Therefore, they do not seek treatment. Many people believe they can deal with their illness themselves.[15] Some patients hold negative views of psychotherapy and pharmacological treatment, while others doubt the efficacy of these treatments. Mental illnesses often carry significant stigma. For those afflicted with mental illness, stigma is a strong deterrent to help-seeking.[16,17] Even when awareness of illness and help-seeking intentions are present, structural barriers such as lack of money, lack of transportation, or inability to take time off from work impede access to treatment.

Compounding the treatment gap is the lack of effectiveness of many current treatments. Only a third of people with depression remit on their first treatment course.[18] Also, difficulties recognizing and classifying mental illnesses hinder prevention, early intervention, and provision of appropriate treatment. It is unlikely that current models of care, which emphasize one-to-one, face-to-face diagnosis and treatment by specialized mental health providers, will be able to curtail the burden of disease of mental illnesses in the foreseeable future. Technology will play a key role in advancing mental health research and care through improved access and effectiveness.

Mental Health Technology

The use of technologies in mental health such as telemedicine, and neuroimaging continues to grow. These increasingly cheap and accessible technologies are the driving force in what has been termed the "Fourth Industrial Revolution."[19] The Fourth Industrial Revolution is characterized by the integration of new technologies across industries and a democratization of information. These new technologies include wearables and other smart sensors devices, mobile technology apps, 3D printing, genomics, virtual reality, robotics, nanotechnology, and neurotechnology. These technologies are accompanied by ways to manage this data such as artificial intelligence (AI), machine learning, and cloud computing that promote rapid data gathering and analytics. The integration of technologies will enable new ways of doing things that will impact both mental health delivery and discovery science.

Other examples of emerging mental health technologies include mobile therapy applications, transcranial direct current stimulation, and pharmacogenomics. Although the evidence base varies for these technologies, the potential to improve prevention and treatment of mental illness is huge. Few of these technologies have used AI or machine learning, which could add further benefit. At first glance, these technologies may seem like amenities, but through personalized care, increased access, efficiency, and effectiveness, they can improve mental health. However, to accelerate technology development and deployment and promote sustainability, substantial financial investment will be required.

The Current State of Funding

Unfortunately, trends in mental health funding have been discouraging. Government and philanthropic organizations are the primary funders of mental health research and care. A comprehensive study by the RAND Corporation[20] identified 1,908 funders with 10 or more manuscript acknowledgments worldwide. Thirty-nine percent of funders were charities, foundations, and nonprofits, 33% of the funders were government bodies, and academia represented 20% of funders, while industry was only 0.06%. Government bodies account for 68% of the total number of funding acknowledgements. For both government and philanthropic funders, a small minority of funders represented a large share of acknowledgements. Industry funders were by far the fewest in number and number of acknowledgements. Industry appeared to support more applied research and less basic research compared other sectors. Although the study did not examine the amount of funding, it suggests limited funding diversity because a small group of funders invested in multiple projects.

The amount of investment in mental health is low. The United States has most data, so it will be the focus. Funding from the National Institute of Mental Health, the main public sector financier of mental health research in the United States, has been stagnant and has not kept up with inflation.[21] Philanthropic funding has increased in amount but decreased in percentage of total health giving.[22] By some estimates, philanthropic funding is less than one percent of total funding for mental health research.[23] As with the aforementioned RAND study, a small number of private foundations, the top 10 funders, accounted for almost half the funding.[22] Similarly, while bilateral donor agencies including USAID have allocated slightly more to mental health over time, the total amount remains low. Among the total development assistance provided between 2006 and 2016, mental health funding accounts for only 0.3%.[24]

Another study of private sector and government investments in research and development (R&D; the activities to create new and adapted products), including federal appropriations, found smaller investments for mental illness and substance use compared to other NCDs.[25] Among NCDs, the private investment in R&D per dollar of disease burden was the smallest for mental illness. For example, the investment for major depressive disorder was $0.40 per $1,000 of economic burden compared to $6.30 for cardiovascular disease and $75.50 for cancer. This amount of funding is insufficient to meet the needs of people with mental illness and their families.

Federal and state investment in mental healthcare is difficult to determine because the final expenditures are often not reported. Using the Substance Abuse and Mental Health Services Administration Community Mental Health Services Block Grant appropriations for states as a proxy for mental healthcare funding, the federal government increased the amount allocated in 2018 after a period of stagnation.[26] Historically, states cut community mental health funding in times of economic recession.[27]

One area with rapid investment growth is digital mental health. Through the third quarter of 2019, $416 million in venture capital has been invested in digital mental health start-ups.[28] While this is only 8% of the total digital health venture capital raised overall during the same time period, it is was one of the few areas where there was growth. This amount is more than double the capital invested in 2017 ($159 million) and a vast increase from $3 million in 2011. Technology companies are increasing also investing in biomedical research.[21] Public and philanthropy funders are increasingly interested in mental health technology as well.[20,29]

In summary, across the public, nonprofit, and private sectors there is an underinvestment in mental health research and care. A greater amount and more reliable funding are necessary. There are promising trends in the investment of mental health technology, and interest appears to be growing in the public and private sectors. To leverage this enthusiasm and stimulate more investment in mental health technology, innovative financing instruments that generate and mobilize funds are necessary.[30]

The remainder of this chapter focuses on financing mechanisms to support mental health technology R&D and care delivery. Investments in these areas are crucial for advancing discovery and delivery science. The financial instruments explored include taxation and cross-sector collaborative (CSC) arrangements including social impact bonds (SIBs) and blended finance.

Earmarked Taxation

Governments use taxation as a primary financing option. A tax is a legally required payment from taxpayers collected by the government. Tax revenues are not returned to the taxpayer, but rather used for communal benefit such as building infrastructure, funding social security insurance, or investing in mental health technology. In other words, the taxation is one mechanism used to fund government expenditures.

Governments can finance health projects through earmarked taxation. Earmarking is the setting aside of a portion of the total revenue.[31] Earmarking is an intention choice to prioritize one area. Revenue earmarking assigns a proportion of a revenue stream to health to raise new funds. Expenditure earmarking designates a proportion of the existing budget to health.

While this sounds simple enough, there is a great deal of nuance in how the earmarking is designed. The design affects the amount of revenue generated and influences whether the tax will be enacted and tolerated by taxpayers. There are several design characteristics to consider. First, is the source of the revenue existing or created because a new tax may require more time to design and implement? What is taxed has consequences. A direct tax is directly paid to the government and is mostly income or asset based, while indirect taxes paid to the government through an intermediary is often based on purchase of goods or services (i.e., consumption tax). For example, an indirect tax on unhealthy goods like alcohol or sugar is called a "sin tax." The primary function of sin taxes is to decrease unhealthy behaviors. Also, who is taxed and who is responsible for the revenue generated is important. Once the revenue is collected, the monetary amount allocated to the designated expenditure, the flexibility in its use, who it allocated to, and who will benefit needs is significant. No matter the design, there will be political consequences because someone must pay for it.

The benefits of earmarking include protecting a revenue stream for a designated purpose and building accountability as well as public support by making it easier to link taxes with a specific benefit. Unlike tax credits, participation is mandatory, which makes the revenues generated more predictable. But depending on how the earmarking is designed, the revenue generated can be unpredictable. For example, if tanning salons are taxed, but most salons go out of business because of a recession, then the revenue generated would dramatically decrease. Another downside is rigidity in budgeting, which can constrain the government's ability to invest in other priorities. Relatedly, there is a risk of lack of coordination across the interdisciplinary programs necessary to make the investment successful.

A few states have used earmarked taxes to finance mental health and substance use. In California, the Mental Health Services Act has funded mental health technology. The act, enacted in 2004, imposes a statewide one percent income tax on household income in excess of $1 million. Annually, around $2 billion in revenues in generated.[32] Because mental health services in California are provided at the county level, the revenues are provided to counties. The counties use revenues to address local needs with stipulations to fund five major categories: 20% allocated to prevention and early intervention, 10% to workforce training, 10% to community program planning and administration, 10% to capital improvement and technology, and 5% to innovation. The technological needs to assist delivery of services and innovation allocations created an opportunity to invest in mental health technology.

Funded and proposed technology projects have varied. Kern, Mono, Orange, Sacramento, Tehama, and Los Angeles counties have collectively invested over $68 million in innovation projects on virtual peer support for people with mental illness and their families, standalone online and mobile app evidence-based interventions, AI-based therapy avatars, telepsychiatry, transcranial magnetic stimulation, and use of passive data from smartphones for digital phenotyping and intervention.[33] Many of these technologies are being provided as a suite to detect distress in real time and provide immediate access to care. Infrastructural supports like electronic health records and data warehouses have also been funded.

The Mental Health Services Act case provides lessons on the use of earmarked taxes. First, the revenue stream is important. In California the tax on income was advantageous because the high number of millionaires in the state. Because earmarked taxes on income or payroll generally generate more revenue than consumption taxes, it may be a better design for mental health technology investment.[31] Despite the large amount of revenue generated, a lack of oversight and planning led to $2.5 billion in unspent funds.[34] Also, during the economic recession there was a large decrease in funding, which means the revenue stream is not always reliable.

Nevertheless, this financing option is worth implementing in other states. Only Washington State, California, Illinois, Colorado, and Missouri have passed legislation for this financing instrument.[32] Some design recommendations for this financing instrument are[31]

1. A not too narrow or broad purpose for expenditures.
2. A strong, but flexible link between revenue and expenditures.
3. Flexibility to reallocate funds for emerging priorities.
4. Transparency of how funds are used and regular audits.
5. A clear timeline for when the earmark would need to be reapproved.

Cross-Sector Collaborations

Improving mental health will require cooperation across the public, nonprofit, and private sectors. Augmentation of traditional funding sources is needed to close the mental health funding gap. Cross-sector financing is the use of resources from a variety of public, nonprofit, and private sources to solve healthcare problems in a way they one sector could not do alone. The public sector usually refers to government. The nonprofit sector includes nongovernment organizations (publicly funded) and nonprofit organizations (publicly and privately funded), and the private sector includes for-profit organizations.

Cross-sector financing is based CSCs. The term *cross-sector collaborations* is used rather than *public–private partnerships* because the distinction between the public, private, and nonprofit sectors is increasingly blurred and the level of engagement across sectors is variable. Specifically, collaborations exist on a continuum from "partnerships" characterized by high levels of trust, engagement, and interdependence as well as more aligned goals to "interactions" with low levels these qualities.[35] Each level of collaboration has its benefits and challenges and one form may be more advantageous depending on the situation or setting.

In CSCs, each sector has its goals and obligations. For the public sector entities, the goal is to lower cost and increase impact. Nonprofits have similar goals to the public sector. The difference is that the public sector is accountable to constituents and nonprofits charities to donors as well as board members in the case of private nonprofits. Private sector goals are broad and could include a better public image, entry into a new market, and so on. Meeting these goals can lead to short- and long-term competitive advantage.[36] Private sector entities' widened goal to generate social and environmental returns in addition to financial returns through money and investment capital is termed *impact investing*. Ultimately, the private sector has an obligation to its shareholders. In CSCs, the private sector is leveraged not only for financing, but quality and efficiency. In mental health technology, there is power differential such that the private sector is the main producer of technology. Still often in CSCs, the public or nonprofit sector sets the agenda. Balancing these power differentials through shared objectives and goals promotes successful collaboration.

With these factors in mind, CSCs provide a more sustainable financing for mental health. The use of multiple revenue streams can help generate more funds and decreases the financial risk for each collaborator. While the financial risk is shared, the level of risk for each collaborator varies. The balance of risk sharing is important for successful collaboration. Ultimately, the financing instrument used will depend on the need. In SIBs, the financial risk is primarily on the private sector, whereas for other financial instruments the risk is primarily on the public and nonprofit sector.

Social Impact Bonds

An SIB is a performance-based contract between different stakeholders. In this arrangement, the government contracts with an intermediary (usually a nonprofit organization) to address a healthcare need. The government and intermediary work to define the intervention structure and metrics of success. The intermediary then recruits investors who provide capital to third-party service provider. The service provider in turn provides the government desired services to the target population. The government repays the capital with a return to the investor if predetermined success metrics are realized. The investor does not receive a financial return if metrics are not met. The financial risk is therefore shifted from the government (i.e., taxpayers) to philanthropic or private sector investors. Roles in SIBs include the following:

- *Government*—Determines the healthcare issue to focus on and pays based on intervention success.
- *Intermediary*—An organization that brings together stakeholders, raises capital to provide and evaluate an intervention of interest, and manages financial flows. The intermediary may or may not deliver the intervention.
- *Investors*—Impact investors or philanthropists that provide capital to finance the intervention of interest.
- *Service provider*—Nonprofit or charity that receives capital and implements the program.
- *Independent evaluator*—Determines if the metrics of success have been achieved.

The increased emphasis on evidence-based programs with measurable outcomes, demand for more government accountability, and impact investing made SIBs popular.[37] Since the first SIB in 2010, more than 130 SIBs have been implemented worldwide.[38] As of 2017, Rizzello and colleagues[39] found 9 out of 36 health-related SIBs started or in development were focused on mental health. Programs targeted elder loneliness, supported employment, dementia prevention, mental illness, and substance use. These SIBs are based in the United States, Canada, New Zealand, Australia, and Japan.

No SIBs explicitly mention mental health technology. This may be explained by the recency of the evidence base for mental health technologies. In general, interventions with a strong evidence base are preferred.[40] Therefore, because internet-delivered interventions for adult depression have a comprehensive evidence base, it is used as an example in line with identified criteria for SIB success.[41]

1. The intervention must address a problem of interest to the public sector.
   - As mentioned in the first section of this chapter, there is a large treatment gap in mental health. Worldwide, only 16.5% of people with depression receive minimally adequate treatment within a year.[9] Increasing access to evidence-based interventions is necessary.
2. The intervention must have a strong research evidence base in terms of effectiveness in clearly identified population(s).
   - A meta-analysis of 32 randomized controlled trials of internet interventions for adult depression[42] found they are comparable to care as usual, waitlist, placebo treatments, and no treatment with an effect size of 0.67 (95% confidence interval: 0.51 to 0.81).
3. The intervention must be economically attractive to the public sector.
   - The cost-effectiveness of internet interventions for depression has been demonstrated for both guided and unguided interventions.[43,44]
4. Outcomes must be expressed as metrics that are clearly defined and quantifiable.
   - Outcomes measures for depression are well established and do not differ for internet interventions. Common measures include Patient Health Questionnaire 9, Beck Depression Inventory-II, and Center for Epidemiologic Studies Depression Scale.

5. Outcomes must be achievable in a reasonable and clearly understood time period.
   - Most studies have found positive outcomes over the course of weeks to six months.[45] This is less than the one to two years stated in the criteria.[41]
6. The evidence-based interventions should be able to be implemented without significant administrative challenges.
   - Since internet interventions are based on evidence-based treatments and do not deter from protocol, there is high treatment fidelity. These interventions can reduce the work burden for healthcare providers[42] and can be delivered effectively with guided nonprofessional[46] support or without human support. For guided interventions, most support provided is encouragement and occurs asynchronously with minimal burden.[47]
7. An intervention's implementation should face no significant political or stakeholder challenges.
   - Although there are concerns about user data and privacy, several organizations and government agencies offer internet interventions for depression. There is high acceptance among people with depression for internet interventions.[48]

While internet interventions for depression are a promising example, there are disadvantages to SIBs, which may limit their viability. Risk may be unattractive to the private sector investors. Having multiple investors share risk makes investment more appealing. Another downside of SIBs is the time and resources involved in their set-up and implementation. The competing interests and high stakes for stakeholders require this proper structuring. These challenges may explain why private sector investment in SIB remains low.[49] More flexible financial instruments may be more fruitful for creating CSCs.

Blended Finance

In the financing instruments discussed thus far, one sector solely provided the funding or the funding sources remained separate. With the increased collaboration between sectors, there has been a move toward blended finance. Blended finance is the strategic use of public and philanthropic funding to mobilize private sector investment. Because of the increased private sector investment in mental health technology, it is an opportune time to use blended finance instruments for mental health technology.

Blended finance often takes the form of concessional capital where government and philanthropies provide capital (e.g., debt, equity, guarantees, and insurance) to shield private investors if the investee disputes or defaults. Alternatively, financing could occur at market rate if market opportunity incentives like intellectual property are provided. Overall, these incentives derisk private sector investing, promoting funding for underfunded areas like mental health. Blended finance instruments can take multiple forms.[50] Because many mental health technologies are still in development, blended finance instruments specific to R&D will be discussed. Investees range from universities and government entities to private sector small- and medium-sized enterprises. Common instruments include the following:

Grant—Capital provided without an expectation of repayment.

Concessional capital—The public/philanthropic capital has a lower priority of being repaid compared to the private investor if the investee defaults. This capital typically is either equity, where capital provided in exchange for ownership in the company, or debt, where capital provided that must be returned with interest.

Guarantees—The guarantor (e.g., the World Bank) takes on full or partial responsibility for an investee's repayment in the cause of defaults, disputes, etc. In addition to mitigating risk for private sector investors/lenders, the guarantor's good credit rating may decrease the interest rate for borrowers.

Technical assistance—Provision of training, instruction, or other supports to investees directly or indirectly through funding (e.g., an incubator) to develop sound business models and build capacity. Although a nonfinancial instrument, technical assistance can increase investors' confidence that the project will be successful.

A blended finance project usually includes more than one instrument. Determining the optimal mix can be complex and is project specific. An umbrella organization with experience in blended finance to organize financing efforts and manage legal and regularity constraints is crucial. In global health, development institutions including multilateral development banks and National Development Finance Institutions have served this role. Blended financing can also be used to pool funds to invest in a portfolio of projects.

Although blended financial instruments are well described, their use is mental health is limited. How might blending financing for mental health technology look? Consider the hypothetic case of a small biomedical company that discovered that individual microbiome composition determines antidepressant medication efficacy. Having completed the National Institutes of Health Small Business Innovation Research Phase II program,[51] the company continues to receive technical assistance from the National Institutes of Health. The technical assistance could focus on increasing understanding of the clinical environment, where the technology would initially be deployed, and associated regulations. A pharmaceutical company is interested in investing in the company as part of their impact investing initiative but is hesitant because depression is a small part of their portfolio. A nonprofit organization invests $2 million in concessional debt to the company. With both the technical assistance and concessional capital in place, the pharmaceutical company invests $8 million in debt at market rate. This hypothetic case is an example of how public and philanthropic blended finance instruments attracted private sector early-stage funding by derisking the investment.

The closest example of blended financing for mental health technology is the European Union Innovative Medicines Initiative (IMI). IMI brings together cross-sector partners to accelerate development and access to novel medicines and treatments, particularly in areas of unmet need.[52] IMI partnership focuses on R&D. Both psychiatric and neurocognitive disorders are current IMI health priorities. The IMI is financed at $3.276 billion with half the funding from the public sector, specifically the EU research and innovation program called Horizon 2020.[53,54] The pharmaceutical industry (i.e., European Federation of Pharmaceutical Industries and

Associations [EFPIA]) and other industries or organizations active in health research, called Associated Partners, fund the other half through in-kind contributions such as researcher time or access to facilities. In this collaboration, the private and philanthropic partners provide technical assistance (i.e., in-kind contributions) rather than direct investments, which makes it unique blended financing case. EFPIA and Associated Partners do not receive EU funding, but through intellectual property agreements they have exclusive access to precompetitive discoveries that could be leveraged for future market advantage. The IMI lays out their objectives and goals in a transparent fashion on their website. They also have multiple checks in place to dissuade conflicts of interest.

Funding is distributed to investees using a challenges model. First, an IMI topical group, private sector partner (i.e., an EFPIA company), an Associated Partner, or a third-party identifies a potential topic for a challenge. If EFPIA partners are willing to work collaboratively together and with other stakeholders on the identified topic, topic text is drafted. There is the review by public sector partners including the European Commission before a call for proposals is issued. Successfully applicants are granted funding.

The Remote Assessment of Disease and Relapse–Central Nervous System (RADAR-CNS) is an IMI funded technology project.[55] The project aims to develop remote assessment biomarkers via smartphone and wearables to predict relapse and deterioration in depression, epilepsy, and multiple sclerosis. The cross-sector collaboration between pharmaceutical, biotech, and academic researchers produced RADAR-BASE, an open source mHealth platform to aggregate smartphone and wearable technology data.[55] The inclusion of patients and family members' input project management is exemplary and appears in several IMI projects.

Although promising, there are challenges with blending financing. Organizing the correct set of stakeholders can be difficult and time-consuming. A significant challenge after aggregating funders is the lack of transparency on the process and results.[56] This makes blended finance hard to evaluate. This occurs, in part, because project details are considered business sensitive information. Also, because of the multiple stakeholders involved, it makes it difficult to determine the contribution of individual investments. The difficulties with evaluation and lack of examples leaves little practical guidance for interested groups. Indeed, blended financing has not garnered as much private sector investment as expected, and the healthcare sector is among the least funded.[57]

Conclusion

The health and economic burden of mental illness is huge. The emerging mental health technology revolution offers a unique opportunity to address this burden. To succeed, a shift from long-standing underfunding to commensurate financing of mental health research and treatment is warranted. Fortunately, several financial instruments across the public, nonprofit, and private sectors exist to expand and sustain the role of mental health technology. Hopefully, the financial instruments described in this chapter and others will foster greater stakeholder willingness invest in mental health technology.

References

1. James SL, Abate D, Abate KH, et al. Global, regional, and national incidence, prevalence, and years lived with disability for 354 diseases and injuries for 195 countries and territories, 1990–2017: a systematic analysis for the Global Burden of Disease Study 2017. *The Lancet.* 2018;392(10159):1789–1858.
2. Vigo D, Thornicroft G, Atun R. Estimating the true global burden of mental illness. *The Lancet Psychiatry.* 2016;3(2):171–178 https://doi.org/10.1016/s2215-0366(15)00505-2.
3. Whiteford HA, Degenhardt L, Rehm J, et al. Global burden of disease attributable to mental and substance use disorders: findings from the Global Burden of Disease Study 2010. *The Lancet.* 2013;382(9904):1575–1586 https://doi.org/10.1016/s0140-6736(13)61611-6.
4. Ngo VK, Rubinstein A, Ganju V, et al. Grand challenges: integrating mental health care into the non-communicable disease agenda. *PLoS Medicine.* 2013;10(5):e1001443 https://doi.org/10.1371/journal.pmed.1001443.
5. Woolf SH, Schoomaker H. Life expectancy and mortality rates in the united states, 1959–2017. *JAMA.* 2019;322(20):1996–2016 https://doi.org/10.1001/jama.2019.16932.
6. Roehrig C. Mental disorders top the list of the most costly conditions in the United States: $201 billion. *Health Affairs.* 2016;35(6):1130–1135 https://doi.org/10.1377/hlthaff.2015.1659.
7. Wang PS, Aguilar-Gaxiola S, Alonso J, et al. Use of mental health services for anxiety, mood, and substance disorders in 17 countries in the WHO world mental health surveys. *The Lancet.* 2007;370(9590):841–850 https://doi.org/10.1016/s0140-6736(07)61414-7.
8. Kohn R, Saxena S, Levav I, Saraceno B. The treatment gap in mental health care. *Bulletin of the World Health Organization.* 2004;82:858–866.
9. Thornicroft G, Chatterji S, Evans-Lacko S, et al. Undertreatment of people with major depressive disorder in 21 countries. *The British Journal of Psychiatry.* 2017;210(2):119–124 https://doi.org/10.1192/bjp.bp.116.188078.
10. Alonso J, Liu Z, Evans-Lacko S, et al. Treatment gap for anxiety disorders is global: Results of the World Mental Health Surveys in 21 countries. *Depression and Anxiety.* 2018;35(3):195–208.
11. McLeod JD, Fettes DL. Trajectories of failure: The educational careers of children with mental health problems. *American Journal of Sociology.* 2007;113(3):653–701 https://doi.org/10.1086/521849.
12. Kim-Cohen J, Caspi A, Moffitt TE, Harrington H, Milne BJ, Poulton R. Prior juvenile diagnoses in adults with mental disorder: developmental follow-back of a prospective-longitudinal cohort. *Archives of General Psychiatry.* 2003;60(7):709–717 https://doi.org/10.1001/archpsyc.60.7.709.
13. Kakuma R, Minas H, Van Ginneken N, et al. Human resources for mental health care: current situation and strategies for action. *The Lancet.* 2011;378(9803):1654–1663 https://doi.org/10.1016/s0140-6736(11)61093-3.
14. Saraceno B, van Ommeren M, Batniji R, et al. Barriers to improvement of mental health services in low-income and middle-income countries. *The Lancet.* 2007;370(9593):1164–1174 https://doi.org/10.1016/s0140-6736(07)61263-x.

15. Andrade LH, Alonso J, Mneimneh Z, et al. Barriers to mental health treatment: results from the WHO World Mental Health surveys. *Psychological Medicine*. 2014;44(6):1303–1317 https://doi.org/10.1017/s0033291713001943.

16. Corrigan PW, Druss BG, Perlick DA. The impact of mental illness stigma on seeking and participating in mental health care. *Psychological Science in the Public Interest*. 2014;15(2):37–70 https://doi.org/10.1177/1529100614531398.

17. Sartorius N. Stigma and mental health. *The Lancet*. 2007;370(9590):810–811 https://doi.org/10.1016/s0140-6736(07)61245-8.

18. Rush AJ, Trivedi MH, Wisniewski SR, et al. Acute and longer-term outcomes in depressed outpatients requiring one or several treatment steps: a STAR* D report. *American Journal of Psychiatry*. 2006;163(11):1905–1917 https://doi.org/10.1176/ajp.2006.163.11.1905.

19. Schwab K. *The Fourth Industrial Revolution*. New York: Knopf Doubleday; 2017.

20. Pollitt A, Cochrane G, Kirtley A, et al. Project ecosystem: Mapping the global mental health research funding system. *RAND*; 2016 https://www.rand.org/pubs/research_reports/RR1271.html

21. Insel TR. Join the disruptors of health science. *Nature News*. 2017;551(7678):23 https://doi.org/10.1038/551023a.

22. Brousseau RT, Hyman AD. What do we really know about foundations' funding of mental health? *Health Affairs*. 2009;28(4):1210–1214 https://doi.org/10.1377/hlthaff.28.4.1210.

23. Chevreul K, McDaid D, Farmer CM, et al. Public and nonprofit funding for research on mental disorders in France, the United Kingdom, and the United States. *Journal of Clinical Psychiatry*. 2012;73(7):e906–e912 https://doi.org/10.4088/jcp.11r07418.

24. Liese BH, Gribble RS, Wickremsinhe MN. International funding for mental health: A review of the last decade. *International Health*. 2019;11(5):361–369 https://doi.org/10.1093/inthealth/ihz040.

25. MacEwan JP, Seabury S, Aigbogun MS, et al. Pharmaceutical innovation in the treatment of schizophrenia and mental disorders compared with other diseases. *Innovations in Clinical Neuroscience*. 2016;13(7–8):17.

26. Department of Health and Human Services. Tracking spending–increasing accountability. https://taggs.hhs.gov/. Accessed November 2, 2019.

27. Larrison CR, Hack-Ritzo S, Koerner BD, Schoppelrey SL, Ackerson BJ, Korr WS. Economic grand rounds: state budget cuts, health care reform, and a crisis in rural community mental health agencies. *Psychiatric Services*. 2011;62(11):1255–1257 https://doi.org/10.1176/ps.62.11.pss6211_1255.

28. Day S. Q3 2019: Digital health funding moderates after particularly strong first half. *Rock Health*, 2019; https://rockhealth.com/reports/q3-2019-digital-health-funding-moderates-after-particularly-strong-first-half/.

29. Bobb A. A new frame of mind: Philanthropy's role in mental health's evolving landscape. *Philanthropy Roundtable*; 2019. https://www.philanthropyroundtable.org/docs/default-source/default-document-library/mental-health-briefing_release.pdf?sfvrsn=e643ab40_0

30. Atun R, Silva S, Knaul FM. Innovative financing instruments for global health 2002–15: A systematic analysis. *The Lancet Global Health*. 2017;5(7):e720–e726 https://doi.org/10.1016/s2214-109x(17)30198-5.

31. Cashin C, Sparkes S, Bloom D. Earmarking for health: From theory to practice. *World Health Organization*; 2017. https://www.who.int/health_financing/documents/earmarking-for-health/en/

32. Purtle J, Stadnick NA. Earmarked taxes as a policy strategy to increase funding for behavioral health services. *Psychiatric Services*. 2020;71(1):100–104. https://doi.org/10.1176/appi.ps.201900332.

33. Mental Health Services Oversight and Accountability Commission. Innovation approved projects FY 2018/2019. 2019; https://mhsoac.ca.gov/what-we-do/innovation/approved-projects.

34. California State Auditor. Mental Health Services Act: The state could better ensure the effective use of Mental Health Services Act funding. 2018; http://www.auditor.ca.gov/pdfs/reports/2017-117.pdf.

35. Johnston LM, Finegood DT. Cross-sector partnerships and public health: Challenges and opportunities for addressing obesity and noncommunicable diseases through engagement with the private sector. *Annual Review of Public Health.* 2015;36:255–271 https://doi.org/10.1146/annurev-publhealth-031914-122802.

36. Porter ME, Kramer MR. *Creating shared value. Harvard Business Review.* 2011;11:30.

37. Gustafsson-Wright E, Gardiner S. *Policy recommendations for the applications of impact bonds.* Washington, DC: Brookings Institution; 2015.

38. Social Finance Inc. Impact Bond Global Database. 2019; http://sibdatabase.socialfinance.org.uk/.

39. Rizzello A, Caridà R, Trotta A, Ferraro G, Carè R. The use of payment by results in healthcare: A review and proposal. In: La Torre M, Calderini M, eds. *Social Impact Investing Beyond the SIB.* Cham, Switzerland: Springer; 2018:69–113.

40. Lantz PM, Rosenbaum S, Ku L, Iovan S. Pay for success and population health: Early results from eleven projects reveal challenges and promise. *Health Affairs.* 2016;35(11):2053–2061 https://doi.org/10.1377/hlthaff.2016.0713.

41. Lantz P, Iovan S. When does pay-for-success make sense. *Stanford Social Innovation Review.* 2017;2:2018.

42. Andrews G, Basu A, Cuijpers P, et al. Computer therapy for the anxiety and depression disorders is effective, acceptable and practical health care: An updated meta-analysis. *Journal of Anxiety Disorders.* 2018;55:70–78 https://doi.org/10.1016/j.janxdis.2018.01.001.

43. Paganini S, Teigelkoetter W, Buntrock C, Baumeister H. Economic evaluations of internet- and mobile-based interventions for the treatment and prevention of depression: A systematic review. *Journal of Affective Disorders.* 2018;225:733–755 https://doi.org/10.1016/j.jad.2017.07.018.

44. Donker T, Blankers M, Hedman E, Ljotsson B, Petrie K, Christensen H. Economic evaluations of Internet interventions for mental health: A systematic review. *Psychological Medicine.* 2015;45(16):3357–3376 https://doi.org/10.1017/s0033291715001427.

45. Karyotaki E, Riper H, Twisk J, et al. Efficacy of self-guided internet-based cognitive behavioral therapy in the treatment of depressive symptoms: A meta-analysis of individual participant data. *JAMA Psychiatry.* 2017;74(4):351–359 https://doi.org/10.1001/jamapsychiatry.2017.0044.

46. Titov N, Andrews G, Davies M, McIntyre K, Robinson E, Solley K. Internet treatment for depression: A randomized controlled trial comparing clinician vs. technician assistance. *PloS One.* 2010;5(6):e10939 https://doi.org/10.1371/journal.pone.0010939.

47. Sánchez-Ortiz VC, Munro C, Startup H, Treasure J, Schmidt U. The role of email guidance in Internet-based cognitive-behavioural self-care treatment for bulimia nervosa. *European Eating Disorders Review.* 2011;19(4):342–348 https://doi.org/10.1002/erv.1074.

48. Renn BN, Hoeft TJ, Lee HS, Bauer AM, Areán PA. Preference for in-person psychotherapy versus digital psychotherapy options for depression: survey of adults in the US. *NPJ Digital Medicine.* 2019;2(1):6 https://doi.org/10.1038/s41746-019-0077-1.

49. Rizzello A, Carè R. Insight into the social impact bond market: An analysis of investors. *ACRN Oxford Journal of Finance and Risk Perspectives.* 2016;5(3):145–171.

50. World Economic Forum. *Blended finance Vol. 1: A primer for development finance and philanthropic funders.* Paper presented at World Economic Forum, Geneva, 2015.

51. U.S. Department of Health and Human Services. Three-phase program. 2016; https://sbir.nih.gov/about/three-phase-program.

52. Innovative Medicines Initiative. Strategic research agenda. 2019; https://www.imi.europa.eu/about-imi/strategic-research-agenda.

53. Innovative Medicines Initiative. The IMI funding model. 2019; https://www.imi.europa.eu/about-imi/imi-funding-model.

54. Faure J-E, Dyląg T, Norstedt I, Matthiessen L. The European Innovative Medicines Initiative: Progress to date. *Pharmaceutical medicine*. 2018;32(4):243–249 https://doi.org/10.1007/s40290-018-0241-y.

55. Ranjan Y, Rashid Z, Stewart C, et al. RADAR-Base: Open source mobile health platform for collecting, monitoring, and analyzing data using sensors, wearables, and mobile devices. *JMIR mHealth and uHealth*. 2019;7(8):e11734.

56. Organisation for Economic Co-operation and Development. The next step in blended finance: Addressing the evidence gap in development performance and results. 2018; https://www.oecd.org/dac/financing-sustainable-development/development-finance-topics/OECD-Blended%20Finance-Evidence-Gap-report.pdf.

57. Larrea J. The state of blended finance 2019: Reflections from the CEO. 2019; convergence.finance/news-and-events/news/2l8EWsMCFluc60m06fW658/view.

35

Convergence Mental Health

Barriers, Solutions, and Actionable Avenues for Philanthropic Investment

James A. Randall and Cara M. Altimus

Introduction

Global Mental Health Crisis Necessitates New Scientific Approaches

In 2017, the National Institute of Mental Health found that an estimated one in five U.S. adults lived with a mental illness (approximately 46.6 million people).[1] Younger individuals (aged 18–25) reported higher prevalence of mental illness than their older peers and often receive mental health services at lower rates.[2]

The high rates of mental illness incidence contributes to high healthcare costs and economic impacts globally. Researchers have suggested that by 2020, the United States will spend approximately $238 billion on mental health services each year.[3] Globally, *The Lancet*'s Commission on Global Mental Health and Sustainable Development reported that mental health conditions "cause more years lived with disability (32.4% [of total across all noncommunicable diseases]) than any other health condition and nearly as many disability-adjusted life-years (13.0%) as cardiovascular disease (13.5%)."[4]

While the global effect is staggering, so is the economic impact: it is estimated that more than 12 billion working days are lost each year to mental health conditions, likely costing the global economy $16 trillion in lost economic output between 2011 and 2030.[4] These figures are staggering and are more impactful than cancer, diabetes, and respiratory diseases combined. Thus, not only does mental illness impact interpersonal dynamics and each person individually, but it also has a profound impact on the United States and global economies.

These high costs exist in a broader context of rising healthcare costs. In 2017, the U.S. healthcare system cost $3.5 trillion, accounting for 17.9% of the United States gross domestic product. The Centers for Medicare and Medicaid Services estimate that costs will continue to rise and that by 2026, the healthcare system will cost over $5.7 trillion, or 19.7% of the gross domestic product.[5] Traditional factors lending to this increased cost in healthcare, such as implementing new medical innovations, defensive medicine, and the treatment of chronic diseases may all be grouped together under the premise of reactive medicine. Much of the healthcare delivered in the United States is reactive, rather than proactive, treating disease after it develops, rather than preventing it from developing in the first place.

Mental healthcare presents specific challenges that contribute to reactive medicine approaches. Specifically, physicians lack objective diagnostic and theragnostic tools across conditions, which results in high rates of misdiagnosis. However, research continues to show that differences in neural function underlies these conditions and that distinction of patients using physiologically based markers will be necessary to appropriately identify, diagnosis, and treat mental illness.

Precision medicine and convergence science approaches are beginning to be applied to mental health and hold incredible promise for addressing the rapidly increasing cost of healthcare, mental healthcare delivery, and the toll that mental health takes on an individual. The ultimate goal of precision health and convergence mental health is not to simply treat illness after onset, but rather prevent it from arising in the first place by using an individual's unique genetic, social, and medical characteristics to most properly and expertly prevent illness from arising in the first place. Precision mental health could deliver healthcare to each person using their individual, unique characteristics, rather than being based on a collective average.

New and emerging technologies, such as digital health tracking, genomic sequencing, telehealth, and digital therapeutics aid in facilitating the national transition from reactive, "sick care" toward proactive "healthcare." In effort to have a more individualized conversation with a medical or mental healthcare provider to address the unique root of an issue, new technologies help in establishing and understanding an individual's

- Physiological and mental health baseline;
- Environment and behavior and how those may manifest as pathological and mental health changes;
- Genetic predisposition to disease and mental health disorders; and
- Risk of developing disease.

Step 1: Improving Science for Quantitative Diagnostic Tools

New and emerging technologies hold significant promise in preventing, diagnosing, and treating mental health disorders. Such new innovations drive progress in precision health and have the potential to track an individual's mental and/or physical health trends over time, enabling providers to work with the individual to use their information in guiding prevention and treatment plans.

Genetic Approaches

Genetic testing is becoming an increasingly popular method for assessing one's risk of developing disease or mental health disorders and in treating them. Direct-to-consumer genetic testing kits from companies like Helix, Novogene, and 23andMe provide the opportunity for individuals to easily determine their genetic profile. These companies and others like them ask participants to collect a biological sample—generally a saliva sample—and will then assess that individual's risk for a number of factors, such as the likelihood of inheriting specific genetic disorders or assessing the risk of epigenetic-based disease development for diseases like type 2 diabetes.

Mental health and genetics, however, have a more complex relationship. Mental health follows a different model than the traditional often unifactorial cause of genetic disease, where mutations within a specific gene or set of genes cause specific and predictable biological changes that manifest as disease. Geneticists instead posit that while mental illness may have a genetic root, these genetic roots are multifaceted, spanning a wide variety of genetic loci. The field of epigenetics, for example, demonstrates that there is a complex relationship between genes and the environment and that sometimes disease or illness is the result of not just genetic causes, but also from the impact of the environment on genes.[6] While future research may identify specific genes that drive identifiable changes of brain function that result in mental illness, current dogma suggests that genetic differences confer risk of disease and when in the presence of environmental, family, or lifestyle differences may result in disease development.

Although the field is still nascent, investigating the risk of developing disease and mental illness based on genetics (especially through direct-to-consumer testing) holds significant promise, especially with regard to mental health. Information from easy-to-use testing may better facilitate conversations between provider and patient and may thus facilitate a transition from reactive mental healthcare to proactive mental healthcare. Ultimately, understanding the genetic contributors of mental illness and lending the tool to do so to providers and consumers holds promise in the field. The following are some identified positives and negatives of giving consumers access to such tools:

Positives

- Understands risk of developing disorder.
- Allows individuals to take pre-emptive measures for dealing with mental health disorders.
- Allows for an open conversation with mental health provider about addressing issues before they arise.
- Mitigates health disparities associated with differences in access.

Negatives

- Creates unnecessary risk, anxiety.
- Has weaker or insufficient evidence for underrepresented populations.

Expanding Brain Imaging

Brain imaging has been incorporated into clinical practice for over 40 years. Scanning tools, such as magnetic resonance imaging and positron emission topography, among others, are useful in noninvasively investigating the brain. Clinically, these strategies are largely useful in diagnosing the presence of any structural abnormalities and for characterizing tumors, inflammation, and other organic processes.[7]

The use and study of brain imaging techniques for psychiatric conditions has been difficult thus far. Consequently, brain imaging is not yet used for clinical diagnosis; however, researchers and clinicians have learned a lot from these imaging studies, which can be used to inform future research. Brain imaging studies have further highlighted that within defined mental health conditions, there are likely specific unique subtypes that may have differing underlying mechanisms which result in similar or overlapping symptomatic profiles.

An imaging study of more than 1,000 individuals diagnosed with depression found four different subtypes and could use the grouping to predict who would respond to a specific treatment.[8] Additionally, the use of imaging highlights that several specific regions of the brain show abnormal activity across a number of disorders, demonstrating both the potential for common underlying mechanisms and the need for further work on differential diagnosis.

Looking forward, brain imaging provides unique data that in combination with other data types such as genetic information, activity data, or other biological markers may fundamentally change the understanding of how psychiatric conditions are classified. Therefore, using brain imaging as a tool for diagnosing or finding biomarkers of mental illness likely requires significantly more clinical development.

Integration of Digital Health Trackers

Digital health trackers highlight individuals' unique health profiles based on both biology and lifestyle. Digital health trackers range in appearance and method but often incorporate everyday technology, like smartwatches and smartphones. The applications on the devices or the devices themselves regularly collect information—either autonomously or input manually by the user—about an individual's lifestyle, food choices, and physiological activity.

Digital health tracking technologies hold promise in the mental health space by regularly capturing a user's energy level, mood, emotions, medication interactions, or biomarker indicators of certain mental health disorders (such as increased perspiration denoting anxiety), among others. The type of information to be collected can be decided through a discussion between a provider and a user, ultimately delivering a clearer, more individualized picture of a person. The individualized aspect of care may then be used to track progress over time and foster more targeted interventions or implementation of better preventative measures.

Circadian Rhythms and Digital Health Trackers

Circadian rhythms have been implicated in the regulation of certain genes, which may impact the quality of sleep and cognitive performance. Recent evidence suggests a link between the circadian rhythm-based gene activation and mood disorders, which may help explain some of the linkages between season-based light sensitivity and disrupted sleep patterns with major depressive disorder. Digital health trackers, through the use of applications and wearable technologies, have the opportunity to track these cycles, measure light exposure and the like, and perhaps give a clearer picture as to how a person experiences mood disorders and where strategic intervention may be offered.

Digital Therapeutics and Telehealth

The rising arena of telehealth facilitates better access to not just physical care, but also mental healthcare. Telehealth enables access to mental healthcare resources for individuals in remote, underserved areas, for individuals in areas where mental health sources are limited, and for individuals wary of receiving mental healthcare services face to face. Private organizations sometimes form partnerships with workplaces or with educational establishments to provide easier-to-access mental healthcare with increased convenience.

Telehealth's ease of use holds promise in increasing access to mental healthcare resources in not just the United States, but also around the world. As it gains popularity, insurers in the United States, including Medicare, are beginning to reimburse for this service. By increasing access, telehealth promises to eventually lower the cost of healthcare by facilitating better primary and mental healthcare delivery and by avoiding medical and mental health complications stemming from a lack of prevention. As it grows, telehealth may even be able to link to digital health technologies to relay information to clinicians in real time. The following are some positives and negatives for the consumer:

Positives

- Mitigates health disparities associated with geographically-based access differences.
- Facilitates better and more ubiquitous access to care.
- Increases the personalization of healthcare delivery.
- Fosters better dialogue between consumer and clinician.
- As it gains popularity, the incentive for insurance to reimburse increases.
- Holds promise for the integration of digital health tracking.

Negatives

- Can be cost-prohibitive.
- Requires access to internet and smart technologies.
- In some cases, requires access to employment.
- Does little to address stigma surrounding mental health.

Advancing the Science of Peripheral Systems

Several hypotheses have emerged in identifying biomarkers for the onset of mental health. Biomarkers are helpful not only for clinicians to more confidently diagnose mental illness, but also for enterprise. Enterprises may develop products, which after rigorous Food and Drug Administration (FDA) testing and authorization, can use these biomarkers to identify the presence, onset, or progressive development of disease. The identification of which will help clinicians and consumers to integrate technology with their healthcare and ultimately better prevent the onset of disease. What follows are several of the leading biomarker hypotheses, which have therapeutic and industry potential.

Inflammation
Inflammation is the body's defense mechanism when it becomes attacked or invaded by some foreign insult, whether a germ or a physical foreign body, like a splinter. When an invader is detected, the body releases a number of hormones to recruit responder cells to the area. The nearby blood vessels swell, diverting blood to the affected areas. The swollen blood vessels, in addition to the recruited white blood cells—the body's chief fighter—cause the affected area to seem swollen and red.

While inflammation was originally thought to only be associated with defense against out-of-body insults, new research suggests that general inflammation, more specifically inflammation in the brain, is correlated with the presentation of major depressive disorder (MDD).

When the body begins fighting an infection, it recruits many organ systems outside of the affected area. When the body initiates this systemic response, individuals often begin presenting with cognitive and behavioral changes, many of which parallel depression-like symptoms, including needing excessive sleep, slowed reaction times, and loss of appetite. Long-term exposure to the body's systemic inflammatory reaction is now thought to correlate with the onset of MDD.

More specifically, the research, while nascent, has shown that some individuals living with depression have elevated blood-levels of inflammatory agents.[9] When the brain initiates its inflammatory response, imaging shows that certain cells, called microglia, are overactive in the prefrontal cortex; that same immune overactivity is sometimes seen in individuals living with MDD. Finally, some of the same symptoms of depression (fatigue, social disinterest, and failure to concentrate) are present when the immune system activates to fight infection.

This research, while currently localized to MDD, shows promise in fostering a more biological understanding of mental health and holds promise as a means to better therapeutically treat mental health disorders. Furthermore, this budding biological field of mental health is prime with opportunity for investment and research, including in the development of new devices, which may better diagnose and treat mental health disorders.

Stress Response

When the body encounters some stressor, it activates the stress pathway; more specifically, it activates the hypothalamic–pituitary–adrenal (HPA) axis. Under normal circumstances, the body encounters an acute stressor, activates the pathway, and subsequently deactivates it once the stress has passed. In some cases, however, the HPA axis remains active over a longer period of time or is continuously activated as a result of encountering chronic stressors. It is this chronic HPA activation, or hyperactivation of the pathway, that is thought to be a major biological contributor in the etiology of several mental health disorders, including MDD.[10]

HPA axis activation is thus implicated in the recruitment of many of the believed biological causes of mental health disorders. As such, it has potential as an area of advanced biological research and investment.

Microbiota

When thinking of biological systems related to mental health, the gut and its microbiome rarely come to mind. Recent research, however, suggests that it should. Among the newer approaches to mental health is the microbiota–gut–brain axis.[11] The gut microbiome plays an integral role in the body's stress response, being activated by the HPA axis, so abnormal microbiomes may be linked to anxiety and stress disorders.

A mouse study conducted almost two decades ago and repeated in 2015 showed that when mice without any bacteria in their gut received microbiome transplants from other mice, the recipient mice adopted some of the same behavioral characteristics as the donor mice.[12] The linkage suggests that the microbiome plays an integral role in development, including perhaps in the onset of psychological illness.[13]

With budding research into the field of gut–brain science comes revolutionary opportunity to invest and develop new treatment and diagnostic modalities for mental health, furthering the importance of understanding each consumer as an individual and incorporating that individuality into their treatment.

Step 2: Matching Therapeutic and Interventional Strategies

Early Success: Chronotype and Bipolar Disorder

Broadly, a chronotype is defined by how a person spends their day sleeping and working. While the circadian rhythm dictates sleep-wake cycles, the chronotype dictates an individual's productivity and sleep period timing. In other words, the chronotype is when a person prefers to carry out their daily activities ranked on a scale of morningness to eveningness.

Evidence suggests that there is a link between the disruption of one's circadian rhythm/chronotype and experiencing bipolar symptoms.[14] Daily melatonin and cortisol levels were delayed in individuals experiencing bipolar compared to individuals who do not display bipolar symptoms; additionally, there was a clear association between alterations in circadian rhythms and depression. Individuals with bipolar tend to qualify more as evening type as well.

Thus treatments targeting not just biochemical pathways, but also circadian rhythm cycles may be effective moving forward, suggesting a pressing need to treat not just pharmacologically, but also appropriately for each individual. Studies investigating the utility of chronotherapeutic interventions in individuals with bipolar disorder have been effective, with some studies reporting that sleep deprivation in conjunction with intensive light therapy have been as effective, if not more effective than standard treatment for depression.[14] Chronotherapy, while new, may yet prove to be an innovative and noninvasive approach to addressing mood disorders and demonstrates that therapeutic interventions must match the individual characteristics of the individual experiencing the symptoms. It holds promise as an interdisciplinary field with opportunity for investment from multiple interrelated stakeholders.

Early Success: Ketamine and Depression

Ketamine is a key anesthetic that the World Health Organization considers an essential medicine. Ketamine use is sometimes stigmatized, however, due to its recreational use as a hallucinogen. As its perception teeters between being essential and being stigmatized, new clinical evidence suggests that ketamine treatment (administered by medical professionals in controlled dosages) can dramatically and expeditiously reduce symptoms of depression, especially in individuals with treatment-resistant depression.

New self-administered ketamine nasal spray treatments, which were approved by the FDA on March 5, 2019, have seen significant reduction in depression symptoms in as few as two days. Ketamine as a therapeutic thus holds significant promise in treating both acute depressive episodes and in treating long-term depressive symptoms.

Recent IV-infused ketamine trials have even shown complete alleviation of depressive symptoms and suicidal ideation within minutes of infusion.

Ketamine holds promise as a new mover in the mental health field. Ketamine has the potential to treat acute depressive episodes, moving the medical dogma toward acute care, rather than trial-and-error chronic care.

Barriers and Opportunities to Precision Mental Health

In 2017, the Milken Institute Center for Strategic Philanthropy conducted a landscape analysis through interviews with key opinion leaders in the field, a systems-based analysis, and a funder's summit in effort to better understand the barriers to more broadly implementing precision health-based interventions. However, the barriers to implementation of precision health approaches are broadly relevant to the study of convergence mental health.

Broadly, four barriers were described as follows:

1. Insufficient scientific evidence;
2. Insufficient data sharing between relevant health partners;
3. Lack of field-wide coordination; and
4. Difficulties with access, including: insurance, providers, and availability of practice.

Barrier 1: Insufficient Scientific Evidence

Evidence is the foundation for which all scientific endeavors, including convergence mental health, are based. The integration of technologies and the renewed focus on the individual, as opposed to a standardized or generalized person, must pair evidence with decisions and treatment plans tailored to every distinct individual. The purpose of evidence is to facilitate objectivity by allaying conflicts of interest, mitigating human error, and providing the most appropriate care for each individual. In pursuit of this mission of objectivity and ubiquitous application, there must be more evidence in areas related to convergence mental health to substantiate it.

Funding
As the field of convergence mental health grows and more evidence becomes available, so too will the number of funders and stakeholders. Funders unanimously cite inadequate scientific evidence as a major barrier toward more proactive and integrated healthcare delivery. The science surrounding the field to date is missing, largely due to heterogeneous populations, insufficient frequency of physiological measurements, and a large majority of available data being taken from individuals following a diagnosis. While much of the present science misses key underserved populations and may be small in scale, organizations like the National Institutes of Health (NIH) have made efforts to champion these studies so desperately needed in the field, a key example being their All of Us campaign. Once the science becomes more robust, donors may become more involved and help move the field forward.

Quantifying Health
Given its complexity, health and mental health are inherently difficult to measure; add on the stigma associated with mental health, and the task becomes yet more difficult. Health and mental health are completely individualized, with each person's experience novel and unlike someone else's, thus it becomes difficult to standardize measurements not only between persons but within persons as well. To effectively treat and provide individualized care, clinicians must be able to compare a person's health and mental health to a baseline. Currently physicians rely on self-reported changes in energy and mood, but when disorders such as bipolar disorder and schizophrenia are associated with impaired self-awareness or anosognosia, individuals may not have the capacity to recognize that differences in their own energy and mood are problematic.

Reactive healthcare makes measuring health over time difficult and comparing to an individual's baseline even more so. More streamlined mental health metrics will not only make it easier for clinicians and consumers alike to track their health, but also for digital health trackers to have suitable standards to facilitate that health tracking. Better data sharing and better quantification metrics will allow both providers and consumers to make better use of their health information, track the information over time, and make more informed healthcare decisions.

Having a better sense of what one's health looks like and how it changes over time will allow individuals to better advocate for themselves and have a better sense of what defines "sick" and what defines "healthy." To achieve this, interest groups will need to develop better individual health monitoring devices, which can be validated against FDA-approved metrics and which can collect data points outside of clinical care visits.

Opportunities for private and public entities to promote the development and standardization of health tools are as follows.

1. Include convergence mental health and precision health tools in current and future longitudinal research studies in effort to both standardize and evaluate effectiveness;.
2. Develop partnerships between nonprofit, government, and for-profit organizations to standardize technology and ensure that tools are safe to use in clinical settings, ensuring that all data collected by convergence mental health tools are streamlined with little to no doubt of their validity.
3. Support comparative effectiveness trials of different types of non-invasive health monitoring and measurement tools.
4. Develop standardized practices among device manufacturers.
5. Coordinate a nonprofit effort to develop a convergence mental health or precision health seal of approval, signifying that a newly developed tool passes industry standards for clinical practice after FDA approval.

Understanding the Multifaceted Contributions of Genes, Environment, and Lifestyle to Mental Health

Given health and mental health's intricate relations with environment, lifestyle, and genetics, practitioners must have a way to effectively quantify these factors. Research exploring the impact of these factors on health may elucidate more tangible health and preventative benefits, enabling better advocacy in the political arena and between provider and consumer. Ultimately, these factors will facilitate better individualized care delivery in addition to lowering the cost of care delivery. Paths to facilitate the inclusion of these factors in health include the following.

1. Develop new products with providers in mind to gather data for use in clinical practice. For example, companies could make data from tools like FitBit, Sworkit, or the Apple Watch more accessible to providers to facilitate treatment plans.
2. Ensure that newly developed devices are to FDA medical device standards for more ubiquitous use in the clinic.
3. Fund pathways to support the validation of convergence mental health tools to be used in the clinic.
4. Expand upon data and findings from large national studies like NIH's All of Us program; partnerships could collect additional data types and test new tools.

Health Economics

In the current healthcare model, health costs and associated economics are not factored into the development of new interventions or coverage of those interventions. Large healthcare payers, such as the Centers for Medicare and Medicaid and private insurers, need to see evidence of return on investment to invest in convergence mental health and important new interventions. These payers must see merit in shifting toward value-based care, which better research on cost can provide.

Should nonprofits, for-profits, and government-based organizations support health economics research, key interest groups may better understand the long-term economic impact of using precision health and convergence mental health tools, moving the field into the mainstream, ultimately attracting the attention of private donors.

Barrier 2: Insufficient Data Sharing Between Health Partners

Private entities and organizations have little incentive to share their health information. Health information to many companies is proprietary and a blossoming business arena. Some business models have even morphed into the monetization of health data. Data repositories do exist, but are often fragmented within each scientific field; some examples of isolated databases include the Influenza Research Database, FlyBase, ChEMBL, and the NOMAD Repository. As the call for broader repositories becomes amplified, there is still continued need for collaboration among research entities. Of the many related data sharing issues, three key problems exist:

1. Data collaboration;
2. The need for large data sets and the technology infrastructure necessary to facilitate cooperation; and
3. Data privacy.

Data Collaboration and Consolidation

To effectively understand the impact of how interrelated factors, like lifestyle, environment, genetics, and economics impact health, researchers require significant amounts of data. Data on these factors exist, although are largely fragmented; consolidation of data can thus be incentivized through better cooperation and data sharing. Without collaboration, innovative breakthroughs will take longer and in some cases, may never become apparent. There is, however, a major solution apparent in this arena, which may be facilitated by third-party investors: provide funds specifically for the purpose of gathering, storing, analyzing, and sharing data.

Missing Large, Cumulative Data Sets, and Tech Infrastructure for Cooperation

Current infrastructure available to facilitate information data sharing is sparse and the infrastructure that exists must abide by stringent, albeit necessary Health Insurance Portability and Accessibility Act (HIPAA) guidelines to protect consumer privacy. While some companies have taken collaborative steps to create cloud-based data sharing modalities, there is still not enough infrastructure given inadequate support.

Most biobanks and electronic health records contain vast amounts of consumer data, although very little of it is available to researchers. Should these data become de-identified and available to researchers, investigators may uncover key metrics related to quantifying health, including identifying associations between mental health and a multitude of psychosociocultural factors.

There are solutions available to combat the lack of open data available for cooperation:

1. Create specialized data platforms to facilitate data sharing and expand existing platforms and policies.
2. Organization partnerships with funding offered to groups doing work related to the development of or expansion of data collaboration efforts.
3. Expand data collection efforts, such as NIH's All of Us program, which aim to increase representativeness of data through large-scale population recruitment and purposeful inclusion of otherwise underrepresented groups in medicine and mental health.
4. Facilitate partnerships among academic institutions and health systems to combine data sets, keep data open to access, and create larger, multidisciplinary data sets.

Maintain the Privacy and Confidentiality of Data

Landmark U.S. legislation in the form of HIPAA and the Genetic Information Nondiscrimination Act provided healthcare consumers with a right to privacy. However, some of the new influx of devices and innovations—including their vague categorization as medical device-adjacent tools—have called into question what should be considered HIPAA protected. Thus, not all information remains private; significant difficulties still remain in terms of which devices keep this information private and which do not.

Social media and nonmedical devices can circumnavigate most laws and regulations concerning healthcare consumer privacy, which is especially concerning considering the frequency of attacks on this information. New innovations seeking to enhance health and mental health must thus be capable of navigating these constant threats and new regulations.

An emerging solution in the fight to maintain privacy is blockchain. Blockchain is a decentralized database of sorts that stores information at many isolated points, meaning that if a hacker attempts to steal information, he or she can be easily identified. Additionally, it is exceedingly difficult to steal a complete file or data series using blockchain. Thus, its implementation in securing health information may prove significantly useful.

Barrier 3: Fieldwide Coordination

Health-based technology fields are constantly changing, with new players entering regularly. However, given the lack of infrastructure, direct collaboration, and data sharing, progress is slow. Furthermore, there is no current coordinated effort to sustain advocacy, coordinate research, or engage stakeholders.[15] The aforementioned issues, as well as other related ones, fall broadly into four key gaps to coordination:

1. Education;
2. Advocacy;
3. Research coordination efforts; and
4. Consumer input.

The most efficient solution to address all four major gaps is to found an organization that focuses exclusively on convergence mental health. Such an organization would bring together stakeholders who could guide the field, being transformative in addressing unmet gaps or coordination issues pertaining to convergence mental health. Currently established organizations with mental health-focused mission could aid in the effort via more targeted efforts as well. A convergence health-focused organization, however, could close the four major gaps by addressing many of the convergence mental health coordination issues through the following:

1. Create educational materials and develop related provider outreach programs.
2. Unite the many health-focused, health technology-focused, and consumer advocacy organizations.
3. Fund efforts to coordinate research.
4. Develop a forum for public and consumer engagement in addition to funding efforts to gather consumer input.

Barrier 4: Access—Insurance, Providers, and Practice

Mental health disorders, while being some of the most common disorders impacting people around the world, are still commonly undiagnosed and untreated. Contributors to the unfortunate phenomenon include stigma, lack of effective therapies, and inadequate mental health resources. A report from the Global Health Observatory supposes that 45% of the world's population have only one psychiatrist per 100,000 people.[16] Clearly there is a need for better access to mental healthcare, which may be facilitated in the United States through better reimbursement practices.

Insurance and Reimbursement
Most recent data suggest that as many as 10% of adults with diagnosed mental illnesses are uninsured. While the implementation of the Affordable Care Act is estimated to have reduced that percentage by 1.9%, there are still a significant number of individuals who have a mental illness but whom are uninsured.[17] Regardless of insurance status, almost 60% of estimated individuals with mental illness do not receive treatment; additionally, given the stigmatized nature of mental illness, the percentage of individuals with a mental health disorder who do not seek treatment is likely much greater.

Even for individuals with insurance, a survey by the National Alliance on Mental Illness found that over half of the mental health providers that individuals with insurance contacted were not accepting new patients or would not accept their insurance; one-third even reported that they more broadly had significant difficulty finding any mental health provider who would accept their insurance.[18]

Mental health services are reimbursed at different rates than are their physical health counterparts. One study focused on MDD found that for every US$1 that insurance companies reimbursed primary healthcare physicians for services rendered, mental health professionals were only reimbursed 83 cents.[19] The inequity in pay partly explains why psychiatrists accept insurance at a lower rate than do other providers.

When healthcare providers stop taking insurance, socioeconomically disadvantaged populations suffer. Many become subjected to a cyclical lack of treatment, perpetuating mental health issues, and driving an increased need for providers, who remain largely unaffordable.

Congress, seeking to alleviate some of the issues surrounding mental healthcare access, passed the Mental Health Parity and Addiction Equity Act in 2008. This landmark piece of legislation was further amended by the Affordable Care Act and sought to prevent health insurers from limiting mental healthcare benefits at an inequitable rate compared to physical health benefits. Insurers could no longer impose annual or lifetime limits on mental health benefits, although the congressional act did not actually require insurers to provide mental health or substance use disorder coverage.

Despite many of the issues surrounding access to care, some broad solutions exist:

1. Medicare, Medicaid, and private insurers become obligated to reimburse for mental healthcare in the same way and at the same rate that they do for physical healthcare services.
2. Foster greater collaboration between advocacy, government, and private interest organizations to transition the public dialogue surrounding mental health disorders to where they are discussed with the same considerations as physical health disorders.

Mental Health Care Practice and Stigma

Stigma remains one of the greatest and most pressing barriers facing better mental healthcare. Stigma disincentivizes health-seeking behavior, stereotyping and prejudicing those who decide to seek treatment. Studies suggest that the more individuals endorse the stigmatization of mental health, the less likely they are to seek treatment.[20]

Current clinical practice and subsequent treatment of many mental health disorders mandate that such disorders be classified along binary means, rather than as a continuum. There remains a conflict between clinical categories of mental health and the experience of those living within those categories and beyond. Moreover, experience of mental health and clinical characterization of mental health can be at odds.[21]

Take for example the age of onset for MDD. Current dogma suggests that fewer than one percent of MDD cases observe pediatric onset (before age 12); however, findings from a Milken Institute survey instead suggest that upwards of 50% to 80%

of individuals begin experiencing MDD symptoms before the age of 18, with approximately 25% of their survey respondents indicating that symptoms began before age 12. Thus there is a significant proportion of the MDD population that is being overlooked and is not being characterized or treated by mental healthcare professionals.[21]

Overall, there is a discrepancy between how clinicians view mental illness and how people living with mental health disorders describe their experience. Practice must be configured to meet the needs of those who experience problems. Additionally, recognizing and thwarting the effects of stigma will be useful. There are several potential solutions moving forward:

1. Coordinate government, drug development, clinician, and lived experience perspectives to develop better descriptions, interventions, and therapeutics for a number of mental health disorders, which incorporate a whole person and their lived experiences.
2. Develop more concurrent descriptions, interventions, and therapeutics for individuals living with mental health disorders, based on the lived experience perspectives and incorporation of the whole person.
3. Modify healthcare policy to better reflect access to pediatric health, specifically pediatric mental health.
4. Foster provider education, which includes lived experience, as a means to reduce stigma and lend credence to individuals living with mental health disorders.

Why Philanthropy Is Important

Historically, funding of the scientific enterprise has been left to government bodies and commercial industries, especially in the United States. This trend leads back to several important realities, one of which is the significant level of capital investment and infrastructure required to support meaningful academic research and clinical development. Governments can often provide consistent funding to a breadth of research topics, while industry can move new therapies from benchtop to population.

Nevertheless, problems can emerge when only government and industry distribute the wealth in science. For instance, government funds can be slow to respond, given bureaucracy and priority changes after elections. Additionally, government funders are usually risk averse, typically favoring more "accepted" research and thereby leaving little room for creativity or untested ideas. On the other side, commercial players—from pharmaceutical giants to emerging biotechnology firms—are beholden to their investors who can also be wary of uncertainty. Similarly, when the financial or research bottom line is not met on funded projects, private investors may divest regardless of how successful—or needed—the research itself may be. The combination of these two realities can lead to stagnation in scientific innovation, that is, an inability to react quickly to a changing climate and gaps in funding to address complex problems.

Philanthropic capital can fill the gaps where commercial and government funds fall short. Foundations and philanthropists alike can fund cutting-edge research and novel hypotheses, providing the seed that might spark a field-altering discovery or spawn a new branch of science. In addition, they can move quickly in response to immediate needs, whether because of defunding through other mechanisms or a crisis. An infusion of philanthropic funds can derisk a sector and demonstrate proof of concept. Philanthropy can act where other entities cannot—bridging sectors despite partisanship, bottom lines, or policy stances—and provide support where most needed.

Philanthropy, however, has limitations. In the United States, philanthropic capital represents a small percentage of overall scientific funding—merely 2% to 4%, depending on how it is counted. Therefore, this capital must be invested as wisely as possible to ensure that it reaps the desired dividends.

Using a systems-based approach and a cross-sectoral vantage point, philanthropy can be used strategically to solve some of the most challenging problems in science and beyond.

References

1. Bose J, Hedden SL, Lipari RN, Park-Lee E. Key substance use and mental health indicators in the United States: Results from the 2017 National Survey on Drug Use and Health. *Substance Abuse and Mental Health Services Administration.* September 2018. https://www.samhsa.gov/data/sites/default/files/cbhsq-reports/NSDUHFFR2017/NSDUHFFR2017.pdf.
2. Merikangas KR, He J-P, Burstein M, et al. Lifetime prevalence of mental disorders in U.S. adolescents: results from the National Comorbidity Survey Replication—Adolescent Supplement (NCS-A). *J Am Acad Child Adolesc Psychiatry.* 2010;49(10):980-989. doi:10.1016/j.jaac.2010.05.017
3. Levit K, RIchardson J, Frankel S, et al. Substance Abuse and Mental Health Services Administration. Projections of national expenditures for treatment of mental and substance use disorders, 2010–2020. *Substance Abuse and Mental Health Services Administration.* October 2014. https://store.samhsa.gov/product/Projections-of-National-Expenditures-for-Treatment-of-Mental-and-Substance-Use-Disorders-2010-2020/SMA14-4883.
4. Patel V, Saxena S, Lund C, et al. The Lancet Commission on global mental health and sustainable development. *Lancet.* 2018;392(10157):1553-1598. doi:10.1016/S0140-6736(18)31612-X
5. Martin AB, Hartman M, Washington B, Catlin A; The National Health Expenditure Accounts Team. National health care spending in 2017: growth slows to post–great recession rates; share of GDP stabilizes. *Health Aff.* 2018;38(1):10.1377/hlthaff.2018.05085. doi:10.1377/hlthaff.2018.05085
6. Hyman SE. The genetics of mental illness: implications for practice. *Bull World Health Org.* 2000;78(4): 455-463.
7. Falkai P, Schmitt A, Andreasen N. Forty years of structural brain imaging in mental disorders: is it clinically useful or not? *Dialogues Clin Neurosci.* 2018;20(3):179-186.
8. Drysdale AT, Grosenick L, Downar J, et al. Resting-state connectivity biomarkers define neurophysiological subtypes of depression. *Nature Med.* 2017;23(1):28-38. doi:10.1038/nm.4246
9. Zunszain PA, Hepgul N, Pariante CM. Inflammation and depression. In: Cowen PJ, Sharp T, Lau JYF, eds. *Behavioral Neurobiology of Depression and Its Treatment.* Berlin: Springer; 2013:135-151. doi:10.1007/7854_2012_211

10. Lamers F, Vogelzangs N, Merikangas KR, de Jonge P, Beekman ATF, Penninx BWJH. Evidence for a differential role of HPA-axis function, inflammation and metabolic syndrome in melancholic versus atypical depression. *Mol Psychiatry.* 2013;18(6):692-699. doi:10.1038/mp.2012.144

11. Malan-Muller S, Valles-Colomer M, Raes J, Lowry CA, Seedat S, Hemmings SMJ. The gut microbiome and mental health: implications for anxiety- and trauma-related disorders. *OMICS.* 2018;22(2):90-107. doi:10.1089/omi.2017.0077

12. De Palma G, Blennerhassett P, Lu J, et al. Microbiota and host determinants of behavioural phenotype in maternally separated mice. *Nature Comm.* 2015;6(1):1-13. doi:10.1038/ncomms8735

13. Schmidt C. Mental health: thinking from the gut. *Nature.* 2015;518(7540):S12-S15. doi:10.1038/518S13a

14. Melo MCA, Abreu RLC, Linhares Neto VB, de Bruin PFC, de Bruin VMS. Chronotype and circadian rhythm in bipolar disorder: a systematic review. *Sleep Med Rev.* 2017;34:46-58. doi:10.1016/j.smrv.2016.06.007

15. Randall JA, Altimus C, Hsiao YL, Briggs L. Next generation prevention: a giving smarter guide. *Milken Institute.* January 2019. https://milkeninstitute.org/sites/default/files/reports-pdf/Next-Gen-Prevention-GSG-FINAL2.pdf.

16. Global Health Observatory. Global Health Observatory data repository: by category/human resources—data by country. *World Health Organization.* http://apps.who.int/gho/data/node.main.MHHR?lang=en. Accessed November 28, 2019.

17. Hellebuyck M, Halpern M, Nguyen T, Fritze D. The state of mental health in America. *Mental Health America.* 2018. https://mhanational.org/sites/default/files/2019-09/2019%20MH%20in%20America%20Final.pdf.

18. Diehl S, Honberg R, Kimball A, Douglas D, Medoff D. The doctor is out: continuing disparities in access to mental and physical health care. *National Alliance on Mental Illness.* November 2017. https://www.nami.org/About-NAMI/Publications-Reports/Public-Policy-Reports/The-Doctor-is-Out/DoctorIsOut.pdf.

19. Davenport S. Melek S, Perlman D, Addiction and mental health vs. physical health: analyzing disparities in network use and provider reimbursement rates. *Milliman.* November 30, 2017. https://careers.milliman.com/en/insight/addiction-and-mental-health-vs-physical-health-analyzing-disparities-in-network-use-and.

20. Corrigan P. How stigma interferes with mental health care. *Am Psychologist.* 2004;59(7):614-625. doi:10.1037/0003-066X.59.7.614

21. Altimus C. Supporting wellness: initial findings from a survey of lived experience and research priorities of depression and bipolar. *Milken Institute.* March 2019. https://milkeninstitute.org/reports/supporting-wellness-initial-findings-survey-lived-experience-and-research-priorities.

36

Trans-Sectoral Neuroscience Innovation for the 21st Century

The BrainMind Model

*Michael McCullough, Laura Roberts, Diana Saville, Calvin Nguyen,
Bo Shao, Juan Enriquez, and Reid Hoffman*

Introduction

Today, the rapid development of tools facilitating discovery and translation of brain research is giving rise to a paradigm shift in neuroscience. Our growing capacity to develop technologies and drugs that impact the human brain offers the opportunity to alleviate suffering and elevate human potential like never before. Patients suffering from neurological conditions or mental health disorders are finally afforded options and the hope of relief; even people who are ostensibly happy and healthy have an opportunity to level up their mood, cognitive capacity, and mental well-being.

While this period of unprecedented advancements unfolds before us, the current infrastructure supporting translation of discoveries in neuroscience to the broader public is optimized for profit instead of human impact. As a result, many ideas that could relieve suffering and positively impact humanity will take an untold number of years before reaching the public, or worse yet, they will fail to ever reach the patients who might benefit from them. Yet, opportunities abound to facilitate the translation of high-impact ideas out of the lab: fostering increased collaboration between the brightest minds in neuroscience, evaluating and organizing academic ideas to form a roadmap of progress, and building infrastructure to support translation are each important dimensions of this goal. The most powerful approach is to coordinate and focus the energy, talent, and resources that already exist today. BrainMind is a nonprofit platform and community that aims to achieve just that. By cultivating a community of scientists, entrepreneurs, investors, philanthropists, ethicists, and institutions, BrainMind is poised to create a collaborative ecosystem geared toward translating powerful ideas in brain and mind science from academia to the world.

A Watershed Moment in the Science of the Brain and the Mind

The US Brain Research through Advancing Innovative Neurotechnologies (BRAIN) Initiative was formed in 2013 as a public–private collaboration to facilitate progress in neuroscience. At the time, President Obama stated that "as humans, we can identify galaxies light years away, we can study particles smaller than an atom. But we still haven't unlocked the mystery of the three pounds of matter that sits between our ears." Unlocking the secrets of the brain and the mind has long felt out of reach, if not impossible. However, with the rapid development of novel technologies such as optogenetics—which uses light to selectively control precise neural activity—as well as imaging platforms such as CLARITY—which makes brain tissue transparent to facilitate highly detailed imaging of the protein and nucleic acid structures within the brain—these mysteries are ever closer to being understood. More recent developments such as lattice light-sheet microscopy, when paired with expansion microscopy, are now facilitating 3D imaging of the brain at a large scale without losing the critical nanoscale information. Advancements in data processing capacity and machine learning mean that the amount of information that we are able to access, evaluate, and manipulate with respect to the brain is unprecedented. Additionally, several technologies that are not inherently new are being developed with machine-learning advancements for innovative neurotechnological purposes. Examples include developing portable dry electroencephalograms to measure brain activity during learning, sports, and everyday activities; functional near-infrared spectroscopy to measure oxygenated hemoglobin in the brain-, eye-, and gesture-tracking technology to improve virtual reality technology; and magnetic resonance imaging being developed for use in emergency rooms for on-the-spot diagnosis and care of patients suffering from stroke and other maladies. These tools and other emergent neurotechnologies are becoming pervasive in academia, and more slowly trickling in to clinical and even commercial use, creating significant opportunities to improve brain health and positively impact humanity.

In this watershed moment in the field of neuroscience, BrainMind is needed for three reasons: first, the incentive structure in academia hinders translation of ideas beyond the lab; second, there is an overreliance on the venture model for translating ideas in brain science, as well as a lack of coordination in philanthropic funding, leaving many important ideas undersupported; and, third, there is a practical and ethical imperative to build a community focused on impact over profit, especially in brain science.

Incentives in Academia Stymie Translation

One of the greatest challenges facing translation of brain science outside the lab is the incentive structures in academia. Most principle investigators are necessarily focused on capturing grant funding for their research. Researchers focus on producing data, partly for progress, but also to build a compelling story to publish in peer-reviewed journals. Publishing papers enables grant funding, and grants not only support the infrastructure of the lab and research but also secure one's position in academia, especially for postdoctoral fellows and faculty.

To facilitate translation of research, researchers must utilize the technology transfer structure within the university. While these structures help to move ideas out of the lab, the vast majority of researchers do not have the expertise or interest to drive their research into commercial or clinical applications. Given that this effort takes time from the demands of research, grant-writing, teaching responsibilities, and running a lab, many scientists are not motivated or positioned to pursue this on their own. Furthermore, researchers do not receive tenure for commercializing their research or for bringing their discoveries to widespread clinical use. Our view isn't that scientists should leave their jobs to build companies, but rather that we can build a better system for translating ideas out of the lab that supports both scientists and entrepreneurs. Within the BrainMind ecosystem, support can be mobilized from entrepreneurs, technologist, investors, and philanthropic organizations to encourage translation without conflicting with the needs and interests of researchers themselves.

Traditional Funding Structures Fail to Facilitate Translation and Impact

As a society, we make enormous investment into biomedical research at early stages; $171.8 billion was directed in 2016 alone.[1] While these investments have been climbing over the years—albeit at a slower rate since 2015—the dollars spent on research and development (R&D) are dwarfed by the enormous amount of money spent on healthcare in the United States as a whole. Investment in R&D accounts for only ~4.9% of all healthcare spending, corresponding to less than 5 cents on every dollar spent toward health. Economic stimulation in early-stage research has produced wonders in modern medicine, catalyzing scientific innovation that generates new ventures—creating more wealth to drive further R&D—and benefiting millions of people across the country and the globe. However, focusing solely on early-stage research funding is not the most effective strategy for bringing ideas to clinical and commercial use. With public health crises such as the COVID-19 pandemic, opioid addiction and increased prevalence of mental health problems, bolstering support for translational medicine will yield a more streamlined development of research and ideas that translate into real-world impact, with a huge benefit to patients and taxpayers alike.

Not only is there a bias of philanthropic and government funding toward early-stage research, the current infrastructure guiding funding for translational science is shaped by traditional economic pressures. In the United States, we spend approximately 10 times more resources annually toward developing academic neuroscience than we do translating this research into effective real-world use. Only a fraction of impactful ideas from neuroscience—those with promise for 3× economic returns or higher within five years—successfully move into venture-backed positions. Even impact investing funds aim for market-rate returns.[2] Ideas that are potentially self-sustaining or modestly profitable (1×–3× return on investment) rarely find funding outside of the lab. We lose out on potentially self-sustaining and impactful applications of brain science simply due to a lack of dedicated investment structures and incomplete incentive schemes. BrainMind maintains that this is not a problem of resources, rather, a problem of how, when, and where those resources are deployed.

For decades, philanthropic organizations have had the ability to invest directly in for-profit companies via program-related investments, mission-related investments, recoverable grants, and loans. Additionally, a portion of the $121 billion in donor-advised funds[3] could be leveraged to do the same. However, very few foundations or donor-advised funds invest in scientific innovation beyond the academic stage. The net outcome is that many of these approaches are dramatically underutilized as a tool in philanthropy, and philanthropy achieves less impact than it could.[4,5] Collectively, these foundations control investment mechanisms and sources of capital on the order of hundreds of billions of dollars, which could potentially be redirected into projects that facilitate the translation of brain science in particular.

Philanthropy is not the only mechanism that could be utilized more effectively. In 2013, Carolynn Levy of Y Combinator created a set of standard legal documents called the *Simple Agreement for Future Equity* (SAFE). These documents streamlined raising capital in early-stage funding rounds, saving start-ups valuable resources in the way of time and money. These documents also made the investing ecosystem more accessible to small investors by reducing legal and administrative friction in early investment stages. SAFE is now a widely used standard document for start-ups that has undoubtedly increased the amount of funding for early stage companies. Foundations would greatly benefit from a similar simple, uniform standard document for conducting early-stage funding rounds, akin to SAFE. Utilizing a nonprofit SAFE would unlock capital from foundations and other nonprofit investors as well as decrease cost, time, and uncertainty. Additionally, a structure of this sort would enable cooperation between nonprofit and for-profit funding sources and smooth the funding continuum for all life science companies, not just nonprofits.

Models for Translating Research Outside of the Lab

As in any cutting-edge domain, few ideas are both highly impactful and highly profitable. Few institutions and entities have set up effective means to support translation outside the constraints of market pressure. Current models of translation that decouple market pressures from the maturation of impactful ideas offer examples of how build infrastructure to better support the translation of neuroscience. For example, the Allen Institute for Brain Science is a privately funded institute that generates deep data sets of high quality that reveal which genes are expressed, when, and where in the brain. These data sets are publicly available for anyone to mine, use, or publish. While this effort has facilitated significant discoveries, it would be considered a failure to a venture capitalist. These kinds of data are extremely difficult to generate investment interest for without any specific problem detailed or financial outcome promised. The Allen Institute's targets for performance are focused on the quality of the science and rigor of methodology rather than publications or economic benefit. This uncoupling of science from the traditional incentive schemes in academia and economic incentive allows for massive impact.

Using a different strategy, the Wyss Institute for Biologically Inspired Engineering at Harvard University approaches translation through a mechanism they call the

"Innovation Funnel." In this model, they preserve the creative freedom of academics—and thus the breeding ground for bright ideas—and pair their scientists with staff focused on product development, prototyping, and maturation of technologies. This structure allows them to derisk novel technologies as they are emerging from the lab and also provides the key support needed to guide these ideas into a commercial sector. Entrepreneurs-in-residence, intellectual property experts, and dedicated development staff all facilitate this transition, making the Wyss Institute a leader and a model for effective translation.

Finally, many universities house offices of technology transfer that support the movement of discoveries out of the academic setting and into the world. The most notable, in this regard, is Stanford University, which is attributed with the first Office of Technology Licensing in 1970 by Niels Reimers. University administrators and patent attorneys work in concert to support the development of ideas into commercial prospects, actively marketing the intellectual property arising from Stanford labs. Many universities now emulate this model, bringing in dedicated staff whose role it is to guide the maturation, funding, and business structures around new technologies and discoveries so that they can have a positive impact in the world.

BrainMind Reorients Current Resources for Optimized Translation of Impactful Ideas

BrainMind was built on the premise that the resources needed to transform good ideas in brain science into applied tools and services are already plentiful. Intelligent reorganization of existing resources (capital, good will, and expertise) will be sufficient to realize a more harmonious and productive infrastructure to translate these ideas to applied uses. The BrainMind approach can be summarized as a three-step process:

1. *Convene a high quality, powerful community:* Build a community of influential experts and stakeholders who are keen to assess and support ideas in brain science based on the potential human impact.
2. *Curate ideas:* Organize an effective roadmap informed by expert advisors to filter, select, and develop the most impactful ideas in brain research.
3. *Cultivate impact:* Thoughtfully harness the energy, capital, and expertise of the BrainMind ecosystem to rapidly translate ideas from the bench to clinical or consumer applications.

The Conference: An Early Model for Building a Roadmap to Drive Coordinated Progress

In the autumn of 1911, classical physics was disrupted at a foundational level. The study of quantum mechanics emerged as observations were made that could not be reconciled with the approach of classical physics, creating a rift between physicists as well as new questions around the power of the atom and the nature of matter itself. Informed by his intuition, a successful, science-leaning industrialist named Ernest Solvay used his network and wealth to convene the world's most talented physicists in an invitation-only global meeting of historic proportions. The Solvay Conference was created with the aim to examine the problem of having two disparate approaches in the field and to put together a roadmap for how to move forward.

The 1911 Solvay Conference marked the start of a powerful collaboration between the private, public, and academic sectors that has lasted over a century. The thesis behind the first meeting was simple: collect the best minds—including, at the time, Albert Einstein and Niels Bohr—and organize around the most important ideas in physics to facilitate progress and impact. To Solvay, an entrepreneur and patent holder in his own right, advancing the field required a collective but focused gestation of ideas, compared to the isolated—albeit brilliant—work being done in the lonely halls of academia. Solvay's efforts guided the emergence of a powerful community that has impacted innovation in the physical sciences tremendously in the years since.

While Solvay aimed to reconcile two competing approaches to physics, BrainMind hopes to unify and coordinate a multisectoral network that will allow for rapid gestation of critical discoveries and technologies so they can rapidly translate outside of academia. As John F. Kennedy said, "by defining our goals more clearly, by making it seem more manageable and less remote, we help all people to see it, to draw hope from it, and to move irresistibly toward it." He believed that the common fate of humanity was both a moral vision and a practical one. BrainMind is working toward creating a practical plan to drive progress in brain science, in part through convening annual summits designed to cultivate momentum and meaningful collaborations in furthering the science of the brain, the mind, and the tools and techniques required to master both. Just as the Solvay Conference has continued to anchor the global physics community for over a century, BrainMind aims to anchor translational brain science and provide resources to maximize the highest possible good that may arise from the discoveries in this space.

BrainMind Summits Convene the Community and Infrastructure for Rapid Translation of Innovative Brain Science

In the fall of 2018, BrainMind convened its first invite-only summit in collaboration with the Stanford Department of Psychiatry and Behavioral Sciences. The following spring, BrainMind joined forces with the Massachusetts Institute of Technology (MIT) Media Lab, the Picower Institute, and the McGovern Institute at MIT for its second summit. These meetings collected renowned neuroscientists, biotechnology venture capitalists, industry titans, tech entrepreneurs, prominent brain science-focused philanthropists and foundations, angel investors, and US policymakers into one room for talks and dialogue to drive forward the BrainMind vision and build the roadmap for effective progress.

Those invited to join the ecosystem share two characteristics: a passion for optimizing brain health and significant leadership or expertise in their respective careers. The core advisory council guides the growth of the ecosystem, working carefully to curate new members. The most influential neuroscientists, entrepreneurs, and funders supporting brain research make up the ranks of the BrainMind community, including scientists who have been honored with the Kyoto Prize, Breakthrough Prize, and Nobel Prize. Leaders of the BRAIN Initiative are active participants, as are major philanthropists and foundations. The collective resources present at each of these BrainMind summits has exceeded $200 billion, with sizeable additional capital and networks one degree removed. In addition, venture capitalists from the Midas List, founders and founding team members of many Fortune 100 tech companies, leadership from the US government, and other sincere and talented people have all come together with the shared vision of driving brain research forward and rapidly translating innovative ideas to maximize impact. Institutional partners include Stanford University, the MIT, and Oxford University. Many social entrepreneurs who have created some of the nation's most successful, self-sustaining, and impactful nonprofits are active participants as well. Economically liberated entrepreneurs, engineers, and board members make exceptional leaders for nascent companies forming through BrainMind, bringing their expertise and experience to accelerate translation of research with shared upside and credit for all parties. A critical aspect of this network is the inclusion of ethicists, philosophers, and policymakers who will serve to guide discoveries forward with an eye toward moral and ethical boundaries while considering the greatest possible impact.

With such a lofty goal, great care is taken to cultivate the core members, with special attention paid to ensure that all stakeholders have a voice in the community. This emphasis on inclusion applies not only to the interdisciplinary nature of the BrainMind ecosystem, but also to elevating underrepresented groups within each discipline. To support the participation of its members, BrainMind created a philanthropically funded program that supports event participation and childcare expense reimbursement for speakers and community members from underrepresented groups. Members of the BrainMind ecosystem are committed to the bringing-to-scale of the science behind the brain and the mind, with an eye toward systemic cooperation between stakeholders. BrainMind is structured around a shared vision and energizing all of the parts and resources required to bring this vision to fruition for the highest possible good.

Curating Ideas into a Refined Roadmap

The curation of ideas in neuroscience relies on the brilliant minds gathered in the BrainMind ecosystem. Following the example set by Bill Newsome in the BRAIN Initiative, whose roadmap was organized around better theories, better maps of the brain, and better tools to stimulate and read the brain, we aim to crystallize key nodes of innovation that are poised for high impact in the coming decade. Through collaborative efforts forged in summits and informal meetings, these experts are called upon to vet and perform diligence on the wide array of ideas stemming from academic neuroscience labs, as well as agree on the major pillars of progress in neuroscience. BrainMind has recruited many of the nation's top venture capitalists to help screen and assess opportunities in brain science, allowing all stakeholders in the BrainMind ecosystem to benefit from their expertise. The goal of this exercise is to have a document that lays out the foundation for how we will marshal our energy and resources to drive progress and translation.

Current focus areas for BrainMind include prevention and wellness-focused innovations, research tools that will enable faster discovery at scale, technologies for mapping the brain, large-scale efforts to generate and share data, AI research in relationship to neuroscience, educational neuroscience, and other areas of neuroscience focused on human flourishing.

Cultivating Impact

In addition to developing a roadmap to chart a path forward, we need a set of filters to ensure that the valuable energy and resources in the BrainMind ecosystem are aimed at best-in-class ideas. One critical consideration is examining where we structurally underinvest in brain science. Currently, prevention of disease is critically underinvested because it does not generate an attractive market-rate return. On average healthcare insurers keep their patients for short periods (<3 years). For most chronic diseases, current incentives support "kicking the cost can down the road" to other insurers or Medicare. Similarly, technologies that promote mental wellness, technologies aimed at small patient populations, and projects that require coordinated research efforts involving multiple institutions are consistently underinvested.

To achieve impact, BrainMind has created structures and recruited talent to help support the development of neuroscience ideas beyond academia (see Figure 36.1). Part of this process is the creation of commonly agreed upon documents that guide philanthropic funding of for-profit companies. BrainMind is working to create new company structures that support a moderately profitable and highly impactful hybrid company model—similar to B-Corp structures or companies that are nonprofit–for-profit hybrids. Using charitable investing rather than philanthropic gifts on early-stage projects is a robust strategy to optimize the utilization of capital for brain science translation. Because charitable investments follow ventures through their entire life cycle, funds are eventually recycled into creating more impact. If philanthropic funds are invested rather than donated, philanthropists would dramatically increase their impact and the number of projects funded.

Venture capital commits $23 billion annually to facilitate the translation of brain science out of academia and into the full service of humanity.[6,7] Unfortunately, many powerful ideas in brain science are not compelling ventures because they fail to meet optimized venture capital criteria. Businesses that meet the self-sustaining threshold of one to two times returns are a failure in this context. However, for a grantmaking foundation, this would be considered a big win. Because the supply of capital from the philanthropic sector is an order of magnitude larger than the annual venture capital

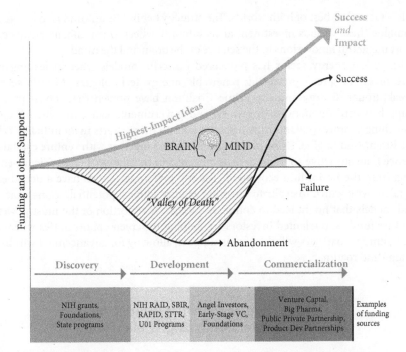

Figure 36.1 BrainMind Supports the most impactful underfunded ideas in brain science. There is ample capital in the health and medicine space for early idea formation. At the far end of the funnel, the economic focus of venture capital filters out many impactful ideas and supports only the minority which promise significant returns. There is comparatively little support in the middle ground. Most impactful technologies that are mature enough to leave the lab will not meet venture criteria. These potentially self-sustaining impactful technologies struggle for funding and end up trapped in what is called the "valley of death." BrainMind is building the community and infrastructure to support these ideas and bring them out of the lab to benefit humanity.

Adapted from Steinmetz KL, and Spack EG. The basics of preclinical drug development for neurodegenerative disease indications. *BMC Neurology.* 2009(Suppl 1):S2.

investment, this difference in perspective is quite powerful. Informed by this distinction, BrainMind has organized funding structures to support impactful brain science ideas that are capable of being self-sustaining.

While utilizing philanthropy as a mechanism for funding ideas that have lower-than-average rates of return, it is important to consider how to bolster the development of these ideas along their full development timeline. Typical philanthropic efforts to translate research are uncoupled from venture capital and the ecosystem that stimulates more rapid translation and improves the likelihood of success. By uniting partnerships across venture and philanthropy, taking advantage of the infrastructure of venture capital and the capital of philanthropic foundations, BrainMind is leveraging the best of both worlds. The strategy behind BrainMind is to curate and combine these various investment arms into a flywheel to continually advance the most impactful innovations in the science of the brain and the mind.

The clean energy sector has pioneered powerful models wherein leading venture investors screen promising renewable energy technologies. Models such as Breakthrough Energy and the Prime Coalition have proven that robust partnerships between foundations, investors, and governments can exist. BrainMind is launching venture–philanthropy fusion similar to these efforts in an initiative called the BrainMind Engine. Using philanthropic dollars together with venture capital diligence is an attractive solution to drive progress in translational brain science emerging from the BrainMind ecosystem. The top investment funds have a deep bench of talent with which to evaluate scientific validity, clinical potential, teams, markets, and models that might lead to company success. A collection of the most powerful venture funds and talented investors are helping to screen opportunities where our philanthropic partners will then focus support, allowing for advancement within the BrainMind roadmap.

Case Studies From the BrainMind Ecosystem: Catalyzing Translation

The investment approaches implemented within the BrainMind ecosystem are designed to support the full spectrum of idea formation across neuroscience, from gestation in research to commercial application. One example of how BrainMind has catalyzed translation is the support generated for a Stanford scientist's work using hypnotherapy to help people quit smoking. Hypnotherapy has been used for over 40 years to help thousands of patients stop smoking and manage their chronic pain. Half of patients quit smoking after one face-to-face therapy session. Lacking a recurring revenue business model, there was little investor interest to deploy this life-altering therapy. Additionally, this intervention was difficult to scale because the professional services model requires time-intensive training and expensive certification of therapists. This breakthrough was restricted to use in the lab for years until a BrainMind angel investor and entrepreneur met the scientist at a BrainMind Summit at Stanford. That night, the investor coded an Alexa Skill that could be invoked by any of the 100 million Alexa-enabled devices in the world. Any of the millions of smokers in the world can now tell their enabled devices "I'm craving a cigarette" and receive the hypnotherapy.

BrainMind leadership has been making carefully crafted introductions between entrepreneurs and scientists within the ecosystem to encourage similar collaborations. Two entrepreneurs joined the BrainMind ecosystem with an interest in neuroscience and expanding their professional pursuits beyond their respective product manager roles at one of the largest marketplace technology companies in Silicon Valley. Through BrainMind they met a prolific nanotechnology inventor who invited them into his Stanford lab to catalog and analyze the highest quality ideas from his group. With the entrepreneurs' top-quality expertise in machine-learning and product development, and the nanotech scientist's expertise, the three of them generated a product prototype within five months and raised millions to commercialize the technology.

As another example, after making a significant leap in progress decoding speech from thoughts to help locked-in patients to communicate, a neurosurgeon and professor at University of California at San Francisco was ready to create custom hardware so that this could help more patients. An introduction to serial hardware technology entrepreneur and investor connected this scientist to resources that enabled him to expedite his product design timeline from one year down to three weeks. As a team, they are rapidly prototyping to create technology that will accelerate the pace of the research in a first-in-class partnership. This connection fostered by BrainMind enabled this technology to be developed more rapidly for applicable use within a structure that would both attract top engineering talent and help to fund the lab's future research.

In early 2020, catalyzed by interactions at a 2019 BrainMind Summit, a group of scientists and social entrepreneurs including a neuroscientist from the University of British Columbia, and a media entrepreneur developed a project to advance progress in understanding Alzheimer's disease and dementia. Building upon a growing, highly interactive patient–caregiver community, they are designing a product to apply machine learning and natural language processing to crowdsourced, patient-focused information from thousands of ethnically and socioeconomically diverse families that could be critical to the better stratification, understanding, and treatment of dementia. The collaborative project promises to deepen understanding of phases of neurodegenerative disease, create a new platform for big data in health, and bring interventions more rapidly to patients and their caregivers.

Many powerful ideas will never produce significant revenue; however, if they produce impact and are able to be self-sustaining, we must support their progress.[1] To see these companies flourish novel company structures will be required, including hybrid models that foster synergy between philanthropists and more traditional investors. BrainMind is catalyzing progress by aligning incentives across its parts: community members who run labs are able to share in the value they create by doing what they are good at; promising ideas are vetted and championed by the investors and entrepreneurs who can build the companies; and impact-focused funding vehicles realize modest returns. Collectively, the BrainMind ecosystem is supporting a healthier and more efficient environment to translate innovative discoveries and technologies in neuroscience for the benefit of humanity.

The Ethical Imperative

In April of 2019, *Nature* magazine published findings from Nenad Sestan's lab describing the revival of disembodied brains of pigs four hours after their death.[8] This result stunned the academic community and beyond, with many bioethicists citing the profound ethical implications this work brought forward. The result was so impactful that *Nature* magazine named Sestan in their "Nature Top 10" people who mattered in 2019. Appropriately, Professor Sestan and his team immediately engaged with bioethicists to move forward with this research in a way that is sensitive to the murky ethical domain into which they stumbled. This is just one example of the many discoveries and innovations that have emerged from the last few years in neuroscience and research focused on the brain and the mind that require rigorous ethical consideration and debate.

The next decade of progress in brain science has the potential to reshape humanity. The pairing of new tools in neuroscience with innovations from other fields, such as machine learning and cheaper computing, is beginning to allow access to and manipulation of activity in both the brain and the mind—a nascent power with great potential for both benefit and harm. This inflection point in neuroscience is comparable to cracking the genetic code or the splitting of the atom, both being historical moments for science whose aftermath profoundly reshaped humanity. Like the Solvay Conference, we have a responsibility to gather together and thoughtfully consider how we are moving these technologies forward and work to understand the moral and ethical implications as we do. BrainMind is convening international advisory board meetings with leading neuroethicists, policymakers, and key leaders from the BrainMind ecosystem to discuss and implement strategies so that these technologies and BrainMind programs are developed within a thoughtful ethical framework.

The Path Forward for BrainMind

As of January 2020, the BrainMind community spanned over 2,500 members across sectors including research, medicine, entrepreneurship, investing, philanthropy, and policy. Those most involved within the ecosystem directly engage with research and entrepreneurial activity in brain science. This community is growing to include more interdisciplinary voices and promote cross-fertilization of ideas and connectivity, including experts in statistics, clinical psychiatry, ethics, computer science, philosophy of mind, and economics, to name a few. These members convene for annual summits, as well as single-day events on prioritized topics such as neuroethics, consciousness, and meditation, wherein experts lead discussions with members of the ecosystem. The goal of these gatherings is to create opportunities for ecosystem members to connect and create synergy and momentum behind some of the most important, risky, and novel ideas in this domain. The more this community grows with more powerful interlocking networks, the more rapidly brain science will move forward both in terms of discovery and in translation for the broader good. The BrainMind ecosystem is poised to contribute to brain science and benefit humanity, regardless of financial return.

The BrainMind Summits at Stanford, MIT, and Oxford are nonprofit efforts.

If you are interested in applying to join the BrainMind ecosystem, please visit www.brainmind.org/application.

References

1. U.S. investments in medical and health research and development 2013–2016. *Research!America*. Fall 2017. https://www.researchamerica.org/sites/default/files/RA-2017_InvestmentReport.pdf [Accessed February 11, 2019].
2. Global Impact Investors Network. Annual impact investor survey 2018. July 16, 2018. https://thegiin.org/assets/2018_GIIN_Annual_Impact_Investor_Survey_webfile.pdf
3. Heisman E, Hastings A, Hoyes E, Brown M. 2018 donor-advised fund report. *NPTrust*. 2019. https://www.nptrust.org/reports/daf-report/ [Accessed February 11, 2019].
4. Henriques R, Nath A, Cote-Ackah C, Rosqueta K. "Program Related Investments." *Center for High Impact Philanthropy, University of Pennsylvania*. April 2016. https://www.impact.upenn.edu/wp-content/uploads/2016/04/160415PRIFINALAH-print.pdf
5. Macpherson R, Kearney S, Murray F. Donor-advised funds: an underutilized philanthropic vehicle to support innovation in science and engineering. *MIT Sloan School of Management*. June 2017. https://innovation.mit.edu/assets/MIT-PRIME_DAF.pdf [Accessed February 11, 2019].
6. 4Q 2018 PitchBook-NVCA Venture Monitor. *Pitchbook/National Venture Capital Association*. January 9, 2019. https://pitchbook.com/news/reports/4q-2018-pitchbook-nvca-venture-monitor
7. Jenni, P. Viewpoint: the strength of worldwide collaboration. *Cern Courier*. July 23, 2014. https://cerncourier.com/viewpoint-the-strength-of-worldwide-collaboration/ [Accessed February 11, 2019].
8. Vrselja Z, Daniele SG, Silbereis J et al. Restoration of brain circulation and cellular functions hours post-mortem. *Nature*. 2019;568:336-343 https://doi.org/10.1038/s41586-019-1099-1.

SECTION VIII
CONCLUSION

37

A Roadmap Toward Convergence
Mental Health

Overcoming Barriers From Research, to Initial Commercialization, to Scaling Up Market Penetration

Erin Smith, Helen Lavretsky, Charles F. Reynolds III, Michael Berk, and Harris A. Eyre

Disclosures

HE reports ownership of shares in CNSdose LLC. HL has a research grant from Allergan. MB reports personal fees from Servier, Lundbeck, Grunbiotics, Controversias Barcelona, HealthEd, ANZOS, Livanova, Janssen, Catalyst, Norwegian Psych Assocation, Otsuka, allergan, Bioconcepts, RANZCP, outside the submitted work. In addition, MB has a patent Modulation of Physiological processes and agents useful for same. issued, and a patent Modulation of diseases of the central nervous system and related disorders pending. ES reports ownership of shares in Prodrome Labs Inc. ES has a research grant from the Michael J. Fox Foundation and a patent Detection system and methods for neurological diseases pending. No other relevant disclosures to report.

Grant Support

HL reports grant support by NIH grant AT009198. MB reports grants from NHMRC Principal Research Fellowship (APP1059660 and APP1156072). No other authors report relevant grant support.

Introduction

In an ancient Indian parable of the blind men and the elephant, there is a group of blind men who have never come across an elephant. They learn to conceptualize what an elephant is like via touch. However, each man feels a different part of the elephant's body and subsequently has a radically different description and understanding of the creature. The man who feels the ears comes to believe the elephant is like a huge fan, whereas the man who feels the tail thinks the elephant resembles a deadly snake.

Unless we can foster a convergence science approach, we may fall prey to a similar dilemma. We may come to understand only disparate elements of complex global mental health crisis but fail to see the larger, systematic solutions.

The shift toward convergence mental health will be underpinned by developments in three main areas: (i) research, (ii) initial commercialization, and (iii) scaling up market penetration. We particularly focus on the research phase in this chapter, as it is the most salient and where the most work is happening right now. However, to forge the path for convergence mental health forward, it is also necessary to think about and lay the groundwork for commercialization and scaling up. These latter elements are particularly relevant for translation of innovations and discoveries, which is critical to prevent stagnation in mental healthcare. The National Academies of Science, Engineering and Medicine report on convergence science provides a robust framework for work in these areas and is a source of inspiration across this section [1,2].

Research

Convergence mental health will require advancements in research and scientific progress. The main research barriers and challenges are in the following areas: informational, leadership, structural and organizational, and education and workforce development. This section addresses each of these areas and provides recommendations for moving forward.

Informational

Challenges
The research community lacks unified understanding about convergence science. The most rudimentary elements—from shared vocabulary to coherent frameworks—remain largely absent. There is a lack of information about what convergence science is and how effective implementation may benefit mental healthcare. Due to lack of common language surrounding the topic, approaching even a conversation around the topic of convergence science is difficult. This is especially problematic as convergence science requires transdisciplinary collaborations; to effectively collaborate among divergent sectors, shared understanding and language is needed.

Recommendations
Shared language coupled with a unified roadmap for the future of mental healthcare is needed to foster collaborations. A convergence science approach will provide the backbone of this roadmap; it will form the connections between the disparate nodes necessary to achieve the future of mental healthcare. A potential roadmap for how the

Table 37.1. Roadmap for Convergence Science Approach

Potential Opportunity	Future Actions
Build the case for convergence	• Convene focused workshops on case topics to assemble the missing pieces that could support convergence in those specific scientific areas • Build agreement on what is meant by "convergence," including how transdisciplinary research and team science contribute to it, as well as where it differs from or extends beyond these concepts • Develop and collate stories to help internal and external audiences understand what convergence enables
Create networks and communities of practice among those interested in convergence	• Establish a "convergence acceleration forum" across universities, institutes, national laboratories, and industry to convene periodic discussions that share ongoing challenges and identify effective practices and transferable elements • Create a peer community of university provosts or senior research officers to address challenges unique to university structures • Create a peer community or association of convergence center and institute directors to compare cross-sectional strategies and identify transferable elements that foster convergence • Connect interested faculty, technical staff, and trainees within a university
Design structures that support and incentivize convergence	• Establish "incubators" to provide momentum for the development of convergence centers. Services and support could include creation of "advisory teams" to help researchers launch effective convergent projects. The teams might draw on expertise in areas such as team science, transdisciplinary research, innovation studies, and organizational change • Establish research instrumentation hubs with expert staff scientists, supported through novel funding mechanisms • Consider the advantages and disadvantages of various financial support models
Develop criteria for success reflective of convergence	• Articulate promising proposal review processes and criteria for evaluating convergent funding submissions • Identify outcome metrics of success for the results of convergent research • Explore strategies to address challenges in publication of convergent manuscripts • Collate effective practices and criteria for research advancement, including academic promotion and tenure and parallel career paths beyond the traditional tenure track • Discuss expanded metrics of success for departments and institutions that will recognize both disciplinary scholarship and convergence

Source: Adapted with permission from NASEM (National Academies of Sciences, Engineering, and Medicine). 2019. Fostering the Culture of Convergence in Research: Proceedings of a Workshop. Washington, DC: The National Academies Press.

informational barriers could be addressed to lay the groundwork for a convergence mental health approach is provided in Table 37.1.

Leadership

Challenges

Robust leadership is needed to bring about the adoption of a convergence science approach to mental healthcare. Momentum from leadership is necessary to drive culture change, navigate challenges associated with transdisciplinary collaborations, and enhance productivity and focus. For convergence mental health to be adopted, leadership must also extend beyond the confinements of managerial tasks and not be exclusively for people in positions of power. Established principal investigators and emerging researchers alike must be supported, making leadership horizontal versus vertical. Further, scientists should not be put in leadership positions without sufficient support. Within corporate organizations and civil service, employees often receive continuous leadership training through workshops and courses. However, in academia, leadership development and support are often absent. A recent Nature survey of 3,200 scientists found a stark leadership training gap [3]. In the survey, two-thirds of researchers who head laboratories said they had not had training in managing people or running a lab in the past year—and the majority of those said they wanted some training [3]. Among the researchers who had received training, five-sixths found it useful [3]. To help labs do better science, better leadership training and support is needed.

Recommendations

For the effective adoption and integration of convergence science, leadership is needed in two forms: (i) organizations and institutions that function as vision-setting bodies and (ii) individuals and groups within institutions who directly and indirectly serve as a sort of organizational gyroscope [4].

Vision-setting bodies are needed as North Stars for convergence science. One current exemplar organization is One Mind. One Mind is a lived-experience–led mental health nonprofit focused on helping people with brain illness and injury recover so that they can succeed in their lives, aiming to achieve healthy brains for all [5]. One Mind has catalyzed comprehensive action, spanning from funding breakthrough science from emerging scientists to scaling implementation of innovations for patients to transforming societal culture and alleviating stigma. One Mind functions as a hub of transdisciplinary collaborations and convergence science, depicting the impact that is possible through this approach.

Within organizations, leadership skills need to be prioritized and continuously developed. Peter Hirst, the associate dean of executive education at the Massachusetts Institute of Technology (MIT) Sloan School of Management in Cambridge, Massachusetts, suggests it is valuable for scientists to learn about business concepts [6]. After all, the unifying entity is human beings; whether you are leading a business or an academic lab, you depend on people to work together to achieve things. In the business world, U.S. corporations spend about US$14 billion each year on educating their employees in leadership and management [7]. However, any sort of training or class in leadership skills remains largely void in academia. Lack of leadership training is especially problematic as research teams dealing with unproductive interpersonal issues, lack of motivation, and unnecessary conflict waste time and incur large costs in terms of money, productivity, and retention of talent [8]. Leading people is hard, as people are not entirely rational [9]. However, leading people is unnecessarily hard when there is lack of enough support. Akin to continuously updating and developing technical skills, continuously learning how to be an effective leader is key for scientific discovery. Learning how to get many people to work together effectively is especially critical for convergence science, as collaboration is the fiber of transdisciplinarity. CERN, ENCODE, and the Human Genome Project depict what is possible through effective leadership in convergence science.

For the past 45 years, the most popular business-school elective at Stanford University has been a class entitled "Organizational Behavior 374: Interpersonal Dynamics" [10]. This course seeks to instill in future business leaders the self-awareness to build more effective relationships and communicate more openly with colleagues. What would it look like if a course was adapted from Interpersonal Dynamics specifically for scientists and researchers? How would that learning transform the productivity, innovation, and teamwork within the research ecosystem and help foster convergence science? What other continuous leadership training would be beneficial for the research ecosystem?

Structural and Organization

Challenges
For effective adoption of convergence science, research institutions must be willing to overcome current structural and institutional limitations. Structural and organizational changes have the potential to cause enormous impacts and ripple effects. Despite the importance of the health of the research ecosystem on the overall health and progress of society, critical evaluation of how science is practiced and funded remains limited. The following questions must be posed and deliberated [11,12]: What incentives are necessary to support a convergence science ecosystem, specifically within mental healthcare? How should scientists be selected and funded? How can collaborations most effectively be achieved and produce the most innovative outputs? What are the optimal structures for identifying and training the new generation of future scientists? Should other countries organize their scientific bodies along the lines of those in the United States or instead pursue deliberate variation?

The research system must not be ran solely by conventional thought or remain unexamined. For example, a subtle shift has occurred since the 1980s. According to recent reports by the National Institute of Health, in 1980, 12 times more funding went to early-career scientists (under 40) than to late-career scientists (over 50) [13]. Today, those figures have switched, with five times more money going to scientists aged 50 or older. Better understanding the implications of this shift—and other changes within research—is needed. Evaluation of the optimal allocation and structure of science funding is needed, especially those that fall outside of the conventional realm such as prizes, fellowships, or sabbaticals [11]. Beyond funding challenges, the larger research ecosystem must be systemically evaluated and addressed to ensure that scientists are being encouraged to take risks and think outside of the box.

Recommendations

Structural and organization changes can help facilitate convergence science approaches. Structures that embrace the following principles are especially important: support productive competition while enabling collaboration; are nimble in addressing a topic and that can be repositioned when needed; maintain critical shared facilities; and address the role of financial incentives for convergence research.

We must also be willing to rethink the work environment and culture that underpin modern research structures and organizations. We must ensure that distractions, meetings, being quick to respond to never-ending emails, and other proxies for productivity are not replacing the high-focus environments and priorities necessary to produce the deep thinking required for high-impact scientific breakthroughs. Adopting methodologies from other industries, such as the agile practices like daily standups and sprints from start-ups to lean practices like the Kanban system from manufacturing,-may aid in creative approaches to research.

Architecture is also an untapped into area of potential for transforming scientific output and progress. Consider the Eudaimonia Machine, a precise workspace layout by architect David Dewane that was popularized in *Deep Work* by Cal Newport [14,15]. The Eudaimonia Machine is inspired by Aristotle's concept of *eudaimonia*, meaning a state of achieving your full human potential. Dewane's scheme consists of five subsequent rooms that require passing through one room to get to the next. Each room is intended to trigger a different mental state. The first room is the gallery, which contains examples of work produced in the building, intended to inspire others and create a culture of healthy stress and motivating peer pressure. After the gallery is the salon. The salon, largely inspired by 18th-century Enlightenment ideals, is a breeding ground for intense curiosity and intellectual debate. Beyond the salon is the library—the "hard drive of the machine." This room contains archives of all work previously produced in the building, while providing resources and information for new projects. Next is the office space, containing the typical whiteboards and cubicles with desk. This room is designated for low-intensity activity and administrative work. Finally, the last room is a collection of deep work chambers that enable total focus and uninterrupted work. The Eudaimonia Machine provides a powerful depiction of how design could be applied to the research ecosystem and optimize productivity, collaborations, and scientific discoveries.

The Francis Crick Institute in London depicts a tangible example of how architectural design can transform research environments [16]. The internal structure of the building is not arranged along disciplinary lines, but rather along interdisciplinary interest groups, aimed at mixing scientific staff in different fields. The deliberate construction and design of the building, including break out spaces, transparent partitions, open spaces, etc., has helped the Crick become a global hub for biomedical innovation. More research is needed to explore how design might transform the research environment and could be applied to future convergence mental health institutions.

The design and culture of the Francis Crick Institute provides an intellectual playground for biomedical research. The shift toward convergence mental health will require a fundamental change in the culture of brain and mind research, akin to that undergone by the Francis Crick Institute. Research will shift from silos to playing fields of convergent activity to solve problems. Embracing the elements of play, experimentation, and creativity are vital. Sociological and psychological studies have demonstrated that during ideation, creative play helps increase flexibility (number of different categories of relevant responses), originality (the uniqueness of a response), and fluency (number of ideas) [17]. There are many facets and usages of play including idea generation, exploration, and entering flow state. Further, financial incentives for convergence "play" are critical. Support from philanthropists who want to foster high-risk, high-reward activity is needed to facilitate a structure where people engaged in convergence science for mental health can feel secure and have the support necessary for vital discoveries (see the Road Ahead section for a more in-depth analysis and suggestions about funding options).

Education and Workforce Development

Challenges
The demands of a today's global problems—especially the mental health crisis—necessitate a fundamental shift in approaching education and workforce development. Research is increasingly organized around single, specialized disciplines. However, today's problems are too complex and nuanced to be addressed by a single domain. Instead, convergence scientists must be equipped to have deep expertise in their field, while also having literacy and understanding across broad range of disciplines necessary for transdisciplinary collaborations. Further, the implications of the pressure to specialize earlier and earlier within research communities needs to be examined. There is a lack of understanding about how this shift is impacting innovation and discoveries over the lifetime of a scientist.

Recommendations
Education and workforce development aims to make the research ecosystem function better by teaching people to think better. To train convergence scientists to think better, three changes are needed: (a) a model thinking movement, (b) unconventional experiences and knowledge, and (c) rethinking traditional educational pathways.

To understand how convergence science training may be achieved, it is helpful to look at a parallel example from the 20th century. In the 1940s, two University of Chicago educators, Robert Maynard Hutchins and Mortimer Adler, had a shared vision to reform higher education. To combat the increasingly specialized nature of higher education, they proposed that the best way to get a liberal education—both in and outside of the university—was to meet and discuss the writings of the world's great thinkers and enduring ideas found in literature [18]. Subsequently, the Great Books movement was born. Today, millions of people have been impacted by the Great Books programs. Akin to the impact the Great Books program has had on higher education, the research ecosystem stands in need of a similar movement. More specifically, a model thinking movement that fosters unique cognitive styles and approaches is needed.

Models provide lenses to observe the world in a specific way and are robust tools for thinking about and approaching problems. Exposure to a vast array of models fosters divergent thinking and equips people with tools to more intelligently address complex problems and phenomenon [19]. Models stem from a broad array of ideas and fields—ranging from business, computer science, politics, physics, etc. Models enable people to see the full complexity and multidimensionality of a problem, preventing intellectual echo chambers. Often when approaching a problem, the models that do the best are those that include a diverse ensemble of formal models from multiple domains, validating a central tenant of convergence science [20]. Similar to approaching the ebbs and flows of life with the big ideas and concepts gleaned from the Great Books, learning to approach scientific complexities and problems through the lens of the big ideas and concepts gleaned from a diverse set of models will lead to clearer, more intelligent thinking and cognitive diversity. Model thinking will underpin a convergence approach and transdisciplinary view necessary for advancing innovation.

Additionally, more transdisciplinary programs are needed. Within universities, the Brainstorm Lab at Stanford University launched the first U.S. university course on mental health innovation (Psyc 240: Designing for the 2 Billion: Leading Innovation in Mental Health) [21]. Started in 2018, this course brings together diverse groups of students from multiple faculties, including Stanford's School of Medicine, Graduate School of Business, Law School, School of Engineering, School of Education, and College. This is intended to educate the emerging leaders of multiple stakeholder fields relevant to mental health as well as increase the educational value of cross-sector dialogue and collaboration [22]. During the class, students learn about mental health, care delivery, technology, and start-ups. They apply frameworks to assessing the impact of current innovations and develop their own ideas for solving mental health problems. Further, students are paired with faculty to improve the clinical validity and marketability of the idea. Within medicine, the Icahn School of Medicine at Mount Sinai is working to promote a convergence science approach and provide innovative learning [23]. Some of their programs include FlexMed and FlexGrad, which allows college sophomores in any major to apply for early acceptance into their MD or PhD and MD/PhD programs. They also offer a variety of experiential programs and dual degree tracks, including a partnership with Google Life Sciences. Further, the curriculum includes build in flex time, which is time that can be devoted to self-directed, individualized learning and discovery, patient-centered experiential learning, community participation, and other essentials for future practitioners and thought leaders. The ability to have custom choices and forge an individual path forward is a critical component of a transdisciplinary approach, promoting flexibility and collaboration over competition and rigidity.

Within academia, the Schmidt Futures Science Fellowship provides an innovative blueprint for training the next generation of scientific leaders. Founded in 2018, the Schmidt Futures Science Fellowship is equipping the next generation of scientific leaders to navigate the new era of science and technology and change the world for the better [24]. Understanding that research is increasingly global and can affect a wide range of pressing societal challenges, the Schmidt Science Fellows undergo a program designed to help the them draw insights across numerous different disciplines, be able to apply new techniques, and possess a broad worldview informed by the intersections between science and the rest of society. Through a combination of group sessions at some of the world's leading universities and a special postdoctoral study in a field different from their existing expertise, fellows are exposed to new topics, divergent ways of thinking, and new people that will guide their future paths to success and maximize their long-term impact on the world.

Another program that provides a model for convergence leadership training is the Knight-Hennessy Scholars at Stanford University [25]. Established in 2016, the program is training the next generation of leaders to find creative solutions to complex global issues. A primary focus is learning how to collaborate and innovate across disciplines and break down traditional academic silos, which will be essential to discover new solutions that will advance humanity. Knight-Hennessy Scholars will be equipped with the intellectual nimbleness and creativity necessary to address the most pressing, multifaceted global problems, including the mental health crisis.

Further, education and training for researchers needs to expand to incorporate unconventional topics and skills, which could include design thinking, entrepreneurship, cryptography, etc. Creative educational opportunities, such as mini-fellowships or exchanges, may help facilitate divergent thinking. Start-up accelerators such as Y Combinator and Techstars have great track records at catalyzing progress among entrepreneurs. What would it look like if a similar entrepreneurial bootcamp was adapted or created for scientists? How would this educational training help transform scientific output and discoveries?

Lastly, traditional education pathways as the sole means of involvement in research must be reconsidered. Many academic majors remain insular, while innovation often flows from the confluence of disparate knowledge banks. To develop innovative solutions, a diverse array of solvers is needed. Collective intelligence, including from citizen scientists, must be leveraged. Bansho is the Japanese method of collective problem-solving [26] and may provide a framework for education and training modules for convergence science researchers. Further, in 2001, InnoCentive was founded by Alph Bingham to crowdsource solutions to the most intractable solutions [27]. As a space for dialogue between specialists and industry outsiders was created, fresh ideas to persistent questions were found, including a chemist from Illinois, John Davies, who was able to use an idea from his earlier career in construction to help solve the cleanup of the Exxon Valdez oil spill on Alaska's coast [28]. Other organizations have utilized the InnoCentive model, including Kaggle, which is dedicated to problems in machine learning [29]. Organizations centered around collective intelligence may be key to overcome the intellectual silos found in traditional education pathways and to solve the seemingly intractable global mental health problems.

Initial Commercialization

Mental health and wellness technology companies are in infancy stages. According to recent CB Insights reports, venture capital-backed deals in mental health and wellness start-ups emerged in 2012, and funding to mental health tech start-ups has risen annually and reached nearly US$200 million in 2016 [30]. The pathway for research and technology in the mental health space to undergo initial commercialization is in a formative period; a clear roadmap has yet to be established. To understand the challenges and opportunity to advance convergence mental health from research to initial commercialization, we must better understand where the sector currently is and where it is heading.

Current State

Initial commercialization of mental health and wellness technology is critical to advance brain science discoveries and translate these findings from the lab to make them readily available and accessible. As such, the existing landscape for commercialization has centered around six main areas that have experienced major research and technological advancements [31]: computerized cognitive behavioral therapy (CCBT), telepsychiatry, provider tools, consumer tools, hardware, and applied artificial intelligence (AI).

Computerized Cognitive Behavioral Therapy

CCBT leverages mobile interfaces to deliver programs focused on changing unhelpful thoughts, beliefs, attitudes, and behaviors. With the traditional healthcare system unable to handle the unprecedented rate of people with undiagnosed and untreated mental conditions, digital delivery of these treatments helps widen accessibility from a geographical and financial perspective and opens a previously untapped market for digital healthcare providers [32]. Among the major players in the CCBT space are Headspace, Akili, and Happify. Founded in 2010, the Headspace app is designed for short-form meditation therapy, offering progressive learning pathways and thematic meditation series and the opportunity for social engagement by allowing the user to connect with and track the progress of "buddies" [33]. Headspace is also seeking to develop the world's first prescription meditation app as a U.S. Food and Drug Administration–cleared treatment option for chronic diseases. Founded in 2011, Akili develops prescription video games that deliver sensor and motor stimuli to target and activate specific cognitive neural systems in the brain [34]. Their prescription games work via adaptive algorithms that automatically adjust the level of challenge to train certain parts of the brain and improve cognitive deficits, allowing patient progress to be continuously monitored by clinicians and caregivers [35]. Akili provides solutions for attention-deficit/hyperactivity disorder and other cognitive disorders and its development pipeline includes solutions for major depressive disorder and multiple sclerosis. Founded in 2012, Happify is a self-help platform for effective, evidence-based solutions for better mental health and well-being for employers, health plans, and pharmaceutical companies [36]. The app assesses users and personalizes the treatment experiences, measures progress, and provides enterprise insights reporting analytics on the whole population of users.

Telepsychiatry

Telepsychiatry start-ups are providing the delivery of psychiatric assessment and care through remote communications technology, usually videoconferencing [37]. With an escalating shortage of psychiatrists and lack of access to affordable treatment, telepsychiatry solutions are especially pertinent [38]. In the telepsychiatry space, major start-ups include AbleTo, Talkspace, and Ginger. Founded in 2008, AbleTo provides a telepsychiatry platform for short-term treatments [39]. AbleTo works with self-insured employers and health plans to identify those in need and use automated assessments to determine need and then provides personal programs with a specialist. Talkspace was founded in 2012 and provides an online psychotherapy platform that matches patients with therapists using proprietary algorithms and allows teletherapy and 24/7 text access [40]. Founded in 2011 as a spinout from MIT Media Lab, Ginger provides a direct counseling service through a chat application that can be accessed instantaneously by members [41]. The platform also has algorithms that analyze the words patients use to better understand the patient's situation and provide personalized recommendations.

Provider Tools

Provider tool start-ups seek to build a new generation of software to help the operational efficiency of therapists or to empower interoperability between practitioners and other key stakeholders of the medical ecosystem. As physician burnout is a "public health crisis that urgently demands action," provider tools are vital [42]. Major companies include Quartet Health, SimplePractice, and Mindstrong. Founded in 2014, Quartet Health provides a platform that pairs primary care doctors with mental health providers, enabling integration of physical and mental health [43]. Its collaborative technology and range of services bring together physicians, mental health providers, and insurance companies to improve health outcomes and drive down costs. Founded in 2012, SimplePractice provides a cloud-based practice management solution and electronic health record software for mental health practices, enabling health and wellness professions to run their practice more efficiently [44]. Founded in 2014, Mindstrong has designed a novel care model for mental health built on a foundation of continuous measurements and AI informed telehealth services. Mindstrong has been a notable pioneer in developing digital biomarkers of brain function from human–computer interactions captured passively from a mobile device, creating a digital "fire alarm" for mental distress [45].

Consumer Tools

Consumer tool start-ups help build nontherapeutic mobile products to improve mental health and wellness through daily personal goals, connecting and facilitating communication between patients and other peers through vertical networks or creating educational content. Consumer tool start-ups help highlight the shift in care modalities and preventative health in the mental health continuum. Among the major players in the space are Thrive Global and WEConnect. Founded in 2016, Thrive Global provides behavior change technology and media to individuals and organizations around the world with the hope of ending the stress and burnout epidemic [46]. WEConnect provides a modern solution for substance use disorder [47]. By establishing individual plans, connecting individuals with a larger community of fellow patients and care providers, and rewarding patients who adhere to their treatment plans, WEConnect helps create sustainable behavior changes and improve outcomes for substance use disorders.

Hardware
Hardware start-ups leverage connected hardware to capture biometric data and help patients or therapists with monitoring or to build more immersive therapeutic content. Hardware start-ups help turn a wide array of technology—from virtual reality headsets to smart wristbands to other sensor enabled devices—into powerful healthcare tools. Major companies include AppliedVR, Pivot, and Muse™. Founded in 2015, AppliedVR provides a virtual reality platform for healthcare and digital therapeutics that improves clinical outcomes for patients with serious health conditions [48]. Founded in 2015, Pivot leverages technology, human coaching, and behavioral science to help people quit smoking for good [49]. A core, unifying element of Pivot's program is a breath sensor that measures exhaled carbon monoxide, an objective measure tied to smoking behavior. Muse™ is an electroencephalogram headband that uses biofeedback to help deepen relaxation in meditations aimed at sleep, performance, stress reduction, etc. [50]. Muse™ depicts how technology may enhance therapeutic options such as meditation.

Applied AI
Applied AI start-ups leverage conversational intelligence, predictive analytics, or machine learning at the core of the product to provide a more personalized and efficient approach to prevention, treatment, or diagnosis. Applied AI start-ups demonstrate the technological advancements and applications that mark the future of healthcare. Key companies in the applied AI space include Neurotrack, Spring Health, and Woebot. Founded in 2012, Neurotrack has developed the first cognitive health program to manage mental health and reduce the risk of future cognitive decline [51]. At the core of their technology is a clinically validated assessment that measures cognition using eye movements and recommendations to preserve and enhance memory. Founded in 2016, Spring Health applies precision medicine to mental healthcare, helping to accurately predict the right, individualized treatment and accelerate recovery [52]. By working with employer healthcare plans, Spring Health enables early detection of many common mental conditions—including attention deficits, anxiety, depression, and eating disorders—and leverages predictive

models to identify the best treatment option and direct patients to the right therapist in its provider network. Woebot was founded in 2017 and provides an AI-powered chatbot that delivers cognitive behavioral therapy to users [53]. Woebot especially helps people think through tough situations with the help of step-by-step guidance, tracks users' mood, and provides evidence-based lessons, exercises, and stories from clinicians [54]. Woebot demonstrates how AI may be used to supplement clinical care and allow 24/7 access and care.

Understanding Venture Capital and Formative Partnerships
Venture capital continues to play a formative role in shaping the mental health and wellness technology landscape. Top investors include Google Ventures, Oak HC/FT, Y Combinator, and Khosla Ventures [30,55], demonstrating the flock toward mental and behavioral health. Further, corporate partnerships and participation have been formative in molding the mental health space. For example, partnerships with Aetna and Blue Cross Blue Shield have enabled AbleTo rapidly expand and develop. Payers and large employers such as those partnered with AbleTo are able to integrate behavioral health services into their plans and shape the delivery and accessibility of mental health resources [56]. Biotech partnerships, such as Amgen Merck and Akili have helped provide funding and key resources, supporting and expanding clinal development and testing and building out the commercial infrastructure [57]. Major tech companies are also playing a critical role, such as Google's partnership with Quartet in 2016, which marked Google Venture's first investment in a mental health start-up [58]. Among hospital systems, Cedars-Sinai has helped bring the shift/adoption of virtual reality medicine through partnering with AppliedVR [59].

The Road Ahead

One of the key challenges of initial commercialization of mental health technology is lack of funding pathways. For example, philanthropic and government grants support innovation in the lab with zero return. Venture and impact investment dollars support high-return company ideas. This leaves a gap in the funding landscape, as less profitable ideas—even those that could revolutionize the field or have a major impact on public health—have no clear funding source. BrainMind is currently one organization tackling this problem and is coordinating support for the most impactful basic science and for self-sustaining companies and nonprofits that could benefit humanity the most. Finding strategies to overcome this "valley of death" (the solution development period after the discovery phase and before the commercialization phase) will be critical to ensure brain sciences discoveries from the lab are translated to become readily available and accessible (see Figure 37.1). Unconventional funding mechanisms, such as the Healthy Brain Financing Initiative for the US$10 billion social impact bond to fund accelerated global research on mental health, are especially critical. Further, while business models have

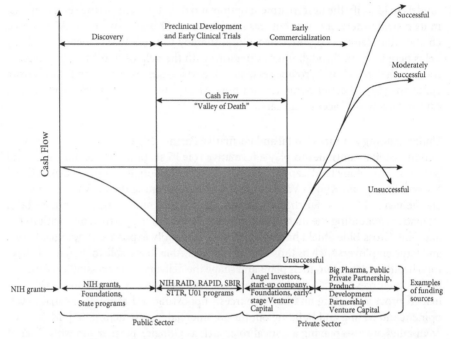

Figure 37.1 Valley of death phase
Adapted from Steinmetz and Spack [60].

been established for companies that fit within the six major categories of the current mental health technology landscape (CCBT, telepsychiatry, provider tools, consumer tools, hardware, and applied AI), we must ensure that innovative business models that support initial commercialization are developed for new discoveries that fall outside of these categories.

Beyond funding challenges, developing the leadership pipeline to support initial commercialization of mental health and wellness technology is crucial. Tom Insel demonstrates the multiplier effect convergence mental health leaders can have. As a noted neuroscientist and psychiatrist, Insel was previously the director of the National Institute of Mental Health and a former Verily leader. He went on to cofound the mental health company Mindstrong and serves as the "mental health czar" for the state of California under Governor Gavin Newsom [61]. Insel's nonlinear career path and dedication have helped weave together the previously disparate nodes necessary for convergence mental health and pave a path for future leaders that can translate research to initial commercialization, ensuring that the discoveries that could most benefit humanity are developed and readily available and accessible.

The responsible innovation in mental health (RIMH) model is also key to successful commercialization [62]. It helps to guide and monitor the implementation of new products and services in mental health. We recently conceptualized RIMH as being critical in risk management of mental health innovations (i.e., risk anticipation, risk detection, risk surveillance, and risk mitigation). We note the helpful principles from the OECD Recommendation on Responsible Innovation in Neurotechnology [63]: these principles include promoting responsible innovation, prioritizing safety assessment, promoting inclusivity, fostering scientific collaborations, enabling societal deliberations, enabling capacity of oversight and advisory bodies, safeguarding personal brain and mental health data, promoting cultures of stewardship and trust across the public and private sector, and anticipating and monitoring potential unintended use and/or misuse of technologies.

Scaling Up Market Penetration

The final area of development necessary for advancing convergence mental health is scaling up market penetration. This stage is important to overcome the second innovation capital gap, bridging development and validation and scale and impact (see Figure 37.2).

GeneSight® provides one of the limited examples of a mental health company at this stage. GeneSight Psychotropic is a pharmacogenomic test that helps clinicians select medications based on patients' individual genetic profile [64]. Over 1 million people have taken the GeneSight test to improve health outcomes. As the research behind the GeneSight test and other mental health technologies continues, it is necessary to consider what burden of evidence is needed for something to become the new standard of care [65]. This question is explored in depth in the fundamentals of the Oxford evidence-based medicine pyramid and is central to determining which technologies, and at which point, enter the scaling up market penetration stage. Also, further development of formal regulatory approval of digital mental health apps and technology is needed to support companies at this stage and ensure the safety of higher risk software in the mental health space.

IDEATION AND FORMULATION DEVELOPMENT AND VALIDATION   SCALE AND IMPACT

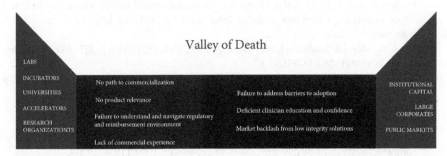

Figure 37.2 Current innovation capital gap.

Scaling up market penetration is the final layer in the convergence mental health funnel. However, there are limited data points and examples of mental health technology that has progressed to this stage, largely due to unaddressed challenges in the initial two stages that were previously discussed (research and initial commercialization). As the challenges of these preliminary stages are addressed, organizations will be better prepared for entering the scaling up market penetration stage.

Conclusion

The promotion of convergence approaches to mental health are important for improving patient outcomes. To support the shift toward convergence mental health, developments in research, initial commercialization, and scaling up market penetration are needed. Each stage of development has its own unique set of challenges and barriers that are addressed throughout the chapter. Though the pathway will be difficult, these steps are critical to advance brain science discoveries and translate findings from the lab to make them readily available and accessible. Ultimately, the promise of convergence science approaches is to engender a social movement on behalf of those living with or at risk for mental health conditions, ensuring greater health justice for all people by doing good in the service of what makes us human.

References

1. National Academies of Sciences, Engineering, and Medicine. *Fostering the culture of convergence in research: Proceedings of a workshop.* 2019: Washington, DC: The National Academies Press. https://doi.org/10.17226/25271
2. National Research Council, *Convergence: Facilitating transdisciplinary integration of life sciences, physical sciences, engineering, and beyond.* 2014: National Academies Press.
3. Van Noorden, R., Some hard numbers on science's leadership problems. *Nature*, 2018. 557(7705): p. 294–296 https://doi.org/10.1038/d41586-018-05143-8.
4. Jensen, D., The many faces of leadership. December 16, 2015; https://www.sciencemag.org/careers/2015/12/many-faces-leadership.
5. Fischer, P. and A. L. Ai, International terrorism and mental health: recent research and future directions. *J Interpers Violence*, 2008. 23(3): p. 339–361 https://doi.org/10.1177/0886260507312292.
6. Kwok, R., How lab heads can learn to lead. *Nature*, 2018. 557(7705): p. 457–459 https://doi.org/10.1038/d41586-018-05156-3.
7. Leiserson, C. E. and C. McVinney, Lifelong learning: Science professors need leadership training. *Nature*, 2015. 523(7560): p. 279–281 https://doi.org/10.1038/523279a.
8. Stephan, P. E. and R. G. Ehrenberg, *Science and the university.* 2007: Univ of Wisconsin Press.
9. Kahneman, D., *Thinking, fast and slow.* 2011: Macmillan.
10. Gee, K., Stanford pushes executives to get "touchy feely." May 1, 2019; https://www.wsj.com/articles/stanford-pushes-executives-to-get-touchy-feely-11556719200.
11. Collison, P. and T. Cowen, We need a new science of progress. *The Atlantic*, 2019.
12. Collison, P. and M. Nielsen, Science is getting less bang for its buck. *The Atlantic*, November 16, 2018.

13. Dolgin, E., The young and the restless. *Nature*, 2017. **551**(7678): p. S15–S18 https://doi.org/10.1038/551s15a.

14. Newport, C., *Deep work: Rules for focused success in a distracted world*. 2016: Hachette UK.

15. Keller, H., Is story's new design the optimal work space? *The Architectural Digest*, March 20, 2018.

16. The Francis Crick Institute, [Home page]. https://www.crick.ac.uk/ [Accessed December 19, 2019].

17. O'Neil, A., et al., A shared framework for the common mental disorders and Non-Communicable Disease: key considerations for disease prevention and control. *BMC Psychiatry*, 2015. **15**: p. 15 https://doi.org/10.1186/s12888-015-0394-0.

18. The Great Books Foundation, Our story. https://www.greatbooks.org/what-we-do/history/ [Accessed December 17, 2019].

19. Page, S. E., *The model thinker: What you need to know to make data work for you*. 2018: Hachette UK.

20. Parrish, S. and R. Beaubien, *The great mental models: General thinking concepts*. 2019: Latticework.

21. Vasan, N., et al., Technological ventures offer new hope for the future of psychiatry. *Psychiatr Times*, 2017. **34**(12).

22. Vasan, N., Grand Rounds Presentation at Department of Psychiatry, Stanford University: D-School for Mental Health: Launching the 1st University Course on Mental Health Innovation. 2018. http://med.stanford.edu/psychiatry/education/grand_rounds.html

23. Icahn School of Medicine at Mount Sinai, Pioneering education in the 21st century. https://icahn.mssm.edu/education/pioneering [Accessed December 28, 2019].

24. Schmidt Futures, Schmidt Futures Science Fellows. https://schmidtfutures.com/our-work/schmidt-science-fellows/. [Accessed January 1, 2020].

25. UNESCO, Science, technology and innovation policy. http://www.unesco.org/new/en/natural-sciences/science-technology/science-policy-and-society/science-diplomacy/ [Accessed January November 14, 2020].

26. Bansho, O. M. *Classrooms*. 2019: Editor. https://ottawabansho.wordpress.com/bansho-in-the-class/

27. Holford, M. and R. W. Nichols, The challenge of building science diplomacy capabilities for early career academic investigators. *Science & Diplomacy*. January 29, 2018; https://www.sciencediplomacy.org/perspective/2018/EACIs.

28. Epstein, D., *Range: Why generalists triumph in a specialized world*. 2019: Riverhead Books.

29. Katz, R., et al., Defining health diplomacy: Changing demands in the era of globalization. *Milbank Q*, 2011. **89**(3): p. 503–523 https://doi.org/10.1111/j.1468-0009.2011.00637.x.

30. Prendergass, J., *Mental health and wellness technology*. 2017: CB Insights.

31. Gaussen, E., *Mapping out the mental health startup ecosystem*. 2018.

32. World Economic Forum, Centre for the Fourth Industrial Revolution. [Home page]. https://www.weforum.org/centre-for-the-fourth-industrial-revolution [Accessed August 8, 2019].

33. Miremadi, T., A model for science and technology diplomacy: How to align the rationales of foreign policy and science. *SSRN*. March 28, 2016; https://ssrn.com/abstract=2737347

34. Leijten, J., Exploring the future of innovation diplomacy. *Eur J Future Res*, 2017. **5**(20) https://doi.org/10.1007/s40309-017-0122-8.

35. Nanalyze, What is computerized cognitive behavioral therapy? February 14, 2019; https://www.nanalyze.com/2019/02/computerized-cognitive-behavioral-therapy/.

36. Bound, K. and T. Saunders, Innovation policy toolkit: Tradecraft for innovation diplomats. *Nesta*. https://www.nesta.org.uk/toolkit/innovation-policy-toolkit-tradecraft-for-innovation-diplomats/ [Accessed November 11, 2018].

37. Fernandes, B. S., et al., The new field of "precision psychiatry." *BMC Med*, 2017. 15(1): p. 80 https://doi.org/10.1186/s12916-017-0849-x.

38. Weiner, S., Addressing the escalating psychiatrist shortage. *AAMC News,* February 12, 2018; https://www.aamc.org/news-insights/addressing-escalating-psychiatrist-shortage.

39. AbleTo, [Home page]. https://www.ableto.com/.

40. Udenrigsministeriet, TechPlomacy. http://techamb.um.dk/en/techplomacy/. [Accessed January 30, 2019].

41. Ginger. [Home page]. https://www.ginger.io/ [Accessed December 28, 2019].

42. Jha, A., A. Ilif, and A. Chaoui, A crisis in health care: A call to action on physician burnout. *Massachusetts Medical Society.* March 28, 2019; http://www.massmed.org/Publications/ Research,-Studies,-and-Reports/A-Crisis-in-Health-Care--A-Call-to-Action-on--Physician-Burnout/#.XzbZ3p5Kg2w.

43. Kramer, A. D., J. E. Guillory, and J. T. Hancock, Experimental evidence of massive-scale emotional contagion through social networks. *Proc Natl Acad Sci U S A*, 2014. 111(24): p. 8788–8790.

44. Arjadi, R., et al., Internet-based behavioural activation with lay counsellor support versus online minimal psychoeducation without support for treatment of depression: A random-ised controlled trial in Indonesia. *Lancet Psychiatry*, 2018. 5(9): p. 707–716 https://doi.org/ 10.1016/s2215-0366(18)30223-2.

45. Carey, B., California tests a digital "fire alarm" for mental distress. *New York Times.* June 17, 2019.

46. Arandjelovic, K., et al., The role of depression pharmacogenetic decision support tools in shared decision making. *J Neural Transm (Vienna)*, 2019. 126(1): p. 87–94.

47. Bousman, C. A. and M. Hopwood, Commercial pharmacogenetic-based decision-support tools in psychiatry. *Lancet Psychiatry*, 2016. 3(6): p. 585–590 https://doi.org/10.1016/ s2215-0366(16)00017-1.

48. Rosenblat, J. D., Y. Lee, and R. S. McIntyre, The effect of pharmacogenomic testing on re-sponse and remission rates in the acute treatment of major depressive disorder: A meta-analysis. *J Affect Disord*, 2018. 241: p. 484–491 https://doi.org/10.1016/j.jad.2018.08.056.

49. Gliddon, E., et al., Evaluating discussion board engagement in the MoodSwings online self-help program for bipolar disorder: Protocol for an observational prospective cohort study. *BMC Psychiatry*, 2015. 15: p. 243 https://doi.org/10.1186/s12888-015-0630-7.

50. Berk, L., et al., Evaluation of the acceptability and usefulness of an information website for caregivers of people with bipolar disorder. *BMC Med*, 2013. 11: p. 162 https://doi.org/ 10.1186/1741-7015-11-162.

51. Insel, T., et al., Research domain criteria (RDoC): Toward a new classification framework for research on mental disorders. *Am J Psychiatry*, 2010. 167(7): p. 748–751 https://doi.org/ 10.1176/appi.ajp.2010.09091379.

52. National Institute of Mental Health, Research domain criteria (RDoC). https://www.nimh. nih.gov/research/research-funded-by-nimh/rdoc/index.shtml [Accessed September 9, 2015].

53. Insel, T. R. and B. N. Cuthbert, Medicine: Brain disorders? Precisely. *Science*, 2015. 348(6234): p. 499–500 https://doi.org/10.1126/science.aab2358.

54. Nanalyze, 10 uses of artificial intelligence in mental health. March 10, 2019: https://www. nanalyze.com/2019/03/artificial-intelligence-mental-health/.

55. Landi, H., *Venture capital investment in AI and mental health startups surges in Q2: report.* 2019: FierceHealthcare.

56. Baum, S., Payers, large employers are pushing to integrate behavioral health services into member plans. *Med City News.* February 21, 2017; https://medcitynews.com/2017/

02/payers-large-employers-are-pushing-to-integrate-behavioral-health-services-into-member-plans/

57. Akili adds Amgen Ventures and M Ventures* to Series B financing, increasing round to $42.4 million. *Business Wire*. July 20, 2016; https://www.businesswire.com/news/home/20160719006692/en/Akili-Adds-Amgen-Ventures-Ventures*-Series-Financing.

58. GV leads $40M Series B in Quartet, its first investment in a mental healthcare startup. *TechCrunch*. April 15, 2016; https://techcrunch.com/2016/04/15/gv-leads-40m-series-b-in-quartet-its-first-investment-in-a-mental-healthcare-startup/.

59. Spiegel, B., Cedars-Sinai study finds virtual reality therapy helps decrease pain in hospitalized patients. *Cedars-Sinai*. March 29, 2017; https://www.cedars-sinai.org/newsroom/cedars-sinai-study-finds-virtual-reality-therapy-helps-decrease-pain-in-hospitalized-patients/.

60. Steinmetz, K. L. and E. G. Spack, The basics of preclinical drug development for neurodegenerative disease indications. *BMC Neurol*, 2009. 9(Suppl 1): p. S2 https://doi.org/10.1186/1471-2377-9-s1-s2.

61. Sheridan, K., California names former Google scientist as the state's "mental health czar." STAT. May 22, 2019; https://www.statnews.com/2019/05/22/tom-insel-california-mental-health-czar/.

62. Eyre, H. A., et al., Leveraging responsible innovation to steward mental health technology development lancet *Psychiatry*, 2020. Accepted; In Press.

63. OECD, Recommendation of the Council on Responsible Innovation in Neurotechnology, OECD/LEGAL/0457. 2020; https://www.oecd.org/science/recommendation-on-responsible-innovation-in-neurotechnology.htm

64. GeneSight, [Home page]. https://genesight.com/ [Accessed December 28, 2019].

65. Oxford Centre for Evidence-based Medicine—Levels of evidence (March 2009), March 2009; https://www.cebm.net/2009/06/oxford-centre-evidence-based-medicine-levels-evidence-march-2009/

Index

For the benefit of digital users, indexed terms that span two pages (e.g., 52–53) may, on occasion, appear on only one of those pages.

Tables, figures and boxes are indicated by *t*, *f* and *b* following the page number